PTEXAM: The Complete Study Guide

SCOREBUILDERS
Your Source for Examination Preparation

Scott M. Giles PT, DPT, MBA

President, Scorebuilders
Clinical Associate Professor
Department of Physical Therapy
University of New England

Scorebuilders
P.O. Box 7242
Scarborough, Maine 04070-7242

Toll Free: (866) PTEXAMS
Phone: (207) 885-0304
Fax: (207) 883-8377
Web site: www.scorebuilders.com

Acknowledgments

Contributors

Therese C. Giles PT, MS
Vice President, Scorebuilders

I would like to thank my wife, Therese, from the bottom of my heart for her many valuable contributions during the entire project.   Her substantial contributions to the academic review and clinical application templates sections were a critical component of the project. Thank you for being my teammate and best friend.

Jon Stuart MBA
President, Mindcom

I would like to thank Jon for his technical expertise and willingness to create and adapt the CD-ROM to the many nuances associated with the current National Physical Therapy Examination.

Special Thanks

To my children Meghan, Erin, and Alexander. Thanks for your hard work on the project and tolerating the many long nights when Dad had to do "work." You are all an ongoing source of inspiration for me. Love always.

To Kathy Lavigne for her numerous contributions to the project.

To Michael Anthony for his graphic design expertise and patience.

To Gwenn Hoyt and Kelly Stuart for their creative expertise and guidance.

To the hundreds of students from academic programs throughout the country that served as reviewers throughout the project.

Introduction

PTEXAM: The Complete Study Guide

Preparing for a comprehensive examination that potentially encompasses all elements of a physical therapy academic program can be an overwhelming task. Students are often exhausted after completing a rigorous academic program and suddenly are faced with the daunting task of taking a comprehensive examination. Anxiety, economics, and a strong desire to practice as a physical therapist only increase a candidate's sense of urgency. Often when faced with such an overwhelming task the reaction is to either procrastinate or to wander aimlessly through study sessions without real direction or focus.

Our text *PTEXAM: The Complete Study Guide* provides candidates with a number of powerful study tools each designed to prepare candidates for the breadth and depth associated with the current National Physical Therapy Examination. A brief description of each unit in the study guide is listed below.

Unit One: National Physical Therapy Examination

The section provides candidates with information on the purpose, development, scoring, and administration of the National Physical Therapy Examination. Candidates are introduced to a systematic approach to answering multiple-choice questions and are exposed to recent developments in item construction.

Unit Two: Academic Review

The section provides candidates with an efficient method to review didactic information from a physical therapy curriculum. The academic review avoids attempting to cover every aspect of a physical therapist's academic training and instead focuses on the most essential information necessary to maximize examination performance. Since the examination is designed to assess entry-level practice it is likely that candidates will encounter the information presented in the academic review frequently on the actual examination. Mastery of the information presented in the academic review can significantly increase students' scores on the National Physical Therapy Examination.

Unit Three: Clinical Application Templates

The section includes a description of the physical therapy management of 50 commonly encountered medical diagnoses on the National Physical Therapy Examination. By utilizing the clinical application templates candidates can expand their applied clinical knowledge while at the same time reinforcing existing knowledge. Since the majority of examination questions are presented in an applied manner it is essential that students possess requisite knowledge related to these medical diagnoses. As candidates become increasingly familiar with the information they will be better able to make informed decisions when answering challenging multiple-choice questions.

Unit Four: Content Outline Examination

The section provides a detailed analysis of each of the content areas of the National Physical Therapy Examination. By exploring the categories and subcategories of each of the content areas candidates gain a better understanding of the breadth and depth of the current examination. A 200 question sample examination consisting of 20 examination questions in 10 different content areas provides students with their first opportunity to answer a full-length examination. An answer key located at the conclusion of the examination includes the correct answer, an explanation supporting the correct answer, and a cited resource with page number.

Unit Five: Paper and Pencil Examinations

The section consists of two, 200 question sample examinations offered in a traditional paper and pencil format. The examinations provide students with the opportunity to refine their test taking skills and to assess their current preparedness for the examination. An answer key located at the conclusion of each of the examinations includes the correct answer, an explanation supporting the correct answer, and a cited resource with page number.

Unit Six: Computer-Based Examinations

The section consists of two, 200 question sample examinations located on a CD-ROM. The examinations were developed based on selected specifications from the current content outline and are designed to expose candidates to the nuances of computer-based testing. Candidates are able to generate a detailed performance analysis summary that identifies current strengths and weaknesses according to selected clinical practice and content outline areas. An answer key located in Unit Six includes the correct answer, an explanation supporting the correct answer, a cited resource with page number, and the clinical practice and content outline area.

*Additional resources to assist candidates with their preparation for the National Physical Therapy Examination are located at the conclusion of the text.

Author's Note

Congratulations on your decision to purchase *PTEXAM: The Complete Study Guide*. Leave no stone unturned in your preparation for this important examination and strive to make your examination score reflect your academic knowledge. Candidates that have a firm grasp of didactic information combined with a meaningful study plan emphasizing applied knowledge are often richly rewarded on this challenging examination. We are confident that our text will be a valuable component of your comprehensive study program. Although undoubtedly there will be many magical moments in your life, you will never forget the moment when you become licensed as a physical therapist. Best of luck on the examination and in your future career endeavors!

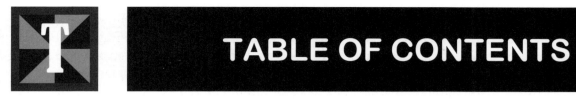

TABLE OF CONTENTS

Unit Three: Clinical Application Templates... 239

Unit Four: Content Outline 343

Unit One
National Physical Therapy Examination

The National Physical Therapy Examination is a 250 question (200 scored, 50 pre-test), multiple-choice examination designed to determine if candidates possess the minimal competency necessary to practice as physical therapists.

The examination is created under the auspices of the Federation of State Boards of Physical Therapy (FSBPT). According to the <u>National Physical Therapy Examination Candidate Handbook</u>, the examination program serves two important purposes:

1. Provide examination services to regulatory authorities charged with the regulation of physical therapists and physical therapist assistants.

2. Provide a common element in the evaluation of candidates so that standards will be comparable from jurisdiction to jurisdiction.

There are two primary methods to obtain a license to practice as a physical therapist in the United States. They are termed examination and endorsement. Licensure by examination is obtained after a candidate meets or exceeds the minimum scoring requirement on the National Physical Therapy Examination and has satisfied all other state requirements. This form of obtaining licensure is the traditional method for candidates seeking initial licensure.

Licensure by endorsement makes it possible for candidates who have already been licensed in a state by virtue of an examination to potentially gain licensure in another state without retaking the examination. Examination scores can be transferred to any physical therapy state licensing agency via the Federation of State Boards of Physical Therapy Score Transfer Service. The web site address for the Federation of State Boards of Physical Therapy is available in the Appendix.

Although the National Physical Therapy Examination is 250 questions, 50 of the questions serve only as pre-test items and are not officially scored. The pre-test items allow new examination questions to be evaluated throughout the year and eliminate lengthy delays in score reporting when new examinations are introduced. Candidates are unable to differentiate between pre-test and scored items on the examination.

The 250 questions are administered to candidates in five sections consisting of 50 questions each. Each section contains scored items and pre-test items, although the number of pre-test and scored items in each section may vary slightly. Candidates have five hours to complete the five sections at their own pace. Since the sections are not timed individually it is important for candidates to effectively manage their allotted time as they progress through each of the five sections. Candidates have the opportunity to take one scheduled break during the examination. Additional breaks can be taken at the conclusion of a given section, however, the elapsed time will not stop.

Candidates are unable to return to previously completed sections once a new section is initiated. The academic content is randomized within each section and scoring is based only on the number of questions a candidate answers correctly out of the 200 scored items. As a result, each of the examinations in *PTEXAM: The Complete Study Guide* consists of only 200 questions (four sections, each consisting of 50 questions). Candidates will have four hours to complete each of the 200 question sample examinations.

The FSBPT publishes the content categories of the examination. The categories are based on the tasks and roles that comprise the practice of physical therapy. Although listed here, the content outline will be discussed in detail in Unit Four.

Examination Content Outline

I. Examination
History and Systems Review

Tests and Measures Group I
1. Strength, ROM, Posture, Body Structures, Prosthetic & Orthotic Devices
2. Cognition, Nerve, Reflex and Sensory Integrity, Neurodevelopment

Tests and Measures Group II
1. Cardiovascular/Pulmonary System
2. Integumentary System
3. Functional Status/Community Integration

II. Evaluation, Diagnosis, Prognosis, and Outcomes
Evaluation and Diagnosis
Prognosis and Outcomes

III. Intervention
Non-Procedural Intervention
1. Coordination of Care
2. Communication
3. Documentation
4. Patient/Family/Client-related instructions

Procedural Intervention
Group I: Exercise and manual therapy
Group II: Transfer and functional activities, gait training, assistive and adaptive devices, and modification of the environment
Group III: Physical agents and modalities, airway clearance techniques, wound care, and promoting health and wellness

IV. Standards of Care
1. Maintaining patient autonomy, confidentiality, and obtaining informed consent

2. Recognizing scope of physical therapy practice, including limitations of the PT role that necessitate referral to other disciplines
3. Utilizing body mechanics/positioning
4. Considering the patient's cultural background, social history, home situation, and geographic barriers, etc.
5. Safety, CPR, emergency care, first aid, standard precautions

According to the FSBPT, the involvement of a large representative group of practicing physical therapists and other professionals at each stage of examination development ensures that the examinations are relevant to the practice of physical therapy. Individual physical therapists are responsible for writing examination questions. The physical therapists involved are required to attend item-writing workshops that are taught by experienced testing professionals. Questions, once completed, are analyzed independently to make sure they are reflective of the current examination content outline. Examination questions tend to focus on decision making and not rote memorization of fact. Successful candidates on the examination must demonstrate the ability to apply knowledge in a safe and effective manner.

Examination Scoring

The questions on the examination are multiple-choice with four possible answers to each question. Each option is listed as 1, 2, 3, 4. Options such as "none of the above", "all of the above", and "1 and 2 only" are not included on the examination. Candidates are asked to identify the best answer to each of the questions. Each question has only one best answer while the other possible answers serve as distracters. A candidate's score is determined based on the number of scored questions answered correctly. Since there is no penalty for questions answered incorrectly it is imperative that candidates answer all of the available questions. A candidate's cumulative score is termed the total raw score. The maximum total raw score for the National Physical Therapy Examination is 200.

Criterion-referenced scoring is used to determine passing scores on the National Physical Therapy Examination. Passing scores are based on the judgment of selected experts on the minimum number of questions that should be answered correctly by a minimally qualified candidate. Criterion-referenced passing scores are determined independently of candidate performance and are designed to reflect the difficulty level of each examination. For example, if a given examination were judged to be particularly difficult, the criterion-referenced passing score would be lower than the criterion-referenced passing score for another examination that was judged to be less difficult. All state licensing agencies have adopted the FSBPT criterion-referenced passing score and therefore do not individually determine passing scores at the state level. As a result, a passing score for a given examination will always be the same in all jurisdictions.

Since the minimum passing score varies based on the difficulty level of each examination it is impossible to determine an automatic passing score. Criterion-referenced passing scores often range from 138 - 152. If the criterion-referenced passing score was established as 147 for a given examination, a total raw score of greater than or equal to 147 would be considered a passing score, while a total raw score of less than 147 would be considered a failing score. Within a given examination cycle, criterion-referenced passing scores usually fluctuate in a relatively small range, perhaps by as few as five questions.

An individual examination score is often reported to candidates in the form of a scaled score. Scaled scores range from 200 - 800 with the minimum passing score always being equal to a scaled score of 600. Scaled scores are necessary as a method of equating examinations with different criterion-referenced passing scores. A few state licensing agencies use a slightly different scaled score system where the minimum passing score is equivalent to a scaled score of 75.

Applying for the Examination

Candidates planning to take the examination should request an application from the state licensing agency in the jurisdiction where they intend to practice as a physical therapist. Candidates are not permitted to apply for the examination in more than one jurisdiction at a time. The address of each agency, phone number, and web site are provided in the Appendix. Some of the state licensing agencies now offer online registration through the Federation of State Boards of Physical Therapy. Please consult individual state requirements prior to taking advantage of this option.

Each state licensing agency can establish its own criteria to be eligible to sit for the National Physical Therapy Examination. A variety of items may be required as part of the application process. These items often include a photograph, a notarized birth certificate, an official transcript from an accredited school, professional reference letters, and a check or money order for the required application, examination, and licensing fees. Candidates should recognize that even a small departure from the established eligibility criteria could lead to a significant delay in processing a candidate's application. To avoid such delays, it is prudent to read the application carefully and to inquire as to the status of the application approximately two weeks after the completed application has been submitted.

Foreign trained therapists are often subjected to a myriad of requirements before they are eligible to become licensed in the United States. Since the requirements vary significantly by state, it is recommended that candidates contact the state licensing agency within the state they intend to practice. The state licensing agency can provide detailed information on their individual requirements.

There are two general requirements for foreign trained therapists that seem to be consistent in all states:

1. Applicants are required to submit their educational credentials for evaluation of their equivalence to the United States trained applicant.

2. Applicants must meet or exceed the minimum scoring requirement on the National Physical Therapy Examination.

Other state requirements can include, but are not limited to, the following:

- Demonstrate proficiency in written and spoken English
- Submit letters of reference
- Obtain a valid visa and resident alien card
- Complete an internship or period of supervised practice
- Appear for an interview
- Attain the equivalent of a United States grade of "C" or higher in all professional coursework

Some states offer candidates with verifiable employment the opportunity to practice prior to being licensed by issuing a temporary license. Typically, candidates are required to have a completed application on file and have met all other qualifications for licensure before being considered for the temporary license. In most states temporary licenses are revoked if a candidate receives notification they were unsuccessful on the National Physical Therapy Examination.

In addition to the National Physical Therapy Examination, a significant number of states require candidates to successfully complete a jurisprudence examination. This type of examination is based on the state rules and regulations governing physical therapy practice. The examination can include multiple-choice items, short-answer questions or fill in the blanks. States can administer the examination using computer-based testing or even as a take home examination.

After the necessary application forms have been completed, the information is returned along with any necessary fees to the state licensing agency or an identified intermediary. Once approved, the state licensing agency forwards eligibility information to the FSBPT. The FSBPT then issues candidates an "authorization to test" letter that includes instructions on how to schedule an appointment to take the examination. Candidates must sit for the examination within 60 days of the date on their letter. It is important to schedule an appointment relatively early in the 60 day window in order to ensure availability at a local Prometric Testing Center. Once an examination appointment is scheduled candidates retain the right to reschedule or cancel the appointment as long as it is done by noon, two business days prior to the scheduled date. Failure to take the examination within the designated 60 day period will require a candidate to go through the application process again.

Candidates should schedule their examination at a time consistent with their optimal level of functioning. For example, if a candidate tends to be a "morning person" it would be prudent to schedule the examination early in the morning. Candidates with significant anxiety related to the examination may also want an early appointment in order to avoid worrying about the examination throughout the day. If candidates are not familiar with the exact location of the examination site, it may be desirable to travel to the site before the actual examination date. The trip will provide candidates with an accurate idea of the time necessary to travel to the site and avoid the possibility of getting lost and subsequently being late for the examination.

Examination Administration

The examination is offered on computer at Prometric Testing Centers within the United States or at selected testing facilities in Canada. A list of participating Prometric Testing Centers by state is located in the Appendix. Testing is typically offered Monday through Saturday from 9:00 AM - 6:00 PM. Within each Prometric Testing Center candidates can concentrate on the examination without environmental distracters. Private, modular booths provide adequate work space with proper lighting and ventilation. All Prometric Testing Centers are fully accessible and in compliance with the Americans with Disabilities Act. Candidates requesting accommodation for a documented disability must do so through the state licensing agency. Candidates are not limited to the testing centers within the state they are applying for licensure. For example, a candidate that has recently graduated from a physical therapy program in Maine could apply for licensure in California and take the required examination while still residing in Maine.

It is important to note that computer skills are not necessary with computer-based testing. Prior to beginning the examination, candidates utilize a tutorial that explains topics such as selecting answers and navigating within the examination. Time spent on the computer tutorial does not count toward the allotted time for the actual examination. The tutorial typically takes candidates less than 10 minutes and if necessary candidates can go through the tutorial a second time.

Once within the actual examination candidates can move freely between examination questions. Candidates have the option of entering their answers using a computer keyboard or mouse. Candidates can go back to previously answered or unanswered questions and make any desired changes within a given section of 50 questions. Once a candidate exits a given section they are unable to return to the questions within the section. Paper and pencil are not permitted in the Prometric Centers, however, candidates are given an erasable note board or an electronic writing board to utilize during the examination.

The FSBPT is responsible for scoring the examination and reporting results to the individual state licensing agencies. The state licensing agencies then notify candidates as to their performance on the examination. Formal notification typically occurs through the mail, however, many state licensing agencies have web sites that allow candidates to determine their licensing status online. In most instances, candidates' scores are available within 3-10 business days.

If a candidate successfully completes the examination, in most cases they have fulfilled the final requirement for licensure. Conversely, if a candidate is unsuccessful on the examination, they are required to reapply to the state licensing agency. With computer-based testing there is no mandatory waiting period before retaking the examination, however, some states limit the number of times a candidate can take the examination as well as mandate remedial coursework. In all states, candidates are prohibited from taking the examination more than three times in a 12 month period.

Candidates that were unsuccessful on the National Physical Therapy Examination can receive role feedback from the FSBPT. The role feedback report compares individual examination performance according to the content outline and selected areas of clinical practice with that of other candidates exposed to the same examination. Additional information on role feedback is available through the FSBPT.

Test Taking Skills

Test taking skills are specific skills that allow individuals to utilize the characteristics and format of a selected examination in order to maximize their performance. These skills can be valuable when taking an examination such as the National Physical Therapy Examination. Despite the importance of this topic, very little, if any, academic time is set aside to address test taking skills. The good news is that test taking skills can be learned and that through dedication, desire, and determination, these skills can serve to improve examination performance.

The National Physical Therapy Examination consists of multiple-choice questions with four potentially correct answers to each question. Candidates are instructed to select the "best answer" to complete each question. Before exploring selected test taking strategies, we need to identify the various components of a multiple-choice question. Multiple-choice questions can be dissected into specific identifiable components:

Item: An item refers to an individual multiple-choice question and the corresponding potential answers. The National Physical Therapy Examination contains 200 scored items and 50 pre-test items. Each item consists of a stem and four options. Items may vary considerably in content and length, but should utilize a consistent format.

Stem: The stem refers to the statement that asks the question. Typically, the stem conveys to the reader the necessary information needed to respond correctly to the question. In addition to the necessary information, many times extraneous information is included in the stem. This information, when not recognized by the candidate as unnecessary, often can serve as a significant distracter.

The stem commonly takes on the form of a complete sentence or an incomplete sentence. The stem can be expressed in a positive or negative form. A positive form requires a candidate to identify correct information, while a negative form requires a candidate to identify incorrect information. It is important to scrutinize each stem, since a single key word such as "not", "except", or "least" can turn a positive stem into a negative stem. Failure to identify this can lead to the identification of an incorrect answer.

Options: The options refer to the potential answers to the question asked. One option in each item will be the "best answer," while the others are considered distracters. Options can take on a variety of forms, including a single word, a group of words, an incomplete sentence, a complete sentence, or a group of sentences. The method for analyzing each option does not change, regardless of form.

Approach for Answering Multiple-Choice Questions

On the National Physical Therapy Examination there are 250 items (200 scored, 50 pre-test) that candidates must answer within a five hour time period. Due to the length of the examination and the time constraints associated with it, candidates need to approach the examination in a systematic and organized fashion. Loss of control during the examination will yield poor results that are not reflective of a candidate's actual knowledge. To assist candidates to minimize the impact of this potential pitfall, we will introduce a systematic approach to utilize when answering sample examination items.

The following six-step approach is recommended as a method for answering examination items:

1. Read the stem carefully
2. Identify or underline relevant words or groups of words
3. Make a mental note of or circle command words that indicate the desired action
4. Attempt to generate an answer to the question
5. Examine each option completely before moving to the next option
6. If necessary, utilize deductive reasoning strategies

The six-step approach can be used effectively on paper and pencil as well as computer-based examinations. For example, as candidates are getting used to the six-step approach they should engage in formal activities such as "underlining" and "circling", however, once they are comfortable with the approach they should transition to a less formal process. Often this is best accomplished by mental processes such as "identifying" or "making mental notes."

The six-step approach begins with a candidate reading the stem. Candidates should sift through the presented information and attempt to extract the necessary components. Relevant words or groups of words should be identified. Perhaps the most important step in the six-step approach is to have candidates attempt to generate an answer to each question based on the identified command words. This is the only opportunity a candidate will have to objectively evaluate the question prior to exposing each of the options. Once a candidate exposes the options they are no longer able to examine the question in a fully objective manner and instead become more likely to have their interpretation of the question influenced by a presented option. If for some reason a candidate is unable to generate a specific answer, they should attempt to think about the general topic and recall related information. Once a possible answer is generated, candidates should then begin to examine each option one at a time. It is important to read the entire option, since one word can often make a potentially correct answer incorrect. If the generated answer is consistent with one of the available options, the candidate should give the option strong consideration; however, since more than one option can be correct it is imperative to analyze each presented option.

If candidates finish analyzing an item and are still unable to select one of the available options they should consider using a deductive reasoning strategy. Deductive reasoning strategies allow candidates to improve examination scores without direct knowledge of subject matter. This type of strategy should be applied only when candidates are unable to identify the correct response using academic knowledge. Deductive reasoning strategies often allow candidates to eliminate one or more of the potential answers. Elimination of any option significantly increases the probability of identifying the correct answer. On the National Physical Therapy Examination, eliminating one option increases the chance of selecting a correct answer from 25% to 33%. Eliminating two options increases the chance of selecting a correct answer to 50%. On the surface this may not seem terribly significant, however, on an examination such as the National Physical Therapy Examination this can often be the difference between a passing and a failing score. Selected deductive reasoning strategies that can be used effectively on the National Physical Therapy Examination are presented.

Absurd options
Many times a multiple-choice item will include an option that is not consistent with what the stem is asking or with the other options. In many cases, this option can be eliminated. Rapid elimination of specific options will allow candidates to spend additional time analyzing other more viable options.

Similar options
When two or more options have a similar meaning or express the same fact, they often imply each other's incorrectness. For this reason, candidates can often eliminate both options.

Obtainable information
There is a great deal of factual material that candidates must sift through when taking the National Physical Therapy Examination. In some instances, the material can provide candidates with valuable information that can assist them when answering other examination questions.

Degree of qualification
Particularly in the sciences, there seems to be many exceptions to general rules. Therefore, specific wording such as "always" or "never" often over qualify an option.

Activity One

In this activity, three sample questions are presented. Candidates should attempt to identify the best answer to each question by utilizing the six-step approach.

An analysis section immediately follows each of the three sample questions. The analysis section begins by showing the sample question with key terms underlined and command words in bold type. A brief narrative follows, which describes how the six-step approach can be applied to the sample question.

An answer key located at the conclusion of the exercise indicates the best answer and an explanation for each question.

Sample Question One:
A physical therapist instructs a patient with a Foley catheter in ambulation activities. During ambulation the therapist should position the collection bag:

1. above the level of the patient's bladder
2. below the level of the patient's bladder
3. above the level of the patient's heart
4. below the level of the patient's heart

Analysis:
A physical therapist instructs a patient with a <u>Foley catheter in ambulation activities</u>. During ambulation the therapist should **position** <u>the collection bag</u>:

1. above the level of the patient's bladder
2. below the level of the patient's bladder
3. above the level of the patient's heart
4. below the level of the patient's heart

A candidate should attempt to generate an answer to the question after reading the stem and identifying the pertinent information and command words. The candidate should then begin to reveal each of the available options one at a time. If a generated answer is consistent with one of the available options, there is a high probability that the answer is correct.

If a candidate was not able to generate an answer, they should expose the first option and give it careful consideration before moving on to the next option. They should progress through the remaining options in a similar manner. Candidates should remember it is possible to have more than one option that satisfactorily answers the question. It is then the candidate's responsibility to select the best answer from the viable options.

Sample Question Two:

A group of physical therapists attempts to determine the relationship between two variables on an examination form. Which of the following correlation coefficients would indicate the strongest relationship?

1. +.86
2. +.45
3. -.34
4. -.89

Analysis:

A group of physical therapists attempts to determine <u>the relationship between two variables</u> on an examination form. Which of the following <u>correlation coefficients</u> would indicate the **strongest relationship**?

1. +.86
2. +.45
3. -.34
4. -.89

After reading the stem and identifying the pertinent information and command words, a candidate should recognize that it is virtually impossible to generate an answer prior to viewing the available options. A candidate should, however, begin to think about correlation coefficients and determining the strength of the relationship between variables. The candidate should then begin to expose each of the available options and attempt to identify the correct response.

Although the six-step approach does not directly supply a candidate with the correct response, by carefully reading the stem, a candidate can avoid an unnecessary mistake. In this item, the stem asks the candidate to identify the correlation coefficient that indicates the strongest relationship between the two variables. If a candidate does not read the question carefully, they may make an assumption that the stem is asking for the strongest positive relationship and subsequently answer the question incorrectly.

It is important that a candidate answer each item based only on the given information. By making even small assumptions or by not reading each item carefully, a candidate can make careless mistakes.

Sample Question Three:
A physical therapist completes an isokinetic examination on an 18-year-old male rehabilitating from a medial meniscectomy. The therapist notes that the patient generates 140 ft/lbs of force using the uninvolved quadriceps at 60 degrees per second. Assuming a normal ratio of hamstrings to quadriceps strength, which of the following would be an acceptable hamstrings value at 60 degrees per second?

1. 64 ft/lbs
2. 84 ft/lbs
3. 114 ft/lbs
4. 116 ft/lbs

Analysis:
A physical therapist completes <u>an isokinetic examination</u> on an <u>18-year-old male</u> <u>rehabilitating from a medial meniscectomy</u>. The therapist notes that the patient generates <u>140 ft/lbs of force using the uninvolved quadriceps at 60 degrees per second</u>. Assuming <u>a normal ratio of hamstrings to quadriceps strength</u>, which of the following would be **an acceptable hamstrings value** <u>at 60 degrees per second</u>?

1. 64 ft/lbs
2. 84 ft/lbs
3. 114 ft/lbs
4. 116 ft/lbs

For the purpose of discussion, let's assume a candidate has no idea of the normal ratio of quadriceps/hamstrings strength at 60 degrees/second. Lack of specific academic knowledge will result in a candidate not being able to identify the correct answer using the first five steps of the six-step approach. However, by utilizing deductive reasoning strategies, a candidate can significantly increase their chances of identifying the best answer without applying direct academic knowledge.

In this item, the stem asks a candidate to identify a value that would be representative of a normal quadriceps/hamstrings ratio at 60 degrees/second. As with many measurements in physical therapy, precise normal values are difficult to ascertain, and therefore often are expressed in ranges. Since options 3 and 4 are so close in value they likely imply each other's incorrectness and can therefore be eliminated. Although in this example deductive reasoning strategies were not able to identify the correct answer, they were able to eliminate two of the four possible options. By eliminating two options, a candidate now has a 50% chance of identifying the best answer, even without utilizing any direct academic or clinical knowledge.

Activity One – Answer Key

1. Correct Answer: 2
   Explanation: The effect of gravity necessitates the collection bag being below the level of the patient's bladder. (Pierson p. 267)

2. Correct Answer: 4
   Explanation: Correlation coefficients range from +1.00 to -1.00. Since the question does not ask for a positive or negative correlation, the strongest relationship is indicated by -.89. (Currier p. 265)

3. Correct Answer: 2
   Explanation: A gross estimate of quadriceps:hamstrings ratio is 3:2. Option 2, 84 ft/lbs is therefore most consistent with the expressed ratio. (Hamill p. 236)

Recent Developments in Item Construction

There have been a number of changes in item construction on the National Physical Therapy Examination within the past few years, most notably the introduction of graphically enhanced items. Although representing a relatively small percentage of the total examination, candidates need to be comfortable answering this type of item. Graphically enhanced items will be incorporated into each of the sample examinations.

Graphically Enhanced Items
Graphically enhanced items consist of figures, diagrams, pictures or other static images that are combined with traditional text in an examination item.

Activity Two

Two graphically enhanced items are presented. Candidates should attempt to identify the best answer to each question. An answer key located at the conclusion of the exercise indicates the best answer and an explanation for each question.

The following image should be used to answer question 1:

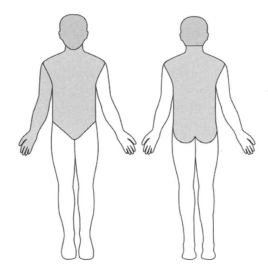

1. A 32-year-old male sustained extensive burns after lighting himself on fire during a suicide attempt. The shaded portion of the body diagrams represents the areas affected by the burns. Using the rule of nines, what percentage of the patient's body was involved?

   1. 40.5%
   2. 44.0%
   3. 49.5%
   4. 54.5%

The following image should be used to answer question 2:

2. A physical therapist instructs a patient to complete an exercise activity using a piece of elastic band as pictured. The patient is a 14-year-old female rehabilitating from a lower extremity injury sustained in a soccer contest. The therapist's primary objective for the activity is to:

   1. strengthen the right hip abductor muscles
   2. strengthen the right hip adductor muscles
   3. stretch the right hip abductor muscles
   4. stretch the right hip adductor muscles

Activity Two – Answer Key

1. Correct Answer: 3
   Explanation: The percentage of the body surface burned in an adult can be calculated using the rule of nines: anterior thorax (18%) + posterior thorax (18%) + head (9%) + anterior arm (4.5%) = 49.5%. (O'Sullivan p. 852)

2. Correct Answer: 2
   Explanation: Successful completion of the activity requires the adductor muscles to exert a force greater than the tension supplied by the elastic band while moving into hip adduction. Muscles acting to adduct the hip include the adductor longus, adductor brevis, adductor magnus, gracilis, and pectineus. (Magee p. 615)

Time Constraints

Like many objective examinations, candidates have a specific allotted time to complete the National Physical Therapy Examination. For physical therapists, the available time is five hours. Since the examination consists of 250 questions, candidates will have 72 seconds available to answer each question. This number, although correct when viewing the examination as a whole, can be misleading. There will be many questions that a candidate will be able to answer in much less than 72 seconds, whereas other questions will take somewhat longer. The key to success lies in progressing through the examination in a consistent and predictable manner.

Although 72 seconds per question does not seem like a great deal of time, the majority of candidates will have ample time to complete the examination. Despite this fact, it is important to pay attention to the elapsed time during the examination. It also is important to know your test taking history. Are you typically one of the first, one of the last, or somewhere in the middle of individuals completing an examination? This information is important as you plan your test taking strategy. In order to make sure your pace is appropriate during practice sessions and during the actual examination, it is important to formally check on the elapsed time, at a very minimum, when completing each section of 50 questions. This action will allow candidates to assess their progress and modify their pace, if necessary.

Preparing for the Examination

The simple thought of preparing for a comprehensive examination such as the National Physical Therapy Examination can be overwhelming. Many candidates ask themselves how it is possible to prepare adequately for an examination that encompasses up to three years of professional coursework. To further complicate matters the majority of candidates take the National Physical Therapy Examination shortly after graduation. This can be a very anxious and unsettled time. Candidates often are actively seeking employment or are attempting to adjust to a new job. As a result, it is critical that candidates outline a well thought out and deliberate study plan for the examination.

One of the largest advantages of taking an examination such as the National Physical Therapy Examination is that it does not require candidates to demonstrate mastery of new material. On the surface this may not seem like a significant advantage, but since candidates are, in effect, only reviewing or relearning previously presented information, their level of attainment should be significantly greater. Many candidates fail to utilize this advantage. Candidates who attempt to learn large quantities of new information, instead of focusing on understanding and applying basic concepts, often do themselves a tremendous disservice. It is true that there undoubtedly will be questions that contain information that was not part of a selected curriculum, but to attempt to study this new information in any significant detail would be a large mistake for most candidates. Instead, candidates should focus on reviewing or relearning basic concepts that are an integral component of all accredited physical therapy programs. It is this type of information that will make up the vast majority of the examination. Individuals who take this common sense approach optimize their chances of success.

In physical therapy academic programs, candidates constantly are learning new information on a variety of topics. Although students typically exhibit mastery of selected material during a scheduled examination, they do not always retain the information for later use. Often times, simply reviewing information is enough for candidates to relearn the material; however, in some cases, a more in-depth approach is necessary.

It is recommended that students pay particular attention to their practice-oriented professional coursework. Practice-oriented professional coursework includes, but is not limited to, study of the musculoskeletal, neuromuscular, cardiopulmonary, and integumentary systems. In addition, candidates usually have coursework in patient care skills, physical agents, administration, ethics, research, and education. Each of these topics are important components of the content outline for the National Physical Therapy Examination.

Special attention must be taken not to become bogged down in one specific area for any significant amount of time. General concepts that are understood should be scanned quickly, while other concepts that are more difficult for a candidate should be read carefully. Concepts that remain unclear after being reviewed should be written down for future study sessions.

Other foundational coursework encountered earlier in the professional curriculum can be consulted as needed during various study sessions. This type of coursework often includes, but is not limited to anatomy and physiology, neuroanatomy, exercise physiology, and kinesiology. It is important to limit the amount of time spent reviewing this type of foundational coursework. Candidates often can make better use of their allotted time by reviewing coursework encountered later in the curriculum that may be more practice-oriented. By reviewing practice-oriented information, candidates not only keep their studying consistent with the format of the examination, but also at the same time indirectly review much of the information presented in the foundational coursework.

Before beginning to study, develop specific goals for each study session. Ideally, these goals should be established on a weekly basis. Establishing goals will ensure that candidates cover the desired material and will serve as a mechanism to keep them on schedule with their study plan. Candidates should be realistic with the goals they establish and should not attempt to cover more material than is possible in a particular study session.

Unit Two

Academic Review

The National Physical Therapy Examination is a generalist examination that attempts to determine if candidates possess the minimal qualifications necessary to practice as an entry-level physical therapist. The examination requires candidates to exhibit familiarity with the management of commonly encountered medical diagnoses and then apply the information to challenging clinically-oriented multiple-choice questions. In order to accomplish the objective it is essential that candidates have a firm understanding of basic didactic information included in a physical therapy academic program.

The academic review unit of *PTEXAM: The Complete Study Guide* is designed to provide candidates with an efficient method to review didactic information. The academic review avoids attempting to cover every aspect of a physical therapy curriculum and instead focuses on the most essential information necessary to maximize examination performance. The unit presents information arranged in eleven distinct chapters. A detailed listing of the content of each chapter is located in the table of contents. The majority of information presented in the academic review should be familiar to candidates, however, due to the sheer volume of information included in a physical therapy academic program there will be many didactic areas that will need to be reviewed prior to the examination.

Candidates should remember that the examination is designed to reflect current clinical practice and as a result topics that are commonly encountered in clinical practice will represent a vast majority of the actual questions on any version of the examination. Candidates should make sure that they are thoroughly familiar with foundational information prior to expanding the breadth and depth of their academic review. This pragmatic approach allows candidates to significantly increase the utility of their study sessions and increase their examination score.

A prime example of this basic premise is as follows. Assume that a candidate is reviewing orthopedic special tests by utilizing the textbook Orthopedic Assessment by David Magee. The textbook offers a complete description of hundreds of special tests organized by area of the body. Although the textbook is a wonderful resource for students and faculty the sheer volume of special tests makes it impractical to attempt to review all of the presented information related to special tests. In contrast, the academic review section of *PTEXAM: The Complete Study Guide* offers a summary of the most commonly encountered special tests organized by body part and by specific condition that the test is designed to identify.

Candidates have numerous resources that they can rely on for additional information such as the textbook by Magee, however, as this example illustrates candidates must have a firm grasp on the basics before expanding the scope of their academic review.

Chapter One
Foundational Science

Anatomy and Physiology

Joint Classification

Fibrous Joints (Synarthroses)

Fibrous joints are composed of bones that are united by fibrous tissue and are nonsynovial. Movement is minimal to none with the amount of movement permitted at the joint dependent on the length of the fibers uniting the bones.

Suture – (e.g., sagittal suture of the skull)
- Union of two bones by a ligament or membrane
- Immovable joint
- Eventual fusion is termed a synostosis

Syndesmosis – (e.g., the tibia and fibula with interosseous membrane)
- Bone connected to bone by a dense fibrous membrane or cord
- Very little motion

Gomphosis – (e.g., a tooth in its socket)
- Two bony surfaces connect as a peg in a hole
- The teeth and corresponding sockets in the mandible/maxilla are the only gomphosis joints in the body
- The periodontal membrane is the fibrous component of the joint

Cartilaginous Joints (Amphiarthroses)

Cartilaginous joints have a hyaline cartilage or fibrocartilage that connects one bone to another. These are slightly moveable joints.

Synchondrosis – (e.g., sternum and true rib articulation)
- Hyaline cartilage
- Cartilage adjoins two ossifying centers of bone
- Provides stability during growth
- May ossify to a synostosis once growth is completed
- Slight motion

Symphysis – (e.g., pubic symphysis)
- Generally located at the midline of the body
- Two bones covered with hyaline cartilage
- Two bones connected by fibrocartilage
- Slight motion

Synovial Joints (Diarthroses)

Synovial joints provide free movement between the bones they join. They have five distinguishing characteristics: joint cavity, articular cartilage, synovial membrane, synovial fluid, and fibrous capsule. The joints are the most complex and vulnerable to injury and are further classified by the type of movement and by the shape of articulating bones.

Uniaxial joint – one motion around a single axis in one plane of the body
- Hinge (ginglymus) – elbow joint
- Pivot (trochoid) – atlantoaxial joint

Biaxial joint – movement occurs in two planes and around two axes through the convex/concave surfaces
- Condyloid – metacarpophalangeal joint of a finger
- Saddle – carpometacarpal joint of the thumb

Multi-axial joint – movement occurs in three planes and around three axes
- Plane (gliding) – carpal joints
- Ball and socket – hip joint

Specific Joints

Shoulder

The shoulder complex consists of four separate articulations.

- **Sternoclavicular joint:** Composed of the clavicle articulating with the manubrium of the sternum.

- **Acromioclavicular joint:** Composed of the lateral end of the clavicle articulating with the acromion of the scapula.

- **Glenohumeral joint:** Classified as a ball and socket joint, in which the round head of the humerus articulates with the shallow glenoid cavity of the scapula. The capsule of the glenohumeral joint is reinforced by the superior glenohumeral ligament, middle glenohumeral ligament, inferior glenohumeral ligament, and the coracohumeral ligament.

- **Scapulothoracic articulation:** Composed of the articulation between the scapula and the posterior rib cage. The articulation is not considered to be a joint since it lacks connection by fibrous, cartilaginous or synovial tissue.

Elbow

The elbow is classified as a hinge joint. It is composed of the humerus, ulna, and radius. Flexion and extension occur at the articulation of the trochlea with the semilunar notch of the ulna. The joint capsule is reinforced by the ulnar collateral ligament and the radial collateral ligament.

Wrist and Hand

The wrist complex consists of the radiocarpal and midcarpal joints. Motions at the wrist include flexion, extension, radial and ulnar deviation. The hand consists of the metacarpophalangeal joints, the proximal and distal interphalangeal joints, and the carpometacarpal joints.

Hip

The hip is classified as a ball and socket joint. It is formed by the articulation of the femur with the innominate bone. The head of the femur inserts into a deep socket called the acetabulum.

Stability is provided to the hip joint by the following:
- Acetabulum
- Iliofemoral ligament
- Pubofemoral ligament
- Ischiofemoral ligament

Knee

The knee is classified as a hinge joint. It is formed by the articulation of the tibia with the femur. The knee is extremely weak in terms of its bony arrangement.

Stability is provided to the knee joint by the following ligaments:
- Anterior cruciate ligament
- Posterior cruciate ligament
- Medial collateral ligament
- Lateral collateral ligament
- Deep medial capsular ligament

Ankle

The ankle is classified as a hinge joint which is formed by the articulation of the tibia and fibula with the talus. The distal ends of the tibia and fibula form a mortise that borders the talus. The bony arrangement provides the ankle with good lateral stability.

The ankle is structurally strong secondary to the bony and ligamentous arrangement.

Medial Ligaments:
- Deltoid

Lateral Ligaments:
- Anterior tibiofibular
- Anterior talofibular
- Calcaneofibular
- Lateral talocalcaneal
- Posterior talofibular

Joint Receptors

Free Nerve Endings

Location:	Joint capsule, ligaments, synovium, fat pads
Sensitivity:	One type sensitive to non-noxious mechanical stress; other type sensitive to noxious mechanical or biochemical stimuli
Primary Distribution:	All joints

Golgi Ligament Endings

Location:	Ligaments, adjacent to ligaments' bony attachment
Sensitivity:	Tension or stretch on ligaments
Primary Distribution:	Majority of joints

Golgi-Mazzoni Corpuscles

Location:	Joint capsule
Sensitivity:	Compression of joint capsule
Primary Distribution:	Knee joint, joint capsule

Pacinian Corpuscles

Location:	Fibrous layer of joint capsule
Sensitivity:	High frequency vibration, acceleration, and high velocity changes in joint position
Primary Distribution:	All joints

Ruffini Endings

Location:	Fibrous layer of joint capsule
Sensitivity:	Stretching of joint capsule, amplitude, and velocity of joint position
Primary Distribution:	Greater density in proximal joints particularly in capsular regions

Muscle Action

Head

Temporomandibular Joint

Depress:
- Lateral pterygoid
- Suprahyoid
- Infrahyoid

Elevate:
- Temporalis
- Masseter
- Medial pterygoid

Protrusion:
- Masseter
- Lateral pterygoid
- Medial pterygoid

Side to Side:
- Medial pterygoid
- Lateral pterygoid
- Masseter
- Temporalis

Retrusion:
- Temporalis
- Masseter
- Digastric

Spine

Cervical Intervertebral Joints

Flexion:
- Sternocleidomastoid
- Longus coli
- Scalenus muscles

Extension:
- Splenius cervicis
- Semispinalis cervicis
- Iliocostalis cervicis
- Longissimus cervicis
- Multifidus
- Trapezius

Rotation and Lateral Bending:
- Sternocleidomastoid
- Scalenus muscles
- Splenius cervicis
- Longissimus cervicis
- Iliocostalis cervicis
- Levator scapulae
- Multifidus

Thoracic and Lumbar Intervertebral Joints

Flexion:
- Rectus abdominis
- Internal oblique
- External oblique

Extension:
- Erector spinae

Rotation and Lateral Bending:
- Psoas major
- Quadratus lumborum
- External oblique
- Internal oblique
- Multifidus
- Quadratus lumborum
- Multifidus
- Longissimus thoracis
- Iliocostalis thoracis
- Rotatores

Upper Extremity

Scapula

Elevation:
- Upper trapezius
- Levator scapulae

Depression:
- Latissimus dorsi
- Pectoralis major
- Pectoralis minor
- Lower trapezius

Protraction:
- Serratus anterior
- Pectoralis major
- Pectoralis minor

Retraction:
- Trapezius
- Rhomboids

Upward Rotation:
- Upper trapezius
- Serratus anterior
- Lower trapezius

Downward Rotation:
- Rhomboids
- Levator scapulae
- Pectoralis minor

Shoulder Joint

Flexion:
- Anterior deltoid
- Coracobrachialis
- Pectoralis major
- Biceps brachii
- Supraspinatus

Extension:
- Latissimus dorsi
- Subscapularis
- Posterior deltoid
- Teres major

Abduction:
- Middle deltoid
- Supraspinatus
- Infraspinatus

Adduction:
- Pectoralis major
- Latissimus dorsi
- Teres major

Lateral Rotation:
- Teres minor
- Infraspinatus
- Posterior deltoid

Medial Rotation:
- Subscapularis
- Teres major
- Pectoralis major
- Latissimus dorsi
- Anterior deltoid

Elbow Joint

Flexion:
- Biceps brachii
- Brachialis
- Brachioradialis

Extension:
- Triceps brachii
- Anconeus

Radioulnar Joint

Supination:
- Biceps brachii
- Supinator

Pronation:
- Pronator teres
- Pronator quadratus

Wrist Joint

Flexion:
- Flexor carpi radialis
- Flexor carpi ulnaris
- Palmaris longus

Extension:
- Extensor carpi radialis longus
- Extensor carpi radialis brevis
- Extensor carpi ulnaris

Radial Deviation:
- Extensor carpi radialis
- Flexor carpi radialis
- Extensor pollicis longus and brevis

Ulnar Deviation:
- Extensor carpi ulnaris
- Flexor carpi ulnaris

Lower Extremity

Hip Joint

Flexion:
- Iliopsoas
- Sartorius
- Rectus femoris
- Pectineus

Extension:
- Gluteus maximus and medius
- Semitendinosus
- Semimembranosus
- Biceps femoris

Abduction:
- Gluteus medius
- Gluteus minimus
- Piriformis
- Obturator internus

Adduction:
- Adductor magnus
- Adductor longus
- Adductor brevis
- Gracilis

Medial Rotation:
- Tensor fasciae latae
- Gluteus medius
- Gluteus minimus
- Pectineus
- Adductor longus

Lateral Rotation:
- Gluteus maximus
- Obturator externus
- Obturator internus
- Piriformis
- Gemelli
- Sartorius

Knee Joint

Flexion:
- Biceps femoris
- Semitendinosus
- Semimembranosus
- Sartorius

Extension:
- Rectus femoris
- Vastus lateralis
- Vastus intermedius
- Vastus medialis

Medial Rotation of Flexed Leg:
- Sartorius
- Popliteus
- Semitendinosus
- Semimembranosus

Lateral Rotation of Flexed Leg:
- Biceps femoris

Ankle Joint

Plantar Flexion:
- Gastrocnemius
- Soleus
- Peroneus longus
- Peroneus brevis
- Plantaris
- Flexor hallucis
- Tibialis posterior

Dorsiflexion:
- Tibialis anterior
- Extensor hallucis longus
- Extensor digitorum longus
- Peroneus tertius

Inversion:
- Tibialis posterior
- Tibialis anterior
- Flexor digitorum longus

Eversion:
- Peroneus longus
- Peroneus brevis
- Peroneus tertius

Nerve Root Dermatomes, Myotomes, Reflexes, and Paresthetic Areas

Nerve Root	Dermatome*	Muscle Weakness (Myotome)	Reflexes Affected	Paresthesias
C1	Vertex of skull	None	None	None
C2	Temple, forehead, occiput	Longus colli, sternocleidomastoid, rectus capitis	None	None
C3	Entire neck, posterior cheek, temporal area, prolongation forward under mandible	Trapezius, splenius capitis	None	Cheek, side of neck
C4	Shoulder area, clavicular area, upper scapular area	Trapezius, levator scapulae	None	Horizontal band along clavicle and upper scapula
C5	Deltoid area, anterior aspect of entire arm to base of thumb	Supraspinatus, infraspinatus, deltoid, biceps	Biceps, brachioradialis	None
C6	Anterior arm, radial side of hand to thumb and index finger	Biceps, supinator, wrist extensors	Biceps, brachioradialis	Thumb and index finger
C7	Lateral arm and forearm to index, long, and ring fingers	Triceps, wrist flexors (rarely, wrist extensors)	Triceps	Index, long, and ring fingers
C8	Medial arm and forearm to long, ring, and little fingers	Ulnar deviators, thumb extensors, thumb adductors (rarely, triceps)	Triceps	Little finger alone or with two adjacent fingers; not ring or long fingers, alone or together (C7)
T1	Medial side of forearm to base of little finger	Disk lesions at upper two thoracic levels do not appear to give rise to root weakness. Weakness of intrinsic muscles of the hand is due to other pathology (e.g., thoracic outlet pressure, neoplasm of lung, and ulnar nerve lesion). Dural and nerve root stress has T1 elbow flexion with arm horizontal. T1 and T2 scapulae forward and backward on chest wall. Neck flexion at any thoracic level.		
T2	Medial side of upper arm to medial elbow, pectoral and midscapular areas			
T3 – T12	T3-T6, upper thorax; T5-T7, costal margin; T8-T12, abdomen and lumbar region	Articular and dural signs and root pain are common. Root signs (cutaneous analgesia) are rare and have such indefinite area that they have little localizing value. Weakness is not detectable.		
L1	Back, over trochanter and groin	None	None	Groin; after holding posture, which causes pain
L2	Back, front of thigh to knee	Psoas, hip adductors	None	Occasionally anterior thigh
L3	Back, upper buttock, anterior thigh and knee, medial lower leg	Psoas, quadriceps, thigh atrophy	Knee jerk sluggish, PKB positive, pain on full SLR	Medial knee, anterior lower leg
L4	Medial buttock, lateral thigh, medial leg, dorsum of foot, big toe	Tibialis anterior, extensor hallucis	SLR limited neck flexion pain, weak or absent knee jerk, side flexion limited	Medial aspect of calf and ankle
L5	Buttock, posterior and lateral thigh, lateral aspect of leg, dorsum of foot, medial half of sole, first, second, and third toes	Extensor hallucis, peroneals, gluteus medius, dorsiflexors, hamstring and calf atrophy	SLR limited one side, neck flexion painful, ankle decreased, crossed-leg raising pain	Lateral aspect of leg, medial three toes
S1	Buttock, thigh, and leg posterior	Calf and hamstring, wasting of gluteals, peroneals, plantar flexors	SLR limited, Achilles reflex weak or absent	Lateral two toes, lateral foot, lateral leg to knee, plantar aspect of foot

Nerve Root Dermatomes, Myotomes, Reflexes, and Paresthetic Areas (cont.)

Nerve Root	Dermatome*	Muscle Weakness (Myotome)	Reflexes Affected	Paresthesias (cont.)
S2	Same as S1	Same as S1 except peroneals	Same as S1	Lateral leg, knee, and heel
S3	Groin, medial thigh to knee	None	None	None
S4	Perineum, genitals, lower sacrum	Bladder, rectum	None	Saddle area, genitals, anus, impotence, massive posterior herniation

*In any part of which pain may be felt.
 PKB = prone knee bending; SLR = straight leg raising.

From Magee, DJ: Orthopedic Physical Assessment. W.B. Saunders Company, Philadelphia 2002, p.16, with permission.

Muscle stretch reflexes

☐ Biceps	C5-6
☐ Supinator (brachioradialis)	C5-6
☐ Triceps	C6-8
☐ Knee	L2-4
☐ Ankle	L5-S2

Cutaneous reflexes

■ Abdominal - Upper	T8-10
☐ Abdominal - Lower	T10-12
■ Cremasteric	L1
☐ Plantar	L4-S2
■ Anal	S2-5

Nerves of the Brachial Plexus

Origin	Nerves	Muscles
From the rami of the plexus:	Dorsal scapular	Rhomboids
		Levator scapulae
	Long thoracic	Serratus anterior
From the trunks of the plexus:	Nerve to subclavius	Subclavius
	Suprascapular	Infraspinatus
		Supraspinatus
From the lateral cord of the plexus:	Lateral pectoral	Pectoralis major
		Pectoralis minor
	Musculocutaneous	Coracobrachialis
		Biceps brachii
		Brachialis
	Lateral root of the median	Flexor muscles in the forearm, except flexor carpi ulnaris, and five muscles in the hand
From the medial cord of the plexus:	Medial pectoral	Pectoralis major
		Pectoralis minor
	Ulnar	1 ½ muscles of the forearm and most small muscles of the hand
	Medial root of the median	Flexor muscles in the forearm, except flexor carpi ulnaris, and five muscles in the hand
From the posterior cord of the plexus:	Upper subscapular	Subscapularis
	Thoracodorsal	Latissimus dorsi
	Lower subscapular	Subscapularis
		Teres major
	Axillary	Deltoid
		Teres minor
	Radial	Brachioradialis and the extensor muscles of the forearm

Lower Extremity Innervation

Lumbar Plexus:	Sciatic Nerve (Tibial Division):
Psoas major	Semitendinosus
Psoas minor	Soleus
	Popliteus
	Semimembranosus
	Plantaris
	Tibialis posterior
	Gastrocnemius
	Biceps femoris (long head)
	Flexor hallucis longus
	Flexor digitorum longus

Sacral Plexus:	Sciatic Nerve (Common Peroneal Division):
Piriformis	Biceps femoris
Superior gemelli	(short head)
Obturator internus	
Inferior gemelli	
Quadratus femoris	

Inferior Gluteal Nerve:	Deep Peroneal Nerve:
Gluteus maximus	Extensor digitorum longus
	Tibialis anterior

Superior Gluteal Nerve:	Superficial Peroneal Nerve:
Gluteus medius	Peroneus longus
Tensor fasciae latae	Peroneus brevis
Gluteus minimus	

Femoral Nerve:	Medial Plantar Nerve:
Iliacus	Abductor hallucis
Vastus lateralis	Lumbricale I
Rectus femoris	Flexor digitorum brevis
Vastus medialis	Flexor hallucis longus
Sartorius	
Vastus intermedius	
Pectineus	

Obturator Nerve:	Lateral Plantar Nerve:
Adductor longus	Abductor digiti minimi
Gracilis	Dorsal interossei
Adductor brevis	Quadratus plantae
Obturator externus	Adductor hallucis
Adductor magnus	Lumbricale II, III, IV
	Plantar interossei
	Flexor digiti minimi brevis

Neuroanatomy

Cranial Nerves and Methods of Testing

Nerve	Afferent (Sensory)	Efferent (Motor)	Test
Olfactory	Smell: Nose		Identify familiar odors (e.g., chocolate, coffee)
Optic	Sight: Eye		Test visual fields
Oculomotor		Voluntary motor: Levator of eyelid; superior, medial, and inferior recti; inferior oblique muscle of eyeball Autonomic: Smooth muscle of eyeball	Upward, downward, and medial gaze Reaction to light
Trochlear		Voluntary motor: Superior oblique muscle of eyeball	Downward and lateral gaze
Trigeminal	Touch, pain: Skin of face, mucous membranes of nose, sinuses, mouth, anterior tongue	Voluntary motor: Muscles of mastication	Corneal reflex Face sensation Clench teeth; push down on chin to separate jaws
Abducens		Voluntary motor: Lateral rectus muscle of eyeball	Lateral gaze
Facial	Taste: Anterior tongue	Voluntary motor: Facial muscles Autonomic: Lacrimal, submandibular, and sublingual glands	Close eyes tight Smile and show teeth Whistle and puff cheeks Identify familiar tastes (e.g., sweet, sour)
Vestibulocochlear (acoustic nerve)	Hearing: Ear Balance: Ear		Hear watch ticking Hearing tests Balance and coordination test
Glossopharyngeal	Touch, pain: Posterior tongue, pharynx Taste: Posterior tongue	Voluntary motor: Unimportant muscle of pharynx Autonomic: Parotid gland	Gag reflex Ability to swallow
Vagus	Touch, pain: Pharynx, larynx, bronchi Taste: Tongue, epiglottis	Voluntary motor: Muscles of palate, pharynx, and larynx Autonomic: Thoracic and abdominal viscera	Gag reflex Ability to swallow Say "Ahhh"
Accessory		Voluntary motor: Sternocleidomastoid and trapezius muscle	Resisted shoulder shrug
Hypoglossal		Voluntary motor: Muscles of tongue	Tongue protrusion (if injured, tongue deviates toward injured side)

From Magee, DJ: Orthopedic Physical Assessment. W.B. Saunders Company, Philadelphia 2002, p.69, with permission.

Kinesiology

Planes of the Body

Motions are described as occurring around three cardinal planes of the body (frontal, sagittal, transverse). Movement in the cardinal planes occurs around three corresponding axes (anterior-posterior, medial-lateral, vertical).

Frontal plane
The frontal plane divides the body into anterior and posterior sections. Motions in the frontal plane such as abduction and adduction occur around an anterior-posterior axis.

Sagittal plane
The sagittal plane divides the body into right and left sections. Motions in the sagittal plane such as flexion and extension occur around a medial-lateral axis.

Transverse plane
The transverse plane divides the body into upper and lower sections. Motions in the transverse plane such as medial and lateral rotation occur around a vertical axis.

Classes of Levers

Class 1 Lever
A class 1 lever has the axis of rotation (fulcrum) between the effort (force) and resistance (load). There are very few class 1 levers in the body. A class 1 lever is illustrated with the triceps brachii force on the olecranon with an external counter force pushing on the forearm. Another example of a class 1 lever is a seesaw.

Class 2 Lever
A class 2 lever has the resistance (load) between the axis of rotation (fulcrum) and the effort (force). The length of the effort arm is always longer than the resistance arm. In most instances, gravity is the effort and muscle activity is the resistance, however, there are class 2 levers that the muscle is the effort when the distal attachment is on a weight bearing segment. An example of a class 2 lever is a wheelbarrow.

Class 3 Lever
A class 3 lever has the effort (force) between the axis of rotation (fulcrum) and the resistance (load). The length of the effort arm is always shorter than the length of the resistance arm. Shoulder abduction with weight at the wrist is a class 3 lever. Class 3 levers usually permit large movements at rapid speeds and are the most common type of lever in the body. An example of a class 3 lever is elbow flexion.

Exercise Physiology

Energy Systems

ATP-PC or Phosphagen System
Anaerobic Glycolysis or Lactic Acid System
Aerobic or Oxygen System

Anaerobic Metabolism

ATP-PC System
This energy system is used for ATP production during high intensity, short duration exercise such as sprinting 100 meters. Phosphocreatine decomposes and releases a large amount of energy that is used to construct ATP. There is two to three times more phosphocreatine in cells of muscles than ATP. This process occurs almost instantaneously allowing for ready and available energy needed by the muscles. The system provides energy for muscle contraction for up to 15 seconds.

The phosphagen system represents the most rapidly available source of ATP for use by the muscle. Reasons for this rapid availability are as follows:
- It does not depend on a long series of chemical reactions.
- It does not depend on transporting the oxygen we breathe to the working muscles.
- Both ATP and PC are stored directly within the contractile mechanisms of the muscle.

Anaerobic Glycolysis
This energy system is a major supplier of ATP during high intensity, short duration activities such as sprinting 400 or 800 meters. Stored glycogen is split into glucose,

and through glycolysis, split again into pyruvic acid. The energy released during this process forms ATP. The process does not require oxygen. This system is nearly 50% slower than the phosphocreatine system and can provide a person with 30 to 40 seconds of muscle contraction.

- Anaerobic glycolysis results in the formation of lactic acid, which causes muscular fatigue.
- It does not require the presence of oxygen.
- It uses only carbohydrates (glycogen and glucose).
- It releases enough energy for the resynthesis of only small amounts of ATP.

Aerobic Metabolism

The aerobic system is used predominantly during low intensity, long duration exercise such as running a marathon. The oxygen system yields by far the most ATP, but it requires several series of complex chemical reactions. This system provides energy through the oxidation of food. The combination of fatty acids, amino acids, and glucose with oxygen releases energy that forms ATP. This system will provide energy as long as there are nutrients to utilize.

Muscle Physiology

Classification of Muscle Fibers	
Type I:	**Type II:**
Aerobic	Anaerobic
Red	White
Tonic	Phasic
Slow twitch	Fast twitch
Slow-oxidative	Fast-glycolytic

Functional Characteristics of Muscle Fibers	
Type I:	**Type II:**
Low fatigability	High fatigability
High capillary density	Low capillary density
High myoglobin content	Low myoglobin content
Smaller fibers	Larger fibers
Extensive blood supply	Less blood supply
Large amount of mitochondria	Fewer mitochondria
Example: marathon, swimming	**Example:** high jump, sprinting

Muscle Receptors

Muscle Spindle
Muscle spindles are distributed throughout the belly of the muscle. They function to send information to the nervous system about muscle length and/or the rate of change of its length. The muscle spindle is important in the control of posture and with the help of the gamma system, involuntary movements.

Golgi Tendon Organ
Golgi tendon organs are encapsulated sensory receptors through which the muscle tendons pass immediately beyond their attachment to the muscle fibers. They are very sensitive to tension especially when produced from an active muscle contraction. They function to transmit information about tension or the rate of change of tension within the muscle.

An average of 10-15 muscle fibers are usually connected in series with each golgi tendon organ. The golgi tendon organ is stimulated through the tension produced by muscle fibers. Golgi tendon organs provide the nervous system with instantaneous information on the degree of tension in each small muscle segment.

Resistive Training

Types of Muscular Contraction

Concentric: A concentric contraction occurs when the muscle shortens while developing tension.

Eccentric: An eccentric contraction occurs when the muscle lengthens while developing tension.

Isometric: An isometric contraction occurs when tension develops but there is no change in the length of the muscle.

Isotonic: An isotonic contraction occurs when the muscle shortens or lengthens while resisting a constant load.

Isokinetic: An isokinetic contraction occurs when the tension developed by the muscle, while shortening or lengthening at a constant speed, is maximal over the full range of motion.

Open-Chain versus Closed-Chain Activities

Open-Chain: Open-chain activities involve the distal segment, usually the hand or foot, moving freely in space. An example of an open-chain activity is kicking a ball with the lower extremity.

Closed-Chain: Closed-chain activities involve the body moving over a fixed distal segment. An example of a closed-chain activity is a squat lift.

Resistive and Overload Training

Isometric Exercise
Muscular force is generated without a change in muscle length. Isometric exercises are often performed against an immovable object. Submaximal isometric exercises are traditionally used in rehabilitation programs.

Isotonic Exercise
Muscular contraction in which the muscle exerts a constant tension. This can also be thought of as muscle movement with a constant load. Isotonic exercises are performed against resistance often employing equipment such as handheld weights.

Isokinetic Exercise
Exercise with a constant maximal speed and variable load. In isokinetic exercise the reaction force is identical to the force applied to the equipment. Cybex, Biodex, and Lido are a few of the companies making isokinetic exercise equipment.

Exercise Programs

DeLorme	Protocol
First Set	10 repetitions x 50% of 10 repetition maximum
Second Set	10 repetitions x 75% of 10 repetition maximum
Third Set	10 repetitions x 100% of 10 repetition maximum

Oxford Technique	Protocol
First Set	10 repetitions x 100% of 10 repetition maximum
Second Set	10 repetitions x 75% of 10 repetition maximum
Third Set	10 repetitions x 50% of 10 repetition maximum

Chapter Two
Musculoskeletal

Orthopedics

Upper Quarter Screening

The upper quarter screen provides a rapid assessment of mobility and neurologic function of the cervical spine and upper extremities. The screen is traditionally performed with the patient in sitting.

The following is an example of the components of an upper extremity screening:

Posture
- Postural assessment

Range of Motion
- Active range of motion of the cervical spine
- Active range of motion of the upper extremities
- Passive overpressure of the cervical spine and upper extremities, if the patient does not exhibit signs and symptoms of pathology

Resistive Testing (C1 – T1)

Resistive Test	Innervation Level
Cervical rotation	C1
Shoulder elevation	C2 – C4
Shoulder abduction	C5
Elbow flexion	C5 – C6
Wrist extension	C6
Elbow extension	C7
Wrist flexion	C7
Thumb extension	C8
Finger adduction	T1

Dermatome Testing (C2 – T1)

Area of Skin	Innervation Level
Posterior head	C2
Posterior-lateral neck	C3
Acromioclavicular joint	C4
Lateral Arm	C5
Lateral forearm and thumb	C6
Palmar distal phalanx – middle finger	C7
Little finger and ulnar border of the hand	C8
Medial forearm	T1

Reflex Testing (C5 – C7)

Reflex	Innervation Level
Biceps	C5
Brachioradialis	C6
Triceps	C7

Lower Quarter Screening

The lower quarter screen provides a rapid assessment of mobility and neurologic function of the lumbosacral spine and lower extremities. The screen is traditionally performed with the patient in standing or sitting.

The following is an example of the components of a lower extremity screening:

Posture
- Postural assessment

Range of Motion
- Active range of motion of the lumbosacral spine
- Active range of motion of the lower extremities
- Passive overpressure of the lumbosacral spine and lower extremities, if the patient does not exhibit signs and symptoms of pathology

Functional Testing (L4 – S1)

Functional Test	Innervation Level
Heel walking	L4 – L5
Toe walking	S1
Straight leg raise	L4 – S1

Resistive Testing (L1 – S1)

Resistive Test	Innervation Level
Hip flexion	L1 – L2
Knee extension	L3 – L4
Ankle dorsiflexion	L4 – L5
Great toe extension	L5
Ankle plantar flexion	S1

Reflex Testing (L4 – S1)

Reflex	Innervation Level
Patella	L4
Achilles	S1

Dermatome Testing (L2 – S5)

Area of Skin	Innervation Level
Anterior thigh	L2
Middle third of anterior thigh	L3
Patella and medial malleolus	L4
Fibular head and dorsum of foot	L5

Dermatome Testing (L2 – S5) (continued)

Area of Skin	Innervation Level
Lateral and plantar aspect of foot	S1
Medial aspect of posterior thigh	S2
Perianal area	S3 – S5

Scanning Examination to Rule Out Referral of Symptoms from Other Tissues

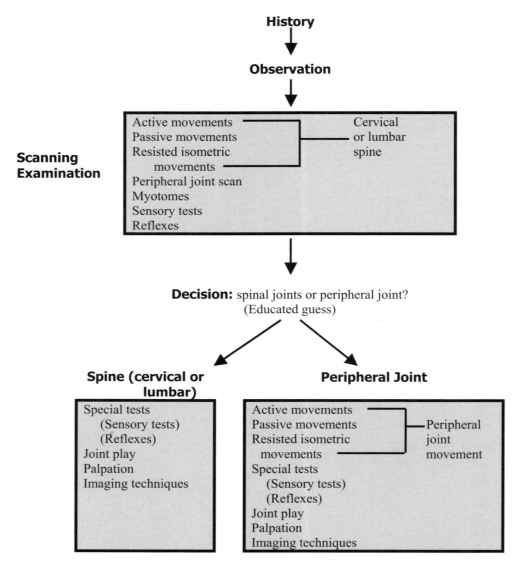

From Magee, DJ: Orthopedic Physical Assessment. W.B. Saunders Company, Philadelphia 2002, p.15, with permission.

Posture

Good and Faulty Posture: Summary Chart

Good Posture	Part	Faulty Posture
In standing, the longitudinal arch has the shape of a half dome. Barefoot or in shoes without heels, the feet toe-out slightly. In shoes with heels the feet are parallel. In walking with or without shoes, the feet are parallel and the weight is transferred from the heel along the outer border to the ball of the foot. In sprinting the feet are parallel or toe-in slightly. The weight is on the balls of the feet and toes because the heels do not come in contact with the ground.	**Foot**	Low longitudinal arch or flat foot. Low metatarsal arch, usually indicated by calluses under the ball of the foot. Weight borne on the inner side of the foot (pronation). "Ankle rolls in." Weight borne on the outer border of the foot (supination). "Ankle rolls out." Toeing-out while walking, or while standing in shoes with heels ("slue-footed"). Toeing-in while walking or standing ("pigeon-toed").
Toes should be straight, that is, neither curled downward nor bent upward. They should extend forward in line with the foot and not be squeezed together or overlap.	**Toes**	Toes bend up at the first joint and down at the middle joints so that the weight rests on the tips of the toes (hammer toes). This fault is often associated with wearing shoes that are too short. Big toe slants inward toward the midline of the foot (hallux valgus). "Bunion." This fault is often associated with wearing shoes that are too narrow and pointed at the toes.
Legs are straight up and down. Kneecaps face straight ahead when feet are in good position. Looking at the knees from the side, the knees are straight, i.e., neither bent forward nor locked backward.	**Knees and Legs**	Knees touch when feet are apart (knock-knees). Knees are apart when feet touch (bowlegs). Knee curves slightly backward (hyperextended knee). "Back-knee." Knee bends slightly forward, that is, it is not as straight as it should be (flexed knee). Kneecaps face slightly toward each other (medially rotated femurs). Kneecaps face slightly outward (laterally rotated femurs).
Ideally, the body weight is borne evenly on both feet, and the hips are level. One side is not more prominent than the other as seen from front or back, nor is one hip more forward or backward than the other as seen from the side. The spine does not curve to the left or the right side. (A *slight* deviation to the left in right-handed individuals and to the right in left-handed individuals is not uncommon. Also, a tendency toward a *slightly* low right shoulder and *slightly* high right hip is frequently found in right-handed people, and vice versa for left-handed people).	**Hips, Pelvis, and Spine Back View**	One hip is higher than the other (lateral pelvic tilt). Sometimes it is not really much higher but appears so because a sideways sway of the body has made it more prominent. (Tailors and dressmakers often notice a lateral tilt because the hemline of skirts or length of trousers must be adjusted to the difference.) The hips are rotated so that one is farther forward than the other (clockwise or counter clockwise rotation).

Good and Faulty Posture: Summary Chart (continued)

Good Posture	Part	Faulty Posture
The front of the pelvis and the thighs are in a straight line. The buttocks are not prominent in back but slope slightly downward. The spine has four natural curves. In the neck and lower back the curve is forward, in the upper back and lowest part of the spine (sacral region) it is backward. The sacral curve is a fixed curve while the other three are flexible.	**Spine and Pelvis Side View**	The low back arches forward too much (lordosis). The pelvis tilts forward too much. The front of the thigh forms an angle with the pelvis when this tilt is present. The normal forward curve in the low back has straightened. The pelvis tips backward as in swayback and flat-back postures. Increased backward curve in the upper back (kyphosis or round upper back). Increased forward curve in the neck. Almost always accompanied by round upper back and seen as a forward head. Lateral curve of the spine (scoliosis); toward one side (C-curve), toward both sides (S-curve).
In young children up to about the age of 10, the abdomen normally protrudes somewhat. In older children and adults it should be flat.	**Abdomen**	Entire abdomen protrudes. Lower part of the abdomen protrudes while the upper part is pulled in.
A good position of the chest is one in which it is slightly up and slightly forward (while the back remains in good alignment). The chest appears to be in a position about halfway between that of a full inspiration and a forced expiration.	**Chest**	Depressed, or "hollow-chest" position. Lifted and held up too high, brought about by arching the back. Ribs more prominent on one side than on the other. Lower ribs flaring out or protruding.
Arms hang relaxed at the sides with palms of the hands facing toward the body. Elbows are slightly bent, so forearms hang slightly forward. Shoulders are level and neither one is more forward or backward than the other when seen from the side. Shoulder blades lie flat against the rib cage. They are neither too close together or too wide apart. In adults, a separation of about 4 inches is average.	**Arms and Shoulders**	Arms held stiffly in any position forward, backward, or out from the body. Arms turned so that palms of hands face backward. One shoulder higher than the other. Both shoulders hiked-up. One or both shoulders drooping forward or sloping. Shoulders rotated either clockwise or counterclockwise. Shoulder blades pulled back too hard. Shoulder blades too far apart. Shoulder blades too prominent, standing out from the rib cage (winged scapulae).
Head is held erect in a position of good balance.	**Head**	Chin up too high. Head protruding forward. Head tilted or rotated to one side.

From Kendall F, McCreary E, Provance P: Muscle Testing and Function. Lippencott, William & Wilkins, Baltimore 1993, p.115-116, with permission

Body Composition

Body composition is defined as the relative percentage of body weight that is comprised of fat and fat-free tissue. There are multiple methods for testing the percentage of body fat including hydrostatic weighing, skinfold measurements, plethysmography, body mass index, and bioelectrical impedance analysis. A healthy range of body fat is 12-18% for males and 18-23% for females.

Densitometry

Hydrostatic Weighing: This method calculates the density of the body by immersing a person in water and measuring the amount of water that becomes displaced. The percentage of body fat is then determined calculating the measured amount of water displaced in an equation based on Archimedes' principle. This method is the most widely used laboratory procedure to determine body density. Limitations of this method include the need to account for residual lung volume during submersion and evaluating patients that must tolerate water submersion during the testing. The standard error for this method is estimated at 2 to 2.5%.

Plethysmography: This method calculates the density of the body utilizing the amount of air displacement during testing within a specialized closed chamber. The change in pressure within the chamber is measured and converted to the percentage of body fat using a standardized equation.

Anthropometry

Skinfold Measurement: This method determines the overall percentage of body fat through the measurement of nine standardized sites. The correlation relies on the theory that the amount of subcutaneous fat is proportional to the total fat in the body. Limitations of this method include the requisite of an experienced examiner as well as variance from the standards based on gender, age, and ethnicity. Accuracy of measurement is within +/-3% with appropriate technique and equipment.

Skinfold Measurement Procedure
✓ All measurements should be taken on the right side of the body
✓ Take multiple measurements at each site to ensure accuracy and retest if the difference is greater than one to two millimeters
✓ Skinfold calipers should be positioned one centimeter away from the examiner's fingers when pinching the side, positioned perpendicular to the skinfold, and centered between the base and top of the fold
✓ Wait one to two seconds before reading the caliper
✓ Maintain pinching of the site during the reading of the caliper

Standard Skinfold Sites

▪ Abdominal	▪ Midaxillary
▪ Triceps *	▪ Subscapular *
▪ Biceps	▪ Suprailiac
▪ Chest/pectoral	▪ Thigh
▪ Medial calf	

There are seven-site and three-site formulas to calculate the percentage of body fat using particular sites. There are also specific formulas for gender, sport, ethnicity, and age.
* Indicates the most popular sites

Other Techniques

Body Mass Index (BMI)
This formula is designed to assess risk potential for obesity-related health issues by calculating an estimated percentage of body fat. The formula divides body weight in kilograms by height in meters squared (kg/m^2). There is evidence that an increase in BMI is associated with an increase in mortality rate secondary to heart disease, diabetes, and cancer. Limitation of this formula is that it does not measure proportional composition of the body or percentage of fat. The standard error with estimating percent fat using BMI is approximately 5%.

BMI Classification System
< 18.5 kg/m^2 underweight
$20 - 24.9$ kg/m^2 desirable
$25 - 29.9$ kg/m^2 overweight
$30 - 34.9$ kg/m^2 grade 1 obesity
$35 - 39.9$ kg/m^2 grade 2 obesity
> 40 kg/m^2 grade 3 obesity

Bioelectrical Impedance Analysis (BIA)
This method of assessing body composition uses a small electrical current and measures the resistance or opposition to the current flow. This technique is based on the principle that resistance to electrical current is inversely related to the composition of water within the body. The formula of $height^2/resistance$ is used for the general population while population-specific equations are also available. The standard error compares to the accuracy of skinfold measurements at approximately +/- 3%. Limitations include the requisite for the subjects to be properly hydrated as well as following all guidelines for the testing protocol.

BIA Protocol
✓ Abstain from eating or drinking within four hours prior to testing
✓ Abstain from vigorous physical activity within 12 hours prior to testing
✓ Urinate within 30 minutes prior to testing
✓ Avoid alcohol consumption for 48 hours prior to testing
✓ Avoid excessive water intake prior to testing

Positioning of a Joint

Descriptions of Specific Positions

	Loose Packed	Close Packed
Stress on joint	Minimal	Maximal
Congruency of joint	Minimal	Full
Ligament position	Great laxity	Full tightness
Joint surface	No volitional separation	Compressed

Resting (Loose Packed) Position of Joints

Joint:	Position:
Facet (spine)	Midway between flexion and extension
Temporomandibular	Mouth slightly open (freeway space)
Glenohumeral	55° abduction, 30° horizontal adduction
Acromioclavicular	Arm resting by side in normal physiological position
Ulnohumeral (elbow)	70° flexion, 10° supination
Radiohumeral	Full extension, full supination
Proximal radioulnar	70° flexion, 35° supination
Distal radioulnar	10° supination
Radiocarpal (wrist)	Neutral with slight ulnar deviation
Carpometacarpal	Midway between abduction - adduction and flexion - extension
Metacarpophalangeal	Slight flexion
Interphalangeal	Slight flexion
Hip	30° flexion, 30° abduction, slight lateral rotation
Knee	25° flexion
Talocrural (ankle)	10° plantar flexion, midway between maximum inversion and eversion
Subtalar	Midway between extremes of range of movement
Midtarsal	Midway between extremes of range of movement
Tarsometatarsal	Midway between extremes of range of movement
Metatarsophalangeal	Neutral
Interphalangeal	Slight flexion

From Magee, DJ: Orthopedic Physical Assessment. W.B. Saunders Company, Philadelphia 2002, p.50, with permission.

Close Packed Position of Joints

Joint:	Position:
Facet (spine)	Extension
Temporomandibular	Clenched teeth
Glenohumeral	Abduction and lateral rotation
Acromioclavicular	Arm abducted to 90°
Sternoclavicular	Maximum shoulder elevation
Ulnohumeral (elbow)	Extension
Radiohumeral	Elbow flexed 90°, forearm supinated 5°
Proximal radioulnar	5° supination
Distal radioulnar	5° supination
Radiocarpal (wrist)	Extension with radial deviation
Metacarpophalangeal (fingers)	Full flexion
Metacarpophalangeal (thumb)	Full opposition
Interphalangeal	Full extension
Hip	Full extension, medial rotation
Knee	Full extension, lateral rotation of tibia
Talocrural (ankle)	Maximum dorsiflexion
Subtalar	Supination
Midtarsal	Supination
Tarsometatarsal	Supination
Metatarsophalangeal	Full extension
Interphalangeal	Full extension

From Magee, DJ: Orthopedic Physical Assessment. W.B. Saunders Company, Philadelphia 2002, p.50, with permission.

Common Capsular Patterns of Joints

Joint:	Restriction:*
Temporomandibular	Limitation of mouth opening
Atlanto-occipital	Extension, side flexion equally limited
Cervical spine	Side flexion and rotation equally limited, extension
Glenohumeral	Lateral rotation, abduction, medial rotation
Sternoclavicular	Pain at extreme of range of movement

Common Capsular Patterns of Joints (continued)

Joint:	Restriction:*
Acromioclavicular	Pain at extreme of range of movement
Humeroulnar	Flexion, extension
Radiohumeral	Flexion, extension, supination, pronation
Proximal radioulnar	Supination, pronation
Distal radioulnar	Full range of movement, pain at extremes of rotation
Wrist	Flexion and extension equally limited
Trapeziometacarpal	Abduction, extension
Metacarpophalangeal and interphalangeal	Flexion, extension
Thoracic spine	Side flexion and rotation equally limited, extension
Lumbar spine	Side flexion and rotation equally limited, extension
Sacroiliac, symphysis pubis, and sacrococcygeal	Pain when joints are stressed
Hip**	Flexion, abduction, medial rotation (but in some cases medial rotation is most limited)
Knee	Flexion, extension
Tibiofibular	Pain when joint stressed
Talocrural	Plantar flexion, dorsiflexion
Talocalcaneal (subtalar)	Limitation of varus range of movement
Midtarsal	Dorsiflexion, plantar flexion, adduction, medial rotation
First metatarsophalangeal	Extension, flexion
Second to fifth metatarsophalangeal	Variable
Interphalangeal	Flexion, extension

* Movements are listed in order of restriction.
**For the hip, flexion, abduction, and medial rotation are always the movements most limited in a capsular pattern. However, the order of restriction may vary.

From Magee, DJ: Orthopedic Physical Assessment. W.B. Saunders Company, Philadelphia 2002, p.28, with permission.

End-Feel

Normal End-feel

End-feel is the type of resistance that is felt when passively moving a joint through the end range of motion. Certain tissues and joints have a consistent end-feel and are described as firm, hard or soft. Pathology can be identified through noting the type of abnormal end-feel within a particular joint.

- **Firm (stretch)**
  - *Examples:*   Ankle dorsiflexion
    - Finger extension
    - Hip medial rotation
    - Forearm supination
- **Hard (bone to bone)**
  - *Example:*   Elbow extension

- **Soft (soft tissue approximation)**
  - *Examples:*   Elbow flexion
    - Knee flexion

Abnormal End-feel

Abnormal end-feel would consist of any end-feel that is felt at an abnormal or inconsistent point in the range of motion or in a joint that normally presents with a different end-feel.

- **Empty (cannot reach end-feel, usually due to pain)**
  - *Examples:*   Joint inflammation
    - Fracture
    - Bursitis
- **Firm**
  - *Examples:*   Increased tone
    - Tightening of the capsule
    - Ligament shortening
- **Hard**
  - *Examples:*   Fracture
    - Osteoarthritis
    - Osteophyte formation
- **Soft**
  - *Examples:*   Edema
    - Synovitis
    - Ligament instability/tear

Muscle Testing

Manual Muscle Testing Grades

Zero (0/5) — The subject demonstrates no palpable muscle contraction.

Trace (1/5) — The subject's muscle contraction can be palpated, but there is no joint movement.

Poor Minus (2-/5) — The subject does not complete range of motion in a gravity eliminated position.

Poor (2/5) — The subject completes range of motion with gravity eliminated.

Poor Plus (2+/5) — The subject is able to initiate movement against gravity.

Fair Minus (3-/5) — The subject does not complete the range of motion against gravity, but does complete more than half of the range.

Fair (3/5) — The subject completes range of motion against gravity without manual resistance.

Fair Plus (3+/5) — The subject completes range of motion against gravity with only minimal resistance.

Good Minus (4-/5) — The subject completes range of motion against gravity with minimal-moderate resistance.

Good (4/5) — The subject completes range of motion against gravity with moderate resistance.

Good Plus (4+/5) — The subject completes range of motion against gravity with moderate-maximal resistance.

Normal (5/5) — The subject completes range of motion against gravity with maximal resistance.

Positioning for Muscle Testing

Supine

Abdominals	Anterior deltoid*
Biceps	Brachioradialis
Finger flexors	Finger extensors
Iliopsoas	Infraspinatus
Lateral rotators of shoulder*	Medial rotators of shoulder*
Neck flexors	Pectoralis major
Pectoralis minor	Peroneals
Pronators	Sartorius
Serratus anterior	Supinators
Tensor fasciae latae	Teres minor
Thumb muscles	Tibialis anterior
Tibialis posterior	Toe extensors
Toe flexors	Triceps*
Wrist extensors	Wrist flexors

Sidelying

Gluteus medius	Gluteus minimus
Hip adductors	Lateral abdominals

Prone

Back extensors	Gastrocnemius
Gluteus maximus	Hamstrings*
Lateral rotators of the shoulder*	Latissimus dorsi
Lower trapezius	Medial rotators of the shoulder*
Middle trapezius	Neck extensors
Posterior deltoid*	Quadratus lumborum
Rhomboids	Soleus
Teres major	Triceps*

Sitting

Coracobrachialis	Deltoid*
Hip flexors*	Lateral rotators of hip
Medial rotators of hip	Quadriceps
Upper trapezius	Serratus anterior*

Standing

Ankle plantar flexors	Serratus anterior*

*Indicates multiple acceptable positions for muscle testing

Gait

Standard versus Rancho Los Amigos Terminology

	Standard Terminology	**Rancho Los Amigos Terminology**
Stance Phase (60% of gait cycle)	Heel strike	Initial contact
	Foot flat	Loading response
	Midstance	Midstance
	Heel off	Terminal stance
	Toe off	Pre-swing
Swing Phase (40% of gait cycle)	Acceleration	Initial swing
	Midswing	Midswing
	Deceleration	Terminal swing

Standard Terminology
Stance Phase

Heel strike: Heel strike is the instant that the heel touches the ground to begin stance phase.

Foot flat: Foot flat is the point in which the entire foot makes contact with the ground and should occur directly after heel strike.

Midstance: Midstance is the point during the stance phase when the entire body weight is directly over the stance limb.

Heel off: Heel off is the point in which the heel of the stance limb leaves the ground.

Toe off: Toe off is the point in which only the toe of the stance limb remains on the ground.

Swing Phase

Acceleration: Acceleration begins when toe off is complete and the reference limb swings until positioned directly under the body.

Midswing: Mid-swing is the point when the swing limb is directly under the body.

Deceleration: Deceleration begins directly after midswing as the swing limb begins to extend and ends just prior to heel strike.

Rancho Los Amigos Terminology
Stance Phase

Initial contact: Initial contact is the beginning of the stance phase that occurs when the foot touches the ground.

Loading response: Loading response corresponds to the amount of time between initial contact and the beginning of the swing phase for the other leg.

Midstance: Midstance corresponds to the point in stance phase when the other foot is off the floor until the body is directly over the stance limb.

Terminal stance: Terminal stance begins when the stance limb's heel rises and ends when the other foot touches the ground.

Pre-swing: Pre-swing phase begins when the other foot touches the ground and ends when the stance foot reaches toe off.

Swing Phase

Initial swing: Initial swing phase begins when the stance foot lifts from the floor and ends with maximal knee flexion during swing.

Midswing: Midswing phase begins with maximal knee flexion during swing and ends when the tibia is perpendicular with the ground.

Terminal swing: Terminal swing phase begins when the tibia is perpendicular to the floor and ends when the foot touches the ground.

Normal Gait

	SWING 40 %			STANCE 60 %				
	Initial Swing	**Midswing**	**Terminal Swing**	**Initial Contact**	**Loading Response**	**Midstance**	**Terminal Stance**	**Pre-Swing**
Trunk	Erect Neutral	Erect Neutral	Erect Neutral	Erect Neutral	Erect Neutral	Erect Neutral	Erect Neutral	Erect Neutral
Pelvis	Level: Backward Rotation 5°	Level: Neutral Rotation	Level: Forward Rotation 5°	Level: Maintains Forward Rotation	Level: Less Forward Rotation	Level: Neutral Rotation	Level: Backward Rotation 5°	Level: Backward Rotation 5°
Hip	Flexion 20° Neutral: Rotation Abduction Adduction	Flexion 20° - 30° Neutral: Rotation Abduction Adduction	Flexion 30° Neutral: Rotation Abduction Adduction	Flexion 30° Neutral: Rotation Abduction Adduction	Flexion 30° Neutral: Rotation Abduction Adduction	Extending to Neutral Neutral: Rotation Abduction Adduction	Apparent Hyperextension 10° Neutral: Rotation Abduction Adduction	Neutral Extension Neutral: Rotation Abduction Adduction
Knee	Flexion 60°	From 60° to 30° Flexion	Extension to 0°	Full Extension	Flexion 15°	Extending to Neutral	Full Extension	Flexion 35°
Ankle	Plantar Flexion 10°	Neutral	Neutral	Neutral Heel First	Plantar Flexion 15°	From Plantar Flexion to 10° Dorsiflexion	Neutral with Tibia Stable and Heel Off Prior to Initial Contact Opposite Foot	Plantar Flexion 20°
Toes	Neutral	Neutral	Neutral	Neutral	Neutral	Neutral	Neutral IP Extended MP	Neutral IP Extended MP

From Rancho Los Amigos National Rehabilitation Center: Normal and Pathological Gait Syllabus, p.11. Downey, California, with permission.

Range of Motion Requirements for Normal Gait

Hip flexion:	0 – 30 degrees
Hip extension:	0 – 15 degrees
Knee flexion:	0 – 60 degrees
Knee extension:	0 degrees
Ankle dorsiflexion:	0 – 10 degrees
Ankle plantar flexion:	0 – 20 degrees

Peak Muscle Activity During the Gait Cycle

Tibialis anterior: Peak activity is just after heel strike. Responsible for eccentric lowering of the foot into plantar flexion.

Gastroc-soleus group: Peak activity is during late stance phase. Responsible for concentric raising of the heel during toe off.

Quadriceps group: Two periods of peak activity. In periods of single support during early stance phase and just before toe off to initiate swing phase.

Hamstrings group: Peak activity is during late swing phase. Responsible for decelerating the unsupported limb.

Gait Terminology

Base of support: The distance measured between the left and right foot during progression of gait. The distance decreases as cadence increases. The average base of support for an adult is two to four inches.

Cadence: The number of steps an individual will walk over a period of time. The average value for an adult is 110–120 steps per minute.

Degree of toe-out: The angle formed by each foot's line of progression and a line intersecting the center of the heel and second toe. The average degree of toe-out for an adult is seven degrees.

Double support phase: The double support phase refers to the two times during a gait cycle where both feet are on the ground. The time of double support increases as the speed of gait decreases. This phase does not exist with running.

Gait cycle: The gait cycle refers to the sequence of motions that occur from one initial contact of the heel to the next consecutive initial contact of the same heel.

Pelvic rotation: Rotation of the pelvis opposite the thorax in order to maintain balance and regulate speed. The pelvic rotation during gait for an adult is a total of 8 degrees (4 degrees forward with the swing leg and 4 degrees backward with the stance leg).

Single support phase: The single support phase occurs when only one foot is on the ground and occurs twice during a single gait cycle.

Step length: The distance measured between right heel strike and left heel strike. The average step length for an adult is 13 to 16 inches.

Stride: The distance measured between right heel strike and the following right heel strike. The average stride length for an adult is 26 to 32 inches.

Abnormal Gait Patterns

Antalgic: A protective gait pattern where the involved step length is decreased in order to avoid weight bearing on the involved side usually secondary to pain.

Ataxic: A gait pattern characterized by staggering and unsteadiness. There is usually a wide base of support and movements are exaggerated.

Cerebellar: A staggering gait pattern seen in cerebellar disease.

Circumduction: A gait pattern characterized by a circular motion to advance the leg during swing phase; this may be used to compensate for insufficient hip or knee flexion or dorsiflexion.

Double step: A gait pattern in which alternate steps are of a different length or at a different rate.

Equine: A gait pattern characterized by high steps; usually involves excessive activity of the gastrocnemius.

Festinating: A gait pattern where a patient walks on toes as though pushed. It starts slowly, increases, and may continue until the patient grasps an object in order to stop.

Hemiplegic: A gait pattern in which patients abduct the paralyzed limb, swing it around, and bring it forward so the foot comes to the ground in front of them.

Parkinsonian: A gait pattern marked by increased forward flexion of the trunk and knees; gait is shuffling with quick and small steps; festinating may occur.

Scissor: A gait pattern in which the legs cross midline upon advancement.

Spastic: A gait pattern with stiff movement, toes seeming to catch and drag, legs held together, hip and knee joints slightly flexed. Commonly seen in spastic paraplegia.

Steppage: A gait pattern in which the feet and toes are lifted through hip and knee flexion to excessive heights; usually secondary to dorsiflexor weakness. The foot will slap at initial contact with the ground secondary to the decreased control.

Tabetic: A high stepping ataxic gait pattern in which the feet slap the ground.

Trendelenburg: A gait pattern that denotes gluteus medius weakness; excessive lateral trunk flexion and weight shifting over the stance leg.

Vaulting: A gait pattern where the swing leg advances by compensating through the combination of elevation of the pelvis and plantar flexion of the stance leg.

Gait Deviations

Ankle and Foot	*Foot slap*	*Toe down instead of heel strike*	*Clawing of toes*	*Heel lift during midstance*	*No toe o...*
	-- Weak dorsiflexors -- Dorsiflexor paralysis	-- Plantar flexor spasticity -- Plantar flexor contracture -- Weak dorsiflexors -- Dorsiflexor paralysis -- Leg length discrepancy -- Hindfoot pain	-- Toe flexor spasticity -- Positive support reflex	-- Insufficient dorsiflexion range -- Plantar flexor spasticity	-- Forefoot/to... -- Weak plant flexors -- Weak toe f... -- Insufficient plantar flex range of mc...
Knee	*Exaggerated knee flexion at contact*	*Hyperextension in stance*	*Exaggerated knee flexion at terminal stance*	*Insufficient flexion with swing*	*Excessive fle... with swin...*
	-- Weak quadriceps -- Quadriceps paralysis -- Hamstrings spasticity -- Insufficient extension range of motion	-- Compensation for weak quadriceps -- Plantar flexor contracture	-- Knee flexion contracture -- Hip flexion contracture	-- Knee effusion -- Quadriceps extension spasticity -- Plantar flexor spasticity -- Insufficient flexion range of motion	-- Flexor withdrawal reflex -- Lower extre... flexor syner...
Hip	*Insufficient hip flexion at initial contact*	*Insufficient hip extension at stance*	*Circumduction during swing*	*Hip hiking during swing*	*Exaggerated flexion duri... swing*
	-- Weak hip flexors -- Hip flexor paralysis -- Hip extensor spasticity -- Insufficient hip flexion range of motion	-- Insufficient hip extension range of motion -- Hip flexion contracture -- Lower extremity flexor synergy	-- Compensation for weak hip flexors -- Compensation for weak dorsiflexors -- Compensation for weak hamstrings	-- Compensation for weak dorsiflexors -- Compensation for weak knee flexors -- Compensation for extensor synergy pattern	-- Lower extre... flexor syner... -- Compensati... for insuffici... hip flexion ... dorsiflexion

Range of Motion

Average Adult Range of Motion for the Upper and Lower Extremities

Upper Extremity

- **Shoulder:**

Flexion:	0-180
Extension:	0-60
Abduction:	0-180
Medial rotation:	0-70
Lateral rotation:	0-90

- **Elbow:**

Extension:	0
Flexion:	0-150

- **Forearm:**

Pronation:	0-80
Supination:	0-80

- **Wrist:**

Flexion:	0-80
Extension:	0-70
Radial deviation:	0-20
Ulnar deviation:	0-30

- **Thumb:**
  - **--Carpometacarpal**
Abduction	0-70
Flexion	0-15
Extension	0-20
Opposition	Tip of thumb to base of fifth digit

  - **--Metacarpophalangeal**
Flexion	0-50

  - **--Interphalangeal**
Flexion	0-80

- **Digits – Second to Fifth:**
  - **--Metacarpophalangeal**
Flexion	0-90
Hyperextension	0-45

  - **--Proximal interphalangeal**
Flexion	0-100

  - **--Distal interphalangeal**
Flexion	0-90
Hyperextension	0-10

Lower Extremity

- **Hip:**
Flexion	0-120
Extension	0-30
Abduction	0-45
Adduction	0-30
Medial rotation	0-45
Lateral rotation	0-45

- **Knee:**
Flexion	0-135

- **Ankle:**
Dorsiflexion	0-20
Plantar flexion	0-50
Inversion	0-35
Eversion	0-15

- **Subtalar:**
Inversion	0-5
Eversion	0-5

Process for Conducting Goniometric Measurements

1. Place the subject in the recommended testing position.
2. Stabilize the proximal joint segment.
3. Move the distal joint segment through the available range of motion. Make sure that the passive range of motion is performed slowly, the end of the range is attained, and the end-feel determined.
4. Make a clinical estimate of the range of motion.
5. Return the distal joint segment to the starting position.
6. Palpate bony anatomical landmarks.
7. Align the goniometer.
8. Read and record the starting position. Remove the goniometer.
9. Stabilize the proximal joint segment.
10. Move the distal segment through the full range of motion.
11. Replace and realign the goniometer. Palpate the anatomical landmarks again if necessary.
12. Read and record the range of motion.

Adapted from Norkin and White: Measurement of Joint Motion: A Guide to Goniometry. F.A. Davis Company, Philadelphia, 2003, p.35, with permission.

Goniometric Technique

Upper Extremity

Shoulder

Flexion
Axis: acromial process
Stationary arm: midaxillary line of the thorax
Moveable arm: lateral midline of the humerus using the lateral epicondyle of the humerus for reference

Extension
Axis: acromial process
Stationary arm: midaxillary line of the thorax
Moveable arm: lateral midline of the humerus using the lateral epicondyle of the humerus for reference

Abduction
Axis: anterior aspect of the acromial process
Stationary arm: parallel to the midline of the anterior aspect of the sternum
Moveable arm: medial midline of the humerus

Adduction
Axis: anterior aspect of the acromial process
Stationary arm: parallel to the midline of the anterior aspect of the sternum
Moveable arm: medial midline of the humerus

Medial rotation
Axis: olecranon process
Stationary arm: parallel or perpendicular to the floor
Moveable arm: ulna using the olecranon process and ulnar styloid for reference

Lateral rotation
Axis: olecranon process
Stationary arm: parallel or perpendicular to the floor
Moveable arm: ulna using the olecranon process and ulnar styloid process for reference

Elbow

Flexion
Axis: lateral epicondyle of the humerus
Stationary arm: lateral midline of the humerus using the center of the acromial process for reference
Moveable arm: lateral midline of the radius using the radial head and radial styloid process for reference

Extension
Axis: lateral epicondyle of the humerus
Stationary arm: lateral midline of the humerus using the center of the acromial process for reference
Moveable arm: lateral midline of the radius using the radial head and radial styloid process for reference

Forearm

Pronation
Axis: lateral to the ulnar styloid process
Stationary arm: parallel to the anterior midline of the humerus
Moveable arm: dorsal aspect of the forearm, just proximal to the styloid process of the radius and ulna

Supination
Axis: medial to the ulnar styloid process
Stationary arm: parallel to the anterior midline of the humerus
Moveable arm: ventral aspect of the forearm, just proximal to the styloid process of the radius and ulna

Wrist

Flexion
Axis: lateral aspect of the wrist over the triquetrum
Stationary arm: lateral midline of the ulna using the olecranon and ulnar styloid process for reference
Moveable arm: lateral midline of the fifth metacarpal

Extension
Axis: lateral aspect of the wrist over the triquetrum
Stationary arm: lateral midline of the ulna using the olecranon and ulnar styloid process for reference
Moveable arm: lateral midline of the fifth metacarpal

Radial deviation
Axis: over the middle of the dorsal aspect of the wrist over the capitate
Stationary arm: dorsal midline of the forearm using the lateral epicondyle of the humerus for reference
Moveable arm: dorsal midline of the third metacarpal

Ulnar deviation
Axis: over the middle of the dorsal aspect of the wrist over the capitate
Stationary arm: dorsal midline of the forearm using the lateral epicondyle of the humerus for reference
Moveable arm: dorsal midline of the third metacarpal

Thumb

Carpometacarpal flexion
Axis: over the palmar aspect of the first carpometacarpal joint
Stationary arm: ventral midline of the radius using the ventral surface of the radial head and radial styloid process for reference
Moveable arm: ventral midline of the first metacarpal

Carpometacarpal extension
Axis: over the palmar aspect of the first carpometacarpal joint
Stationary arm: ventral midline of the radius using the ventral surface of the radial head and radial styloid process for reference
Moveable arm: ventral midline of the first metacarpal

Carpometacarpal abduction
Axis: over the lateral aspect of the radial styloid process
Stationary arm: lateral midline of the second metacarpal using the center of the second metacarpophalangeal joint for reference
Moveable arm: lateral midline of the first metacarpal using the center of the first metacarpophalangeal joint for reference

Carpometacarpal adduction
Axis: over the lateral aspect of the radial styloid process
Stationary arm: lateral midline of the second metacarpal using the center of the second metacarpophalangeal joint for reference
Moveable arm: lateral midline of the first metacarpal using the center of the first metacarpophalangeal joint for reference

Fingers

Metacarpophalangeal flexion
Axis: over the dorsal aspect of the metacarpophalangeal joint
Stationary arm: over the dorsal midline of the metacarpal
Moveable arm: over the dorsal midline of the proximal phalanx

Metacarpophalangeal extension
Axis: over the dorsal aspect of the metacarpophalangeal joint
Stationary arm: over the dorsal midline of the metacarpal
Moveable arm: over the dorsal midline of the proximal phalanx

Metacarpophalangeal abduction
Axis: over the dorsal aspect of the metacarpophalangeal joint
Stationary arm: over the dorsal midline of the metacarpal
Moveable arm: dorsal midline of the proximal phalanx

Metacarpophalangeal adduction
Axis: over the dorsal aspect of the metacarpophalangeal joint
Stationary arm: over the dorsal midline of the metacarpal
Moveable arm: dorsal midline of the proximal phalanx

Proximal interphalangeal flexion
Axis: over the dorsal aspect of the proximal interphalangeal joint
Stationary arm: over the dorsal midline of the proximal phalanx
Moveable arm: over the dorsal midline of the middle phalanx

Proximal interphalangeal extension
Axis: over the dorsal aspect of the proximal interphalangeal joint
Stationary arm: over the dorsal midline of the proximal phalanx
Moveable arm: over the dorsal midline of the middle phalanx

Distal interphalangeal flexion
Axis: over the dorsal aspect of the distal interphalangeal joint
Stationary arm: over the dorsal midline of the middle phalanx
Moveable arm: over the dorsal midline of the distal phalanx

Distal interphalangeal extension
Axis: over the dorsal aspect of the distal interphalangeal joint
Stationary arm: over the dorsal midline of the middle phalanx
Moveable arm: over the dorsal midline of the distal phalanx

Lower Extremity

Hip

Flexion
Axis: over the lateral aspect of the hip joint using the greater trochanter of the femur for reference
Stationary arm: lateral midline of the pelvis
Moveable arm: lateral midline of the femur using the lateral epicondyle for reference

Extension
Axis: over the lateral aspect of the hip joint using the greater trochanter of the femur for reference
Stationary arm: lateral midline of the pelvis
Moveable arm: lateral midline of the femur using the lateral epicondyle for reference

Abduction
Axis: over the anterior superior iliac spine (ASIS) of the extremity being measured
Stationary arm: align with imaginary horizontal line extending from one ASIS to the other ASIS
Moveable arm: anterior midline of the femur using the midline of the patella for reference

Adduction
Axis: over the anterior superior iliac spine (ASIS) of the extremity being measured
Stationary arm: align with imaginary horizontal line extending from one ASIS to the other ASIS
Moveable arm: anterior midline of the femur using the midline of the patella for reference

Medial rotation
Axis: anterior aspect of the patella
Stationary arm: perpendicular to the floor or parallel to the supporting surface
Moveable arm: anterior midline of the lower leg using the crest of the tibia and a point midway between the two malleoli for reference

Lateral rotation
Axis: anterior aspect of the patella
Stationary arm: perpendicular to the floor or parallel to the supporting surface
Moveable arm: anterior midline of the lower leg using the crest of the tibia and a point midway between the two malleoli for reference

Knee

Flexion
Axis: lateral epicondyle of the femur
Stationary arm: lateral midline of the femur using the greater trochanter for reference
Moveable arm: lateral midline of the fibula using the lateral malleolus and fibular head for reference

Extension
Axis: lateral epicondyle of the femur
Stationary arm: lateral midline of the femur using the greater trochanter for reference
Moveable arm: lateral midline of the fibula using the lateral malleolus and fibular head for reference

Ankle

Dorsiflexion
Axis: lateral aspect of the lateral malleolus
Stationary arm: lateral midline of the fibula using the head of the fibula for reference
Moveable arm: parallel to the lateral aspect of the fifth metatarsal

Plantar flexion
Axis: lateral aspect of the lateral malleolus
Stationary arm: lateral midline of the fibula using the head of the fibula for reference
Moveable arm: parallel to the lateral aspect of the fifth metatarsal

Inversion
Axis: anterior aspect of the ankle midway between the malleoli
Stationary arm: anterior midline of the lower leg using the tibial tuberosity for reference
Moveable arm: anterior midline of the second metatarsal

Eversion
Axis: anterior aspect of the ankle midway between the malleoli
Stationary arm: anterior midline of the lower leg using the tibial tuberosity for reference
Moveable arm: anterior midline of the second metatarsal

Subtalar

Inversion
Axis: posterior aspect of the ankle midway between the malleoli
Stationary arm: posterior midline of the lower leg
Moveable arm: posterior midline of the calcaneus

Eversion
Axis: posterior aspect of the ankle midway between the malleoli
Stationary arm: posterior midline of the lower leg
Moveable arm: posterior midline of the calcaneus

Muscle Insufficiency

A muscle contraction that is less than optimal due to an extremely lengthened or shortened position of the muscle. There are two types of insufficiency:

Active: when a two-joint muscle contracts across both joints simultaneously

Passive: when a two-joint muscle is lengthened over both joints simultaneously

Dynamometry

Dynamometry is the process of measuring forces that are doing work. A dynamometer is a device that measures strength through the use of a load cell or spring loaded gauge. There are various kinds of dynamometers that are used based on treatment objectives. Three types of dynamometry that will be discussed here include the hand-held dynamometer that measures grip strength, the hand-held dynamometer used to measure strength of the extremities through isometric contraction, and the dynamometer used to measure strength through isokinetic contraction. Hand-held dynamometry demonstrates intrarater reliability of > .94. The same dynamometer should be used each session and the same tester should consistently measure the patient.

- **A hand-held dynamometer** can be used to assess the grip strength of a patient. Normally, a patient's dominant grip strength is five to ten pounds greater than the non-dominant grip strength. Hand-held dynamometry is also used to measure muscle group strength by having the patient exert maximal force against the dynamometer. Portable, non-electric units include a hydraulic or spring-load system and display the force on a gauge. Electrical units use load cells or strain gauges and display force digitally.

- **Isometric dynamometry** measures the static strength of a muscle group without any movement. The extremity is restrained by stabilization straps or stabilized with only verbal instruction.
  Benefits include attaining peak and average force data, reaction time data, rate of motor recruitment, and maximal exertion data. This method is relatively safe, simple to use, easy to interpret data, and incurs a relative low cost.
  Disadvantages include the inability to convert data to functional activities, as well as the need for caution with patients with acute orthopedic injury, osteoporosis or hernia. This method is contraindicated for patients with fractures and significant hypertension.

- **Isokinetic dynamometry** measures the strength of a muscle group during a movement with constant, predetermined speed. This device will alter the resistance to accommodate for the change in the length-tension ratio and lever arm throughout the entire arc of motion. The muscle group will therefore maximally contract throughout the motion. Common speeds of motion include 60, 120, and 180 degrees per second.
  Benefits include the ability to test the muscle strength at various speeds, the ability to measure the patient's power, and that the patient will never have more

resistance than they can handle during the isokinetic testing.
Disadvantages include the high cost of operation for the device, limitations in patterns of movement, a higher level of understanding required by the patient, and that this method doesn't truly correlate to function since people do no perform at a constant velocity during daily activities.

Make Test:
A make test is an evaluation procedure where a patient is asked to apply a force against the dynamometer.

Break Test:
A break test is an evaluation procedure where a patient is asked to hold a contraction against pressure that is applied in the opposite direction to the contraction.

Special Tests

Special Tests Outline

Upper Extremity

Shoulder

--**Dislocation**
   Apprehension test for anterior shoulder dislocation
   Apprehension test for posterior shoulder dislocation

--**Biceps Tendon Pathology**
   Ludington's test
   Speed's test
   Yergason's test

--**Rotator Cuff Pathology/Impingement**
   Drop arm test
   Hawkins-Kennedy impingement test
   Neer impingement test
   Supraspinatus test

--**Thoracic Outlet Syndrome**
   Adson maneuver
   Allen test
   Costoclavicular syndrome test
   Roos test
   Wright test (hyperabduction test)

--**Miscellaneous**
   Glenoid labrum tear test

Elbow

--Ligamentous Instability
Varus stress test
Valgus stress test

--Epicondylitis
Cozen's test
Lateral epicondylitis test
Medial epicondylitis test
Mill's test

--Neurological Dysfunction
Tinel's sign

Wrist/Hand

--Ligamentous Instability
Ulnar collateral ligament instability test

--Vascular Insufficiency
Allen test
Capillary refill test

--Contracture/Tightness
Bunnel-Littler test
Tight retinacular ligament test

--Neurological Dysfunction
Froment's sign
Phalen's test
Tinel's sign

--Miscellaneous
Finkelstein test
Grind test
Murphy sign

Lower Extremity

Hip

--Contracture/Tightness
Ely's test
Ober's test
Piriformis test
Thomas test
Tripod sign
90-90 straight leg raise test

--Pediatric Tests
Barlow's test
Ortolani's test

--Miscellaneous
Craig's test
Patrick's test (Faber test)
Quadrant scouring test
Trendelenburg test

Knee

--Ligamentous Instability
Anterior drawer test
Lachman test
Lateral pivot shift test
Posterior drawer test
Posterior sag sign
Slocum test
Valgus stress test
Varus stress test

--Meniscal Pathology
Apley's compression test
Bounce home test
McMurray test

--Swelling
Brush test
Patellar tap test

--Miscellaneous
Clarke's sign
Hughston's plica test
Noble compression test
Patellar apprehension test

Ankle

--Ligamentous Instability
Anterior drawer test
Talar tilt

--Miscellaneous
Homans' sign
Thompson test
Tibial torsion test
True leg length discrepancy test

Spine

Cervical Region

Foraminal compression test
Vertebral artery test

Lumbar/Sacroiliac Region

Sacroiliac joint stress test
Sitting flexion test
Standing flexion test

Descriptions of Special Tests

Upper Extremity

Shoulder

Dislocation

Apprehension test for anterior shoulder dislocation
The patient is positioned in supine with the arm in 90 degrees of abduction. The therapist laterally rotates the patient's shoulder. A positive test is indicated by a look of apprehension or a facial grimace prior to reaching an end point.

Apprehension test for posterior shoulder dislocation
The patient is positioned in supine with the arm in 90 degrees of flexion and medial rotation. The therapist applies a posterior force through the long axis of the humerus. A positive test is indicated by a look of apprehension or a facial grimace prior to reaching an end point.

Biceps Tendon Pathology

Ludington's test
The patient is positioned in sitting and is asked to clasp both hands behind the head with the fingers interlocked. The patient is then asked to alternately contract and relax the biceps muscles. A positive test is indicated by absence of movement in the biceps tendon and may be indicative of a rupture of the long head of the biceps.

Speed's test
The patient is positioned in sitting or standing with the elbow extended and the forearm supinated. The therapist places one hand over the bicipital groove and the other hand on the volar surface of the forearm. The therapist resists active shoulder flexion. A positive test is indicated by pain or tenderness in the bicipital groove region and may be indicative of bicipital tendonitis.

Yergason's test
The patient is positioned in sitting with 90 degrees of elbow flexion and the forearm pronated. The humerus is stabilized against the patient's thorax. The therapist places one hand on the patient's forearm and the other hand over the bicipital groove. The patient is directed to actively supinate and laterally rotate against resistance. A positive test is indicated by pain or tenderness in the bicipital groove and may be indicative of bicipital tendonitis.

Rotator Cuff Pathology/Impingement

Drop arm test
The patient is positioned in sitting or standing with the arm in 90 degrees of abduction. The patient is asked to slowly lower the arm to their side. A positive test is indicated by the patient failing to slowly lower the arm to their side or by the presence of severe pain and may be indicative of a tear in the rotator cuff.

Hawkins-Kennedy impingement test
The patient is positioned in sitting or standing. The therapist flexes the patient's shoulder to 90 degrees and then medially rotates the arm. A positive test is indicated by pain and may be indicative of shoulder impingement involving the supraspinatus tendon.

Neer impingement test
The patient is positioned in sitting or standing. The therapist positions one hand on the posterior aspect of the patient's scapula and the other hand stabilizing the elbow. The therapist elevates the patient's arm through flexion. A positive test is indicated by a facial grimace or pain and may be indicative of shoulder impingement involving the supraspinatus tendon.

Supraspinatus test
The patient is positioned with the arm in 90 degrees of abduction followed by 30 degrees of horizontal adduction with the thumb pointing downward. The therapist resists the patient's attempt to abduct the arm. A positive test is indicated by weakness or pain and may be indicative of a tear of the supraspinatus tendon, impingement or suprascapular nerve involvement.

Thoracic Outlet Syndrome

Adson maneuver
The patient is positioned in sitting or standing. The therapist monitors the radial pulse and asks the patient to rotate his/her head to face the test shoulder. The patient is then asked to extend his/her head while the therapist laterally rotates and extends the patient's shoulder. A positive test is indicated by an absent or diminished radial pulse and may be indicative of thoracic outlet syndrome.

Allen test

The patient is positioned in sitting or standing with the test arm in 90 degrees of abduction, lateral rotation, and elbow flexion. The patient is asked to rotate the head away from the test shoulder while the therapist monitors the radial pulse. A positive test is indicated by an absent or diminished pulse when the head is rotated away from the test shoulder. A positive test may be indicative of thoracic outlet syndrome.

Costoclavicular syndrome test

The patient is positioned in sitting. The therapist monitors the patient's radial pulse and assists the patient to assume a military posture. A positive test is indicated by an absent or diminished radial pulse and may be indicative of thoracic outlet syndrome caused by compression of the subclavian artery between the first rib and the clavicle.

Roos test

The patient is positioned in sitting or standing with the arms positioned in 90 degrees of abduction, lateral rotation, and elbow flexion. The patient is asked to open and close their hands for three minutes. A positive test is indicated by an inability to maintain the test position, weakness of the arms, sensory loss or ischemic pain. A positive test may be indicative of thoracic outlet syndrome.

Wright test (hyperabduction test)

The patient is positioned in sitting or supine. The therapist moves the patient's arm overhead in the frontal plane while monitoring the patient's radial pulse. A positive test is indicted by an absent or diminished radial pulse and may be indicative of compression in the costoclavicular space.

· Miscellaneous

Glenoid labrum tear test

The patient is positioned in supine. The therapist places one hand on the posterior aspect of the patient's humeral head while the other hand stabilizes the humerus proximal to the elbow. The therapist passively abducts and laterally rotates the arm over the patient's head and then proceeds to apply an anterior directed force to the humerus. A positive test is indicated by a clunk or grinding sound and may be indicative of a glenoid labrum tear.

Elbow

· Ligamentous Instability

Varus stress test

The patient is positioned in sitting with the elbow in 20 to 30 degrees of flexion. The therapist places one hand on the elbow and the other hand proximal to the patient's wrist. The therapist applies a varus force to test the lateral collateral ligament while palpating the lateral joint line. A positive test is indicated by increased laxity in the lateral collateral ligament when compared to the contralateral limb, apprehension or pain. A positive test may be indicative of a lateral collateral ligament sprain.

Valgus stress test

The patient is positioned in sitting with the elbow in 20 to 30 degrees of flexion. The therapist places one hand on the elbow and the other hand proximal to the patient's wrist. The therapist applies a valgus force to test the medial collateral ligament while palpating the medial joint line. A positive test is indicated by increased laxity in the medial collateral ligament when compared to the contralateral limb, apprehension or pain. A positive test may be indicative of a medial collateral ligament sprain.

· Epicondylitis

Cozen's test

The patient is positioned in sitting with the elbow in slight flexion. The therapist places his/her thumb on the patient's lateral epicondyle while stabilizing the elbow joint. The patient is asked to make a fist, pronate the forearm, radially deviate, and extend the wrist against resistance. A positive test is indicated by pain in the lateral epicondyle region or muscle weakness and may be indicative of lateral epicondylitis.

Lateral epicondylitis test

The patient is positioned in sitting. The therapist stabilizes the elbow with one hand and places the other hand on the dorsal aspect of the patient's hand distal to the proximal interphalangeal joint. The patient is asked to extend the third digit against resistance. A positive test is indicated by pain in the lateral epicondyle region or muscle weakness and may be indicative of lateral epicondylitis.

Medial epicondylitis test

The patient is positioned in sitting. The therapist palpates the medial epicondyle and supinates the patient's forearm, extends the wrist, and extends the elbow. A positive test is indicated by pain in the medial epicondyle region and may be indicative of medial epicondylitis.

Mill's test

The patient is positioned in sitting. The therapist palpates the lateral epicondyle and pronates the patient's forearm, flexes the wrist, and extends the elbow. A positive test is indicated by pain in the lateral epicondyle region and may be indicative of lateral epicondylitis.

Neurological Dysfunction

Tinel's sign

The patient is positioned in sitting with the elbow in slight flexion. The therapist taps with the index finger between the olecranon process and the medial epicondyle. A positive test is indicated by a tingling sensation in the ulnar nerve distribution of the forearm, hand, and fingers. A positive test may be indicative of ulnar nerve compression or compromise.

Wrist/Hand

· Ligamentous Instability

Ulnar collateral ligament instability test

The patient is positioned in sitting. The therapist holds the patient's thumb in extension and applies a valgus force to the metacarpophalangeal joint of the thumb. A positive test is indicated by excessive valgus movement and may be indicative of a tear of the ulnar collateral and accessory collateral ligaments. This type of injury is referred to as gamekeeper's or skier's thumb.

· Vascular Insufficiency

Allen test

The patient is positioned in sitting or standing. The patient is asked to open and close the hand several times in succession and then maintain the hand in a closed position. The therapist compresses the radial and ulnar arteries. The patient is then asked to relax the hand and the therapist releases the pressure on one of the arteries while observing the color of the hand and fingers. A positive test is indicated by delayed or absent flushing of the radial or ulnar half of the hand and may be indicative of an occlusion in the radial or ulnar artery.

Capillary refill test

The patient is positioned in sitting or standing. The therapist compresses the patient's nailbed and after releasing the pressure notes the amount of time taken for the color to return to the nail. A positive test is indicated by a delayed or muted response (greater than two seconds) and may be indicative of arterial insufficiency.

· Contracture/Tightness

Bunnel-Littler test

The patient is positioned in sitting with the metacarpophalangeal joint held in slight extension. The therapist attempts to move the proximal interphalangeal joint into flexion. If the proximal interphalangeal joint does not flex with the metacarpophalangeal joint extended, there may be a tight intrinsic muscle or capsular tightness. If the proximal interphalangeal joint fully flexes with the metacarpophalangeal joint in slight flexion, there may be intrinsic muscle tightness without capsular tightness.

Tight retinacular ligament test

The patient is positioned in sitting with the proximal interphalangeal joint in neutral and the distal interphalangeal joint flexed. If the therapist is unable to flex the distal interphalangeal joint the retinacular ligaments or capsule may be tight. If the therapist is able to flex the distal interphalangeal joint with the proximal interphalangeal joint in flexion, the retinacular ligaments may be tight and the capsule may be normal.

· Neurological Dysfunction

Froment's sign

The patient is positioned in sitting or standing and is asked to hold a piece of paper between the thumb and index finger. The therapist attempts to pull the paper away from the patient. A positive test is indicated by the patient flexing the distal phalanx of the thumb due to adductor pollicis muscle paralysis. If at the same time the patient hyperextends the metacarpophalangeal joint of the thumb it is termed Jeanne's sign. Both objective findings may be indicative of ulnar nerve compromise or paralysis.

Phalen's test

The patient is positioned in sitting or standing. The therapist flexes the patient's wrists maximally and asks the patient to hold the position for 60 seconds. A positive test is indicated by tingling in the thumb, index finger, middle finger, and lateral half of the ring finger and may be indicative of carpal tunnel syndrome due to median nerve compression.

Tinel's sign
The patient is positioned in sitting or standing. The therapist taps over the volar aspect of the patient's wrist. A positive test is indicated by tingling in the thumb, index finger, middle finger, and lateral half of the ring finger distal to the contact site at the wrist. A positive test may be indicative of carpal tunnel syndrome due to median nerve compression.

Miscellaneous
Finkelstein test
The patient is positioned in sitting or standing and is asked to make a fist with the thumb tucked inside the fingers. The therapist stabilizes the patient's forearm and ulnarly deviates the wrist. A positive test is indicated by pain over the abductor pollicis longus and extensor pollicis brevis tendons at the wrist and may be indicative of tenosynovitis in the thumb (de Quervain's disease).

Grind test
The patient is positioned in sitting or standing. The therapist stabilizes the patient's hand and grasps the patient's thumb on the metacarpal. The therapist applies compression and rotation through the metacarpal. A positive test is indicated by pain and may be indicative of degenerative joint disease in the carpometacarpal joint.

Murphy sign
The patient is positioned in sitting or standing and is asked to make a fist. A positive test is indicated by the patient's third metacarpal remaining level with the second and fourth metacarpals. A positive test may be indicative of a dislocated lunate.

Lower Extremity

Hip

Contracture/Tightness
Ely's test
The patient is positioned in prone while the therapist passively flexes the patient's knee. A positive test is indicated by spontaneous hip flexion occurring simultaneously with knee flexion and may be indicative of a rectus femoris contracture.

Ober's test
The patient is positioned in sidelying with the lower leg flexed at the hip and the knee. The

therapist moves the test leg into hip extension and abduction and then attempts to slowly lower the test leg. A positive test is indicated by an inability of the test leg to adduct and touch the table and may be indicative of a tensor fasciae latae contracture.

Piriformis test
The patient is positioned in sidelying with the test leg positioned toward the ceiling and the hip flexed to 60 degrees. The therapist places one hand on the patient's pelvis and the other hand on the patient's knee. While stabilizing the pelvis, the therapist applies a downward (adduction) force on the knee. A positive test is indicated by pain or tightness, and may be indicative of piriformis tightness or compression on the sciatic nerve caused by the piriformis.

Thomas test
The patient is positioned in supine with the legs fully extended. The patient is asked to bring one of his/her knees to the chest in order to flatten the lumbar spine. The therapist observes the position of the contralateral hip while the patient holds the flexed hip. A positive test is indicated by the straight leg rising from the table and may be indicative of a hip flexion contracture.

Tripod sign
The patient is positioned in sitting with the knees flexed to 90 degrees over the edge of a table. The therapist passively extends one knee. A positive test is indicated by tightness in the hamstrings or extension of the trunk in order to limit the effect of the tight hamstrings.

90-90 straight leg raise test
The patient is positioned in supine and is asked to stabilize the hips in 90 degrees of flexion with the knees relaxed. The therapist instructs the patient to alternately extend each knee as much as possible while maintaining the hips in 90 degrees of flexion. A positive test is indicated by the knee remaining in 20 degrees or more of flexion and is indicative of hamstrings tightness.

Pediatric Tests
Barlow's test
The patient is positioned in supine with the hips flexed to 90 degrees and the knees flexed. The therapist tests each hip individually by stabilizing the femur and pelvis with one hand while the other hand moves the test leg into abduction while applying forward pressure posterior to the greater trochanter. A positive test is indicated by a click or

a clunk and may be indicative of a hip dislocation being reduced. The test is considered to be a variation of Ortolani's test.

Ortolani's test

The patient is positioned in supine with the hips flexed to 90 degrees and the knees flexed. The therapist grasps the legs so that their thumbs are placed along the patient's medial thighs and the fingers are placed on the lateral thighs toward the buttocks. The therapist abducts the infant's hips and gentle pressure is applied to the greater trochanters until resistance is felt at approximately 30 degrees. A positive test is indicated by a click or a clunk and may be indicative of a dislocation being reduced.

Miscellaneous

Craig's test

The patient is positioned in prone with the test knee flexed to 90 degrees. The therapist palpates the posterior aspect of the greater trochanter and medially and laterally rotates the hip until the greater trochanter is parallel with the table. The degree of anteversion corresponds to the angle formed by the lower leg with the perpendicular axis of the table. Normal anteversion for an adult is 8-15 degrees.

Patrick's test (Faber test)

The patient is positioned in supine with the test leg flexed, abducted, and laterally rotated on the opposite leg. The therapist slowly lowers the test leg in abduction toward the table. A positive test is indicated by a failure of the test leg to abduct below the level of the opposite leg and may be indicative of iliopsoas, sacroiliac, or hip joint abnormalities.

Quadrant scouring test

The patient is positioned in supine. The therapist passively flexes and adducts the hip with the knee in maximal flexion. The therapist applies a compressive force through the shaft of the femur while continuing to passively move the patient's hip. A positive test is indicated by grinding, catching or crepitation in the hip and may be indicative of pathologies such as arthritis, avascular necrosis or an osteochondral defect.

Trendelenburg test

The patient is positioned in standing and is asked to stand on one leg for approximately ten seconds. A positive test is indicated by a drop of the pelvis on the unsupported side and may be indicative of

weakness of the gluteus medius muscle on the supported side.

Knee

Ligamentous Instability

Anterior drawer test

The patient is positioned in supine with the knee flexed to 90 degrees and the hip flexed to 45 degrees. The therapist stabilizes the lower leg by sitting on the forefoot. The therapist grasps the patient's proximal tibia with two hands and places their thumbs on the tibial plateau and administers an anterior directed force to the tibia on the femur. A positive test is indicated by excessive anterior translation of the tibia on the femur with a diminished or absent end-point and may be indicative of an anterior cruciate ligament injury.

Lachman test

The patient is positioned in supine with the knee flexed to 20-30 degrees. The therapist stabilizes the distal femur with one hand and places the other hand on the proximal tibia. The therapist applies an anterior directed force to the tibia on the femur. A positive test is indicated by excessive anterior translation of the tibia on the femur with a diminished or absent end-point and may be indicative of an anterior cruciate ligament injury.

Lateral pivot shift test

The patient is positioned in supine with the hip flexed and abducted to 30 degrees with slight medial rotation. The therapist grasps the leg with one hand and places the other hand over the lateral surface of the proximal tibia. The therapist medially rotates the tibia and applies a valgus force to the knee while the knee is slowly flexed. A positive test is indicated by a palpable shift or clunk occurring between 20 and 40 degrees of flexion and is indicative of anterolateral rotary instability. The shift or clunk results from the reduction of the tibia on the femur.

Posterior drawer test

The patient is positioned in supine with the knee flexed to 90 degrees and the hip flexed to 45 degrees. The therapist stabilizes the lower leg by sitting on the forefoot. The therapist grasps the patient's proximal tibia with two hands and places their thumbs on the tibial plateau and administers a posterior directed force to the tibia on the femur. A positive test is indicated by excessive posterior translation of the tibia on the femur with a diminished or absent end-point and may be indicative of a posterior cruciate ligament injury.

Posterior sag sign
The patient is positioned in supine with the knee flexed to 90 degrees and the hip flexed to 45 degrees. A positive test is indicated by the tibia sagging back on the femur and may be indicative of a posterior cruciate ligament injury.

Slocum test
The patient is positioned in supine with the knee flexed to 90 degrees and the hip flexed to 45 degrees. The therapist rotates the patient's foot 30 degrees medially to test anterolateral instability or 15 degrees laterally to test anteromedial instability. The therapist stabilizes the lower leg by sitting on the forefoot. The therapist grasps the patient's proximal tibia with two hands and places their thumbs on the tibial plateau and administers an anterior directed force to the tibia on the femur. A positive test is indicated by movement of the tibia occurring primarily on the lateral side and may be indicative of anterolateral instability.

Valgus stress test
The patient is positioned in supine with the knee flexed to 20-30 degrees. The therapist positions one hand on the medial surface of the patient's ankle and the other hand on the lateral surface of the knee. The therapist applies a valgus force to the knee with the distal hand. A positive test is indicated by excessive valgus movement and may be indicative of a medial collateral ligament sprain. A positive test with the knee in full extension may be indicative of damage to the medial collateral ligament, posterior cruciate ligament, posterior oblique ligament, and posteromedial capsule.

Varus stress test
The patient is positioned in supine with the knee flexed to 20-30 degrees. The therapist positions one hand on the lateral surface of the patient's ankle and the other hand on the medial surface of the knee. The therapist applies a varus force to the knee with the distal hand. A positive test is indicated by excessive varus movement and may be indicative of a lateral collateral ligament sprain. A positive test with the knee in full extension may be indicative of damage to the lateral collateral ligament, posterior cruciate ligament, arcuate complex, and posterolateral capsule.

Meniscal Pathology
Apley's compression test
The patient is positioned in prone with the knee flexed to 90 degrees. The therapist stabilizes the patient's femur using one hand and places the other hand on the patient's heel. The therapist medially and laterally rotates the tibia while applying a compressive force through the tibia. A positive test is indicated by pain or clicking and may be indicative of a meniscal lesion.

Bounce home test
The patient is positioned in supine. The therapist grasps the patient's heel and maximally flexes the knee. The patient's knee is extended passively. A positive test is indicated by incomplete extension or a rubbery end-feel and may be indicative of a meniscal lesion.

McMurray test
The patient is positioned in supine. The therapist grasps the distal leg with one hand and palpates the knee joint line with the other. With the knee fully flexed the therapist medially rotates the tibia and extends the knee. The therapist repeats the same procedure while laterally rotating the tibia. A positive test is indicated by a click or pronounced crepitation felt over the joint line and may be indicative of a posterior meniscal lesion.

Swelling
Brush test
The patient is positioned in supine. The therapist places one hand below the joint line on the medial surface of the patella and strokes proximally with the palm and fingers as far as the suprapatellar pouch. The other hand then strokes down the lateral surface of the patella. A positive test is indicated by a wave of fluid just below the medial distal border of the patella and is indicative of effusion in the knee.

Patellar tap test
The patient is positioned in supine with the knee flexed or extended to a point of discomfort. The therapist applies a slight tap over the patella. A positive test is indicated if the patella appears to be floating and may be indicative of joint effusion.

Miscellaneous
Clarke's sign
The patient is positioned in supine with the knees extended. The therapist applies slight pressure with the web space of their hand over the superior pole of the patella. The therapist then asks the patient to contract the quadriceps muscle while

maintaining pressure on the patella. A positive test is indicated by failure to complete the contraction without pain and may be indicative of patellofemoral dysfunction.

Hughston's plica test
The patient is positioned in supine. The therapist flexes the knee and medially rotates the tibia with one hand while the other hand attempts to move the patella medially and palpate the medial femoral condyle. A positive test is indicated by a popping sound over the medial plica while the knee is passively flexed and extended.

Noble compression test
The patient is positioned in supine with the hip slightly flexed and the knee in 90 degrees of flexion. The therapist places the thumb of one hand over the lateral epicondyle of the femur and the other hand around the patient's ankle. The therapist maintains pressure over the lateral epicondyle while the patient is asked to slowly extend the knee. A positive test is indicated by pain over the lateral femoral epicondyle at approximately 30 degrees of knee flexion and may be indicative of iliotibial band friction syndrome.

Patellar apprehension test
The patient is positioned in supine with the knees extended. The therapist places both thumbs on the medial border of the patella and applies a laterally directed force. A positive test is indicated by a look of apprehension or an attempt to contract the quadriceps in an effort to avoid subluxation and may be indicative of patella subluxation or dislocation.

Ankle

• Ligamentous Instability

Anterior drawer test
The patient is positioned in supine. The therapist stabilizes the distal tibia and fibula with one hand, while the other hand holds the foot in 20 degrees of plantar flexion and draws the talus forward in the ankle mortise. A positive test is indicated by excessive anterior translation of the talus away from the ankle mortise and may be indicative of an anterior talofibular ligament sprain.

Talar tilt
The patient is positioned in sidelying with the knee flexed to 90 degrees. The therapist stabilizes the distal tibia with one hand while grasping the talus with the other hand. The foot is maintained in a

neutral position. The therapist tilts the talus into abduction and adduction. A positive test is indicated by excessive adduction and may be indicative of a calcaneofibular ligament sprain.

• Miscellaneous

Homans' sign
The patient is positioned in supine. The therapist maintains the leg in extension and passively dorsiflexes the patient's foot. A positive test is indicated by pain in the calf and may be indicative of deep vein thrombophlebitis.

Thompson test
The patient is positioned in prone with the feet extended over the edge of a table. The therapist asks the patient to relax and proceeds to squeeze the muscle belly of the gastrocnemius and soleus muscles. A positive test is indicated by the absence of plantar flexion and may be indicative of a ruptured Achilles tendon.

Tibial torsion test
The patient is positioned in sitting with the knees over the edge of a table. The therapist places the thumb and index finger of one hand over the medial and lateral malleolus. The therapist then measures the acute angle formed by the axes of the knee and ankle. Normal lateral rotation of the tibia is considered to be 12-18 degrees in an adult.

True leg length discrepancy test
The patient is positioned in supine with the hips and knees extended and the legs 15 to 20 cm apart with the pelvis in balance with the legs. Using a tape measure the therapist measures from the distal point of the anterior superior iliac spines to the distal point of the medial malleoli. A positive test is indicated by a bilateral variation of greater than one centimeter and may by indicative of a true leg length discrepancy.

Spine

Cervical Region

Foraminal compression test
The patient is positioned in sitting with the head laterally flexed. The therapist places both hands on top of the subject's head and exerts a downward force. A positive test is indicated by pain radiating into the arm toward the flexed side and may be indicative of nerve root compression.

Vertebral artery test

The patient is positioned in supine. The therapist places the patient's head in extension, lateral flexion, and rotation to the ipsilateral side. A positive test is indicated by dizziness, nystagmus, slurred speech or loss of consciousness and may be indicative of compression of the vertebral artery.

Lumbar/Sacroiliac Region

Sacroiliac joint stress test

The patient is positioned in supine. The therapist crosses their arms placing the palms of the hands on the patient's anterior superior iliac spines. The therapist applies a downward and lateral force to the pelvis. A positive test is indicated by unilateral pain in the sacroiliac joint or gluteal area and may be indicative of sacroiliac joint dysfunction.

Sitting flexion test

The patient is positioned in sitting with the knees flexed to 90 degrees and the feet on the floor. The patient's hips should be abducted to allow the patient to bend forward. The therapist places his/her thumbs on the inferior margin of the posterior superior iliac spines and monitors the movement of the bony structures as the patient bends forward and reaches toward the floor. A positive test is indicated by one posterior superior iliac spine moving further in a cranial direction and may be indicative of an articular restriction.

Standing flexion test

The patient is positioned in standing with the feet 12 inches apart. The therapist places his/her thumbs on the inferior margin of the posterior superior iliac spines and monitors the movement of the bony structures as the patient bends forward with the knees extended. A positive test is indicated by one posterior superior iliac spine moving further in a cranial direction and may be indicative of an articular restriction.

Orthotics

Types of Orthoses

Lower Extremity

· Foot Orthotics

A semirigid or rigid insert worn inside a shoe that corrects foot alignment and improves function. May also be used to relieve pain. Foot orthotics are custom molded and are often designed for a specific level of functioning.

· Ankle-foot Orthosis (AFOs)

A metal ankle-foot orthosis consists of two metal uprights connected proximally to a calf band and distally to a mechanical ankle joint and shoe. The ankle joint may have the ability to be locked and not allow any motion, or set to have limited anterior/posterior capability depending on the patient's need. A plastic ankle-foot orthosis is fabricated by a cast mold of the patient's lower extremity. The use of plastic is more cosmetic, lighter, and requires that if a patient presents with edema it does not significantly fluctuate. Proper fit of a plastic ankle-foot orthosis requires that a patient be casted in a subtalar neutral position. A footplate can be incorporated into the ankle-foot orthosis to assist with tone reduction. Solid ankle-foot orthoses control dorsiflexion/plantar flexion and also inversion/eversion with a trim line anterior to the malleoli. They can be fabricated to keep an ankle positioned at 90 degrees or can be fabricated with an articulating ankle joint. This articulation allows the tibia to advance over the foot during the mid to late stance phase of gait. A posterior leaf spring is a plastic AFO with a trim line posterior to the malleoli. Its primary purpose is to assist with dorsiflexion and prevent foot drop. It requires adequate medial/lateral control by the patient. Ankle-foot orthoses can also influence knee control. A floor reaction AFO assists with knee extension during stance through positioning of a calf band and/or positioning at the ankle. Ankle-foot orthoses are commonly prescribed for patients with peripheral neuropathy, nerve lesions or hemiplegia.

· Knee-ankle-foot Orthosis (KAFOs)

Knee-ankle-foot orthoses provide support and stability to the knee and ankle. The orthoses can be fabricated using two metal uprights extending from the foot/shoe to the thigh with calf and thigh bands. Plastic knee-ankle-foot orthoses are fabricated by a cast mold of the patient's lower extremity. A plastic thigh shell is connected to a plastic ankle-foot orthosis through metal uprights lateral and medial to the knee joint. Both types allow for a lock mechanism at the knee that provides stability. The ankle is also held in proper alignment.

· Craig-Scott knee-ankle-foot Orthosis

A knee-ankle-foot orthosis designed specifically for persons with paraplegia. This design allows a person to stand with a posterior lean of the trunk.

- **Hip-knee-ankle-foot Orthosis (HKAFOs)**

A hip-knee-ankle orthosis is indicated for patients with hip, foot, knee, and ankle weakness. It consists of bilateral knee-ankle-foot orthoses with an extension to the hip joints with use of a pelvic band. The orthosis can control rotation at the hip and abduction/adduction. The orthosis is heavy and restricts patients to a swing-to or swing-through gait pattern.

- **Reciprocating gait Orthosis (RGOs)**

Reciprocating gait orthoses are a derivative of the HKAFO and incorporate a cable system to assist with advancement of the lower extremities during gait. When the patient shifts weight onto a selected lower extremity, the cable system advances the opposite lower extremity. The orthoses are used primarily for patients with paraplegia.

- **Parapodiums**

A standing frame designed to allow a patient to sit when necessary. It is a prefabricated frame and ambulation is achieved by shifting weight and rocking the base across the floor. It is primarily used by the pediatric population.

Spine

- **Corset**

A corset is constructed of fabric and may have metal uprights within the material to provide abdominal compression and support. Corsets are utilized to provide pressure and relieve pain associated with mid and low back pathologies.

- **Halo Vest Orthosis**

The halo vest is an invasive cervical thoracic orthosis that provides full restriction of all cervical motion. A metal ring with four posts that attach to a vest is placed on a patient and secured by inserting four pins through the ring into the skull. This orthosis is commonly used with cervical spinal cord injuries to prevent further damage or dislocation during the recovery period. A patient will wear a halo vest until the spine becomes stable.

- **Milwaukee Orthosis**

The Milwaukee orthosis is designed to promote realignment of the spine due to scoliotic curvature. The orthosis is custom made and extends from the pelvis to the upper chest. Corrective padding is applied based on the location and severity of the curve.

- **Taylor Brace**

The Taylor brace is a thoracolumbosacral orthosis that limits trunk flexion and extension through a three-point control design.

- **Thoracolumbosacral Orthosis (TLSO)**

A custom molded TLSO is utilized to prevent all trunk motions and is commonly utilized as a means of post-surgical stabilization. The rigid shell is fabricated from plastics in a bivalve style using straps/velcro to secure the orthosis.

Functions of Orthotics

- Prevent deformity
- Assist function of a weak limb
- Maintain proper alignment of joints
- Inhibit tone
- Protect against injury of a weak joint
- Allow for maximal functional independence
- Facilitate motion

Orthotic Considerations

- Cost
- Energy efficiency
- Cosmesis
- Temporary versus permanent
- Dynamic versus static
- Encourage normal movement

Orthotic Profile

Examination

- Past medical history
- History of current condition
- Social history (caregiver support)
- Medications
- Living environment
- Systems review
- Skin assessment
- Edema/girth measurements
- Postural tone assessment
- Pathological reflex assessment
- Sensation, proprioception, and kinesthesia
- Range of motion
- Motor assessment/strength
- Mobility skills

Intervention

- Ensure continued proper fit
- Donning/doffing orthosis
- Implement progressive wearing schedule
- Patient/caregiver teaching:
- --Skin inspection
- --Care of orthosis
- Mobility training with orthosis

Goals

- Maximize functional mobility skills with orthosis
- Maximize independence with donning/doffing
- Maximize independence with wearing schedule
- Maximize independence with skin inspection
- Maximize competence with care of orthosis

Mobilization

Mobilization is a passive movement technique designed to improve joint function.

Grades of Movement

Grade I	Small amplitude movement performed at the beginning of range.
Grade II	Large amplitude movement performed within the range, but not reaching the limit of the range and not returning to the beginning of range.
Grade III	Large amplitude movement performed to the limit of range.
Grade IV	Small amplitude movement performed at the limit of range.

Mobilization Technique

- The patient should have a general understanding of the purpose of mobilization.
- The patient should be completely relaxed during treatment.
- The therapist should be in a comfortable position while performing mobilization activities.
- The therapist's position should allow for optimal control of movement.
- Explain specific mobilization techniques to the patient prior to beginning treatment.
- Complete a general examination of each patient prior to beginning mobilization activities.
- Use gravity to assist with mobilization whenever possible.

- Mobilization activities are usually performed initially with the joint in a loose packed position.
- Maintain contact with the mobilizing hand as close to the joint space as possible.
- Allow one digit to palpate the joint line when possible.
- Mobilize one joint in one direction at a time.
- Use a mobilization belt or wedge to assist with stabilization when necessary.
- Constantly modify mobilization techniques based on individual patient response.
- Compare the quality and quantity of joint play bilaterally.
- Reassess each patient prior to each treatment session.

Convex-Concave Rule

Determines the direction of decreased joint gliding and the appropriate direction for the mobilizing force.

Convex surface moving on a concave surface:
- Roll and slide occur in the opposite direction
- Mobilizing force should be applied in the opposite direction of the bone movement

Concave surface moving on a convex surface:
- Roll and slide occur in the same direction
- Mobilizing force should be applied in the same direction as the bone movement

Indications: restricted joint mobility, restricted accessory motion, desired neurophysiological effects

Contraindications: active disease, infection, advanced osteoporosis, articular hypermobility, fracture, acute inflammation, muscle guarding, joint replacement

Orthopedic Profile

Examination

- Past medical history
- History of current condition
- --Surgical procedures
- --Precautions/contraindications
- Social history
- Medications
- Living environment
- Systems review
- --Vital signs
- Observation/inspection
- Postural assessment
- Reflex assessment
- Special tests

- Pain
- Range of motion
- Gait
- Mobility skills
- Strength

Intervention

- Exercise training
- Edema control
- Pain management
- Electrotherapeutic modalities
- Physical agents
- Joint mobilization
- Mobility training
- Patient/caregiver teaching:
    - --Precautions/contraindications
    - --Exercise program
    - --Positioning
    - --Competence with an assistive device
    - --Proper body mechanics

Goals

- Maximize functional mobility skills
- Reduce edema to the affected areas
- Maximize strength and endurance
- Maximize range of motion
- Minimize pain
- Maximize proper posture
- Maximize tissue healing
- Maximize patient/caregiver competence with:
    - --Safe use of assistive device
    - --Body mechanics
    - --Home exercise program
- Safe positioning for mobility

Orthopedic Surgical Procedures

Total Hip Replacement (THR)

Surgical Indications:
- Osteoarthritis
- Failed internal fixation of a fracture
- Osteomyelitis
- Rheumatoid arthritis
- Developmental dysplasia
- Avascular necrosis

Surgical Contraindications:
- Poor periarticular support
- Sepsis
- Active infection

Types of Total Hip Replacement:
- *Cemented*
    - --Immediate weight bearing as tolerated
    - --May require more bone tissue removal
    - --May experience loosening of the prosthesis

- *Noncemented*
    - --Toe touch weight bearing for up to six weeks
    - --Longer life expectancy than cemented
    - --Allows a larger amount of bone tissue to remain intact
    - --Allows for continued tissue growth

Potential Post-surgical Complications:
- Deep vein thrombosis
- Dislocation or subluxation of the femoral head
- Pulmonary embolus
- Infection
- Heterotopic ossification
- Sciatic nerve injury
- Periprosthetic fracture

General Post-operative Precautions (Posterolateral approach):
- Use an abduction pillow
- Maintain appropriate weight bearing status
- Avoid hip adduction
- Avoid hip medial rotation
- Avoid hip flexion > 90 degrees
- Do not sit on low surfaces
- Do not bend over towards the ground
- Do not lean over to get up from a chair
- Do not bend over to tie shoes
- Do not pivot towards the surgical side
- Do not cross the legs when sitting or lying down
- Use a pillow between the legs when sidelying

Physical Therapy Intervention:
- ✓ Maintain appropriate weight bearing status
- ✓ Mobility training using hip precautions
- ✓ Early ambulation training
- ✓ Initiate strengthening with isometric exercises and progress as tolerated
- ✓ Implement gentle stretching using hip precautions

Total Knee Replacement (TKR)

Surgical Indications:
- Disabling pain
- Failed conservative treatment
- Impaired mobility due to advanced arthritis

Surgical Contraindications:
- Active infection
- Advanced osteoporosis
- Severe peripheral vascular disease
- Sepsis
- Morbid obesity

Types of Total Knee Replacement:

- *Cemented*
--Immediate weight bearing as tolerated
--Used with older and sedentary patients

- *Hybrid*
--Toe touch weight bearing for up to six weeks
--Cemented tibial component and noncemented femoral and patellar components

- *Noncemented*
--Toe touch weight bearing for up to six weeks
--Femoral, tibial, and patellar components are all noncemented
--Longer life expectancy than cemented
--Preferred for younger patients

Potential Post-surgical Complications:
- Deep vein thrombosis
- Chronic joint effusion
- Periprosthetic fracture
- Restricted range of motion
- Infection
- Pulmonary embolus
- Peroneal nerve palsy

General Post-operative Precautions:
- Maintain appropriate weight bearing status
- Post-surgical use of knee immobilizer for stability

Physical Therapy Intervention:
✓ Maintain appropriate weight bearing status
✓ Mobility training
✓ Early ambulation training with knee immobilizer
✓ Use of a continuous passive motion machine (CPM)
✓ Initiate strengthening with isometric exercises
✓ Initiate passive range of motion to attain 90 degrees of knee flexion and 0 degrees of knee extension
✓ Use compression stockings for excess edema
✓ Wean from the knee immobilizer once the patient gains quadriceps control

Continuous Passive Motion Machine

The continuous passive motion machine (CPM) is a mechanical device designed to provide continuous motion for a particular joint using a predetermined range and speed. Robert Salter first developed this device based on research that continuous passive motion had beneficial healing effects for joints and surrounding soft tissues. Subsequent studies looking at the beneficial effects using a CPM machine versus not using a CPM machine vary in conclusion. Some studies show no significant difference in short-term outcome for CPM use versus an alternate form of early motion. Others show benefits from using the CPM to include earlier motion resulting in shorter hospitalizations. The primary indication for CPM use is to improve range of motion that may have been impaired secondary to a surgical procedure. Any joint may be indicated for CPM use, however, the knee is the most common joint treated with a CPM machine.

Therapeutic Effects:
- May lessen the debilitating effects from immobilization
- May improves the rate of recovery
- May provide a stimulating effect on tissue healing
- May provide a quicker increase in range of motion
- May decrease post-operative pain
- May reduce edema by assisting venous and lymphatic return

Contraindications:
- If the CPM increases a patient's pain
- If the CPM causes unwanted translation of opposing bones
- Particular anticoagulant therapy that may place the patient at risk for an intracompartment hematoma

Treatment Parameters:
✓ CPM can be applied immediately after surgery.
✓ Specific protocols apply for each individual joint regarding time of use and degrees of motion.
✓ The patient must be instructed in the use of the CPM and all associated safety information (including how to stop the machine in case of emergency).
✓ The patient's joint must be positioned to correctly align with the fulcrum of the CPM in order to receive effective and safe treatment.
✓ The patient will usually begin with a small arc of motion and progress approximately 10 degrees per day or as tolerated.
✓ CPMs may be utilized at home after discharge from the hospital, if necessary. A patient or caregiver must be independent with the CPM protocol for home use.

Orthopedic Pathology

Rheumatism

A condition found in a number of disorders characterized by inflammation, degeneration or metabolic derangement of the connective tissue, soreness, joint pain, and stiffness of muscles. Some conditions that present with rheumatism include: osteoarthritis, rheumatoid arthritis, juvenile rheumatoid arthritis, gout, systemic lupus erythematosus, and ankylosing spondylitis.

Physical Therapy Examination:
- Measurement of independence with functional activities
- Measurement of joint inflammation
- Measurement of joint range of motion
- Determination of limiting factors including pain, weakness, and fatigue

Physical Therapy Goals:

Short-Term Goals (Acute or Exacerbation)
- Alleviate pain
- Decrease inflammation
- Maintain strength and endurance to activity
- Provide splinting and/or assistive devices to increase safety

Long-Term Goals
- Patient independence and competence with:
  - Proper body mechanics
  - Reduction of biomechanical stressors
  - Exercise program
- Maximize functional mobility
- Maximize endurance to tolerate activities of daily living
- Demonstrate safety with ambulation and all mobility
- Management of pain

Osteoarthritis

A chronic disease that primarily involves the weight bearing joints. Osteoarthritis causes a degeneration of articular cartilage. Subsequent deformity and thickening of subchondral bone occurs with an outcome of impaired functional status. Any joint may be involved, however, the most commonly affected sites include cervical spine (C5-C6), lumbar spine, hips, and knees. It is common to be diagnosed with osteoarthritis after age 40.

The disease affects men more than women. Risk factors include trauma, repetitive microtrauma, and obesity.

Pathogenesis:
- Cartilage becomes soft and damaged
- Osteophytes form
- Subchondral bone thickens
- Synovitis is mild to moderate

Clinical Presentation:
- Pain present at the affected joint
- Increased pain after exercise
- Joints may become enlarged
- Joint crepitus
- Joint stiffness < 15 minutes
- Bouchard's nodes
- Usually localized to a few joints
- Increased pain with weather changes
- Joint motion limitation
- Heberden's nodes
- Gradual onset

Physical Therapy Intervention:
- ✓ Rest required for the affected joints
- ✓ Patient education on disease process, energy conservation, body mechanics, and joint protection techniques
- ✓ Splinting
- ✓ Use of cold and/or heat
- ✓ Ultrasound, hydrotherapy, paraffin
- ✓ Use of assistive devices to reduce weight bearing on affected joints
- ✓ Weight loss
- ✓ Isometric exercise followed by gradual progression to isotonic exercise
- ✓ Transcutaneous electrical nerve stimulation
- ✓ NSAIDs
- ✓ Orthopedic surgical intervention

Rheumatoid Arthritis

Rheumatoid arthritis is a systemic autoimmune disorder of unknown etiology. The disease presents with a chronic inflammatory reaction in the synovial tissues of a joint that results in erosion of cartilage and supporting structures within the capsule. One to two percent of the American population is affected. Women are affected three times more than men and the most common age of onset falls between thirty and fifty years of age. Onset of rheumatoid arthritis may occur first at any joint, but it is common to find it in the small joints of the hand, foot, wrist, and ankle. This disease has periods of exacerbation and remission.

Pathogenesis:
- Thickening of synovial membrane in affected joints
- Colonization of lymphocytes which synthesize the rheumatoid factor
- Subsequent erosion of cartilage and supporting structures

Clinical Presentation:
- Onset may be gradual or immediate
- Pain and tenderness of affected joints
- Warm joints
- Decrease in appetite
- Boutonniere deformity – DIP extension
- PIP flexion
- Symmetrical polyarthritis
- Morning stiffness > one hour
- Malaise and increased fatigue
- Redness at joints
- Swan neck deformity – DIP flexion
- PIP hyperextension

Physical Therapy Intervention:
- ✓ Complete bed rest or regular rest periods may be indicated
- ✓ NSAIDs or other medications
- ✓ Patient education on disease process, energy conservation, body mechanics, and joint protection techniques
- ✓ Modalities such as hydrotherapy, hot pack, paraffin, or use of cold - avoid deep heat
- ✓ Splinting
- ✓ Use of assistive devices
- ✓ Passive range of motion during acute stage
- ✓ Active range of motion once in the subacute stages
- ✓ Hydrotherapy and isometrics once in the subacute stages
- ✓ Exercise which may include swimming, stationary bicycle, or walking may be indicated
- ✓ Orthopedic intervention
- ✓ Aggressive stretching is contraindicated

Types of Fractures

Avulsion fracture: A portion of a bone becomes fragmented at the site of tendon attachment from a traumatic and sudden stretch of the tendon.

Closed fracture: A break in a bone where the skin over the site remains intact.

Comminuted fracture: A bone that breaks into fragments at the site of injury.

Compound fracture: A break in a bone that protrudes through the skin.

Greenstick fracture: A break on one side of a bone that does not damage the periosteum on the opposite side. This type of fracture is often seen in children.

Nonunion fracture: A break in a bone that has failed to unite and heal after nine to twelve months.

Stress fracture: A break in a bone due to repeated forces to a particular portion of the bone.

Spiral fracture: A break in a bone shaped as an "S" due to torsion and twisting.

Orthopedic Terminology

Bursitis: A condition caused by acute or chronic inflammation of the bursae. Symptoms may include a limitation in active range of motion secondary to pain and swelling.

Contusion: A sudden blow to a part of the body that can result in mild to severe damage to superficial and deep structures. Treatment includes active range of motion, ice, and compression.

Edema: An increased volume of fluid in the soft tissue outside of a joint capsule.

Effusion: An increased volume of fluid within a joint capsule.

Genu valgum: A condition where the knees touch while standing with the feet separated. Genu valgum will increase compression of the lateral condyle and increase stress to the medial structures. Genu valgum is also termed knock-knee.

Genu varum: A condition where there is bowing of the legs with added space between the knees while standing with the feet together. Genu varum will increase compression of the medial tibial condyle and increase stress to the lateral structures. Genu varum is also termed bowleg.

Kyphosis: An excessive curvature of the spine in a posterior direction usually identified in the thoracic spine. Common causes include osteoporosis, compression fractures, and poor posture secondary to paralysis.

Lordosis: An excessive curvature of the spine in an anterior direction usually identified in the cervical or lumbar spine. Common causes include weak abdominal muscles, pregnancy, excessive weight in the abdominal area, and hip flexion contractures.

Myositis ossificans: A condition of heterotopic bone formation that occurs three to four weeks after a contusion or trauma within the soft tissue.

Osteoporosis: The thinning of bone matrix with eventual bone loss and an increased risk for fracture. Osteoporosis is usually found in postmenopausal women. Causative factors for osteoporosis include decreased weight bearing, inactivity, family history, smoking, and drinking. Diagnosis of osteoporosis is made through bone density screening. Medications used to slow the process of osteoporosis include estrogen, calcium, vitamin D, calcitonin, and fluoride.

Q angle: The degree of angulation present when measuring from the midpatella to the anterosuperior iliac spine and to the tibial tubercle. A normal Q angle measured in supine with the knee straight is 13 degrees for a male and is 18 degrees for a female. An excessive Q angle can lead to pathology and abnormal tracking.

Scoliosis: A lateral curvature of the spine. Scoliosis can occur in the cervical, thoracic or lumbar curves. Classifications of scoliosis include idiopathic, non-structural, and structural.

Shoulder dislocation: A true separation of the humerus from the glenoid fossa.

Shoulder separation: A disruption in the stability of the acromioclavicular joint.

Sprain: An acute injury involving a ligament.
- **Grade I** – mild pain and swelling, little to no tear of the ligament
- **Grade II** – moderate pain and swelling, minimal instability of the joint, minimal to moderate tearing of the ligament, decreased range of motion
- **Grade III** – severe pain and swelling, substantial joint instability, total tear of the ligament, substantial decrease in range of motion

Strain: An injury involving the musculotendinous unit that involves a muscle, tendon or their attachments to bone.
- **Grade I** – localized pain, minimal swelling, and tenderness
- **Grade II** – localized pain, moderate swelling, tenderness, and impaired motor function
- **Grade III** – a palpable defect of the muscle, severe pain, and poor motor function

Tendonitis: A condition caused by acute or chronic inflammation of a tendon. Symptoms may include gradual onset, tenderness, swelling, and pain.

Pharmacological Intervention for Pain/Orthopedic Management

Opioid Agents (Narcotics) Provide analgesia for acute severe pain management May produce mood swings, sedation, confusion, and physical dependence	Morphine (MS Contin) Hydromorphone (Dilaudid) Meperidine (Demerol) Codeine (Codeine) Oxycodone (Oxycontin) Naloxone (Narcan) Propoxyphene (Darvon) Fentanyl (Sublimaze)
Nonopioid Agents Provide analgesia and pain relief, produce anti-inflammatory effects, anti-pyretic (reduces fever) properties May produce gastrointestinal distress with long-term use	**Acetylsalicylic Acid** Aspirin (Bayer, Ascriptin) Acetaminophen (Tylenol, Panadol) **Nonsteroidal Anti-inflammatories** Diclofenac (Voltaren) Ibuprofen (Motrin, Advil) Indomethacin (Indocin) Ketorolac (Toradil) Naproxen sodium (Aleve) Celecoxib (Celebrex)

Pharmacological Intervention for Pain/Orthopedic Management(cont.)

Glucocorticoid Agents (corticosteroids)	Cortisol (Hydrocortone) Prednisone (Deltasone, Prednisone) Dexamethasone (Decadron) Prednisolone (Prelone, Pediapred) Methylprednisolone (Medrol)
Produce anti-inflammatory, hormonal, and metabolic effects Suppression of articular and systemic disease processes May produce muscle atrophy, gastrointestinal distress, and glaucoma	

Amputations and Prosthetics

Factors that Influence Vascular Disease

- Hypertension
- Aging
- Diabetes mellitus
- Infection
- Poor nutrition
- Cigarette smoking

Risk Factors for Amputation

- Vascular disease
  - --Atherosclerosis/arteriosclerosis
  - --Venous insufficiency
  - --Buerger's disease
  - --Diabetes mellitus
- Malignancy/tumor
  - --Osteosarcoma
- Congenital deformities
- Infection
- Trauma

Types of Lower Extremity Amputations

Hemicorporectomy: Surgical removal of the pelvis and both lower extremities

Hemipelvectomy: Surgical removal of one half of the pelvis and the lower extremity

Hip Disarticulation: Surgical removal of the lower extremity from the pelvis

Transfemoral: Surgical removal of the lower extremity above the knee joint

Knee Disarticulation: Surgical removal through the knee joint

Transtibial: Surgical removal of the lower extremity below the knee joint

Syme's: Surgical removal of the foot at the ankle joint with removal of the malleoli

Chopart's: Disarticulation at the midtarsal joint

Transmetatarsal: Surgical removal of the midsection of the metatarsals

Considerations for Prosthetic Training

Hemipelvectomy and Hip Disarticulation
- All functions of the hip, knee, ankle, and foot are absent
- Most common cause is malignancy
- Does not allow for activation of the prosthesis through a residual limb
- Prosthetic motion must be initiated through weight bearing

Transfemoral Amputation
- Length of the residual limb with regard to leverage and energy expenditure
- No ability to weight bear through the end of the residual limb
- Susceptible to hip flexion contracture
- Adaptation required for balance, weight of prosthesis, and energy expenditure

Knee Disarticulation
- Loss of all knee, ankle, and foot function
- The residual limb can weight bear through its end
- Susceptible to hip flexion contracture
- Knee axis of the prosthesis is below the natural axis of the knee
- Gait deviations can occur secondary to the malalignment of the knee axis

Transtibial Amputation
- Loss of ankle and foot functions
- Residual limb does not allow for weight bearing at its end
- Weight bearing in the prosthesis should be distributed over the total residual limb
- Patella tendon should be the area of primary weight bearing
- Adaptations required for balance
- Susceptible to knee flexion contracture

Syme's Amputation

- Loss of all foot functions
- Residual limb can weight bear through its end
- Residual limb is bulbous with a non-cosmetic appearance
- Dog ears must be reduced for proper prosthetic fit
- Adaptation required for the increased weight of the prosthesis
- Adaptation required due to diminished toe off during gait

Transmetatarsal and Chopart's Amputation

- Loss of forefoot leverage
- Loss of balance
- Loss of weight bearing surface
- Loss of proprioception
- Tendency to develop equinus deformity

Potential Complications

Neuroma
A neuroma is a bundle of nerve endings that group together and can produce pain due to scar tissue, pressure from the prosthesis or tension on the residual limb.

Phantom Limb
Phantom limb refers to a painless sensation where the patient feels that the limb is still present. This is seen soon after the amputation and will usually subside with desensitization and prosthetic use, however, may continue for extended periods of time for some patients.

Phantom Pain
Phantom pain refers to the patient's perception of some form of painful stimuli. The pain can be continuous or intermittent, local or general, and short-term or permanent. This type of pain can disable the patient and interfere with successful rehabilitation. Treatment options include TENS, ultrasound, icing, relaxation techniques, desensitization techniques, and prosthetic use.

Types of Post-operative Dressings

Rigid (Plaster of Paris)	
Advantages	**Disadvantages**
Allows early ambulation with pylon	Immediate wound inspection is not possible
Promotes circulation and healing	Does not allow for daily dressing change
Stimulates proprioception	Requires professional application

Advantages	**Disadvantages**
Provides protection	
Provides soft tissue support	
Limits edema	

Semi-rigid (Una paste, air splint)	
Advantages	**Disadvantages**
Reduces post-operative edema	Does not protect as well as the rigid dressing
Provides soft tissue support	Requires more changing than rigid dressing
Allows for earlier ambulation	May loosen and allow for development of edema
Provides protection	
Easily changed	

Soft (Ace wrap, shrinker)	
Advantages	**Disadvantages**
Reduces post-operative edema	Tissue healing is interrupted by frequent dressing changes
Provides some protection	Joint range of motion may delay the healing of the incision
Relatively inexpensive	Increased risk of joint contractures
Provides soft tissue support	Less control of residual limb pain
Easily removed for wound inspection	Cannot control the amount of tension in the bandage
Allows for active joint range of motion	Risk of a tourniquet effect

Wrapping Guidelines

- ✓ Elastic wrap should not have any wrinkles
- ✓ Diagonal and angular patterns should be used
- ✓ Do not wrap in circular patterns
- ✓ Provide pressure distally to enhance shaping
- ✓ Anchor wrap above the knee for transtibial amputations
- ✓ Anchor wrap around pelvis for transfemoral amputations
- ✓ Promote full knee extension for transtibial amputations

Wrapping Guidelines (continued)

✓ Promote full hip extension for transfemoral amputations
✓ Secure the wrap with tape; do not use clips as they are unsafe
✓ Use 3-4 inch wrap for transtibial amputations
✓ Use 6 inch wrap for transfemoral amputations
✓ Rewrap frequently to maintain adequate pressure

Components of a Prosthesis

	Transfemoral	Transtibial
Socket:	• Quadrilateral socket • Ischial containment socket	• Patella tendon bearing socket (PTB) • Supracondylar patella tendon socket (PTS) • Supracondylar – suprapatellar socket (SC-SP)
Suspension:	• Complete suction • Partial suction --Silesian bandage --Pelvic belt/band	• Supracondylar cuff • Thigh corset • Supracondylar brim • Rubber sleeve suspension • Waist belt with fork strap
Knee:	• Single axis knee • Polycentric knee **Friction mechanisms:** Constant friction Variable friction Sliding friction Hydraulic friction Pneumatic friction	• Not needed
Shank:	• Exoskeleton – rigid exterior • Endoskeleton – pylon covered with foam	• Same as transfemoral shank

	Transfemoral	Transtibial
Foot:	• Solid ankle cushion heel (SACH) • Stationary attachment flexible endoskeleton (SAFE) • Single axis foot • Multi-axis foot	• Same as transfemoral foot

Gait Deviations

Lateral Bending	
Prosthetic Causes	**Amputee Causes**
Prosthesis may be too short	Poor balance
Improperly shaped lateral wall	Abduction contracture
High medial wall	Improper training
Prosthesis aligned in abduction	Short residual limb
	Weak hip abductors on prosthetic side
	Hypersensitive and painful residual limb

Abducted Gait	
Prosthetic Causes	**Amputee Causes**
Prosthesis may be too long	Abduction contracture
High medial wall	Improper training
Improperly shaped lateral wall	Adductor roll
Prosthesis positioned in abduction	Weak hip flexors and adductors
Inadequate suspension	Pain over lateral residual limb
Excessive knee friction	

Circumducted Gait	
Prosthetic Causes	**Amputee Causes**
Prosthesis may be too long	Abduction contracture
Too much friction in the knee	Improper training
Socket is too small	Weak hip flexors
Excessive plantar flexion of prosthetic foot	Lacks confidence to flex the knee
	Painful anterior distal stump
	Inability to initiate prosthetic knee flexion

Amputation and Prosthetic Profile

Excessive Knee Flexion During Stance	
Prosthetic Causes	**Amputee Causes**
Socket set forward in relation to foot	Knee flexion contracture
Foot set in excessive dorsiflexion	Hip flexion contracture
Stiff heel	Pain anteriorly in residual limb
Prosthesis too long	Decrease in quadriceps strength
	Poor balance

Vaulting	
Prosthetic Causes	**Amputee Causes**
Prosthesis may be too long	Residual limb discomfort
Inadequate socket suspension	Improper training
Excessive alignment stability	Fear of stubbing toe
Foot in excess plantar flexion	Short residual limb
	Painful hip/residual limb

Rotation of Forefoot at Heel Strike	
Prosthetic Causes	**Amputee Causes**
Excessive toe-out built in	Poor muscle control
Loose fitting socket	Improper training
Inadequate suspension	Weak medial rotators
Rigid SACH heel cushion	Short residual limb

Forward Trunk Flexion	
Prosthetic Causes	**Amputee Causes**
Socket too big	Hip flexion contracture
Poor suspension	Weak hip extensors
Knee instability	Pain with ischial weight bearing
	Inability to initiate prosthetic knee flexion

Medial or Lateral Whip	
Prosthetic Causes	**Amputee Causes**
Excessive rotation of the knee	Improper training
Tight socket fit	Weak hip rotators
Valgus in the prosthetic knee	Knee instability
Improper alignment of toe break	

Examination

- Past medical history
- History of current condition
- Social history (caregiver support)
- Medications
- Living environment
- Systems review
- Residual limb assessment
  - --Level of healing
  - --Color
  - --Shape
  - --Pulses
  - --Edema
  - --Girth and length
- Sensation
- Skin assessment
- Range of motion
- Balance
- Endurance
- Pain
  - --Phantom sensation
  - --Phantom pain
  - --Neuroma
- Mobility skills

Preprosthetic Intervention

- Positioning
  - --Prone lying
- Residual limb care
- Patient/caregiver teaching:
  - --Nutrition
  - --Desensitization
  - --Positioning
  - --Wrapping technique
  - --Skin inspection and care
- Range of motion
- Strengthening
- Edema control
- Physical agents
- Electrotherapeutic modalities
- Pain management
- Endurance activities
- Balance activities
- Mobility training
- Gait training
- Wheelchair prescription
- Assistive device training

Prosthetic Intervention

- Proper adjustment/alignment of prosthesis
- Development of wearing schedule
- Skin inspection with prosthetic use
- Donning/doffing prosthesis
- Mobility training with prosthesis

Preprosthetic Goals

- Maximize functional mobility
- Maximize range of motion
- Maximize strength and endurance
- Reduce edema and promote proper shaping
- Maximize independence with wheelchair management and assistive devices
- Maximize balance
- Maximize patient/caregiver competence with:
  - --Skin care and inspection
  - --Wrapping
  - --Desensitization techniques
  - --Positioning

Prosthetic Goals

- Maximize functional mobility using prosthesis
- Maximize independence with donning/doffing prosthesis
- Maximize wearing tolerance of prosthesis
- Maximize competence with prosthetic care and use

Chapter Three
Neuromuscular

Anatomy

Central Nervous System (CNS)
- Brain
- Spinal cord

Peripheral Nervous System (PNS)
- Cranial nerves and their ganglia
- Spinal nerves, their ganglia and plexuses
- Efferent and afferent somatic nerves outside the CNS
- **Autonomic nervous system (ANS)**
  --Sympathetic (fight or flight)
  --Parasympathetic (activated during time of rest)

Brain (Encephalon)
- **Brainstem** (midbrain or mesencephalon, pons, medulla oblongata)
- **Cerebellum**
- **Diencephalon** (hypothalamus, infundibulum, optic chiasm)
- **Cerebral hemispheres** (cortex, white matter, basal nuclei)
  -Two hemispheres, deep white matter, basal ganglia, lateral ventricles

Fissures
- **interhemispheric fissure:** separates the two cerebral hemispheres
- **Sylvian or lateral fissure:** (anterior portion) separates the temporal from frontal lobes; (posterior portion) separates temporal from parietal lobes

Sulci
- **central sulcus:** separates frontal and parietal lobes laterally
- **parieto-occipital sulcus:** separates the parietal and occipital lobes medially
- **calcarine sulcus:** separates the occipital lobe into superior and inferior halves

Meninges
Meninges is the term to describe the three layers of connective tissue covering the brain and spinal cord.
- **dura mater:** outer most meninge, has four folds, lines the periosteum of the skull
- **arachnoid:** the middle meninge, surrounds the brain in a loose manner
- **pia mater:** inner most meninge, covers the contours of the brain, forms choroid plexus in the ventricular system

Ventricular System
The ventricular system is designed to protect and nourish the brain; comprised of four ventricles and multiple foramen that allow the passage of cerebrospinal fluid (CSF). CSF acts as a cushion around the brain and spinal cord and is produced by the choroid plexus of each ventricle.

Dural Spaces
- **epidural space:** space occupied between the skull and outer dura mater
- **subdural space:** space occupied between the dura and arachnoid meninges
- **subarachnoid space:** space occupied between the arachnoid and pia mater that contains CSF and the circulatory system for the cortex

Ascending and Descending Tracts
Corticospinal tract (anterior): pyramidal motor tract responsible for ipsilateral voluntary movement
Corticospinal tract (lateral): pyramidal motor tract responsible for contralateral voluntary fine movement
Fasciculus gracilis: sensory tract for trunk and lower extremity proprioception, vibration, two-point discrimination and graphesthesia
Fasciculus cuneatus: sensory tract for trunk, neck and upper extremity proprioception, vibration, two-point discrimination, and graphesthesia
Rubrospinal tract: extrapyramidal motor tract responsible for motor input of gross postural tone
Spinocerebellar tract (dorsal): sensory tract for ipsilateral and contralateral subconscious proprioception
Spinocerebellar tract (ventral): sensory tract for ipsilateral subconscious proprioception

Spinothalamic tract (lateral): sensory tract for pain, light touch, and temperature

Tectospinal tract: extrapyramidal motor tract responsible for contralateral posture muscle tone associated with auditory/visual stimuli

Vestibulospinal tract: extrapyramidal motor tract responsible for ipsilateral gross postural adjustments subsequent to head movements

Sensory Testing

Light touch	Cotton ball; light pressure with finger
Deep pain	Squeeze the forearm or calf muscle
Superficial pain	Pen cap, paper clip end, pin
Vibration	Tuning fork
Proprioception	Identify a static position of an extremity/part
Kinesthesia	Identify direction and extent of movement of a joint or body part
Temperature	Hot and cold test tubes
Stereognosis	Identify an object without sight
Graphesthesia	Draw a number or letter on the skin with your finger; then identify without sight
Two-point discrimination	Two-point caliper on skin; identify one or two points without sight

Cranial Nerve Testing

The cranial nerves refer to twelve pairs of nerves that have their origin in the brain. The majority of cranial nerves contain both sensory and motor fibers, however, there are several exceptions. Since lesions affecting the cranial nerves produce specific and predictable alterations, it is often prudent to perform cranial nerve testing as part of a neurological examination. The following information is a summary of some of the more common methods of testing selected cranial nerves.

Cranial Nerve I - Olfactory
The patient is positioned in sitting with the eyes closed or blindfolded. The therapist places an item with a familiar odor under the patient's nostril and the patient is asked to identify the odor. A positive test may be indicated by an inability to identify familiar odors.

Cranial Nerve II - Optic
The patient is positioned in standing a selected distance from a chart or diagram. The therapist asks the patient to identify objects or read selected items from the chart or diagram. A positive test may be indicated by an inability to identify objects at a reasonable distance.

Cranial Nerve III - Oculomotor
The patient is positioned in sitting and is asked to follow an object such as a writing utensil with their eyes as it is moved vertically, horizontally, and diagonally. The therapist should make sure the patient does not rotate their head during the testing and should inspect the patient's eyes for asymmetry or ptosis. A positive test is indicated by an identified tracking deficit, asymmetry, or ptosis.

Cranial Nerve IV - Trochlear
The patient is positioned in sitting and asked to follow an object such as a writing utensil with their eyes as it is moved in an inferior direction. The therapist should make sure the patient does not move his head downward. A positive test results by an inability to depress the eyes and/or complaints of diplopia.

Cranial Nerve V - Trigeminal
The patient is positioned in sitting and is asked to close their eyes. The therapist uses a piece of cotton and a safety pin to alternately touch the patient's face. The patient is asked to classify each contact with the face as "sharp" or "dull." A positive test for the sensory component may be identified by impaired or absent sensation or the inability to differentiate between "sharp" or "dull". The motor component is tested by asking the patient to perform mandibular protrusion, retrusion, and lateral deviation. A positive test may be indicated by an impaired ability to move the mandible through the specified motions.

Cranial Nerve VI - Abducens
The patient is positioned in sitting. The therapist asks the patient to abduct their eyes without rotating the head. A positive test may be indicated by an inability to abduct the eyes.

Cranial Nerve VII - Facial
The patient is positioned in sitting and is asked to distinguish between sweet and salty substances placed on the anterior portion of the tongue. A positive test for the sensory component may be identified by an inability to

accurately identify sweet and salty substances. The motor component is tested by performing a manual muscle test of selected muscles involved in facial expression. A positive test for the motor component may be indicated by an inability to mimic selected facial expressions due to muscle impairment.

Cranial Nerve VIII - Vestibulocochlear

The patient is positioned in sitting in a quiet location. The therapist, positioned behind the patient and to one side, slowly brings a ticking watch toward the patient's ear. The therapist records the distance from the ear when the patient is able to identify the ticking sound. The therapist repeats the procedure on the contralateral ear and compares the measurements. A positive test is indicated by an inability to hear the ticking sound at 18-24 inches or a significant bilateral difference. Alternate tests include the Weber and Rinne tests which require a 512 Hz tuning fork.

Cranial Nerve IX - Glossopharyngeal

The patient is positioned in sitting. The therapist touches the pharynx with a tongue depressor. A positive test may be indicated by lack of gagging or an inability to feel the tongue depressor touch the back of the throat. The sensory component is tested by assessing the patient's ability to distinguish objects by taste after they are placed on the posterior portion of the tongue. A positive test for the sensory component may be identified by an inability to accurately identify tasted substances, especially sour and bitter substances, placed on the posterior third of the tongue.

Cranial Nerve X - Vagus

The patient is positioned in sitting. The therapist touches the pharynx with a tongue depressor. A positive test may be indicated by a lack of gagging or an inability to feel the tongue depressor touch the back of the throat. (Same description for Cranial Nerve IX - Glossopharyngeal). If the gag reflex is absent the therapist should carefully assess the movement of the soft palate and uvula.

Cranial Nerve XI - Accessory

The patient is positioned in sitting with the arms at the side. The therapist asks the patient to shrug their shoulders and maintain the position while the therapist applies resistance through the shoulders in the direction of shoulder depression. A positive test may be indicated by an inability to maintain the test position against resistance.

Cranial Nerve XII - Hypoglossal

The patient is positioned in sitting. The therapist asks the patient to protrude the tongue. A positive test may be indicated by an inability to fully protrude the tongue or the tongue deviating to one side during protrusion.

Deep Tendon Reflexes (DTR)

A reflex is a motor response to a sensory stimulation that is used in an assessment to observe the integrity of the nervous system. Deep tendon reflexes (DTR) elicit a muscle contraction when the muscle's tendon is stimulated.

Procedure Guidelines
- ✓ The patient should be relaxed.
- ✓ The muscle should be placed on a slight stretch.
- ✓ A reflex hammer taps the tendon with an anticipated immediate response.
- ✓ Both sides of the body should be assessed.
- ✓ Reflexes can be graded as normal, exaggerated (hyper), or depressed (hypo) or on a scale of 0-4.

Grading

0 = no response
1+ = diminished/depressed response
2+ = active normal response
3+ = brisk/exaggerated response
4+ = very brisk/hyperactive; abnormal response

Common DTR Sites

Biceps tendon	C5-C6 spinal level
Brachioradialis tendon	C5-C6 spinal level
Triceps tendon	C7-C8 spinal level
Patellar tendon	L3-L4 spinal level
Tibialis posterior tendon	L4-L5 spinal level
Achilles tendon	S1-S2 spinal level

DTR Normal Response

Biceps tendon	Contraction of the biceps muscle
Brachioradialis tendon	Elbow flexion and/or forearm pronation
Triceps tendon	Elbow extension or contraction of the triceps muscle
Patellar tendon	Knee Extension
Tibialis posterior tendon	Plantar flexion/inversion of the foot
Achilles tendon	Plantar flexion of the foot

Peripheral Nerves

The peripheral nervous system is the nervous system that lies outside of the brain and spinal cord. The peripheral nervous system (PNS) consists of motor, sensory, and autonomic neurons. These neurons are located in cranial, spinal, and peripheral nerves. The PNS consists of 12 pairs of cranial nerves, 31 pairs of spinal nerves, and all associated ganglia and sensory receptors. Most peripheral nerves contain motor (efferent) and sensory (afferent) components.

A Fibers
- Large fibers
- Myelinated
- High conduction rate
- Contained in the alpha and gamma motor systems
- Sensory components include:
  -Muscle spindle (primary afferent ending): primary for low-threshold stretch
  -Muscle spindle (secondary afferent endings): receptors that respond to change in length
  -Golgi tendon organ: responds to tension/stretch of a tendon
  -Bare nerve endings: joint receptors, mechanoreceptors of soft tissues, exteroceptors of pain, cold, and touch

B Fibers
- Medium fibers
- Myelinated
- Reasonably fast conduction rate
- Pre-ganglionic fibers of the autonomic system

C Fibers
- Small nerve fibers
- Poorly myelinated or unmyelinated
- Slowed conduction rate
- Post-ganglionic fibers of sympathetic system
- Exteroceptors for pain, temperature, and touch

Types of Nerve Injury

Nerve injury can occur through many mechanisms of injury. Possible etiologies include: mechanical (compression injury), crush and percussion (fracture, compartment syndrome), laceration, penetrating trauma (stab wound), stretch (traction injury), high velocity trauma (MVA), and cold (frostbite).

Neurapraxia
- Mildest form of injury
- Conduction block usually due to myelin dysfunction
- Axonal continuity conserved
- Nerve conduction is preserved proximal and distal to the lesion
- Nerve fibers are not damaged
- Recovery will occur within 4-6 weeks

Axonotmesis
- A more severe grade of injury to a peripheral nerve
- Reversible injury to damaged fibers
- Damage occurs to the axons with preservation of the endoneurium (neural connective tissue sheath), epineurium, Schwann cells, and supporting structures
- Distal Wallerian degeneration can occur
- The nerve can regenerate distal to the site of lesion at a rate of one millimeter per day

Neurotmesis
- The most severe grade of injury to a peripheral nerve
- Axon, myelin, connective tissue components are all damaged or transected
- Irreversible injury; no possibility of regeneration
- All motor and sensory loss distal to lesion becomes permanently impaired

Peripheral Nervous System Pathology

Anterior Horn Cell	Peripheral Polyneuropathy
<ul><li>Sensory component intact</li><li>Motor weakness and atrophy</li><li>Fasciculation</li><li>Decreased DTR</li><li>Example: ALS, polio</li></ul>	<ul><li>Sensory impairments; "stocking glove" distribution</li><li>Motor weakness and atrophy; weaker distally than proximally; may have fasciculations</li><li>Decreased DTR</li><li>Example: diabetic peripheral neuropathy</li></ul>
Spinal Roots and Nerves	**Neuromuscular Junction**
<ul><li>Sensory component will have corresponding dermatomal deficits</li><li>Motor weakness in an innervated pattern; may have fasciculations</li><li>Decreased DTR</li><li>Example: herniated disc</li></ul>	<ul><li>Sensory component intact</li><li>Motor fatigue noted</li><li>Normal DTR</li><li>Example: myasthenia gravis</li></ul>
Peripheral Nerve (mononeuropathy)	**Muscle**
<ul><li>Sensory loss along the nerve route</li><li>Motor weakness and atrophy in a peripheral distribution; may have fasciculations</li><li>Example: trauma</li></ul>	<ul><li>Sensory component intact</li><li>Motor weakness; fasciculations are rare</li><li>Normal or decreased DTR</li><li>Example: muscular dystrophy</li></ul>

Upper versus Lower Motor Neuron Disease

	UMND	LMND
Reflexes	Hyperactive	Diminished or absent
Atrophy	Mild from disuse	Present
Fasciculations	Absent	Present
Tone	Hypertonic	Hypotonic to flaccid

Upper Motor Neuron Disease

An upper motor neuron disease is characterized by a lesion found in descending motor tracts within the cerebral motor cortex, internal capsule, brainstem or spinal cord. Symptoms include weakness of involved muscles, hypertonicity, hyperreflexia, mild disuse atrophy, and abnormal reflexes. Damaged tracts are in the lateral white column of the spinal cord.

Examples of upper motor neuron lesions include cerebral palsy, hydrocephalus, CVA, birth injuries, multiple sclerosis, and brain tumors.

Lower Motor Neuron Disease

A lower motor neuron disease is characterized by a lesion that affects nerves or their axons at or below the level of the brainstem, usually within the "final common pathway." The ventral gray column of the spinal cord may also be affected. Symptoms include flaccidity or weakness of the involved muscles, decreased tone, fasciculations, muscle atrophy, and decreased or absent reflexes.

Examples of lower motor neuron lesions include poliomyelitis, tumors involving the spinal cord, trauma, infection, and muscular dystrophy.

Blood Supply to the Brain

Posterior cerebral Artery (PCA)
- Portion of midbrain
- Subthalamic nucleus
- Basal nucleus
- Thalamus
- Inferior temporal lobe
- Occipital and occipitoparietal cortices

Middle cerebral Artery (MCA)
- Most of outer cerebrum
- Basal ganglia
- Posterior and anterior internal capsule
- Putamen
- Pallidum
- Lentiform nucleus

Vertebrobasilar Artery
- Medulla
- Cerebellum
- Pons
- Middle occipital cortex

Cerebral Hemisphere Function

Frontal Lobe
(precentral gyrus, supplementary motor area, prefrontal pole, paracentral lobule, Broca's area)

Responsibilities
- Voluntary motor function
- Advanced motor planning
- Initiation of action
- Cranial nerves III, IV, VI, IX, X, XII
- Interpretation of emotion
- Personality center
- Judgment, conscience
- Planning, motivation
- Bladder & bowel inhibition
- Broca's motor speech center (dominant); appreciation of intonation, understanding gestures (non-dominant)

Impairments
- Contralateral weakness
- Contralateral head and eye paralysis
- Personality changes, antisocial behavior
- Ataxia, primitive reflexes
- Broca's aphasia (language deficits)
- Delayed or poor initiation

Parietal Lobe
(postcentral gyrus, parietal pole, optic radiation, Wernicke's area, Gustatory cortex)

Responsibilities
- Process perceptual and sensory information
- Body schema
- Contralateral pain, posture, touch, and proprioception (to arm, trunk, and leg)
- Perform calculations
- Spatial awareness
- Sensory: speech comprehension center (dominant)
- Appreciation of tone of voice and other emotional language (non-dominant)
- Visual tract
- Taste perception

Impairments
- Agraphia, finger agnosia (dominant)
- Constructional apraxia, dressing apraxia, anosognosia (non-dominant)
- Wernicke's aphasia (receptive)
- Homonymous visual deficits
- Impaired language comprehension
- Impairment in taste

Temporal Lobes
(superior temporal gyrus-auditory cortex, middle/inferior temporal gyri, limbic lobe and olfactory cortex, Wernicke's area)

Responsibilities
-Auditory and limbic processing
-Appreciation of language (dominant)
-Appreciation of music and sound (non-dominant)
-Memory
-Learning
-Affective mood centers (primitive behaviors, visceral emotions)
-Short-term memory
-Same responsibilities for Wernicke's area (as parietal lobe)

Impairments
-Auditory impairment
-Hearing impairment (dominant)
-Impaired appreciation of music (non-dominant)
-Memory deficits
-Learning deficits
-Wernicke's aphasia
-Antisocial behaviors

Occipital Lobe
(optic radiation, striate and parastriate cortices)

Responsibilities
-Primary processing area of visual information
-Visual tract
-Perception of vision

Impairments
-Homonymous hemianopsia
-Impaired extraocular muscle movement

Cerebellum
(anterior, posterior, flocculonodular lobes)

Responsibilities
-Coordination of motor skills
-Postural tone
-Sensory/motor input for trunk and extremities
-Coordination of gait
-Sensory/motor input from eyes and head for coordination of eye/head movement and balance

Impairments
-Ataxia
-Discoordination of trunk and extremities
-Intention tremor
-Balance deficits
-Ipsilateral facial sensory loss
-Dysdiadochokinesia

Diencephalon
***Thalamus** (specific and association nuclei)

Responsibilities
-Cortical arousal
-Memory
-Communicates information to and from the cerebral cortex

***Hypothalamus**
(mamillary bodies, optic chiasm, infundibulum)

Responsibilities
-Controls basic life functions (body temperature, thirst, hunger, sleep/wake cycles)
-Centers for sympathetic and parasympathetic responses
-Regulates anterior pituitary gland

***Epithalamus** (pineal body, posterior commissure)

Responsibilities
-Limbic system association

***Subthalamus**
(substantia nigra, red nuclei)

Responsibilities
-Association for motor control

***Pituitary** (anterior and posterior lobes)

Responsibilities
-Reproductive hormones
-Secretion of ADH/oxytocin

***Internal Capsule**
(tracts connecting thalamus to cortex)

Responsibilities
-Communication between cortex and spinal cord

Brainstem
***Midbrain** (superior cerebellar peduncles, superior/inferior colliculi, reticular formation, cerebral aqueduct, medial/lateral lemniscus, III, IV nuclei)

Responsibilities
-Communication pathways between higher and lower brain centers
-Auditory and visual reflexes

***Pons** (middle cerebellar peduncles, anterior wall of 4th ventricle, respiratory center, V, VI, VII, VIII nuclei)

Responsibilities
-Communication pathways between higher and lower brain centers

***Medulla** (inferior cerebellar peduncles, decussation of pyramidal tracts, inferior olivary nuclei, nucleus cuneatus and gracilis, IX, X, XI, XII nuclei)

Responsibilities
-Center for respiratory, cardiac, and vasomotor homeostasis

Diencephalon	**Brainstem**
Impairments	**Impairments**
-Altered consciousness	-Altered consciousness
-Contralateral hemiparesis, hemiplegia	-Contralateral hemiparesis, hemiplegia
-Dyskinesia	-Cranial nerve injury (palsy)
-Visual deficits	-Altered respiratory pattern
-Headache	-Attention deficits
-Autonomic function	

Hemisphere Specialization/Dominance

Left:	Right:
• Language	• Nonverbal processing
• Sequence and perform movements	• Process information in a holistic manner
• Understand language	• Artistic abilities
• Produce written and spoken language	• General concept comprehension
• Analytical	• Hand-eye coordination
• Controlled	• Spatial relationships
• Logical	• Kinesthetic awareness
• Rational	• Understand music
• Mathematical calculations	• Understand nonverbal communication
• Express positive emotions such as love and happiness	• Mathematical reasoning
• Process verbally coded information in an organized, logical, and sequential manner	• Express negative emotions
	• Body image awareness

Cerebellum

• Balance	• Creative
• Higher level muscular movements	• Pictorial
• Integration and coordination of multijoint movements	• Intuitive
• Initiation, timing, and sequencing of muscle contraction	

Balance

Balance can be defined as "a state of physical equilibrium," "maintenance and control of the center of gravity," and "achieving and maintaining an upright posture." All definitions assume integrated somatosensory, visual, and vestibular information within the central nervous system.

Somatosensory input

Somatosensory receptors are located in the joints, muscles, ligaments, and skin to provide proprioceptive information regarding length, tension, pressure, pain, and joint position. Proprioceptive and tactile input from the ankles, knees, hips, neck, and eye musculature provide balance information to the brain.

Visual input

Visual receptors allow for perceptual acuity regarding verticality, motion of objects and self, environmental orientation, postural sway, and movements of the head/neck. Children rely heavily on this system for maintenance of balance.

Vestibular input

The vestibular system provides the central nervous system with feedback regarding the position and movement of the head with relation to gravity. The labyrinth (which lies within the otic capsule of the temporal bone) consists of three semicircular canals filled with endolymph and two otolith organs. Semicircular canals respond to the movement of fluid with head motion. Otoliths measure the effects of gravity and movement with regard to acceleration/deceleration.

Balance Reflexes

Vestibuloocular reflex (VOR): VOR allows for head/eye movement coordination. This reflex supports gaze stabilization where the eyes can move while the head is fixed; visual tracking can also occur when both the eyes and head are moving.

Vestibulospinal reflex (VSR): VSR attempts to stabilize the body and control movement. The reflex assists with stability while the head is moving as well as coordination of the trunk during upright postures.

Automatic postural strategies: Automatic postural strategies are automatic motor responses that are used to maintain the center of gravity over the base of support. These responses always react or respond to a particular stimulus.

Ankle strategy: The ankle strategy is the first strategy to be elicited by a small range and slow velocity perturbation when the feet are on the ground. Muscle groups contract in a distal to proximal fashion to control postural sway from the ankle joint.

Hip strategy: The hip strategy is elicited by a greater force, challenge or perturbation through the pelvis and hips. The hips will move (in the opposite direction from the head) in order to maintain balance. Muscle groups contract in a proximal to distal fashion in order to counteract the loss of balance.

Suspensory strategy: The suspensory strategy is used to lower the center of gravity during standing or ambulation in order to better control the center of gravity. Examples of this strategy include knee flexion, crouching or squatting. This strategy is often used when both mobility and stability are required during a task (such as surfing).

Stepping strategy: The stepping strategy is elicited through unexpected challenges or perturbations during static standing or when the perturbation produces such a movement that the center of gravity is beyond the base of support. The lower extremities step and/or upper extremities reach to regain a new base of support.

Vertigo

Vertigo is used to describe a sense of movement and rotation of oneself or the surrounding environment. True vertigo is caused by inner ear disease.

Common causes of peripheral vertigo include benign paroxysmal positional vertigo, vestibular neuronitis, Meniere disease, and immune-mediated inner ear disease.

Common causes of central dizziness include migraine headaches and associated syndromes. Other causes include cerebellar lesions, acoustic tumors or demyelination.

Nystagmus

Nystagmus is abnormal eye movement that entails nonvolitional, rhythmic oscillation of the eyes. The speed of movement is faster in one direction than the other direction. A patient with nystagmus will also commonly complain of vertigo.

> **Spontaneous nystagmus:** an imbalance of vestibular signals to the oculomotor neuron that causes a constant drift in one direction that is countered by a quick movement in the opposite direction.
>
> **Peripheral nystagmus:** occurs with a peripheral vestibular lesion and is inhibited when the patient fixates their vision on an object.
>
> **Central nystagmus:** occurs with a central lesion of the brain stem/cerebellum and is not inhibited by visual fixation on an object.

Vestibular Rehabilitation

Vestibular rehabilitation is a therapeutic intervention that can be highly successful for patients with vestibular or central balance system disorders. Exercise protocols for vestibular retraining utilize compensation, adaptation, and plasticity to increase the brain's sensitivity, restore symmetry, improve vestibuloocular control, and subsequently increase motor control and movement.

Goals for Vestibular Rehabilitation

- ✓ Improve balance
- ✓ Improve trunk stability
- ✓ Increase strength and range of motion in order to improve musculoskeletal balance responses and strategies
- ✓ Decrease the rate and risk of falls
- ✓ Minimize dizziness

Balance Testing

Static Standing Tests	Outcome Measurement Tools	Vertigo
• Romberg test • One-legged stance test • Timed standing test • Nudge/push test • Postural Stress test • Motor control test • The Clinical Test for Sensory Interaction on Balance	• Tinetti Performance Oriented Mobility Assessment • Berg Balance Scale • Get up and Go test • Timed Get up and Go test • Gait Assessment Rating Scale • The Dynamic Gait Index	• Hallpike-Dix test • VOR test • Oculomotor tests • Fukuda stepping test • Semicircular canal function • Hamid vestibular stress test
Nystagmus	**Active Standing Tests**	**Other**
• Head-shaking test • Head thrust test • Positional testing • Hallpike-Dix test • Electrooculography • Saccadic test • Gaze test	• The Functional Reach test • The Multi-Directional Reach test • The Sensory Organization test • Gait observation	• The Fregley-Graybiel Ataxia Test Battery • Fugl-Meyer Sensorimotor Assessment of Balance Performance Battery • The Dizziness Handicap Inventory

Pharmacological Intervention for Vestibular Management

Antihistamine Agents -Treats vertigo	Meclizine (Antivert) Dimenhydrinate (Dramamine)
Anticholinergic Agents -Decreases conduction in vestibular-cerebellar pathways	Scopolamine (Isopto) Glycopyrrolate (Robinul)
Benzodiazepine Agents -Treats vertigo and emesis	Diazepam (Valium)
Phenothiazine Agents -Treats emesis	Promethazine (Phenergan) Prochlorperazine (Compazine)
Monoaminergic Agents -Treats vertigo	Ephedrine (Pretz-D)

Vestibuloocular Retraining Therapeutic Guidelines

- ✓ Vestibuloocular reflex (VOR) stimulation exercises
- ✓ Ocular motor exercises
- ✓ Balance exercises
- ✓ Gait exercises
- ✓ Combination exercises (obstacle courses, functioning at the mall)
- ✓ Habituation training exercises (use only with appropriate patients)
- ✓ Individualize each program based on the patient's specific impairments (rehabilitation vs. compensation training)
- ✓ Use of practice, feedback, and repetition are vital for skill refinement
- ✓ Use of gravity, varying surface conditions, visual conditions, and environmental cues should be included in therapeutic planning
- ✓ The center of gravity must be controlled at each stage of treatment
- ✓ Strategy (hip, ankle, stepping, suspense) training that should be implemented during treatment so strategies become automatic responses
- ✓ Forceplate systems, electromyographic biofeedback, optokinetic visual stimulation, and videography are all technical systems that can provide feedback to motor learning during vestibular rehabilitation
- ✓ Foam, mirrors, rocker boards, BAPS boards, Swiss balls, foam roller, trampolines, and wedges are lower "tech" treatment tools that are successfully used for vestibular rehabilitation

Communication Disorders

Aphasia (Dysphasia)

Aphasia is an acquired neurological impairment of processing for receptive and/or expressive language. Aphasia is the result of brain injury, head trauma, CVA, tumor or infection. There are multiple forms of aphasia; diagnosis is based on the site of lesion in the brain and the blood vessels involved. Patients with aphasia are classified based on observation of:
- Fluent versus non-fluent
- Good versus poor comprehension
- Good versus poor repetition

Fluent Aphasia
- Lesion often in temporoparietal lobe of dominant hemisphere
- Word output is functional
- Speech production is functional
- Prosody is acceptable
- "Empty speech" or jargon
- Speech lacks any substance
- Use of paraphasias (substitution of incorrect words)

Wernicke's Aphasia
- Lesion found at the posterior region of the superior temporal gyrus
- Major fluent aphasia
- Also known as receptive aphasia
- Comprehension (reading/auditory) impaired
- Use of paraphasias
- Good articulation
- Use of neologism (fabricated words)
- Impaired writing
- Poor naming ability

Conduction Aphasia
- Lesion of the supramarginal gyrus and arcuate fasciculus
- Major fluent aphasia
- Severe impairment with repetition
- Intact fluency
- Good comprehension
- Speech interrupted by word-finding difficulties
- Reading intact
- Writing impaired

Anomic Aphasia
- Lesion of angular gyrus
- Minor fluent aphasia
- Word finding difficulties with writing and speech
- Functional comprehension
- Good repetition skills
- Speech can seem empty; words regarding content are dropped

Non-fluent Aphasia
- Lesion often in frontal region of the dominant hemisphere
- Poor word output
- Increased effort for producing speech
- Poor articulation
- Dysprosodic speech
- Content of speech is present, but syntactical words are impaired

Broca's Aphasia
- Major non-fluent aphasia
- Also known as "expressive aphasia"
- Most common form of aphasia
- Lesions of the 3rd convolution of the frontal lobe
- Intact auditory and reading comprehension
- Impaired repetition and naming skills
- Frequent frustration regarding language skill errors

Global Aphasia
- Major non-fluent aphasia
- Lesion of frontal, temporal, and parietal lobes
- Comprehension (reading and auditory) is severely impaired
- Impaired naming and writing skills
- Impaired repetition skills
- May involuntarily verbalize; usually without correct context
- May use nonverbal (gestures) skills for communication

Prognosis is dependent on the individual patient, location, and extent of lesion. The following characteristics associated with aphasia are often associated with a poor prognosis: perseveration of speech, severe auditory comprehension impairments, unreliable yes/no answers, and the use of empty speech without recognition of impairments.

Verbal Apraxia
Apraxia is a non-dysarthric and non-aphasic impairment of prosody and articulation of speech. Verbal expression is impaired secondary to deficits in motor planning. A patient is unable to initiate learned movement (articulation of speech) even though they understand the task. Lesions are usually found in the left frontal lobe adjacent to Broca's area.

Dysarthria
Dysarthria is a motor disorder of speech that is caused by an upper motor neuron lesion that affects the muscles that are used to articulate words and sounds. Speech is often noted as "slurred" and there may also be an effect on respiratory or phonatory systems due to the weakness.

Cerebrovascular Accident

Risk Factors for Cerebrovascular Accident

Primary:	Secondary:
- Hypertension	- Obesity
- Heart disease	- High cholesterol
- Diabetes mellitus	- Behaviors related to hypertension
- Cigarette smoking	- Physical inactivity
- Transient ischemic attacks	- Increased alcohol consumption

Types of Cerebrovascular Accidents

Completed Stroke
A CVA that presents with total neurological deficits at the onset.

Stroke in Evolution
A CVA, usually caused by a thrombus, that gradually progresses. Total neurological deficits are not seen for one to two days after onset.

Ischemic Stroke
Once there is a loss of perfusion to a portion of the brain (within just seconds) there is a central area of irreversible infarction surrounded by an area of potential ischemia.
- Embolus
- Thrombus

--Embolus (20% of ischemic CVAs)
Associated with cardiovascular disease, an embolus may be a solid, liquid or gas, and can originate in any part of the body. The embolus travels through the bloodstream to the cerebral arteries causing occlusion of a blood vessel and a resultant infarct. The middle cerebral artery is most commonly affected by an embolus from the internal carotid arteries. Due to the sudden onset of occlusion, tissues distal to the infarct can sustain higher permanent damage than those of thrombotic infarcts. An embolic CVA occurs rapidly with no warning, and often presents with a headache. Common cardiac disorders that can lead to embolism include valvular disease (i.e., rheumatic mitral stenosis), ischemic heart disease, acute myocardial infarction, arrhythmias (i.e., atrial fibrillation), patent foramen ovale, cardiac tumors, and post cardiac catheterization.

--Thrombus
An atherosclerotic plaque develops in an artery and eventually occludes the artery or a branching artery causing an infarct. This type of CVA is extremely

variable in onset where symptoms can appear in minutes or over several days. A thrombotic CVA usually occurs during sleep or upon awakening, after a myocardial infarction or post-surgical procedure.

Hemorrhage (10 - 15% of CVAs)

An abnormal bleeding in the brain due to a rupture in blood supply. The infarct is due to disruption of oxygen to an area of the brain and compression from the accumulation of blood. Hypertension is usually a precipitating factor causing rupture of an aneurysm or arteriovenous malformation. Trauma can also precipitate hemorrhage and subsequent CVA. Characteristics include severe headache, vomiting, high blood pressure, and abrupt onset of symptoms. Hemorrhage usually occurs during the day with symptoms evolving in relation to the speed of the bleed. Approximately 50% of deaths from hemorrhagic stroke occur within the first 48 hours.

Transient Ischemic Attack (TIA)

A transient ischemic attack is usually linked to an atherosclerotic thrombosis. There is a temporary interruption of blood supply to an area. The effects may be similar to a CVA, but symptoms resolve quickly. A TIA most often occurs in the carotid and vertebrobasilar arteries and may indicate future CVA.

Expected Impairment Based on Vascular Involvement

Anterior Cerebral Artery	Posterior Cerebral Artery
• Lower extremity involvement	• Pain and temperature sensory loss
• Loss of bowel and bladder control	• Contralateral hemiplegia (central area)
• Loss of behavioral inhibition	• Ataxia, athetosis or choreiform movement
• Significant mental changes	• Quality of movement is impaired
• May see neglect	• Thalamic pain syndrome
• May see aphasia	• Anomia
• May see apraxia and agraphia	• Prosopagnosia with occipital infarct
• Perseveration	• Hemiballismus
	• Visual agnosia
Vertebral-Basilar Artery	• Homonymous hemianopsia
• Loss of consciousness	• Mild hemiparesis
• Hemiplegia or quadriplegia	• Memory impairment
• Comatose or vegetative state	• Dyschromatopsia
	• Palinopsia, micropsia, macropsia
• Inability to speak	• Alexia, dyslexia

• Locked-in syndrome	• Achromatopsia
• Vertigo, nystagmus	
• Dysphagia	
• Dysarthria	
• Syncope	
• Ataxia	

Middle Cerebral Artery	Lacunar Infarct
• Most common site of a CVA	• Cystic cavity after infarct
• Wernicke's aphasia in dominant hemisphere	• Contralateral weakness
• Homonymous hemianopsia	• Sensory loss
• Apraxia	• Ataxia
• Flat affect in right hemisphere	• Dysarthria
• Superficial MCA – greater face and arm involvement	• Deep regions of the brain:
• Deep MCA – pure motor hemiplegia without sensory impairment	--internal capsule --thalamus --basal ganglia --pons
• Impaired spatial relations	
• Anosognosia in non-dominant hemisphere	
• Impaired body schema	

Characteristics of a Cerebrovascular Accident

Right Hemisphere
- Weakness, paralysis of the left side
- Decreased attention span
- Left hemianopsia
- Decreased awareness and judgment
- Memory deficits
- Left inattention
- Decreased abstract reasoning
- Emotional lability
- Impulsive behaviors
- Decreased spatial orientation

Left Hemisphere
- Weakness, paralysis of the right side
- Increased frustration
- Decreased processing
- Possible aphasia (expressive, receptive, global)
- Possible dysphagia
- Possible motor apraxia (ideomotor and ideational)
- Decreased discrimination between left and right
- Right hemianopsia

Brainstem
- Unstable vital signs
- Decreased consciousness
- Decreased ability to swallow
- Weakness on both sides of the body
- Paralysis on both sides of the body

Cerebellum
- Decreased balance
- Ataxia
- Decreased coordination
- Nausea
- Decreased ability for postural adjustment
- Nystagmus

Synergy Patterns

Upper Limb

	Flexor Synergy	Extensor Synergy
Scapula	Elevation and retraction	Depression and protraction
Shoulder	Abduction and lateral rotation	Medial rotation and adduction
Elbow	Flexion	Extension
Forearm	Supination	Pronation
Wrist	Flexion	Extension
Fingers	Flexion with adduction	Flexion with adduction
Thumb	Flexion and adduction	Adduction and flexion

- The flexor synergy is seen when the patient attempts to lift up their arm or reach for an object.

Lower Limb

	Flexor Synergy	Extensor Synergy
Hip	Abduction and lateral rotation	Extension, medial rotation and adduction
Knee	Flexion	Extension
Ankle	Dorsiflexion with supination	Plantar flexion with inversion
Toes	Extension	Flexion and adduction

- The flexor synergy is characterized by great toe extension and flexion of the remaining toes secondary to spasticity.

When the central nervous system is damaged as with a CVA, the higher centers of the brain are also damaged. The higher centers are responsible for both complex motor patterns and the inhibition of massive gross motor patterns. Synergy patterns result when the higher centers of the brain lose control and the uncontrolled or partially controlled stereotyped patterns of the middle and lower centers emerge.

Theories of Neurological Rehabilitation

Bobath

Neuromuscular Developmental Treatment (NDT)

An approach developed by Karl and Berta Bobath based on the hierarchical model of neurophysiologic function. Abnormal postural reflex activity and abnormal muscle tone is caused by the loss of central nervous system control at the brainstem and spinal cord levels. The concept recognizes that interference of normal function of the brain caused by central nervous system dysfunction leads to a slowing down or cessation of motor development and the inhibition of righting reactions, equilibrium reactions, and automatic movements. The patient should learn to control movement through activities that promote normal movement patterns that integrate function.

Key Terminology

Facilitation: A technique utilized to elicit voluntary muscular contraction.

Inhibition: A technique utilized to decrease excessive tone or movement.

Key points of control: Specific handling of designated areas of the body (shoulder, pelvis, hand, and foot) will influence and facilitate posture, alignment, and control.

Placing: The act of moving an extremity into a position that the patient must hold against gravity.

Reflex inhibiting posture: Designated static positions that Bobath found to inhibit abnormal tonal influences and reflexes.

Intervention
- ✓ Inhibition of abnormal patterns with facilitation of normal patterns
- ✓ Alteration of abnormal tone and influencing isolated active movement

✓ Avoid utilization of abnormal reflexes
✓ Manual contact and handling through key points of control for facilitation and inhibition
✓ Achieve a balance between muscle groups
✓ Use of developmental sequence
✓ Provide the patient with the sensation of normal movement by inhibiting abnormal postural reflex activity
✓ Use of dynamic reflex inhibiting patterns
✓ Use of functional activities with varying levels of difficulty
✓ Treatment should be active and dynamic
✓ Avoid associated reactions
✓ Emphasize the component of rotation during treatment activities
✓ Orientation to midline control by moving in and out of midline with dynamic activity
✓ Compensation techniques are avoided and perceived as unnecessary

Brunnstrom

Movement Therapy in Hemiplegia

Movement therapy in hemiplegia developed by Signe Brunnstrom is based on the hierarchical model by Hughlings Jackson. This approach created and defined the term synergy and initially encouraged the use of synergy patterns during rehabilitation. The belief was to immediately practice synergy patterns and subsequently develop combinations of movement patterns outside of the synergy. Synergies are considered primitive patterns that occur at the spinal cord level as a result of the hierarchical organization of the central nervous system. Reinforcing synergy patterns is rarely utilized now as research has indicated that reinforced synergy patterns are very difficult to change. Brunnstrom developed the *seven stages of recovery*, which are used for evaluation and documentation of patient progress.

Key Terminology

Associated reactions: An involuntary and automatic movement of a body part as a result of an intentional active or resistive movement in another body part.

Homolateral synkinesis: A flexion pattern of the involved upper extremity facilitates flexion of the involved lower extremity.

Limb synergies: A group of muscles that produce a predictable pattern of movement in flexion or extension patterns.

Raimiste's phenomenon: The involved lower extremity will abduct/adduct with applied resistance to the uninvolved lower extremity in the same direction.

Souque's phenomenon: Raising the involved upper extremity above 100 degrees with elbow extension will produce extension and abduction of the fingers.

Stages of recovery: Brunnstrom separates neurological recovery into seven separate stages based on progression through abnormal tone and spasticity. These seven stages of recovery describe tone, reflex activity, and volitional movement.

Seven Stages of Recovery	
Stage 1:	No volitional movement initiated.
Stage 2:	The appearance of basic limb synergies. The beginning of spasticity.
Stage 3:	The synergies are performed voluntarily; spasticity increases.
Stage 4:	Spasticity begins to decrease. Movement patterns are not dictated solely by limb synergies.
Stage 5:	A further decrease in spasticity is noted with independence from limb synergy patterns.
Stage 6:	Isolated joint movements are performed with coordination.
Stage 7:	Normal motor function is restored.

Intervention

✓ Evaluation of strength focuses on patterns of movement rather than straight plane motion at a joint
✓ Sensory examination is required to assist with treating motor deficits
✓ Initially limb synergies are encouraged as a necessary milestone for recovery
✓ Encourage overflow to recruit active movement of the weak side
✓ Use of repetition of task and positive reinforcement
✓ A patient will follow the stages of recovery, but may experience a plateau at any point so that full recovery is not achieved
✓ Movement combinations that deviate from the basic limb synergies should be introduced in stage 4 of recovery

Kabat, Knott, and Voss

Proprioceptive Neuromuscular Facilitation (PNF)

PNF was introduced in the early 1950's using the hierarchical model as its framework. The original goal of treatment was to lay down gross motor patterns within the central nervous system. This approach is based on the premise that stronger parts of the body are utilized to stimulate and strengthen the weaker parts. Normal movement and posture is based on a balance between control of antagonist and agonist muscle groups. Development will follow the normal sequence through a component of motor learning. This theory places great emphasis on manual contacts and correct handling. Short and concise verbal commands are used along with resistance throughout the full movement pattern. The PNF approach utilizes methods that promote or hasten the response of the neuromuscular mechanism through stimulation of the proprioceptors. Movement patterns follow diagonals or spirals that each possess a flexion, extension, and rotatory component and are directed toward or away from midline.

Key Terminology

Chopping: A combination of bilateral upper extremity asymmetrical extensor patterns performed as a closed-chain activity.

Developmental sequence: A progression of motor skill acquisition. The stages of motor control include mobility, stability, controlled mobility, and skill.

Mass movement patterns: The hip, knee, and ankle move into flexion or extension simultaneously.

Overflow: Muscle activation of an involved extremity due to intense action of an uninvolved muscle or group of muscles.

PNF Diagonal Patterns – Upper Extremity Responses

	D1 Flexion Pattern	D1 Extension Pattern	D2 Flexion Pattern	D2 Extension Pattern
Scapula	Elevation Abduction Upward rotation	Depression Adduction Downward rotation	Elevation Adduction Upward rotation	Depression Abduction Downward rotation
Shoulder	Flexion Adduction Lateral rotation	Extension Abduction Medial rotation	Flexion Abduction Lateral rotation	Extension Adduction Medial rotation
Elbow	Flexion or extension	Flexion or extension	Flexion or extension	Flexion or extension
Radioulnar	Supination	Pronation	Supination	Pronation
Wrist	Flexion Radial deviation	Extension Ulnar deviation	Extension Radial deviation	Flexion Ulnar deviation
Thumb	Adduction	Abduction	Extension	Opposition

PNF Diagonal Patterns – Lower Extremity Responses

	D1 Flexion Pattern	D1 Extension Pattern	D2 Flexion Pattern	D2 Extension Pattern
Pelvis	Protraction	Retraction	Elevation	Depression
Hip	Flexion Adduction Lateral rotation	Extension Abduction Medial rotation	Flexion Abduction Medial rotation	Extension Adduction Lateral rotation
Knee	Flexion or extension	Flexion or extension	Flexion or extension	Flexion or extension
Ankle and Toes	Dorsiflexion Inversion	Plantar flexion Eversion	Dorsiflexion Eversion	Plantar flexion Inversion

Intervention

- ✓ A patient learns diagonal patterns of movement
- ✓ Techniques must have accurate timing, specific commands, and correct hand placement
- ✓ Verbal commands must be short and concise
- ✓ Repetition is important in motor learning
- ✓ Resistance given during the movement pattern is greater if the objective is stability, less if the objective is mobility
- ✓ Techniques utilize isometric and isotonic muscle contractions
- ✓ Treatment objectives will dictate the use of techniques through either full movement or at points within the range
- ✓ Developmental sequence is used in conjunction with PNF techniques in order to increase the balance between agonists and antagonists
- ✓ PNF techniques are implemented to progress a patient through the stages of motor control
- ✓ Functional patterns of movement are used to increase control
- ✓ Techniques should be utilized that increase strength or improve relaxation by enhancing irradiation from the stronger to the weaker muscles

Levels of Motor Control

Mobility
The ability to initiate movement through a functional range of motion.

Stability
The ability to maintain a position or posture through cocontraction and tonic holding around a joint. Unsupported sitting with midline control is an example of stability.

Controlled Mobility
The ability to move within a weight bearing position or rotate around a long axis. Activities in prone on elbows or weight shifting in quadruped are examples of controlled mobility.

Skill
The ability to consistently perform functional tasks and manipulate the environment with normal postural reflex mechanisms and balance reactions. Skill activities include ADLs and community locomotion.

PNF Therapeutic Exercises

Technique	Mobility		Stability	Controlled Mobility	Skill		Strength
	Increased ROM	Initiate Movement			Distal Functional Movement	Proximal Dynamic Stability	
Agonistic Reversals				X		X	
Alternating Isometrics			X				X
Contract-Relax	X						
Hold-Relax	X						
Hold-Relax Active Movement		X					
Joint Distraction	X	X					
Normal Timing					X		
Repeated Contractions		X					X
Resisted Progression						X	X
Rhythmic Initiation		X					
Rhythmical Rotation	X	X					
Rhythmic Stabilization	X		X				
Slow Reversal			X	X	X		
Slow Reversal Hold			X	X	X		
Timing for Emphasis							X

PNF Therapeutic Exercise Descriptions*

*Italicized terms indicate level of developmental sequence.

Agonistic Reversals (AR)

Controlled mobility, skill: An isotonic concentric contraction performed against resistance followed by alternating concentric and eccentric contractions with resistance. AR requires use in a slow and sequential manner, and may be used in increments throughout the range to attain maximum control.

Alternating Isometrics (AI)

Stability: Isometric contractions are performed alternating from muscles on one side of the joint to the other side without rest. AI emphasizes endurance or strengthening.

Contract-Relax (CR)

Mobility: A technique used to increase range of motion. As the extremity reaches the point of limitation the patient performs a maximal contraction of the antagonistic muscle group. The therapist resists movement for eight to ten seconds with relaxation to follow. The technique is repeated until no further gains in range of motion are noted during the session.

Hold-Relax (HR)

Mobility: An isometric contraction used to increase range of motion. The contraction is facilitated for all muscle groups at the limiting point in the range of motion. Relaxation occurs and the extremity moves through the newly acquired range to the next point of limitation until no further increases in range of motion occur. The technique is often used for patients that present with pain.

Hold-Relax Active Movement (HRAM)

Mobility: A technique to improve initiation of movement to muscle groups tested at 1/5 or less. An isometric contraction is performed once the extremity is passively placed into a shortened range within the pattern. Overflow and facilitation may be used to assist with the contraction. Upon relaxation the extremity is immediately moved into a lengthened position of the pattern with a quick stretch. The patient is asked to return the extremity to the shortened position through an isotonic contraction.

Joint Distraction

Mobility: A proprioceptive component used to increase range of motion around a joint. Consistent manual traction is provided slowly and usually in combination with mobilization techniques. It can also be used in combination with quick stretch to initiate movement.

Normal Timing (NT)

Skill: A technique used to improve coordination of all components of a task. NT is performed in a distal to proximal sequence. Proximal components are restricted until the distal components are activated and initiate movement. Repetition of the pattern produces a coordinated movement of all components.

Repeated Contractions (RC)

Mobility: A technique used to initiate movement and sustain a contraction through the range of motion. Repeated contractions is used to initiate a movement pattern, throughout a weak movement pattern or at a point of weakness within a movement pattern. The therapist provides a quick stretch followed by isometric or isotonic contractions.

Resisted Progression (RP)

Skill: A technique used to emphasize coordination of proximal components during gait. Resistance is applied to an area such as the pelvis, hips, or extremity during the gait cycle in order to enhance coordination, strength or endurance.

Rhythmic Initiation (RI)

Mobility: A technique used to assist initiating movement when hypertonia exists. Movement progresses from passive ("let me move you"), to active assistive ("help me move you"), to slightly resistive ("move against the resistance"). Movements must be slow and rhythmical to reduce the hypertonia and allow for full range of motion.

Rhythmical Rotation (RR)

Mobility: A passive technique used to decrease hypertonia by slowly rotating an extremity around the longitudinal axis. Relaxation of the extremity will increase range of motion.

Rhythmic Stabilization (RS)

Mobility, stability: A technique used to increase range of motion and coordinate isometric contractions. The technique requires isometric contractions of all muscles around a joint against progressive resistance. The patient should relax and move into the newly acquired range and repeat the technique. If stability is the goal, RS should be applied as a progression from AI in order to simultaneously stabilize all muscle groups around the specific body part.

Slow Reversal (SR)

Stability, controlled mobility, skill: A technique of slow and resisted concentric contractions of agonists and antagonists around a joint without rest between reversals. This technique is used to improve control of movement and posture.

Slow Reversal Hold (SRH)

Stability, controlled mobility, skill: Using slow reversal with the addition of an isometric contraction that is performed at the end of each movement in order to gain stability.

Timing for Emphasis (TE)

Skill: Used to strengthen the weak component of a motor pattern. Isotonic and isometric contractions produce overflow to weak muscles.

Motor Control: A Task-Oriented Approach

Theories of motor control have been documented since the late nineteenth century when Sir Charles Sherrington postulated the reflex theory of motor control. Motor control refers to the ability to produce, regulate, and alter mechanisms that produce movement and control posture. The various theories are based on a specific interpretation of how the brain functions and interacts with other body systems. A task-oriented approach to motor control utilizes a systems theory of motor control that views the entire body as a mechanical system with many interacting subsystems that all work cooperatively in managing internal and environmental influences. The task-oriented approach utilizes an examination that consists of observation of functional performance, analysis of strategies used to accomplish tasks, and assessment of impairments. Treatment attempts to resolve impairments, design and implement effective recovery and compensatory strategies, and retrain using functional activities.

Key Terminology

Compensation: The ability to utilize alternate motor and sensory strategies due to an impairment that limits the normal completion of a task.

Motor learning: The ability to perform a movement as a result of internal processes that interact with the environment and produce a consistent strategy to generate the correct movement.

Plasticity: The ability to modify or change at the synapse level either temporarily or permanently in order to perform a particular function.

Postural control: The ability of the motor and sensory systems to stabilize position and control movement.

Recovery: The ability to utilize previous strategies to return to the same level of functioning.

Strategy: A plan used to produce a specific result or outcome that will influence the structure or system.

Intervention

✓ Models of motor control vary based on the interpretation of brain function
✓ Evaluation determines the degree of impairment
✓ Intervention is designed at the level of impairment
✓ Sensory, motor, and cognitive strategies are used to acquire postural control
✓ Focus is both on recovery and compensatory techniques
✓ Tasks are broken down into components of the task for practice
✓ Sensory, motor, and perceptual input contribute to motor control
✓ Movement is based around a behavioral goal
✓ Variable practice allows for training in a different and changing environment
✓ Type and amount of feedback (visual, verbal) should be evaluated for each individual patient
✓ Emphasis on postural control, alignment, and sequencing of movements is essential
✓ Intervention should create multiple ways to solve a movement disorder
✓ Environmental factors must be considered with intervention, planning, and implementation

Rood

This theory is based on Sherrington and the reflex stimulus model. Rood believed that all motor output was the result of both past and present sensory input. Treatment is based on sensorimotor learning. It takes into account the autonomic nervous system and emotional factors as well as motor ability. Rood used a developmental sequence, which was seen as "key patterns" in the enhancement of motor control. A goal of this approach is to obtain homeostasis in motor output and to activate muscles and perform a task independently of a stimulus. Exercise is seen as a treatment technique only if the response is correct and if it provides sensory feedback that enhances the motor learning of that response. Once a response is obtained during treatment the stimulus should be withdrawn. Rood introduced the use of sensory stimulation to facilitate or inhibit responses such as icing and brushing in order to elicit desired reflex motor responses.

Key Terminology

Heavy work: A method used to develop stability by performing an activity (work) against gravity or resistance. Heavy work focuses on the strengthening of postural muscles.

Light work: A method used to develop controlled movement and skilled function by performing an activity (work) without resistance. Light work focuses on the extremities.

Key patterns: A developmental sequence designed by Rood that directs patients' mobility recovery from synergy patterns through controlled motion.

Sensory Stimulation Techniques	
Facilitation	**Inhibition**
▪ Approximation	▪ Deep pressure
▪ Joint compression	▪ Prolonged stretch
▪ Icing	▪ Warmth
▪ Light tough	▪ Prolonged cold
▪ Quick stretch	▪ Carotid reflex
▪ Resistance	
▪ Tapping	
▪ Traction	

Intervention

- ✓ Use of sensory stimulation to achieve motor output
- ✓ Movement is considered autonomic and noncognitive
- ✓ Homeostasis of all systems is essential
- ✓ Use of techniques such as neutral warmth, maintained pressure, and slow rhythmical stroking to calm a patient
- ✓ Tactile stimulation is used to facilitate normal movement
- ✓ Exercise must provide proper sensory feedback in order to be therapeutic

Pharmacological Intervention for CVA Management

Thrombolytic Agents -Produces anticoagulation effects, destroys thrombus/emboli	Heparin Ximelagatran Alteplase (Activase) Warafarin (Coumadin) Tissue-type plasminogen activator (tPA)
Antiplatelet Agents -Reduce atherosclerotic events and decrease the risk for CVA	Aspirin (Bayer, Ascriptin) Ticlopidine (Ticlid) Clopidogrel (Plavix) Aggrenox Dipyridamole (Persantine)
Cholesterol-lowering Agents -Decrease the triglycerides and low-density lipoproteins in the bloodstream	Atorvastatin (Lipitor) Lovastatin (Mevacaor) Pravastatin (Pravachol) Simvastatin (Zocor) Gemfibrozil (Lopid)
Neuroprotective Agents -Administered only within the acute stage of CVA (within three hours)	N-methyl-D-aspartate (NMDA)

Antiarrhythmic Agents
-Prevention of arrhythmias, ischemia and hypertension
  -Sodium channel blockers
  -Beta-blockers (cardiac medications p. 113)
  -Refractory period alterations
  -Calcium channel blockers (cardiac medications p. 113)
	Sodium channel blockers
	Encainide (Enkaid)
	Lidocaine (Xylocaine)
	Procainamide (Pronestyl)
	Quinidine (Biquin)
	Disopyramide (Norpace)
	Refractory period alterations
	Amlodarone (Cordarone)
	Ibutilide fumarate (Corvert)

Antihypertensive Agents -Assist to lower blood pressure; decrease tension within the circulation system	**Diuretics** Thiazide Furosemide (Lasix) Chlorothiazide (Divril) Bumetanide (Bumex) Amiloride (Midamor) **Beta-blockers** Acebutolol (Sectral) Pindolol (Visken) Ateolol (Tenormin) Propanolol (Inderal) Metoprolol (Lopressor) **Calcium channel blockers** Amlodipine (Norvasc) Diltiazem (Cardizem) Nicardipine (Cardene) Verapamil (Calan) **Alpha-blockers** Phenoxybenzamine (Dibenzyline) Prazosin (Minipress) Terazosin (Hytrin) Doxazosin (Cardura)

Neurological Profile

Examination

- ▪ Past medical history
- ▪ History of current condition
- ▪ Social history (caregiver support)
- ▪ Medications
- ▪ Living environment
- ▪ Systems review
- ▪ Cognitive and language assessment
- ▪ Respiratory assessment
- ▪ Postural tone assessment
- ▪ Righting and equilibrium reaction assessment
- ▪ Pathological reflex assessment
- ▪ Pain

- Sensation, proprioception, and kinesthesia
- Range of motion
- Motor assessment
- Mobility skills

Intervention

- Postural control
- Positioning
- Therapeutic exercise
- Developmental activities training
- Facilitation/inhibition techniques
- Motor function retraining
- Sensory integration
- Wheelchair and orthotic prescription
- Mobility training

Goals

- Maximize functional mobility
- Normalize tonal abnormalities
- Maximize active isolated movement and strength
- Maximize range of motion and joint integrity
- Maximize independence with adaptive equipment
- Maximize static and dynamic balance
- Maximize patient/caregiver competence with:
  --Positioning
  --Use of adaptive equipment and orthotic devices
  --Home exercise programs

Neurological Terminology

Agnosia: The inability to interpret information.

Agraphesthesia: The inability to recognize symbols, letters or numbers traced on the skin.

Agraphia: The inability to write due to a lesion within the brain.

Akinesia: The inability to initiate movement; commonly seen in patients with Parkinson's disease.

Aphasia: The inability to communicate or comprehend due to damage to specific areas of the brain.

Apraxia: The inability to perform purposeful learned movements, although there is no sensory or motor impairment.

Astereognosis: The inability to recognize objects by sense of touch.

Ataxia: The inability to perform coordinated movements.

Athetosis: A condition that presents with involuntary movements combined with instability of posture. Peripheral movements occur without central stability.

Bradykinesia: Movement that is very slow.

Chorea: Movements that are sudden, random, and involuntary.

Clonus: A characteristic of an upper motor neuron lesion; involuntary alternating spasmodic contraction of a muscle precipitated by a quick stretch reflex.

Constructional apraxia: The inability to reproduce geometric figures and designs. This person is visually unable to analyze how to perform a task.

Decerebrate rigidity: A characteristic of a corticospinal lesion at the level of the brainstem that results in extension of the trunk and all extremities.

Decorticate rigidity: A characteristic of a corticospinal lesion at the level of the diencephalon where the trunk and lower extremities are positioned in extension and the upper extremities are positioned in flexion.

Diplopia: Double vision

Dysarthria: Slurred and impaired speech due to a motor deficit of the tongue or other muscles essential for speech.

Dysdiadochokinesia: The inability to perform rapidly alternating movements.

Dysmetria: The inability to control the range of a movement and the force of muscular activity.

Dysphagia: The inability to properly swallow.

Dystonia: Closely related to athetosis, however, there is larger axial muscle involvement rather than appendicular muscles.

Emotional lability: A characteristic of a right hemisphere infarct where there is an inability to control emotions and outbursts of laughing or crying that are inconsistent with the situation.

Hemiballism: An involuntary and violent movement of a large body part.

Hemiparesis: A condition of weakness on one side of the body.

Hemiplegia: A condition of paralysis on one side of the body.

Homonymous hemianopsia: The loss of the right or left half of the field of vision in both eyes.

Ideational apraxia: The inability to formulate an initial motor plan and sequence tasks where the proprioceptive input necessary for movement is impaired.

Ideomotor apraxia: A condition where a person plans a movement or task, but cannot volitionally perform it. Automatic movement may occur, however, a person cannot impose additional movement on command.

Kinesthesia: The ability to perceive the direction and extent of movement of a joint or body part.

Neglect: The inability to interpret stimuli on the left side of the body due to a lesion of the right frontal lobe of the brain.

Perseveration: The state of repeatedly performing the same segment of a task or repeatedly saying the same word/phrase without purpose.

Proprioception: The ability to perceive the static position of a joint or body part.

Rigidity: A state of severe hypertonicity where a sustained muscle contraction does not allow for any movement at a specified joint.

Synergy: A result of brain damage that presents with mass movement patterns that are primitive in nature and coupled with spasticity.

Spinal Cord Injury

Types of Spinal Cord Injury

Complete lesion: A lesion to the spinal cord where there is no preserved motor or sensory function below the level of lesion.

Incomplete lesion: A lesion to the spinal cord with incomplete damage to the cord. There may be scattered motor function, sensory function or both below the level of lesion.

Specific Incomplete Lesions

Anterior Cord Syndrome

An incomplete lesion that results from compression and damage to the anterior part of the spinal cord or anterior spinal artery. The mechanism of injury is usually cervical flexion. There is loss of motor function and pain and temperature sense below the lesion due to damage of the corticospinal and spinothalamic tracts.

Brown-Sequard's Syndrome

An incomplete lesion usually caused by a stab wound, which produces hemisection of the spinal cord. There is paralysis and loss of vibratory and position sense on the same side as the lesion due to the damage to the corticospinal tract and dorsal columns. There is a loss of pain and temperature sense on the opposite side of the lesion from damage to the lateral spinothalamic tract. Pure Brown-Sequard's syndrome is rare since most spinal cord lesions are atypical.

Cauda Equina Injuries

An injury that occurs below the L1 spinal level where the long nerve roots transcend. Cauda equina injuries can be complete, however, are frequently incomplete due to the large number of nerve roots in the area. A cauda equina injury is considered a peripheral nerve injury. Characteristics include flaccidity, areflexia, and impairment of bowel and bladder function. Full recovery is not typical due to the distance needed for axonal regeneration.

Central Cord Syndrome

An incomplete lesion that results from compression and damage to the central portion of the spinal cord. The mechanism of injury is usually cervical hyperextension that damages the spinothalamic tract, corticospinal tract, and dorsal columns. The upper extremities present with greater involvement than the lower extremities and greater motor deficits exist as compared to sensory deficits.

Posterior Cord Syndrome

A relatively rare syndrome that is caused by compression of the posterior spinal artery and is characterized by loss of pain perception, proprioception, two-point discrimination, and stereognosis. Motor function is preserved.

Potential Complications of Spinal Cord Injury

Autonomic Dysreflexia

Autonomic dysreflexia is perhaps the most dangerous complication of spinal cord injury and can occur in patients with lesions above T6. A noxious stimulus below the level of the lesion triggers the autonomic nervous system causing a sudden elevation in blood pressure. Common causes include distended or full bladder, kink or blockage in the catheter, bladder infections, pressure ulcers, extreme temperature changes, tight clothing, or even an ingrown toenail. If not treated, this condition can lead to convulsions, hemorrhage, and death.

Symptoms: High blood pressure, severe headache, blurred vision, stuffy nose, profuse sweating, goose bumps below the level of the lesion, and vasodilation (flushing) above the level of injury

Treatment: The first reaction to this medical crisis is to check the catheter for blockage. The bowel should also be checked for impaction. A patient should remain in a sitting position. Lying a patient down is contraindicated and will only assist to further elevate blood pressure. The patient should be examined for any other irritating stimuli. If the cause remains unknown, the patient should receive immediate medical intervention.

Deep Vein Thrombosis (DVT)

Deep vein thrombosis results from the formation of a blood clot that becomes dislodged and is termed an embolus. This is considered a serious medical condition since the embolus may obstruct a selected artery. A patient with a spinal cord injury has a greater risk of developing a DVT due to the absence or decrease in the normal pumping action by active contractions of muscles in the lower extremities. Homans' sign is a special test designed to confirm the presence of a DVT. Prevention of a DVT should include prophylactic anticoagulant therapy, maintaining a positioning schedule, range of motion, proper positioning to avoid excessive venous stasis, and use of elastic stockings.

Symptoms: Swelling of the lower extremity, pain, sensitivity over the area of the clot, and warmth in the area.

Treatment: Once a DVT is suspected there should be no active or passive movement performed to the involved lower extremity. Bed rest and anticoagulant drug therapy are usually indicated. Surgical procedures can be performed if necessary.

Ectopic Bone

Ectopic bone or heterotopic ossification refers to the spontaneous formation of bone in the soft tissue. It typically occurs adjacent to larger joints such as the knees or the hips. Theories regarding etiology range from tissue hypoxia to abnormal calcium metabolism.

Symptoms: Early symptoms include edema, decreased range of motion, and increased temperature of the involved joint.

Treatment: Drug intervention usually involves diphosphates that inhibit ectopic bone formation. Physical therapy and surgery are often incorporated into treatment. Physical therapy must focus on maintaining functional range of motion and allowing the patient the most independent functional outcome possible.

Orthostatic Hypotension

Orthostatic hypotension or postural hypotension occurs due to a loss of sympathetic control of vasoconstriction in combination with absent or severely reduced muscle tone. Venous pooling is fairly common during the early stages of rehabilitation. A decrease in systolic blood pressure greater than 20 mm Hg after moving from a supine position to a sitting position is typically indicative of orthostatic hypotension.

Symptoms: Complaints of dizziness, light-headedness, nausea, and "blacking out" when going from a horizontal to a vertical position

Treatment: Monitoring vital signs assists with minimizing the effects of orthostatic hypotension. The use of elastic stockings, ace wraps to the lower extremities, and abdominal binders are common. Gradual progression to a vertical position using a tilt table is often indicated. Drug intervention may be indicated in order to increase blood pressure.

Pressure Ulcers

A pressure ulcer is caused by sustained pressure, friction, and/or shearing to a surface. The most common areas susceptible to pressure ulcers are the coccyx, sacrum, ischium, trochanters, elbows, buttocks, malleoli, scapulae, and prominent vertebrae. Pressure ulcers require immediate medical intervention and often can significantly delay the rehabilitation process.

Symptoms: A reddened area that persists; an open area

Treatment: Prevention is of greatest importance. A patient should change position frequently, maintain proper skin care, sit on an appropriate cushion, consistently weight shift, and maintain proper nutrition and hydration. Surgical intervention is often necessary with advanced pressure ulcers.

Spasticity

Spasticity can occasionally be useful to a patient with a spinal cord injury, however, more often serves to interfere with functional activities. Spasticity can be enhanced by both internal and external sources such as stress, decubiti, urinary tract infections, bowel or bladder obstruction, temperature changes or touch.

Symptoms: Increased involuntary contraction of muscle groups, increased tonic stretch reflexes, excessive deep tendon reflexes

Treatment: Medications are usually administered in an attempt to reduce the degree of spasticity (Dantrium, Baclofen, Lioresal). Aggressive treatment includes phenol blocks, rhizotomies, myelotomies, and other surgical intervention. Physical therapy intervention includes positioning, aquatic therapy, weight bearing, functional electrical stimulation, range of motion, resting splints, and inhibitive casting.

Functional Outcomes for Complete Lesions

Functional Skills	Level of Assistance Required (by SCI level groups)			
	High Tetraplegia (C1-C5)	**Mid-Level Tetraplegia (C6)**	**Low Tetraplegia (C7-C8)**	**Paraplegia**
Bed Mobility • Rolling side to side • Rolling supine/prone • Supine/sitting • Scooting all directions	-Dependent (C1-C4) -Moderate to maximal assistance (C5) -Able to verbally direct	-Minimal assistance to modified independent with equipment -Able to verbally direct	-Independent with all	-Independent
Transfers • Bed • Car • Toilet • Bath equipment • Floor • Upright wheelchair	-Dependent (C1-C4) -Maximal assistance with level sliding board transfers (C5) -Able to verbally direct	-Minimal assistance to modified independent for sliding board transfers -Dependent with wheelchair loading in car -Dependent with floor transfers and uprighting wheelchair -Able to verbally direct	-Modified independent to independent with level surface transfer (sliding board or depression) -Moderate assistance to modified independent with car transfer -Maximal to moderate assistance with floor transfers and uprighting wheelchair -Able to verbally direct	-Independent with level surface and car transfers (depression) -Minimal assistance to independent with floor transfers and uprighting wheelchair -Able to verbally direct
Weight Shifts • Pressure relief • Repositioning in wheelchair	-Set-up to modified independent with power recline/tilt weight shift -Dependent with manual recline/tilt/lean weight shift -Able to verbally direct	-Modified independent with power recline/tilt weight shift -Minimal assistance to modified independent with side to side/forward lean weight shift -Able to verbally direct	-Modified independent with side to side/forward lean, or depression weight shift	-Modified independent with depression weight shift

Functional Outcomes for Complete Lesions (continued)

Functional Skills	Level of Assistance Required (by SCI level groups)			
	High Tetraplegia (C1-C5)	Mid-Level Tetraplegia (C6)	Low Tetraplegia (C7-C8)	Paraplegia
Wheelchair Management • Wheel locks • Armrests • Footrests/legrests • Safety strap(s) • Cushion adjustment • Anti-tip levers • Wheelchair maintenance	-Dependent with all -Able to verbally direct	-Some assistance required -Able to verbally direct	-May require assistance with cushion adjustment, anti-tip levers, and wheelchair maintenance -Able to verbally direct	-Independent with all
Wheelchair Mobility • Smooth surfaces • Up/down ramps • Up/down curbs • Rough terrain • Up/down steps (manual wheelchair only)	-Supervision/set-up to modified independent on smooth, ramp, and rough terrain with power wheelchair -Modified independent with manual wheelchair on smooth surface in forward direction (C5) -Maximal assistance to dependent with manual wheelchair in all other situations (C5) -Able to verbally direct	-Modified independent in smooth, ramp, and rough terrain with power wheelchair -Dependent to maximal assistance up/down curb with power wheelchair -Modified independent on smooth surfaces with manual wheelchair -Moderate to minimal assistance on ramps and rough terrain with manual wheelchair -Maximal to moderate assistance up/down curbs with manual wheelchair -Able to verbally direct	-Modified independent on smooth, ramp, and rough terrain with power wheelchair -Dependent to maximal assistance up/down curb with power wheelchair -Modified independent on smooth surfaces and up/down ramps with manual wheelchair -Minimal assistance to modified independent on rough terrain -Moderate to minimal assistance up/down curbs with manual wheelchair -Dependent to maximal assistance up/down steps with manual wheelchair -Can verbally direct	-Minimal assistance to modified independent up/down 6" curbs with manual wheelchair -Modified independent with descending steps with manual wheelchair -Maximal to minimal assistance to ascend steps with manual wheelchair -Able to verbally direct
Gait • Don/doff orthoses • Sit/stand • Smooth surfaces • Up/down ramps • Up/down curbs • Up/down steps • Rough terrain • Safe falling	-Not applicable	-Not applicable	-Not applicable	Abilities range from: ·exercise only with KAFOs* ·household gait with KAFOs ·limited community gait with KAFOs or AFOs* ·functional community ambulation with or without orthoses

Functional Outcomes for Complete Lesions (continued)

Functional Skills	Level of Assistance Required (by SCI level groups)			
	High Tetraplegia (C1-C5)	**Mid-Level Tetraplegia (C6)**	**Low Tetraplegia (C7-C8)**	**Paraplegia**
ROM/Positioning • PROM to trunk, legs, and arms • Pad/position in bed	-Dependent -Able to verbally direct	-Moderate assistance to modified independent with all -Able to verbally direct	-Minimal assistance to modified independent with all -Able to verbally direct	-Independent
Feeding • Drinking • Finger feeding • Utensil feeding	-Dependent (C1-C4) -Minimal assistance with adaptive equipment (C5) -Able to verbally direct	-Modified independent with adaptive equipment	-Modified independent with adaptive equipment (C7)	-Independent
Grooming • Face • Teeth • Hair • Makeup • Shaving face	-Dependent (C1-C4) -Minimal assistance with adaptive equipment for face, teeth, makeup/shaving (C5) -Maximal/moderate assistance for hair grooming (C5) -Able to verbally direct	-Modified independent with adaptive equipment	-Modified independent	-Independent
Dressing • Dressing and undressing (in bed or wheelchair) • Upper body/lower body (in bed or wheelchair)	-Dependent -Able to verbally direct	-Modified independent for upper body in bed or wheelchair -Minimal assistance with lower body dressing in bed -Moderate assistance with lower body undressing in bed -Able to verbally direct	-Modified independent for upper/lower body dressing in bed -Minimal assistance with lower body dressing/undressing in wheelchair (C7) -Modified independent for upper/lower body dressing/undressing in wheelchair (C8) -Able to verbally direct	-Modified independent
Bathing • Bathing and drying off • Upper body and lower body	-Dependent -Able to verbally direct	-Minimal assistance for upper body bathing and drying -Moderate assistance for lower body bathing and drying -Use of shower or tub chair -Able to verbally direct	-Modified independent with all using shower or tub chair	-Modified independent with all on tub bench or tub bottom cushion

Functional Outcomes for Complete Lesions (continued)

Functional Skills	Level of Assistance Required (by SCI level groups)			
	High Tetraplegia (C1-C5)	Mid-Level Tetraplegia (C6)	Low Tetraplegia (C7-C8)	Paraplegia
Bowel/Bladder Problems • Intermittent catheterization • Leg bag care • Condom application • Clean up • In bed/wheelchair (bladder) • Feminine hygiene • Bowel program	-Dependent -Able to verbally direct	**Bladder:** -Minimal assistance for male in bed or wheelchair -Moderate assistance for female in bed **Bowel:** -Moderate assistance with use of equipment -Able to verbally direct	**Bladder:** -Modified independent for male in bed or wheelchair -Modified independent for female in bed; moderate assistance for female in wheelchair **Bowel:** -Minimal assistance to modified independent with use of equipment -Able to direct	**Bladder:** -Modified independent for male and female **Bowel:** -Modified independent for male and female

*KAFO, knee-ankle-foot orthosis; AFO = ankle-foot orthosis

From Umphred DA: Neurological Rehabilitation. Mosby-Year Book, Inc. 1995, p. 502-505, with permission.

Pharmacological Intervention for SCI Management

Corticosteroid Agents -Administered within eight hours after injury to prevent overall decline in white matter within the cord. Allows for enhanced blood flow and reduces post-traumatic ischemia	Methylprednisolone (Adlone, Depo-Medrol, Medrol) Dexamethasone (AK-Dex, Baldex, Decadron) GM-1* ------- *GM-1 is a complex acidic glycolipid administered with methylprednisolone to enhance recovery	**Biphosphonate Agents** -Prevent demineralization and SCI-induced osteoporosis	Pamidronate (Aredia) Cyclical Etidronate (Didronel) Clodronate (Bonetos) Ibandronate (Boniva)
		Agents for Bladder Program	Minipress Probanthine Ditropan Urecholine
Antispasticity Agents	Baclofen (Lioresal) Tizanidine Clonidine (Catapres) Diazepam (Valium) Gabapentin Dantrolene (Dantrium)	**Agents for Bowel Program**	Dulcolax Glycerine Docusate sodium Mylicon Pericolace
Anticonvulsant Agents -Treatment of neurogenic pain	Gabapentin	**Anti-bone Resorption Agents** -Treats heterotopic ossification through inhibiting bone resorption and formation and prevents ossification	Etidronate (Didronel) Alendronate (Fosamax)
Tricyclic Antidepressants -Treatment of neurogenic pain	Amitriptyline (Elavil) Doxepin (Sinequan) Desipramine (norpramin) Clomipramine (Anafranil) Nortriptiline (Pamelor)		
Parathyroid Hormone -Promotes new bone formation and an increase in bone mineral density	Teriparatide (Forteo)	**Anticoagulation Agents** -Prevents deep vein thrombus	Warafarin (Coumadin) Heparin (unfractionated heparin) Enoxaparin (Lovenox)

Spinal Cord Injury Profile

Examination

- Past medical history
- History of current condition
- Social history (caregiver support)
- Medications
- Living environment
- Systems review
- Cognitive assessment
- Skin assessment
- American Spinal Cord Injury Association (ASIA) Standard Neurological Classification
    - --Sensory examination
    - --Motor examination
- American Spinal Cord Injury Association (ASIA) impairment scale
- Respiratory assessment
    - --Cough
    - --Chest expansion
    - --Accessory muscle use
    - --Vital capacity
- Range of motion
- Pain
- Mobility skills

Intervention

- Positioning
- Family/caregiver teaching
- Respiratory training
    - --Assisted cough and secretion clearance
    - --Breathing exercises
- Wheelchair, cushion, and orthotic prescription
- Pressure relief
- Range of motion
- Motor function retraining
- Mobility training
- Gait training (T9 or lower)

Goals

- Maximize functional mobility based on level of injury (please refer to "functional outcome" chart)
- Maximize respiratory function
- Attain functional range of motion for all joints
- Maximize strength of available muscle groups
- Maximize patient/caregiver competence with:
    - --Pressure relief
    - --Positioning
    - --Range of motion
    - --Strengthening
    - --Wheelchair management

Spinal Cord Injury Terminology

Cauda equina injury: A term used to describe injuries that occur below the L1 level of the spine. A cauda equina injury is considered to be a lower motor neuron lesion.

Dermatome: Designated sensory areas based on spinal segment innervation.

Myelotomy: A surgical procedure that severs certain tracts within the spinal cord in order to decrease spasticity and improve function.

Myotome: Designated motor areas based on spinal segment innervation.

Neurectomy: A surgical removal of a segment of a nerve in order to decrease spasticity and improve function.

Neurogenic bladder: The bladder empties reflexively for a patient with an injury above the level of S2. The sacral reflex arc remains intact.

Neurologic level: The lowest segment (most caudal) of the spinal cord with intact strength and sensation. Muscle groups at this level must receive a grade of fair.

Nonreflexive bladder: The bladder is flaccid as a result of a cauda equina or conus medullaris lesion. The sacral reflex arc is damaged.

Paraplegia: A term used to describe injuries that occur at the level of the thoracic, lumbar or sacral spine.

Rhizotomy: A surgical resection of the sensory component of a spinal nerve in order to decrease spasticity and improve function.

Sacral sparing: An incomplete lesion where some of the innermost tracts remain innervated. Characteristics include sensation of the saddle area, movement of the toe flexors, and rectal sphincter contraction.

Spinal shock: A physiologic response that occurs between 30 and 60 minutes after trauma to the spinal cord and can last up to several weeks. Spinal shock presents with total flaccid paralysis and loss of all reflexes below the level of injury.

Tenotomy: A surgical release of a tendon in order to decrease spasticity and improve function.

Tetraplegia (quadriplegia): A term adopted by the American Spinal Cord Injury Association to describe injuries that occur at the level of the cervical spine.

Zone of preservation: A term used to describe poor or trace motor or sensory function for up to three levels below the neurologic level of injury.

Traumatic Brain Injury

Types of Injury

Open Injury
An injury of direct penetration through the skull to the brain. Location, depth of penetration, and pathway determine the extent of brain damage. Examples include gunshot wound, knife or sharp object penetration, skull fragments, and direct trauma.

Closed Injury
An injury to the brain without penetration through the skull. Examples include concussion, contusion, hematoma, injury to extracranial blood vessels, hypoxia, drug overdose, near drowning, and acceleration or deceleration injuries.

Primary Injury
Initial injury to the brain sustained by impact. Examples include skull penetration, skull fractures, and contusions to gray and white matter.

Coup lesion: A direct lesion of the brain under the point of impact. Local brain damage is sustained.

Contrecoup lesion: An injury that results on the opposite side of the brain. The lesion is due to the rebound effect of the brain after impact.

Secondary Injury
Brain damage that occurs as a response to the initial injury. Examples include hematoma, hypoxia, ischemia, increased intracranial pressure, and post-traumatic epilepsy.

Epidural hematoma: A hemorrhage that forms between the skull and dura mater.

Subdural hematoma: A hemorrhage that forms due to venous rupture between the dura and arachnoid.

Acute Diagnostic Management

- **Glasgow Coma Scale:** level of arousal and cerebral cortex function
- **CAT Scan:** observe intracranial structures
- **X-Ray:** fractures
- **MRI:** observe intracranial structures
- **Cerebral angiography:** observe blood vessels and internal anatomy of the brain
- **Evoked potential/electroencephalogram:** localizing structural damage
- **Positron emission tomography:** cerebral metabolism abnormalities
- **Ventriculography:** radiography used to observe cerebral ventricles following cerebrospinal fluid removal
- **Radioisotope imaging:** allows for a two dimensional concentrated view of the brain

Glasgow Coma Scale

A neurological assessment tool used initially after injury to determine arousal and cerebral cortex function. A total score of eight or less correlates to coma in 90% of patients. Scores of 9 to 12 indicate moderate brain injuries and scores from 13 to 15 indicate mild brain injuries.

Glasgow Coma Scale	
Eye Opening	**E**
Spontaneous	4
To speech	3
To pain	2
Nil	1
Best Motor Response	**M**
Obeys commands	6
Localizes pain	5
Withdraws	4
Abnormal flexion	3
Extensor response	2
Nil	1
Verbal Response	**V**
Oriented	5
Confused conversation	4
Inappropriate words	3
Incomprehensible sounds	2
Nil	1

Coma Score (E+M+V) = 3 to 15
From Management of Head Injuries by Bryan Jennett and Graham Teasdale, Copyright-1981 by Oxford University Press, Inc. Used by permission of Oxford University Press, Inc.

Rancho Los Amigos Levels of Cognitive Functioning

I. NO RESPONSE

Patient appears to be in a deep sleep and is completely unresponsive to any stimuli.

II. GENERALIZED RESPONSE

Patient reacts inconsistently and non-purposefully to stimuli in a nonspecific manner. Responses are limited and often the same regardless of stimulus presented. Responses may be physiological changes, gross body movements, and/or vocalization.

III. LOCALIZED RESPONSE

Patient reacts specifically but inconsistently to stimuli. Responses are directly related to the type of stimulus presented. May follow simple commands such as closing the eyes or squeezing the hand in an inconsistent, delayed manner.

IV. CONFUSED-AGITATED

Patient is in a heightened state of activity. Behavior is bizarre and non-purposeful relative to the immediate environment. Does not discriminate among persons or objects; is unable to cooperate directly with treatment efforts. Verbalizations frequently are incoherent and/or inappropriate to the environment; confabulation may be present. Gross attention to environment is very brief; selective attention is often nonexistent. Patient lacks short and long-term recall.

V. CONFUSED-INAPPROPRIATE

Patient is able to respond to simple commands fairly consistently. However, with increased complexity of commands or lack of any external structure, responses are non-purposeful, random, or fragmented. Demonstrates gross attention to the environment but is highly distractible and lacks the ability to focus attention on a specific task. With structure, may be able to converse on a social automatic level for short periods of time. Verbalization is often inappropriate and confabulatory. Memory is severely impaired; often shows inappropriate use of objects; may perform previously learned tasks with structure, but is unable to learn new information.

VI. CONFUSED-APPROPRIATE

Patient shows goal-directed behavior, but is dependent on external input or direction. Follows simple directions consistently and shows carryover for relearned tasks such as self-care. Responses may be incorrect due to memory problems, but they are appropriate to the situation. Past memories show more depth and detail than recent memory.

VII. AUTOMATIC-APPROPRIATE

Patient appears appropriate and oriented within the hospital and home settings; goes through daily routine automatically, but frequently robot-like. Patient shows minimal to no confusion and has shallow recall of activities. Shows carryover for new learning, but at a decreased rate. With structure is able to initiate social or recreational activities; judgment remains impaired.

VIII. PURPOSEFUL-APPROPRIATE

Patient is able to recall and integrate past and recent events and is aware of and responsive to environment. Shows carryover for new learning and needs no supervision once activities are learned. May continue to show a decreased ability relative to premorbid abilities, abstract reasoning, tolerance for stress, and judgment in emergencies or unusual circumstances.

From Professional Staff Association, Rancho Los Amigos Hospital, p.87-88, with permission.

Levels of Consciousness

Coma: A state of unconsciousness and a level of unresponsiveness to all internal and external stimuli.

Stupor: A state of general unresponsiveness with arousal occurring from repeated stimuli.

Obtundity: A state of consciousness that is characterized by a state of sleep, reduced alertness to arousal, and delayed responses to stimuli.

Delirium: A state of consciousness that is characterized by disorientation, confusion, agitation, and loudness.

Clouding of consciousness: A state of consciousness that is characterized by quiet behavior, confusion, poor attention, and delayed responses.

Consciousness: A state of alertness, awareness, orientation, and memory.

Memory Impairments

Anterograde memory: The inability to create new memory. Anterograde memory is usually the last to recover after a comatose state. Contributing factors include poor attention, distractibility, and impaired perception of stimuli.

Post-traumatic amnesia: The time between the injury and when the patient is able to recall recent events. The patient does not recall the injury or events up until this point of recovery. Post-traumatic amnesia is used as an indicator of the extent of damage.

Retrograde amnesia: An inability to remember events prior to the injury. Retrograde amnesia may progressively decrease with recovery.

Treatment Guidelines for Brain Injury

✓ Emphasis on motivation
✓ Promote independence
✓ Therapy should be goal-directed, functional, and recreational
✓ Focus on orientation
✓ Focus on behavior modification activities
✓ The use of repetition may be helpful
✓ Educate patient in compensatory strategies for success
✓ Structure is essential depending on the level of the patient
✓ Avoid overstimulation during therapy
✓ Use of calm voice and simple commands
✓ Perform activities that are both familiar and enjoyable for the patient
✓ Family education and support can enhance and assist in the rehabilitation process
✓ Allow patient to choose activities on occasion
✓ Flexibility in treatment is needed based on patient's immediate needs and state of mind

Pharmacological Intervention for TBI Management

Diuretic Agents -Decreases the volume of fluid in the brain and the intracranial pressure	Mannitol Furosemide Glycerol Urea Osmitrol Resectisol
Antidepressant Agents -Reduce disruptive or aggressive behavior	Elavil Marplan Nardil Pemelor Ritalin Paroxetine (Paxil) Fluoxetine (Prozac) Sertraline (Zoloft)
Anticonvulsant Agents -Prevention of early seizures in head injury	Phenytoin (Dilantin) Carbamazepine (Tegretol) Clonazepam (Klonopin) Phenobarbital Valproic acid (Depakane)

Electrolytes -Adequate stores are needed during the acute phase of head injury	Magnesium sulfate
Calcium Channel Blocker Agents -May improve outcome for traumatic subarachnoid hemorrhage	Nimodipine (Nimotop)
Psychostimulant Agents -Improve alertness and cognition	Methylphenidate (Ritalin) Pemoline (Cylert)
Dopamine Agonist Agents -May improve alertness or with post-traumatic Parkinsonism	Levodopa (Dopar, Larodopa)
Selective Serotonin Reuptake Inhibitor Agents -May benefit patients with head injury and emotional inhibition/impairment	Sertraline (Zoloft) Fluoxetine (Prozac) Paroxetine (Paxil)
Antispasticity Agents -May assist with relaxing increased muscle tone and/or cramping	Tizanidine hydrochloride (Zanaflex) Baclofen (Lioresal) Dantrolene (Dantrium) Diazepam (Valium)

Traumatic Brain Injury Profile

Examination

- Past medical history
- History of current condition
- Social history (caregiver support)
- Medications
- Living environment
- Systems review
- Cognitive and language assessment
- Behavioral assessment
- Safety assessment
- Skin assessment
- Postural tone assessment
- Sensation, proprioception, and kinesthesia
- Range of motion
- Motor assessment
- Endurance assessment
- Mobility skills

Intervention

- Cognitive and orientation training
- Therapeutic exercise
- Positioning
- Sensory integration
- Balance and vestibular training
- Range of motion
- Motor function training
- Wheelchair and adaptive equipment prescription
- Splinting and serial casting
- Mobility training

Goals

- Maximize functional mobility
- Maximize community independence
- Maximize strength
- Maximize range of motion and prevent heterotopic ossification
- Maximize static and dynamic balance
- Maximize endurance
- Maximize patient/caregiver competence with:
    - --Positioning
    - --Use of adaptive equipment and orthotic/splinting devices
    - --Home exercise program

Chapter Four
Cardiopulmonary

Cardiac

Anatomy of the Heart

Apex: Located at the fifth intercostal space at the midclavicular line; this represents the tip of the left ventricle.

Base: Located at the second intercostal space behind the sternum on the posterior aspect of the heart; it lies adjacent to the vertebral bodies of T6 through T9.

Endocardium: A thin layer of tissue that lines the inside surface of the heart and valves.

Epicardium: The outer layer of the cardiac wall that covers the surface to protect against trauma or infection.

Myocardium: The thick layer of muscle of the heart that provides the pumping force for the ventricles.

Pericardium: A double-walled connective tissue sac (fibrous layer and serous layer) that surrounds the heart and protects it from trauma or infection.

Right atrium: Receives venous blood from the superior and inferior vena cava.

Right ventricle: Receives venous blood from the right atrium through the tricuspid valve. Pushes blood into the pulmonary artery and pulmonary circulation.

Left atrium: Receives arterial blood from the pulmonary veins.

Left ventricle: Receives blood from the left atrium. Pushes blood into the aorta and the systemic circulation.

Tricuspid valve: Prevents right ventricular blood from going back into the right atrium.

Pulmonic valve: Prevents blood from returning to the right ventricle.

Mitral valve: Prevents left ventricular blood from returning to the left atrium.

Aortic valve: Prevents the systemic blood from returning to the left ventricle.

Atrioventricular valves: Blood from each atria flows to each ventricle through these valves. The valves close upon ventricular contraction to avoid backflow.

Semilunar valves: Blood from each ventricle flows out of the heart through these valves. The valves close upon the subsequent diastole to avoid backflow of the blood into the heart.

Aorta: Largest artery which carries the total cardiac output. Divisions include the carotids, subclavians, and descending aorta.

- **Ascending aorta:** provides blood to the head, neck, and arms
- **Descending aorta:** provides blood to the lower body and visceral tissues

Superior vena cava: The primary vein that drains venous blood from the head, neck, and upper body into the right atrium.

Inferior vena cava: The primary vein that drains venous blood from the lower body and viscera into the right atrium.

Pulmonary artery: The primary artery that carries blood to the lungs from the right ventricle.

Coronary Arteries

Left coronary artery supplies:
- Left atrium
- Left ventricle (majority)
- Right ventricle (a portion of)
- Interventricular septum (majority)
- AV bundle
- SA node (40-45% of population)

Left coronary artery bifurcates into:
- Left anterior descending artery
- Left circumflex artery

Right coronary artery supplies:
- Right atrium
- Right ventricle (majority)
- Left ventricle (small portion)
- Interventricular septum (small portion)
- AV node and bundle of His (80% population)
- SA node (55-60% population)

Right coronary artery gives branches to:
- Right marginal artery
- Atrioventricular nodal artery (70% population)

Right coronary artery turns into:
- Posterior interventricular artery

Cardiac Conduction System

Sinoatrial Node (SA): The sinoatrial node is located in the right atrium near the superior vena cava and is the primary pacemaker of the heart.

Atrioventricular Node (AV): The atrioventricular node or junctional node is located in the inferior wall of the right atrium close to the tricuspid valve.

Bundle of His: The Bundle of His is a group of fibers that initiates at the atrioventricular node, enters the interventricular system, and splits into the left and right ventricles. The fibers branch into small Purkinje fibers.

Purkinje Fibers: Purkinje fibers compose the last part of the electrical conduction system of the heart. The fibers relay the electrical impulses to the muscle cells of the heart.

Cardiac Reflexes

There are several quick-acting nervous system mechanisms that influence heart rate when triggered. The reflexes are divided into the baroreceptor reflex, Bainbridge reflex, and chemoreceptor reflex.

Baroreceptor Reflex
The baroreceptor reflex is produced by a group of mechanoreceptors that are found within the walls of the heart, intrathoracic vessels, the large arteries (especially the aorta), the carotid arteries, and carotid sinuses. This reflex is activated when pressure rises within the large arteries above 60 mm Hg. The mechanoreceptors that are sensitive to stretch and pressure peak in activity at approximately 180 mm Hg. Activation results in vasodilation secondary to inhibition of the vasomotor centers within the medulla as well as a decrease in heart rate and strength of contraction secondary to vagal stimulation.

Bainbridge Reflex
The Bainbridge reflex occurs when mechanoreceptors embedded within the right atrial myocardium respond to an increase in pressure and stretch (distention of the right atrium). This reflex stimulates the vasomotor centers of the medulla and results in increased sympathetic input and heart rate. This reflex can also influence a decrease in heart rate when the heart is beating too fast.

Chemoreceptor Reflex
The chemoreceptor reflex responds to the need for increased depth and rate of ventilation. Chemoreceptors are located on the carotid and aortic bodies and detect lack of oxygen, thus responding to an increase in arterial CO_2 levels.

Heart Sounds

S1	"lub" mitral and tricuspid valves closing at the onset of systole
S2	"dub" aortic and pulmonic valves closing at the onset of diastole
S3	(ventricular gallop) abnormal in older adults; noncompliant left ventricle; may be associated with congestive heart failure
S4	Pathological sound of vibration of the ventricular wall with ventricular filling and atrial contraction; may be associated with hypertension, stenosis, hypertensive heart disease or myocardial infarction

Cardiac Facts

Cardiac Output
Cardiac output is the amount of blood pumped out of the heart through the aorta each minute. Normal cardiac output for an adult male at rest is 5.6 L/min with women producing 10 to 20% less. A person can increase the cardiac output to upwards of 25 L/min during extensive exercise. Cardiac output = stroke volume (x) heart rate.

Venus Return
Venous return is the amount of blood that comes from the veins to the right atrium each minute. This is similar in volume to the cardiac output.

Stroke Volume
Stroke volume is the amount of blood ejected from the ventricles with each contraction. Many factors can influence stroke volume including "preload" which is influenced by end-diastolic volume, "afterload", and contractility.

Cardiac Index

The cardiac index is the amount of blood pumped out of the heart per minute per square meter of body mass. Normal cardiac index ranges between 2.5 to 40.0 liters/min/meter.

Blood Volume

Blood volume in an adult is usually 7-8% of their body weight. The blood is pumped through the body at 30 cm/sec with a total circulation time of 20 seconds.

Common Circulatory Pulse Locations

Artery	Location
Carotid	Anterior to sternocleidomastoid muscle
Brachial	Medial aspect of arm midway between shoulder and elbow
Radial	At wrist, lateral to flexor carpi radialis tendon
Ulnar	At wrist, between flexor digitorum superficialis and flexor carpi ulnaris tendons
Femoral	In femoral triangle (sartorius, adductor longus, and inguinal ligament)
Popliteal	Posterior aspect of knee (deep and hard to palpate)
Posterior tibial	Posterior aspect of medial malleolus
Dorsalis pedis	Between first and second metatarsal bones on superior aspect

From Magee, DJ: Orthopedic Physical Assessment. W.B. Saunders Company, Philadelphia 2002, p.52, with permission.

Diagnostic Tests for Cardiac Dysfunction

Procedure	Description
Cardiac catheterization (for angiography)	The coronary arteries are injected with a contrast material, and the arterial system can be visualized with cinefluoroscopy: narrowing or occlusion of arteries can be evaluated.
Cardiac catheterization	Catheterization is used to measure intracardiac, transvalve, and pulmonary artery pressures and measure blood gas pressures to determine cardiac output and evaluate shunting.
Continuous hemodynamic monitoring	Pulmonary artery catheterization (Swan-Ganz) provides immediate cardiopulmonary pressure measurements. An invasive bedside (intensive care unit) procedure that evaluates left ventricular function. A balloon-tipped, flow-directed catheter, connected to a transducer and a monitor, is used to allow measurements of pulmonary artery pressure; pulmonary capillary wedge pressure; cardiac output; and mixed venous saturation, which evaluates pulmonary vascular resistance and tissue oxygenation.
Echocardiography a. Transthoracic (TTE)	The reflections of ultrasound waves from cardiac surfaces are analyzed. It is used to evaluate left ventricular systolic function and the structure and function of cardiac walls, valves, and chambers; it can identify abnormal conditions such as tumors or pericardial effusion.
b. Transesophageal (TEE)	Transesophageal echocardiography is performed through the esophagus and stomach by a modified gastroscopy probe with one or two ultrasound transducers at its tip. TEE provides better image resolution and superior images of posterior cardiac structures. Continuous imaging is possible during operations or invasive procedures.
Electrocardiogram (ECG)	Surface electrodes record the electrical activity of the heart. A 12-lead ECG provides 12 views of the heart; it is used to assess cardiac rhythm, to diagnose the location, extent, and acuteness of myocardial ischemia and infarction; and to evaluate changes with activity.
Hemodynamic monitoring	See *Continuous hemodynamic monitoring*

Diagnostic Tests for Cardiac Dysfunction (continued)

Exercise stress tests	Numerous protocols for exercise tests have been used to assess responses to increased workloads with steps, treadmills, or bicycle ergometers. In conjunction with ECG and blood pressure recordings, patients are evaluated for exercise capacity, cardiac dysrhythmias, and diagnosis, prognosis, and management of coronary artery disease.
Holter monitoring	Continuous ambulatory ECG monitoring done by tape recording the cardiac rhythm for up to 24 hours. It is used to evaluate cardiac rhythm, efficacy of medications, transient symptoms that may indicate cardiac disease, and pacemaker function; and to correlate symptoms with activity.
Pharmacologic stress tests	A non-invasive assessment for patients with coronary disease who are unable to achieve adequate cardiac stress with exercise.
a. Dipyridamole thallium	This potent vasodilator markedly enhances blood flow to normally perfused myocardium, whereas myocardium fed by stenotic coronary arteries demonstrates relative hypoperfusion and diminished thallium activity.
b. Dobutamine echocardiography	An incremental infusion is given causing an increase in the myocardial oxygen demand. Simultaneous evaluation of wall motion abnormalities, ECG, and BP are performed.
Phonocardiography	This test records cardiac sounds. It is used to time the events of the cardiac cycle and to confirm auscultatory findings.

Radionuclide angiography	Red blood cells tagged (marked) with a radionuclide are injected into blood. Ventricular wall motion can be evaluated and the ejection fraction determined; abnormal blood flow with valve and congenital defects can be detected. Techniques include gated-pool equilibrium studies and first-pass techniques.
Technetium-99m scanning (hot spot imaging)	Technetium-99m injected into blood is taken up by damaged myocardial tissue; this identifies and localizes acute myocardial infarctions.
Thallium-201 myocardial perfusion imaging (cold spot imaging)	Thallium-201 injected into blood at peak exercise; scanning identifies ischemic and infarcted myocardium, which does not take up thallium-201. It is used to diagnose coronary artery disease and perfusion, particularly when ECG is equivocal.

From Rothstein J, Roy S, Wolf S: The Rehabilitation Specialist's Handbook. F. A. Davis Company Inc, Philadelphia 1998, p.624-626, with permission.

Electrocardiogram

ECG: Measures the electrical activity of the heart

12-lead Electrocardiogram
- Six limb leads (I, II, III, aVR, aVL, aVF)
- Six precordial leads (V1, V2, V3, V4, V5, V6)
- Provides 12 different views of the heart
- Leads I, II, III are bipolar limb leads that form a triangle connecting the right arm, left arm, and left foot; the heart should be at the center of the triangle
- Leads aVR, aVL, aVF are unipolar augmented leads

Precordial Lead Placement
V1 – right of sternum, 4th intercostal space
V2 – left of sternum, 4th intercostal space
V3 – half way between V2 and V4
V4 – midclavicular line in the 5th intercostal space
V5 – halfway between V4 and V6
V6 – Midaxillary line in the 5th intercostal space

P wave: Atrial depolarization

PR interval: Time required for conduction from the SA node to AV node. The time between atrial and ventricular depolarization. This is normally .12 to .2 seconds.

QRS complex: Ventricular depolarization and atrial repolarization.

QT interval: Electrical systole that is measured by the time elapsed from the start of the Q wave to the end of the T wave. This is normally .32 to .40 seconds.

ST segment: Delay before repolarization of the ventricles; useful in assessing myocardial ischemia

T wave: Ventricular repolarization

Pathological Changes in an ECG

Depressed QRS: Heart failure, ischemia, pericardial effusion, obesity, chronic obstructive pulmonary disease

Ectopic foci: a location where abnormal myocardial depolarization originates. This can occur if the rhythmicity of the ectopic pacemaker increases; the rhythmicity of normal pacemakers is inhibited, or if the conduction path from the normal pacemakers to the ectopic foci is blocked. These beats should be monitored.

Elevated QRS: Hypertrophy of the myocardium

Q Wave: Previous myocardial infarction

ST Segment Elevation: Acute myocardial infarction

Atrial fibrillation (A. fib)
- Irregular atrial rhythm
- No rate
- No P waves
- "F" waves absent
- Quivers noted
- Ventricular rhythm varies

Common causes include: hypertension, congestive heart failure, coronary artery disease, rheumatic heart disease, cor pulmonale, pericarditis, and illegal drug use.

Supraventricular tachycardia
- Rate varies between 160 to 250 bpm
- Regular rhythm
- Originates from a location above the AV node
- Will start and stop without cause

Common causes include: mitral valve prolapse, cor pulmonale, digitalis toxicity, and rheumatic heart disease.

Premature atrial contractions (PAC)
- Occur when an ectopic focus in the atrium fires and supersedes the SA node
- The P wave is premature with abnormal configuration
- Rate normal between 60-100 bpm
- Irregular rhythm that can be regularly irregular such as consistently skipping every third beat
- Can be indicative of ischemia or valve pathology

Common causes include: intake of caffeine, emotional stress, smoking and pathologies such as coronary artery disease, electrolyte imbalance, infection, and congestive heart failure.

Ventricular tachycardia (VT)
- Rate usually > 100 bpm
- Rhythm usually regular
- No P wave or it appears after QRS complex with retrograde conduction
- Needs immediate medical attention

Common causes include: post myocardial infarction, rheumatic heart disease, coronary artery disease, and cardiomyopathy.

Ventricular fibrillation
- No regular rate or rhythm
- Emergency
- Need immediate medical intervention

Common causes include: long-term or severe heart disease, post myocardial infarction, hypercalcemia, hypokalemia, and hyperkalemia.

Multifocal ventricular tachycardia
- Rate > 150 bpm
- Irregular rhythm
- No P waves
- QRS complex is wide
- Needs immediate medical intervention

Common causes include: hypokalemia, hypomagnesemia, hypothermia, and drug-induced through antiarrhythmic medications.

Premature ventricular contractions (PVC)
- Occur when an ectopic focus in the ventricles or Purkinje fibers fires and supersedes normal conduction
- Focal PVCs occur from one ectopic foci and have the same waveform
- Multifocal PVCs have multiple ectopic foci that result in different waveforms
- Rate is normal between 60-100 bpm
- The P wave is absent, the ST segment is distorted, and the QRS complex occurs early

Premature ventricular contractions (cont.)

- Irregular rhythm that can be regularly irregular such as consistently skipping every third beat
- A couplet is known as two skips in a row; bigeminy is a skip every other beat; trigeminy is a skip every third beat

Common causes include: intake of caffeine, emotional stress, smoking, pathologies such as coronary artery disease, digitalis toxicity, cardiomyopathy, and myocardial infarction.

Complete heart block (third-degree AV block)

- Regular rhythm
- Atrial rate > ventricular rate
- Needs immediate medical intervention (pacemaker)

Common causes include: infection, electrolyte imbalance, coronary artery disease, anteroseptal myocardial infarction, and impairment with the AV conduction system.

Asystole:

- No rhythm
- Absence of P wave, QRS, and T waves
- Can have abrupt onset
- Needs immediate medical attention

Common causes include: failure of all pacemakers to initiate, conduction system failure, acute myocardial infarction and ventricular rupture.

Comparisons of Right and Left-Sided Heart Failure

Right	Left
Elevated end-diastolic right ventricular pressure	Elevated end-diastolic left ventricular pressure

Systemic congestion:
  -Enlarged liver
  -Ascites
  -Jugular venous distention
  -Dependent (pitting) edema
	Pulmonary congestion:
	  -Pulmonary edema
	  -Dyspnea, orthopnea
	  -Paroxysmal nocturnal dyspnea
	  -Cough
	  -Bronchospasm
	  -(Cardiac asthma)

Fatigue	Fatigue
Oliguria, nocturia	Oliguria
Cyanosis (capillary stasis)	Cyanosis (central)
Pleural effusion (R>L)	Tachycardia
Anorexia and bleeding	
Unexplained weight gain	

Right	Left

Etiology:
  -Mitral stenosis
  -Pulmonary parenchymal or vascular disease
  -Pulmonic or tricuspid valvular disease
  -Infective endocarditis
	Etiology:
	  -Hypertension
	  -Coronary artery disease
	  -Aortic valve disease
	  -Cardiomyopathies
	  -Congenital heart defects
	  -Infective endocarditis
	  -High-output conditions
	  -Various connective tissue disorders

From Rothstein J, Roy S, Wolf S: The Rehabilitation Specialist's Handbook. F. A. Davis Company, Philadelphia 1998, p.654-655, with permission.

Vital Signs

Blood Pressure

Normal blood pressure values are accepted as:
Infants: 70-90 / 45-65 mm Hg
Child: 85-114 / 52-85 mm Hg
Adult: 100-140 / 60-90 mm Hg

Systole: A period of contraction of the cardiac muscle.

Diastole: A period of relaxation of the cardiac muscle.

Atrial systole: A period that is initially comprised of atrial emptying of blood into the ventricles through the pressure gradient between the chambers as well as contraction of the cardiac muscle.

Atrial diastole: A period of atrial filling secondary to pressure from the venous circulation.

Ventricular systole: A period of a ventricular contraction that causes a rapid ejection of blood.

Ventricular diastole: A period of ventricular filling secondary to the pressure gradient from the atria in combination with atrial contraction.

Blood Pressure Classification

Hypertension

Hypertension is defined as a condition where there is an elevated arterial blood pressure both for systole and diastole. Factors that can influence the onset of hypertension include age, level of physical fitness, genetic predisposition, smoking, sedentary life, obesity, and diabetes mellitus.

Hypertension exists if:

Infant > 90/60 mm Hg
Children >120/80 mm Hg
Adults – borderline > 140-159 / 90-99 mm Hg
Adults – moderate > 160-179 / 100-109 mm Hg
Adults – severe > 180/110 mm Hg

Hypotension exists if:

Systolic pressure < 100 mm Hg
- This condition is not dangerous, however, a patient may experience periods of dizziness especially when changing position.

Korotkoff's Sounds

Phase I: the first clear sound detected that indicates systolic pressure

Phase II: the sounds now have a muffle or swishing sound

Phase III: the sounds are louder and clear compared to the initial sounds

Phase IV: the sounds abruptly become muffled, as if a whisper; this is the indication of diastolic pressure

Phase V: the sounds disappear, there is nothing heard through auscultation

Preparation and Procedure

- ✓ Requires sphygmomanometer and stethoscope
- ✓ Ensure proper size cuff for children, adults, and obese patients
- ✓ Width of bladder should equal 40% of the circumference of the midpoint of the extremity (adult: 3-6 inches wide)
- ✓ Values are usually slightly higher when measured in the left upper extremity versus the right upper extremity; be consistent on which side the blood pressure is taken on
- ✓ Expose the antecubital space and palpate the pulse
- ✓ Place arrow on cuff over brachial artery
- ✓ Wrap the cuff above the antecubital space with a snug fit (false readings with occur if too loose)
- ✓ Palpate the brachial pulse, inflate the cuff and note the reading when the pulse disappears
- ✓ Release the cuff and wait 30-60 seconds
- ✓ Inflate the cuff to 20 mm Hg above this reading (where the brachial pulse disappears)
- ✓ Slowly deflate the cuff observing the needle gauge
- ✓ The first Korotkoff's sound indicates the systolic pressure, the last audible sound indicates the diastolic pressure
- ✓ The thigh is an alternate site to obtain a blood pressure reading

Ankle-Brachial Index (ABI)

The ankle-brachial index is a test that measures arterial perfusion using a Doppler unit. Blood pressures are measured in both upper extremities (using the brachial arteries) and lower extremities (using the dorsalis pedis or tibialis posterior artery). The patient is tested in the supine position for all measurements. The highest lower extremity systolic pressure is divided by the brachial systolic pressure. The ratio for normal blood flow is 1.0. A ratio of .9 at rest or .85 after exercise indicates peripheral artery disease.

1.0	Normal
.5 – .9	Arterial occlusion Impairment with wound healing Therapeutic exercise beneficial
< .5	Severe arterial occlusion Exercise is unrealistic Poor to no wound healing

Heart Rate/Pulse

Heart rate indirectly measures the rate of contraction of the left ventricle through a peripheral pulse site.

Normal heart rate values are accepted as:

Infants: 100 to 130 bpm
Child: 80 to 100 bpm
Adult: 60 to 100 bpm

Pulse sites for measurement include: brachial, carotid, dorsal pedal, femoral, popliteal, posterior tibial, radial, and temporal pulses. The carotid and radial pulse sites are the most common sites for measuring a patient's pulse rate.

Bradycardia: a condition of a heart rate consistently below 60 bpm

Tachycardia: a condition of a heart rate consistently above 100 bpm

Strong/regular: adequate force and consistent beats

Weak: poor force with contraction

Irregular: inconsistency during heart rate measurement with regard to strength and beat of the heart

Preparation and Procedure

- ✓ A regular and strong heart beat may be taken for 15 seconds and multiply by four to total the per minute heart rate
- ✓ If there is any form of irregularity the pulse should be taken for a full 60 seconds
- ✓ Find the appropriate pulse site and use a timepiece with a seconds hand (stop watch)

✓ Use the index and middle fingers to measure the heart rate, never the thumb
✓ Assess and document the rhythm as regular or irregular
✓ Assess and document the strength or amplitude of the pulse as strong, medium or weak
✓ An alternate method to obtain heart rate is to auscultate over the apical pulse for one minute

Peripheral Pulse Assessment Grading Systems

0-3 scale
0   absent
1+ weak/thready pulse
2+ normal
3+ full, firm pulse

Pulse Amplitude Classification
0   absent
1+ diminished
2+ normal
3+ moderately increased
4+ markedly increased

Respiratory Rate

Inspiration: to breathe air into the lungs

Expiration: to breathe air out of the lungs

Normal respiration rates are:
Infants: 30 to 50 respirations per minute
Adults: 12 to 18 respirations per minute

Values above 20 respirations or lower than 10 respirations per minute for an adult are considered abnormal

Preparation and Procedures
✓ Observe the patient at rest breathing for 60 seconds
✓ Use a timepiece with a seconds hand (stop watch)
✓ Assess and document the patient's respiration rate, rhythm of respiration, depth of respiration, and any deviation away from quiet respiration
✓ Assess and document if there is any accessory muscle use
✓ An alternate method to measure respiration rate is to place your hand gently over the patient's upper thorax and observe and feel movement with each respiration

Borg's Rate of Perceived Exertion Scale and the Revised 10-Grade Scale

RPE:		10-Grade Rating Scale:	
6		0	Nothing at all
7	Very, very light	0.5	Very, very weak (just noticeable)
8		1.0	Very weak
9	Very light	2.0	Weak (light)
10		3.0	Moderate
11	Fairly light	4.0	Somewhat strong
12		5.0	Strong (heavy)
13	Somewhat hard	6.0	
14		7.0	Very strong
15	Hard	8.0	
16		9.0	
17	Very hard	10.0	Very, very strong (almost maximum)
18			Maximal
19	Very, very hard		

From Borg GAV: Psychophysical Bases of Perceived Exertion. Med Sci Sports Exerc 14:377, 1982, American College of Sports Medicine, with permission.

Metabolic Equivalents (METS)

A MET is the amount of oxygen consumed per kilogram of body weight per minute to perform a given activity. At rest a person consumes 3.5 ml/kg/minute. The following list identifies METS associated with common activities of daily living.

Eating	1
Toileting	1 – 2
Driving a car	1 – 2
Dressing	2
Walking (2 mph)	2 – 2.5
Bathing	2 – 3
Cooking	2 – 3
Light housework	2 – 4
Light gardening	3 – 4
Showering	3.5 – 4
Sexual intercourse	4 – 5
Dancing	4 – 5
Walking (4 mph)	4.5 – 5.5
Swimming	4 – 8
Shoveling snow	6 – 7
Mowing the lawn	6 – 7

Cardiac Pathology

Risk Factors for Cardiac Pathology

Modifiable Factors

- Cholesterol – more than 200 mg/dL
- Hypertension
- Smoking
- Atherogenic diet
- Culture
- Physical inactivity
- Stress

Non-Modifiable Factors

- Age – risk increases with age
- Sex – male > female (after menopause female equal to male)
- Family history
- Culture

Secondary Factors

- Alcohol consumption
- Obesity
- Coping with stress
- Diabetes mellitus
- Peripheral vascular disease

Symptoms of Cardiac Pathology

- Chest pain
- Shortness of breath
- Cardiac arrhythmia (palpitation)
- Fainting
- Claudication
- Cyanosis of lips and nailbeds
- Fatigue
- Edema

Symptoms of Myocardial Infarction

- Severe chest pain
- Chest heaviness
- Radiating pain down one or both arms
- Weakness
- Nausea
- Vomiting
- Diaphoresis
- Shortness of breath

Diagnosis of Myocardial Infarction

- Abnormal ECG
- Elevation in enzyme level
  -- Creatine phosphokinase (CPK)
  -- Aspartate aminotransferase (AST)
  -- Lactate dehydrogenase

Methods to Determine Exercise Intensity

Target Heart Rate Formula

Target heart rate formula is a method for obtaining an appropriate demand on the heart during exercise. The age-adjusted maximum heart rate is determined by subtracting the patient's age from 220. The training heart rate is determined by multiplying the age-adjusted maximum heart rate by the appropriate percentage of intensity that the patient should maintain during exercise. Normal training intensity ranges from 60-90% of the age-adjusted maximum heart rate. A patient with cardiac pathology must have exercise intensity determined from the results of a stress test.

Karvonen's Formula – Heart Rate Reserve Method

The Karvonen formula is a method to obtain an appropriate range for training heart rate. The maximum heart rate is obtained by an exercise stress test (or the age-adjusted maximum heart rate) and the resting heart rate is subtracted from it. This number is termed the heart rate reserve. The heart rate reserve is multiplied by both ends of the prescribed range (e.g., HR reserve x 60% and HR reserve x 80%). The resting heart rate is then added to each of the two numbers to identify the upper and lower limits of the prescribed target heart rate.

Cardiac Rehabilitation

Indications for Cardiac Rehabilitation

• Myocardial infarction	• End-stage renal disease
• Angina (stable)	• Status post pacemaker insertion
• Coronary artery bypass surgery	• Cardiomyopathy
• Compensated heart failure	• Peripheral vascular disease
• Cardiac surgery	• Heart transplant
• High risk for coronary artery disease	• High risk for diabetes
• High risk for high blood pressure	

Relative Contraindications to Stop Exercising during Cardiac Rehabilitation

- Abnormal heart rate that increases > 50 bpm with low-level activity
- Blood pressure that increases > 210 mm Hg systolic during exercise
- Blood pressure that increases > 110 mm Hg diastolic during exercise
- Decrease in systolic pressure > 10 mm Hg during low-level exercise
- Any ST segment changes
- Severe lower extremity claudication
- Angina
- Confusion
- Extreme fatigue
- Ventricular gallop

Contraindications for Cardiac Rehabilitation

- Uncontrolled atrial/ventricular arrhythmias
- Recent diagnosis of embolism
- Resting diastolic pressure > 110 mm Hg
- Thrombophlebitis
- Orthostatic blood pressure (> 20 mm Hg drop)
- Acute infection
- Resting ST segment displacement of > 2 mm
- Unstable angina
- Resting systolic pressure > 200 mm Hg
- Uncompensated congestive heart failure

Absolute Contraindications for Treatment of an Unstable Cardiac Patient

- Third-degree heart block
- Uncompensated congestive heart failure
- PVCs of ventricular tachycardia at rest
- Multifocal PVCs
- Chest pain with ST segment changes
- ECG changes that indicate ischemia
- Dissecting aortic aneurysm

Absolute Contraindications to Exercise Testing

- ECG changes that denote cardiac ischemia
- Recent myocardial infarction < 48 hrs
- Multifocal PVCs
- Uncontrolled heart failure
- Unstable angina
- Uncontrolled cardiac arrhythmias
- Untreated heart block (2nd or 3rd degree)
- Pulmonary embolism
- Acute infection

Benefits of Routine Exercise

- Decrease myocardial oxygen cost
- Decrease heart rate and blood pressure
- Increase maximal oxygen uptake
- Decrease minute ventilation
- Decrease in depression and/or anxiety
- Decrease serum triglycerides
- Decrease risk of heart disease
- Decrease percent body fat
- Improve glucose tolerance
- Increase HDL cholesterol

Description of a Cardiac Rehabilitation Program

Phase I

A Phase I program begins with the physician referral to the cardiac rehabilitation program. Patients are referred to the inpatient program when they are medically stable. Phase I consists of patient and family education, self-care evaluation, continuous monitoring of vital signs, group discussions, and low-level exercise. Exercise activities include active range of motion, ambulation, and self-care. Exercise intensity is often prescribed according to heart rate and by rating on a perceived exertion scale. A Phase I program typically concludes with a low-level exercise test, although this activity may not be appropriate for high-risk clients. The trend toward early hospital discharge following a cardiac event has resulted in Phase I programs averaging 3-5 days.

Phase II

A Phase II program begins immediately after hospitalization and lasts from 2-12 weeks depending on the patient's ability to tolerate the exercise training. Patients are monitored closely during the Phase II program and are supervised during all activities. Goals for a Phase II program include increasing functional capacity through exercise, educating the patient on risk factor modification, and developing independence in self-monitoring. Frequency of visits in a Phase II program averages 2-3 times a week. Patients typically progress to a Phase III program when they are clinically stable, independent with self-monitoring techniques, and do not require ECG monitoring.

Phase III

A Phase III program is often viewed as a continuation of a Phase II program and lasts approximately 6-8 weeks. Exercise training, physical fitness, level of endurance, and risk factor modification are the primary emphasis of the program. Phase III programs often include exercise, education, and counseling. A maximal symptom-limited exercise test is required to assess fitness level and appropriately plan for exercise intensity. The average frequency of the program is once per week.

Phase IV

A Phase IV program lasts throughout the patient's lifetime and is designed to promote optimal health. Requirements for participation in a Phase IV program include independence with self-monitoring of exercise, stable cardiac status, no contraindications to exercise, and at least a 5 MET capacity for activities.

Therapist Role During Inpatient Cardiac Rehabilitation

✓ Provide constant monitoring of heart rate, blood pressure, and ECG interpretation before, during, and after each session
✓ Develop program within the guidelines of the patient's prescribed training heart rate
✓ Use of exertion scales to identify subjective intensity of exercise
✓ Promote proper technique and breathing patterns during exercise
✓ Progress activities based on METs tolerated

Therapist Role During Outpatient Cardiac Rehabilitation

✓ Initially close monitoring of ECG, heart rate, and blood pressure throughout session is required
✓ Constant measurement of vital signs should decrease and self-monitoring of heart rate and perceived exertion by the patient should guide exercise sessions
✓ Development of an exercise program should be based on a symptom-limited treadmill test and determined target heart rate
✓ Exercise should be gradual in progression; the session should generally include warm-up for 5-10 minutes, aerobic activity for 20-60 minutes, and a cool down for 5-10 minutes
✓ Warm-up should include stretching as well as low-intensity activity which will slowly increase heart rate
✓ Exercise may include walking, stationary bicycling, as well as isotonic strengthening (low resistance)
✓ Isometrics are contraindicated

Cardiopulmonary Resuscitation Standards

ABC's

Airway – maintain an open airway
Breathing (rescue breathing) – "Look, listen, and feel"
Circulation (compressions) – check pulse

CPR – Adult (eight years +)

Breathing	Two initial breaths followed by 12/minute
Compressions	100/minute
Depth of compressions	1 ½ to 2 inches
Placement for chest compressions	Lower half of sternum
One-rescuer ratio of compressions:ventilations	15:2
Two-rescuer ratio of compressions:ventilations	15:2

CPR – Child (one to eight years old)

Breathing	Two initial breaths followed by 20/minute
Compressions	100/minute
Depth of compressions	1/3-1/2 the depth of chest
Placement for chest compressions	Lower half of sternum
One-rescuer ratio of compressions:ventilations	5:1
Two-rescuer ratio of compressions:ventilations	5:1

CPR – Infant (less than one year old)

Breathing	Two initial breaths mouth to mouth and nose followed by 20/minute
Compressions	Minimum of 100/minute
Depth of compressions	1/3-1/2 the depth of chest
Placement for chest compressions	Lower half of sternum
One-rescuer ratio of compressions:ventilations	5:1
Two-rescuer ratio of compressions:ventilations	5:1

From American Red Cross: BLS Health Care Providers. American Red Cross, 2002

Continue to perform CPR until:
- Breathing, coughing or other signs of circulation return
- The emergency medical personnel arrive
- You are too exhausted to continue

Automatic External Defibrillator (AED)

An automatic external defibrillator is a portable defibrillation unit that can be used by emergency personnel in the case of cardiac arrest. The units are able to assess whether defibrillation shock is warranted. Research indicates that defibrillation within the first few minutes after cardiac arrest may increase survival 50% from sudden death.

Cardiac Profile

Outcome Measurement Tools

Outcome is the term used to qualitatively describe the end result of a particular intervention including changes (good or bad) that occurred to the health of a person, group or community. Factors that influence outcome include: primary diagnosis, co-morbidities, medical stability, prior physical status, current physical status, age and gender, beliefs, and attitudes.

Measuring outcome data is imperative to continually improve intervention strategies. Outcome data is also a powerful tool for positive feedback for the clinical staff and patient. The measuring tool must be both valid and reliable and the staff administering the tool must be familiar and qualified to do so in order to obtain meaningful and reliable results.

There are several tools utilized to evaluate cardiac or pulmonary dysfunction:

- Borg's Rate of Perceived Exertion Scale
- Six-Minute Walk test
- Minnesota Living with Heart Failure Questionnaire
- Outcomes Institute Angina Type Specification
- Quality of Life after Myocardial Infarction
- Seattle Angina Questionnaire
- Functional Status Questionnaire
- Duke Activity Scale Index
- Living with Asthma Questionnaire
- Pulmonary Functional Status Scale
- Cardiac Depression Scale

✓ **Primary outcomes** include functional and health status.
✓ **Secondary outcomes** include behavioral and clinical changes that impact the patient's life.
✓ Outcomes measure accountability, influence decision-making, and are used for ongoing research purposes.
✓ Measurement tools should be valid and reliable, and provide reproducible information about the specific characteristics that are measured.
✓ Outcome measurement data can influence reimbursement, amount of referrals, daily inpatient census, and staff compliance.

Examination

- Past medical history
- History of current condition
- --Cardiac testing
- Social history (caregiver support)
- Medications
- Living environment
- Risk factors profile
- Systems review
  --Vital signs
  --Auscultation of heart and lung sounds
- Skin assessment
  --Cyanosis
  --Edema
  --Pallor
  --Diaphoresis
- Cognitive assessment
- Pain
- Strength as tolerated
- Endurance
- Mobility skills as tolerated

Intervention

- Patient/caregiver teaching:
  --Risk factor modification
  --Signs and symptoms of pathology
  --Measurement of vital signs
  --Nutrition
- Breathing exercises
- Endurance/exercise training
- Mobility training
- Relaxation techniques

Inpatient Goals

- Maximize self-care skills
- Maximize functional mobility skills
- Maximize endurance
- Maximize patient/caregiver competence with:
  --Safe activity guidelines
  --Modification of risk factors
  --Monitoring of vital signs
  --Breathing exercises
  --Stress management
- Perform low-level exercise test (4-6 METS)
- Maximize energy conservation techniques

Outpatient Goals

- Maximize functional mobility skills
- Maximize endurance
- Maximize aerobic capacity
- Maximize patient/caregiver competence with:
  --Nutritional education
  --Monitoring of vital signs
  --Energy conservation techniques
  --Warning signs of cardiac pathology
  --Home exercise program

Cardiac Pathology

Aneurysm

An aneurysm is a weakening in the wall of a vessel that produces a sac-like area. By definition there is a 50% increase in the normal vessel diameter with weakening of all layers of the arterial (or venous) wall. Etiology can include genetic disposition, trauma or infection. The most common sites include aorta, abdominal aorta, femoral, and popliteal arteries. Surgical repair prior to rupture has a good prognosis; a ruptured aneurysm is a medical emergency with high mortality rates.

Symptoms
-Dependent on site of aneurysm
-Intermittent or constant pain
-Abnormal heart beat
-Serious complications can occur including MI, stroke, renal failure, and embolization

Angina Pectoris

A transient process that occurs when the coronary arteries are unable to supply the heart with adequate oxygen. Sudden onset is common once the myocardial oxygen demand is higher than the supply. Coronary artery disease accounts for 90% of all angina. The four most common types of angina pectoris are as follows:

- **Nocturnal:** Angina that will wake someone up from his or her sleep with the same characteristics as angina from exertion. This may be related to congestive heart failure.
- **Prinzmetal's:** Angina that occurs while at rest secondary to coronary artery disease or spasm. This can be severe and not readily relieved by nitroglycerin.
- **Stable:** Angina that usually occurs at a predictable level of exertion, exercise or stress and responds to rest or nitroglycerin.
- **Unstable:** Angina that can occur at rest or with exertion and has changed intensity, frequency, and/or duration.

Symptoms
-Temporary pain
-Sudden onset
-Pain may radiate
-Usually lasts one to five minutes
-Usually relieved with rest or nitroglycerin

Atherosclerosis

Atherosclerosis is a condition of progressive accumulation of fatty plaques on the inner walls of vessels that ultimately produces stenosis. This process begins in childhood and usually effects medium-sized arteries. Over time the plaque that produces stenosis inside the vessel can also block blood flow. Heart attack or stroke can result from atherosclerosis.

Cardiomyopathy

Cardiomyopathy refers to a group of conditions that affect the myocardium muscle itself, impairing the ability for the heart to contract and relax. Three types of cardiomyopathy are dilated, hypertrophic, and restrictive.

Symptoms
-Dependent on the type of cardiomyopathy
-Symptoms are the same as heart failure
-Neck vein distension
-Fatigue, weakness
-Possible chest pain
-Sudden death (hypertrophic)
-Exercise intolerance

Congestive Heart Failure (CHF)

Congestive heart failure is a condition that usually results from coronary artery disease when the heart is unable to maintain an adequate cardiac output. CHF is characterized by abnormal retention of fluid and results in diminished blood flow to the tissue and congestion of the pulmonary and/or systemic circulation. This is not a disease, but rather a symptom of pathology within the heart muscle itself or the cardiac valves.

Symptoms
-Dependent on type of CHF
-Pulmonary edema
-Dyspnea when lying down (orthopnea)
-Cough (non-productive)
- S3 gallop
-Exertional hypotension
-Weight gain within hours
-Increased resting heart rate
-See chart on page 104 for symptoms

Coronary Artery Disease (CAD)

Coronary artery disease is the narrowing or blockage of the coronary arteries that may produce ischemia and necrosis of the myocardium. There is an inability for vasodilation and as a result the arteries cannot meet the metabolic demands. This will produce ischemia and ultimately necrosis. CAD includes thrombus, vasospasms, and atherosclerosis. CAD results from inheritance, environment, culture, nutrition, and smoking.

Symptoms
-Appear after significant blockage is present > 75%
-Pain in the occluded artery's region
-If untreated, MI or sudden death

Heart Failure

Heart failure is a condition where there is an inability of the heart to maintain a proper cardiac output of four liters per minute while a patient is at rest. The most common etiology associated with heart failure is chronic hypertension.

Infective Endocarditis

Endocarditis causes inflammation of the endothelium that lines the heart and cardiac valves. This condition most commonly damages the mitral valve, then the aortic and tricuspid valves. Endocarditis is commonly caused by bacteria that are normally present in the body. It can also occur after an invasive medical or dental procedure. At-risk individuals can easily prevent endocarditis with antibiotic prophylaxis, however, once infected it is not easily diagnosed or treated.

Symptoms
-May have sudden onset or be asymptomatic for months
-Valvular dysfunction
-May affect organ systems
-Chest pain, CHF, clubbing
-Arthralgia, arthritis, acidosis
-Myalgia, low back pain
-Meningitis, stroke, confusion

Myocardial Infarction (MI)

A myocardial infarction causes irreversible damage to a segment of heart muscle due to prolonged ischemia. The causative factors include narrowing of coronary arteries due to atherosclerotic occlusion, poor coronary perfusion secondary to hemorrhage or occlusion of one of the major coronary arteries.

Symptoms
-Sudden constant pain and/or pressure
-May radiate up neck, down arm
-Shortness of breath
-Profuse perspiration
-Unexplained fatigue

Area of Infarct	Expected Damage
Anterior heart	-Left anterior descending artery -High risk of large infarction -Heart failure -Sudden death
Inferior heart	-Right coronary artery -Right ventricle damage -AV block -Medium infarct possible
Lateral heart and/or Superior heart	-Least area of muscle affected -Usually the least overall damage -Minor impairment or complications

Myocarditis

Myocarditis refers to an uncommon condition of inflammation to the myocardium muscle itself, usually due to infection. This condition can be treated with antimicrobial therapy, however, left untreated can quickly progress to a dilated cardiomyopathy with heart failure.

Symptoms
-Mild, low-level chest pain
-Soreness in the epigastric region
-Fatigue
-Palpitations

Pericarditis

Pericarditis refers to an inflammation of the pericardium (the outer membrane) of the heart. This condition may be acute or chronic (constrictive pericarditis) and can be painful or asymptomatic. Etiology is often unknown; however, causes such as infection, myocardial infarction, radiation therapy, post cardiac surgery, metabolic disorders, and aortic dissection have been linked to this diagnosis. Prognosis is usually good, however, if left untreated a patient can experience shock or death.

Symptoms
-Symptoms are varied and based on the underlying
  etiology
-Auscultation reveals pericardial friction rub
-Pleuretic chest pain
-Diffuse ST segment elevation
-Retrosternal chest pain
-Cough and hoarseness
-Fever, fatigue, and weakness
-Joint pain

Rheumatic Heart Disease

Rheumatic heart disease is the result of damage to the heart secondary to inflammation from rheumatic fever. Rheumatic fever can occur from streptococcal group A bacteria (i.e., strep throat) and is classified as an autoimmune disease. It can affect all connective tissues of the heart, joints, and central nervous system and frequently damages the cardiac valves. Acute rheumatic fever has a low mortality rate; however, recurrent or chronic rheumatic disease has significant influence on long-term outcome and level of disability.

Symptoms
-Carditis with chest pain
-Acute onset of polyarthritis
-Chorea
-Arthralgias and weakness
-Fever
-Palpitations

Cardiac Medications

There are multiple medications that are administered for various cardiac conditions. General classifications of drugs with example medications are listed. The list is designed to serve as a general overview of major cardiac medications.

Pharmacological Intervention for Cardiac Management

Diuretic Agents	
-Increase sodium and water excretion to manage hypertension, congestive heart failure Types: Thiazide, Loop, Potassium sparing	Furosemide (Lasix) Hydrochlorothiazide (Esidrix, microzide, hydrodiuril) Chlorthalidone (Thalitone, Hygroton) Spirondactone (Aldactone) Amiloride (Midamor)

Beta-adrenergic Blocking Agents (Beta-blockers)	
-Decrease the heart's oxygen demand through decreasing heart rate and contractility. Treat angina, arrhythmias, and hypertension	Bisoprolol (Zebeta) Atenolol (Tenormin) Metoprolol (Lopressor) Propanlol (Inderal)
Alpha-adrenergic Blocking Agents -Block post-synaptic alpha 1-adrenergic receptors which dilates arterioles and veins; decreases blood pressure	Prazosin (Minipress) Terazosin (Hytrin) Doxazosin (Cardura)
Angiotensin-converting Enzyme Inhibitor (ACE) Agents -Decrease blood pressure, and afterload in patients with congestive heart failure and hypertension	Captorpril (Capoten) Enalapril (Vasotec) Lisinopril (Prinivil) Fosinopril (Monopril) Benazepril (Lotensin) Ramipril (Altace)
Angiotensin II Receptor Antagonist Agents -Used when patients cannot tolerate ACE inhibitors	Losartan (Cozaar) Diltiazem (Cardizem) Verapamil (Calan)
Nitrates -Decrease ischemia through smooth muscle relaxation of preload and afterload	Nitroglycerin (Nitrostat) Isosorbide dinitrate (Isordil) Erythrityl tetranitrate (Tetranitrol)
Antiarrhythmic Agents -Alter conductivity in order to correct ectopic stimuli or other electrical abnormality	Lidocaine (Xylocaine) Amiodarone (Cordarone) Bretylium tosylate Procainamide (Procanbid)
Calcium Channel Blocker Agents -Decreases the heart's oxygen demand by reducing the flow of calcium. Allows for peripheral vasodilation that further reduces demand on the heart	Amlodipine (Norvasc) Nifedipine (Procardia XL) Verapamil (Calan) Diltiazem (Cardizem)

Pulmonary

Breath Sounds

Normal tracheal and bronchial sounds
These are loud and tubular sounds with a high-pitch noted during inspiration and expiration, pausing between the two components.

Vesicular breath sounds
These are normal, soft, and low-pitched sounds heard over the more distal airways primarily during inspiration. During expiration the soft sound is diminished and only heard during the beginning of expiration.

Abnormal breath sounds
These are sounds that are heard outside of their normal location or phase of respiration.

Adventitous breath sounds
These are abnormal breath sounds heard using a stethoscope with inspiration and/or expiration. These sounds can be continuous or discontinuous sounds.

Wheeze (formally rhonchi)
These are continuous adventitious sounds comprised of a musical nature, constant pitch (high or low) and varying duration. These are usually heard during expiration but may also be present on inspiration. Wheezes are typically a sign of airway obstruction from retained secretions or due to bronchoconstriction or bronchospasm. Wheezes found with inspiration indicate a more severe airway obstruction.

Stridor
A continuous adventitious sound comprised of a very high-pitched wheeze that can be heard with inspiration and expiration and also indicates upper airway obstruction. A stridor that is heard without a stethoscope can indicate an emergency.

Crackle (formally rales)
A discontinuous adventitious sound heard with a stethoscope that "bubbles" or "pops". Crackles typically represent the movement of fluid or secretions during inspiration (wet crackles) or occur from the sudden opening of closed airways (dry crackles). Crackles that occur during the latter half of inspiration typically represent atelectasis, fibrosis, pulmonary edema or pleural effusion. Crackles secondary to the movement of secretions are usually low-pitched and can be heard during inspiration and/or expiration.

Bronchial breath sounds
These sounds are abnormal breath sounds when heard in locations that vesicular sounds are normally present. Pneumonia may produce these sounds.

Decreased or diminished sounds
A less audible sound may indicate severe congestion, emphysema, or hypoventilation.

Absent breath sounds
Absent lung sounds may indicate pneumothorax or lung collapse.

Voice sounds

Egophony, bronchophony, and whispering pectoriloquy are techniques to further assess lung pathology. If there is an abnormal transmission of sound it can further substantiate particular lung abnormalities.

- **Egophony:** While auscultating lung segments the patient repeatedly says the letter "e". If when auscultating the distal segments it sounds like "a", fluid is expected in the air spaces or lung parenchyma.
- **Bronchophony:** While auscultating lung segments throughout the chest the patient repeatedly says "99". If the word is clearly audible in distal lung fields the test is positive for consolidation. If the word is less audible, softer or weaker sounding, the test is positive for hyperinflation.
- **Whispering pectoriloquy:** While auscultating lung segments the patient repeatedly whispers words. The clearly audible and less audible words indicate the same findings as bronchophony testing.

Pulmonary Function Testing

Anatomic dead space volume (VD): The volume of air that occupies the non-respiratory conducting airways.

Expiratory reserve volume (ERV): Maximal volume expired after normal expiration.

Forced expiratory volume (FEV): The amount of air exhaled in the 1st, 2nd, and 3rd second of a forced vital capacity test.

Forced vital capacity (FVC): The amount of air forcefully expired after a maximal inspiration.

Functional residual capacity (FRC): Volume in the lungs after normal exhalation.

Inspiratory capacity (IC): The amount of air that can be inspired after a normal exhalation.

Inspiratory reserve volume (IRV): Maximal volume inspired after normal inspiration.

Minute volume ventilation (VE): The amount of air expired in one minute. This is equal to the product of the tidal volume and the respiratory rate.

Peak expiratory flow (PEF): The maximum flow of air during the beginning of a forced expiratory breath.

Residual volume (RV): Lung volume remaining in the lungs at the end of a maximal expiration.

Tidal volume (TV): Total volume inspired and expired per breath.

Total lung capacity (TLC): Lung volume measured at the end of a maximal inspiration.

Vital capacity (VC): Maximal volume forcefully expired after a maximal inspiration.

Gas Pressure (mm Hg)

Gas	Dry Air	Moist Tracheal Air	Alveolar Gas	Arterial Blood	Mixed Venous Blood
PO_2	159.1	149.2	104.0	100.0	40.0
PCO_2	0.3	0.3	40.0	40.0	46.0
PH_2O	0.0	47.0	47.0	47.0	47.0
PN_2	600.6	563.5	569.0	573.0	573.0
P_{TOTAL}	760.0	760.0	760.0	760.0	760.0

From Rothstein, JM: Rehabilitation Specialist's Handbook. F.A. Davis Company, Philadelphia 1998, p.528, with permission.

Pulmonary Function Reference Values

Values are calculated for an individual patient based on variables such as height, weight, sex, and age. A value is usually considered abnormal if it is less than 80% of the reference value.

Determining Lung Capacities

Total Lung Capacity (TLC) =	Inspiratory Reserve Volume (IRV) + Tidal Volume (TV) + Expiratory Reserve Volume (ERV) + Residual Capacity (RC)
Vital Capacity (VC) =	Inspiratory Reserve Volume (IRV) + Tidal Volume (TV) + Expiratory Reserve Volume (ERV)

Inspiratory Capacity (IC) =	Tidal Volume (TV) + Inspiratory Reserve Volume (IRV)
Functional Residual Capacity (FRC) =	Expiratory Reserve Volume (ERV) + Residual Volume (RV)

Typical Lung Volumes and Capacities

Tidal Volume =	500 mL
Expiratory Reserve Volume =	1000 mL
Vital Capacity =	4000-5000 mL
Inspiratory Capacity =	3000-4000 mL 75-80% of vital capacity 55-60% of total lung capacity

Forced Expiratory Volumes

Forced Expiratory Volume in one second (FEV1):	83% of VC
Forced Expiratory Volume in two seconds (FEV2):	94% of VC
Forced Expiratory Volume in three seconds (FEV3):	97% of VC

Arterial Blood Gases (ABG)

The study of blood gases is used as a tool to determine the effectiveness of alveolar ventilation. Values are expressed as the partial pressure of the gas. PaO_2, the partial pressure of oxygen within the arterial system, is normally 95-100 mm Hg. Supplemental oxygen is usually required for oxygen saturation rates less than 90%. The body cannot carry out vital functions with oxygen saturation less than 70%. $PaCO_2$, the partial pressure of carbon dioxide within the arterial system, is normally 35-45 mm Hg. The range for the acid-base balance or pH is 7.35-7.45. Changes in the $PaCO_2$ directly affect the balance of pH in the body. Prolonged imbalance of the pH in either direction can affect the nervous system and in some cases cause convulsions or coma.

Hypercapnia: an increased amount of CO_2 in the blood.

Hyperkalemia: an increased amount of potassium in the blood.

Hypocapnia: a decreased amount of CO_2 in the blood.

Hypoxemia: when the PaO_2 is less than 80 mm Hg.

Physical Signs Observed in Various Disorders

Condition	Breath Sounds	Adventitious Sounds	Voice Sounds	Inspection	Tactile Fremitus	Percussion
Normal	Nl	None	Muffled, distant, indistinct	Trachea midline, symmetric chest expansion	Nl	Nl
Asthma, acute moderately severe attack	↓, Bronchial, prolonged expiration	Inspiratory plus expiratory wheezes	↓	↑ Use of accessory muscles, tachypnea	↓	Nl-↑
Atelectasis	↓ Or 0	Crackles	↓ Or 0	Trachea deviated to affected side	↓	↓-↓↓
Bronchiectasis	Nl	Crackles	Nl	↓ Expansion AS, tachypnea, clubbing	↑ Rhonchal fremitus	Nl
Bronchitis	Nl, possible prolonged expiration	Crackles, wheezes	Nl	Possible ↓ motion, occasional use of accessory muscles	↓ Bilaterally	↑ Bilaterally
COPD	↓-↓↓, Prolonged expiration	None versus Crackles and wheezes	↓ Or 0 bilaterally	Barrel-shaped chest, moves as a unit, ↑ use of accessory muscles	↓ Bilaterally	↑ Bilaterally
Consolidation	Bronchial	Crackles	Whispered pectoriloquy	↓ Motion AS	↑	↓
Fibrosis ▪ Localized	↓	Crackles	↓	↓ Motion over area	↓ Or 0	↓
▪ Generalized	↓	Crackles	↓	↓ Motion bilaterally	↓ Or 0	↓
Heart failure	Nl	Dependent crackles	Nl	Nl chest expansion, tachypnea	Nl	Nl
Pleural effusion (moderate to large)	↓ Or 0,* Bronchial**	Possible pleural rub	↓*↑**	↓ Motion AS, ↑ RR, trachea deviated to OS	↓ Or 0	↓-↓↓
Pneumothorax (>15%)	↓ Or 0	None	↓ Or 0	↓ Motion AS	↓ Or 0	↑

Nl = normal, ↓ = decreased, ↓↓ = very decreased, ↑ = increased, 0 = absent, AS = on affected side, COPD = chronic obstructive pulmonary disease,
RR = respiratory rate, OS = opposite side; *Over the effusion; **Above the fluid.

From Watchie, J: Cardiopulmonary Physical Therapy: A Clinical Manual. W.B. Saunders Co.

Interpretation of Abnormal Acid-Base Balance

Type	pH	PaCO$_2$	HCO$_3$	Causes	Signs and Symptoms
Respiratory alkalosis	↑	↓	WNL	Alveolar hyperventilation	Dizziness, syncope, tingling, numbness, early tetany
Respiratory acidosis	↓	↑	WNL	Alveolar hypoventilation	Early: anxiety, restlessness, dyspnea, headache; late: confusion, somnolence, coma
Metabolic alkalosis	↑	WNL	↑	Bicarbonate ingestion, vomiting, diuretics, steroids, adrenal disease	Vague symptoms: weakness, mental dullness, possibly early tetany
Metabolic acidosis	↓	WNL	↓	Diabetic, lactic, or uremic acidosis, prolonged diarrhea	Secondary hyperventilation (Kussmaul's breathing), nausea and vomiting, cardiac dysrhythmias, lethargy, and coma

From Rothstein, JM: Rehabilitation Specialist's Handbook. F.A. Davis Company, Philadelphia 1998, p.529, with permission.

Normal Values

pH	7.4
P$_{CO2}$	40 mm Hg
P$_{O2}$	97 mm Hg
HCO$_3$	24 mEq/L
%Sat	95 - 98%

Metabolic alkalosis	pH > 7.5	PaCO$_2$ 35-45 mm Hg
Metabolic acidosis	pH < 7.3	PaCO$_2$ 35-45 mm Hg
Acute alveolar hyperventilation	pH > 7.5	PaCO$_2$ < 30 mm Hg
Acute ventilatory failure	pH < 7.3	PaCO$_2$ > 50 mm Hg

Chest Physical Therapy

Indications for Chest Physical Therapy

- Patients who have acute or chronic respiratory problems
- The inability to expel pulmonary secretions
- An ineffective cough
- Patients with increased secretions
- Patients with pneumonia
- Patients with atelectasis
- Patients with neurological impairments that cause swallowing difficulties

Contraindications for Postural Drainage

- Congestive heart failure
- Significant pulmonary edema
- Significant pleural effusion
- Pneumothorax
- Cardiac arrhythmia
- History of recent myocardial infarction
- Unstable angina
- Pulmonary embolism

Contraindications for Percussion

- Over a fracture
- Over a spinal fusion site
- Over osteoporotic bone
- Unstable angina
- Low platelet count
- Anticoagulation therapy
- Pulmonary embolism

Guidelines for Chest Physical Therapy

- ✓ Treatment should be administered prior to eating or at least one hour after meals.
- ✓ Percuss and vibrate over each segment to be treated for at least 3-5 minutes.
- ✓ Cough after each segment is treated.
- ✓ Allow for a rest period after each segment is treated.
- ✓ Review breathing exercises in each drainage position.
- ✓ Treatment should not exceed 45-60 minutes secondary to patient fatigue.

Goals for Chest Physical Therapy

✓ Mobilize secretions
✓ Expel secretions
✓ Improve breathing patterns
✓ Improve ventilation throughout all lobes
✓ Improve overall function

Technique

Percussion

Percussion is a technique using cupped hands that strike over a particular lung segment in alternating fashion during inspiration and expiration in order to mobilize secretions. This rhythmic sequence should last for several minutes and should not be painful.

Vibration

Vibration is a technique using both hands (one on top of another) directly over the chest wall to provide pressure and manual vibration during exhalation. Vibration should be used in conjunction with percussion and only during expiration. Pressure should be applied in the same direction as chest wall movement during expiration.

Positioning

Trendelenburg position

The Trendelenburg position places the person in a "head down" position in supine with the bottom of the bed inclined to approximately 45°. This position is ideal to assist with secretion drainage from the lower lobes of the lungs. It can also assist with increasing blood pressure in the case of hypotension. Patients with congestive heart failure, pulmonary edema, hypertension, shortness of breath or other circulatory problems will not tolerate this position.

Reverse Trendelenburg position

The reverse Trendelenburg position places a person in supine with their head raised above their trunk and lower extremities. This position is opposite of the Trendelenburg position, resulting in its name. This position may be used with patients diagnosed with hypertension or other cardiac conditions. This position also decreases the weight of the abdominal contents on the diaphragm providing it with less resistance to movement during breathing.

Semi-Fowler's position

The semi-Fowler's position places a patient in supine with the head of the bed elevated to 45° and pillows under the patient's knees for support and maintenance of a proper lumbar curve. This position is used quite often for patients with congestive heart failure or other cardiac conditions.

Bronchial Drainage

Upper Lobes

- **Apical Segment: Left and Right Anterior**
  Sitting: Lean back against a pillow; clap above the clavicles between the neck and shoulder.

- **Apical Segment: Left and Right Posterior**
  Sitting: Lean forward onto a pillow; clap on both sides of the back above the scapula. Fingers should be positioned slightly over the shoulder.

- **Anterior Segment: Left and Right**
  Supine: Lie flat on back with pillow under knees for comfort; clap on both sides just below the clavicles and above the nipple line.

- **Left Posterior Segment**
  Side: Lie on right side with head and shoulders elevated on pillows. Make 1/4 turn forward; clap over the left scapula.

- **Right Posterior Segment**
  Side: Lie on left side. Place a pillow in front from the shoulders to the hips and roll slightly forward onto it; clap over the right scapula.

- **Left Lingula**
  Side: Elevate bottom of bed 14-16 inches. Lie on right side. Place pillow behind from the shoulders to the hips and roll slightly back onto it; clap over left nipple.

Middle Lobe

- **Right Middle Lobe**
  Side: Elevate bottom of bed 14-16 inches. Lie on left side. Place pillow behind from the shoulders to the hips and roll slightly back onto it; clap over selected lobe.

Lower Lobes

- **Superior Segments: Left and Right**
  Prone: Lie flat on stomach; place pillow under the stomach area for added comfort and clap over the middle back at the tip of the scapula.

- **Lateral Basal Segment: Left and Right**
  Side: Elevate bottom of bed 20 inches. Lie on opposing side; clap at lower ribs. A pillow under the waist may help to keep the spine straight.

- **Anterior Basal Segment: Left and Right**
  Supine: Elevate bottom of bed 18-20 inches. Lie on back and place a pillow under the knees; clap at the lower ribs on both sides.

- **Posterior Basal Segment: Left and Right**
  Prone: Elevate bottom of bed 18-20 inches. Lie on stomach and place pillow under the hips; clap at the lower ribs on both sides.

Breathing Exercises

Inspiratory Muscle Training
Inspiratory muscle training attempts to increase ventilating capacity and decrease dyspnea through the strengthening of the diaphragm and intercostal muscles. This is commonly used with patients that exhibit decreased chest expansion, shortness of breath, bradypnea, and decreased breath sounds.

Treatment Protocol:
- ✓ Teach the patient proper use of inspiratory muscles
- ✓ Two to four sessions of 30 to 60 minutes of deep breathing concentrating on proper diaphragmatic breathing
- ✓ Use "sniffing" to increase awareness regarding the proper use of the diaphragm when breathing
- ✓ Strength training through resisted inhalation (for patients that have tidal volumes > 500 ml)
- ✓ Strength training through active breathing exercises (for patients that have tidal volumes < 500 ml)

Goals for Breathing Retraining
- ✓ Improve overall ventilation and respiration
- ✓ Decrease accumulation of secretions and prevent complications
- ✓ Decrease the work of breathing
- ✓ Improve the efficiency of coughing
- ✓ Strengthening respiratory muscles
- ✓ Improve chest wall mobility

Diaphragmatic Breathing
Diaphragmatic breathing attempts to enhance movement of the diaphragm upon inspiration and expiration and diminish accessory muscle use.
- Position the patient in bed with head and trunk elevated 45 degrees.
- Place dominant hand over the rectus abdominis muscles.
- Place non-dominant hand over the sternum.
- Direct the patient to inspire slowly and feel the dominant hand rise.
- Instruct the patient to control both inspiration and expiration.
- The non-dominant hand should have only minimal movement.

Incentive Spirometry
Incentive spirometry is used to increase inspiration using a device that provides immediate feedback to the patient regarding performance. This type of intervention is commonly utilized to treat patients status post surgery in order to strengthen weak inspiratory muscles and to prevent alveolar collapse.
- Position the patient in a comfortable setting.
- Instruct the patient to breathe into the spirometer.
- Instruct the patient to perform a maximal exhalation into the spirometer.
- Repeat 7 to 10 times per session and repeat the session 3-4 times per day.
- Increase volume expectations on regular intervals until the patient is within normal range.

Low-frequency Breathing
Low-frequency breathing is slow deep breathing designed to improve alveolar ventilation and oxygenation.
- Instruct the patient to breathe slowly, taking long and deep breaths.
- Ensure that the patient is not at risk for hyperventilation.

Pursed-lip Breathing
Pursed-lip breathing attempts to improve ventilation by decreasing the respiratory rate and increasing the tidal volume. This technique assists with shortness of breath that is commonly encountered in patients with COPD.
- Position the patient in a comfortable setting.
- Instruct the patient to avoid using the abdominal muscles.
- Instruct the patient to place a hand over the abdominal muscles while breathing.
- Slowly inhale.
- Relax and loosely purse lips during exhalation.
- Expiration should be twice as long as inspiration.

Segmental Breathing
- Segmental breathing is used to prevent accumulation of fluid and to increase chest mobility by directing inspired air to predetermined areas.
- Position the patient in a comfortable setting based on the targeted lung segment.
- Place hands on target area and apply pressure downward and inward during exhalation.
- Apply a quick stretch immediately before inspiration.
- Instruct the patient to slowly inspire air into the target lung area under your hands. Give mild resistance during inspiration.
- Observe accessory muscles during exercise in order to limit their use.

Pulmonary Profile

Examination

- Past medical history
- History of current condition
  - --Pulmonary function testing
  - --Arterial blood gases
- Social history (caregiver support)
- Medications
- Living environment
- Systems review
  - --Pulse oximetry
  - --Auscultation of the lungs
  - --Vital signs
  - --Cough
- Observation of breathing/use of accessory muscles
- Postural assessment
- Cognitive assessment
- Pain
- Strength
- Endurance
- Mobility skills

Intervention

- Breathing exercises
- Coughing techniques
- Postural drainage, chest physical therapy
- Endurance/exercise training
- Relaxation techniques
- Patient/caregiver teaching:
  - --Energy conservation
  - --Breathing techniques
  - --Coughing techniques
  - --Stress management
  - --Measurement of vital signs
- Mobility training

Goals

- Maximize independence in secretion clearance
- Maximize self-care skills
- Maximize functional mobility skills
- Maximize aerobic capacity
- Maximize independence with performing and monitoring home exercise program
- Maximize patient/caregiver competence with:
  - --Energy conservation techniques
  - --Breathing techniques
  - --Stress management techniques

Pulmonary Pathology

Asthma

Asthma is a reversible, obstructive lung condition characterized by increased responsiveness of the trachea and bronchi to stimuli, inflammation, and overproduction of mucous glands with widespread narrowing of the airways. Asthma attacks may be mild or life threatening. Clinical symptoms include increased respiration rate, prolonged expiration time with wheezing, increased use of accessory muscles, episodes of dyspnea, and a non-productive cough. Immediate medical intervention and the use of bronchodilators may be warranted.

Bronchiectasis

Bronchiectasis is a progressive obstructive lung disease that produces abnormal dilation of a bronchus. This is an irreversible condition that is usually associated with chronic infections, aspiration, cystic fibrosis or immune system impairment. The bronchial walls weaken over time secondary to infection and allow for permanent dilation of bronchi and bronchioles. Symptoms include a consistent productive cough, hemoptysis, weight loss, anemia, crackles, wheezes, and loud breath sounds.

Chronic Bronchitis

Chronic bronchitis is characterized by increased mucus secretions from the bronchioles as well as structural changes to the bronchi. A productive cough is usually present for three months during two consecutive years. The major impairments include hypertrophy of the mucus secreting glands and insufficient oxygenation of the alveoli due to mucus blockage. Clinical symptoms include increased pulmonary artery pressure, thick sputum, increased use of accessory muscles, persistent cough, wheezing, dyspnea, and cyanosis. Patients with chronic bronchitis are often called "blue bloaters".

Chronic Obstructive Pulmonary Disease (COPD)

Chronic obstructive pulmonary disease is characterized by increased resistance to the passage of air in and out of the lungs due to narrowing of the bronchial tree. COPD symptoms include dyspnea, chronic productive cough, and excessive mucus production. Progression of the disease includes alveolar destruction and subsequent increases in the amount of air that remains in the lungs. Patients with COPD have an overall increased total lung capacity with a significant increase in residual volume. The disease is diagnosed by determining the amount of air forcibly expired from the lungs in one second. Chronic obstructive pulmonary disease includes bronchitis, emphysema, asthma, and bronchiectasis.

Cor Pulmonale

Cor pulmonale is considered to be a medical emergency. There is a sudden dilatation of the right ventricle of the heart secondary to a pulmonary embolus. Right-sided heart failure will occur if the condition is not treated. As the condition progresses symptoms resemble congestive heart failure. Clinical symptoms include chronic cough, chest pain, distal swelling (bilateral), dyspnea, fatigue, and weakness.

Emphysema

Emphysema is a condition that develops from a long history of chronic bronchitis. The alveolar walls present with significant pathology and the air spaces are permanently over inflated. Expiration is difficult and dead space increases within the lungs. Emphysema is categorized as centrilobular, panlobular or paraseptal. Clinical symptoms include dyspnea, chronic cough, orthopnea, barrel chest, increased use of accessory muscles, and increased respiration rate.

Restrictive Pulmonary Disease

Restrictive pulmonary disease is characterized by the lungs' failure to fully expand due to a weakened diaphragm, structural inability of the chest wall to expand, and a decrease in the elasticity of lung tissue. Clinical symptoms include shortness of breath, a persistent non-productive cough, and increased respiratory rate. There may be chronic inflammation of the alveoli or plaques that develop and result in progressive fibrosis and a decreased lung capacity. Restrictive pulmonary disease results in a decrease in all lung volumes. Restrictive pulmonary diseases include scoliosis, atelectasis, pneumonia, and adult respiratory distress syndrome.

Tuberculosis (TB)

Tuberculosis is a bacterial infection that is transmitted in an airborne fashion (coughing, sneezing, and speaking). The lungs are primarily involved, however, TB can occur in kidneys, lymph nodes, and meninges. Lesions in the lungs can be seen with x-ray. Clinical symptoms include fatigue, weight loss, loss of appetite, low-grade fever, productive cough, chest discomfort, and dyspnea. Treatment includes anti-tuberculosis drug therapy. Prevention of TB through immunization is recommended for children.

Pulmonary Medications

Pharmacological Intervention for Pulmonary Management

Bronchodilator Agents -Relieve bronchospasm, increase size of the airway, and reduce resistance and subsequent obstruction. -Three subsets: anticholinergic, beta-adrenergic, methylxanthine	Albuterol (Proventil) Epinephrine (Primatene Mist) Pirbuterol acetate (Maxair) Salmeterol (Serevent) Aminophylline (Phyllocontin) Theophylline (Slo-bid)
Inhaled Corticosteroid Agents -Control inflammation of the airways; decrease bronchospasm and stabilize inflammatory response in the respiratory tract	Beclomethasone (Vanceril) Budesonide (Pulmicort) Fluticasone propionate (Flovent) Dexamethasone (Decadron)
Mucolytic Agents -Thin mucous secretions by altering the composition and consistency of mucus	Acetylcysteine (Mucosil) Dornase alpha (Pulmozyme)
Expectorant Agents -Increase removal of mucus through transport from the lungs	Guaifenesin (Anti-Tuss) Iodinated glycerol (Iophen) Terpin hydrate
Antiasthmatic Agents -Stabilize mast cells; inhibit the release of inflammatory medications	Cromolyn sodium (Intal) Nedocromil sodium (Tilade)

Chapter Five
Integumentary

Integumentary System

The integumentary system consists of the dermal and epidermal layers of skin, hair follicles, nails, sebaceous glands, and sweat glands.

Key Functions of the Integumentary System

- Excretion of sweat
- Protection
- Sensation
- Thermoregulation
- Vitamin D synthesis

Ulcers

Type of Ulcers

Arterial insufficiency ulcers
Wounds resulting from arterial insufficiency occur secondary to ischemia from inadequate circulation of oxygenated blood often due to complicating factors such as atherosclerosis. (See Table)

Venous insufficiency ulcers
Wounds resulting from venous insufficiency occur secondary to inadequate functioning of the venous system resulting in inadequate circulation and eventual tissue damage and ulceration. (See Table)

Pressure ulcers
Pressure ulcers, often called decubitus ulcers, result from sustained or prolonged pressure at levels greater than the level of capillary pressure on the tissue. Pressure against the skin over a bony prominence results in localized ischemia and/or tissue necrosis. Factors contributing to pressure ulcers include shear, moisture, heat, friction, medication, muscle atrophy, malnutrition, and debilitating medical conditions.

Neuropathic ulcers
Neuropathic ulcers are a secondary complication usually associated with a combination of ischemia and neuropathy. Most often neuropathic ulcers are associated with diabetes. Neuropathic ulcers are frequently found on the plantar surface of the foot, often beneath the metatarsal heads. The wound is typically well defined by a prominent callus rim. The wound has good granulation tissue and little or no drainage. Patients rarely report pain with neuropathic ulcers in part due to altered sensation. Pedal pulses are most often diminished or absent. The distal limb may appear to be shiny and appear somewhat cool to touch. The periwound skin often appears to be dry or cracked.

Characteristics of Arterial and Venous Insufficiency Ulcers

	Arterial Ulcers	Venous Ulcers
Location	Lower one-third of leg, toes, web spaces (distal toes, dorsal foot, lateral malleolus)	Proximal to the medial malleolus
Appearance	Smooth edges, well defined; lack granulation tissue; tend to be deep	Irregular shape; shallow
Pain	Severe	Mild to moderate
Pedal Pulses	Diminished or absent	Normal
Edema	Normal	Increased
Skin Temperature	Decreased	Normal
Tissue Changes	Thin and shiny; hair loss; yellow nails	Flaking, dry skin; brownish discoloration
Miscellaneous	Leg elevation increases pain	Leg elevation lessens pain

Intervention and Treatment Recommendations

Intervention for arterial insufficiency ulcers focuses on:
- Cleansing the ulcer
- Rest
- Reducing risk factors
- Limb protection

General Recommendations
- ✓ Wash and dry feet thoroughly
- ✓ Avoid unnecessary leg elevation
- ✓ Inspect legs and feet daily
- ✓ Wear appropriately sized shoes with clean, seamless socks
- ✓ Use bandages as necessary and avoid any unnecessary pressure
- ✓ Avoid using heating pads or soaking feet in hot water

Intervention for venous insufficiency ulcers focuses on:
- Cleansing the ulcer
- Compression to control edema

General Recommendations
- ✓ Elevate legs above heart when resting or sleeping
- ✓ Attempt active exercise including frequent range of motion
- ✓ Inspect legs and feet daily
- ✓ Wear appropriately sized shoes with clean, seamless socks
- ✓ Use bandages as necessary and avoid scratching or other forms of direct contact

Types of Dressings

Hydrocolloids

Hydrocolloid dressings consist of gel-forming polymers such as gelatin, pectin, and carboxymethylcullulose with a strong film or foam adhesive backing. The dressings vary in permeability, thickness, and transparency. Hydrocolloids absorb exudate by swelling into a gel-like mass and vary from being occlusive to semi-permeable. The dressing does not attach to the actual wound itself and is instead anchored to intact skin surrounding the wound.

Indications: Hydrocolloids are useful for partial and full-thickness wounds. The dressings can be used effectively with granular or necrotic wounds.

Advantages
- Provides a moist environment for wound healing
- Enables autolytic debridement
- Offers protection from microbial contamination
- Provides moderate absorption
- Does not require a secondary dressing
- Provides a waterproof surface

Disadvantages
- May traumatize surrounding intact skin upon removal
- May tend to roll in areas of excessive friction
- Cannot be used on infected wounds

Hydrogels

Hydrogels consist of varying amounts of water and varying amounts of gel-forming materials such as glycerin. The dressings are available in sheet form or amorphous form.

Indications: Hydrogels are commonly used on superficial and partial-thickness wounds (e.g., abrasions, blisters, pressure ulcers) that have minimal drainage. Rather than absorb drainage, hydrogels are moisture retentive.

Advantages
- Provides a moist environment for wound healing
- Enables autolytic debridement
- May reduce pressure and diminish pain
- Can be used as a coupling agent for ultrasound
- Minimally adheres to wound

Disadvantages
- Potential for dressings to dehydrate
- Cannot be used on wounds with significant drainage
- Typically requires a secondary dressing

Foam Dressings

Foam dressings are composed from a hydrophilic polyurethane base. The dressings are hydrophilic at the wound contact surface and are hydrophobic on the outer surface. The dressings allow exudates to be absorbed into the foam through the hydrophilic layer. The dressings are most commonly available in sheets or pads with varying degrees of thickness. Semi-permeable foam dressings are produced in adhesive and non-adhesive forms. Non-adhesive forms require a secondary dressing.

Indications: Foam dressings are used to provide protection over partial and full-thickness wounds with varying levels of exudate. They can also be used as secondary dressings over amorphous hydrogels.

Advantages
- Provides a moist environment for wound healing
- Available in adhesive and non-adhesive forms

- Provides prophylactic protection and cushioning
- Encourages autolytic debridement
- Provides moderate absorption

Disadvantages
- May tend to roll in areas of excessive friction
- Adhesive form may traumatize periwound area upon removal
- Lack of transparency makes inspection of wound difficult

Transparent Film

Film dressings are thin membranes made from transparent polyurethane with water resistant adhesives. The dressings are permeable to vapor and oxygen, but are mostly impermeable to bacteria and water. They are highly elastic, conform to a variety of body contours, and allow easy visual inspection of the wound since they are transparent.

Indications: Film dressings are useful for superficial wounds (scalds, abrasions, lacerations) or partial-thickness wounds with minimal drainage.

Advantages
- Provides a moist environment for wound healing
- Enables autolytic debridement
- Allows visualization of the wound
- Resistant to shearing and frictional forces
- Cost effective over time

Disadvantages
- Excessive accumulation of exudates can result in periwound maceration
- Adhesive may traumatize periwound area upon removal
- Cannot be used on infected wounds

Gauze

Gauze dressings are manufactured from yarn or thread and are the most readily available dressing used in an inpatient environment. Gauze dressings come in many shapes and sizes (e.g., sheets, squares, rolls, packing strips). Impregnated gauze is a variation of woven gauze in which various materials such as petrolatum, zinc or antimicrobials have been added.

Indications: Gauze dressings are commonly used on infected or non-infected wounds of any size. The dressings can be used for wet-to-wet, wet-to-moist or wet-to-dry debridement.

Advantages
- Readily available, cost effective dressings
- Can be used alone or in combination with other dressings or topical agents
- Can modify number of layers to accommodate for changing wound status
- Can be used on infected or uninfected wounds

Disadvantages
- Has a tendency to adhere to wound bed
- Highly permeable and therefore requires frequent dressing changes (prolonged use decreases cost effectiveness)
- Increased infection rate compared to occlusive dressings

Alginates

Alginate dressings consist of calcium salt of alganic acid that is extracted from seaweed. Alginates are highly permeable and non-occlusive. As a result, they require a secondary dressing. Alginate dressings are based on the interaction of calcium ions in the dressing and the sodium ions in the wound exudate.

Indications: Alginates are typically used on partial and full-thickness draining wounds such as pressure wounds or venous insufficiency ulcers. Alginates are often used on infected wounds due to the likelihood of excessive drainage.

Advantages
- High absorptive capacity
- Enables autolytic debridement
- Offers protection from microbial contamination
- Can be used on infected or uninfected wounds
- Non-adhering to wound

Disadvantages
- May require frequent dressing changes based on level of exudate
- Requires a secondary dressing
- Cannot be used on wounds with an exposed tendon, joint capsule or bone

Occlusion and Moisture

Occlusion refers to the ability of a dressing to transmit moisture, vapor or gases from the wound bed to the atmosphere. A truly occlusive substance would be completely impermeable, while a truly non-occlusive substance would be completely permeable.

Dressings are classified according to this continuum. The following list of dressings is arranged from most occlusive to non-occlusive:

- Hydrocolloids, hydrogels, semi-permeable foam, semi-permeable film, impregnated gauze, alginates, and traditional gauze

Dressings can also be classified by their ability to retain moisture. The following list of dressings is arranged from most moisture retentive to least moisture retentive:

- Alginates, semi-permeable foam, hydrocolloids, hydrogels, semi-permeable films

Primary Versus Secondary Dressings

A **primary dressing** comes into direct contact with the wound.

A **secondary dressing** is placed directly over the primary dressing to provide protection, absorption, and/or occlusion.

Red-Yellow-Black System

Color	Wound Description	Goals
Red	Pink granulation tissue	Protect wound; maintain moist environment
Yellow	Moist yellow slough	Debride necrotic tissue; Absorb drainage
Black	Black, thick eschar firmly adhered	Debride necrotic tissue

Selective Debridement

Selective debridement involves removing only nonviable tissues from a wound. Selective debridement is most often performed by sharp debridement, enzymatic debridement, and autolytic debridement.

Sharp Debridement

Sharp debridement requires the use of scalpel, scissors, and/or forceps to selectively remove devitalized tissues, foreign materials or debris from a wound. Sharp debridement is most often used for wounds with large amounts of thick, adherent, necrotic tissue; however, it is also used in the presence of cellulitis or sepsis. Sharp debridement is the most expedient form of removing necrotic tissue. Physical therapists are permitted to perform sharp debridement in the majority of states.

Enzymatic Debridement

Enzymatic debridement refers to the topical application of enzymes to the surface of necrotic tissue. Enzymatic debridement can be used on infected and non-infected wounds with necrotic tissue. This type of debridement may be used in wounds that have not responded to autolytic debridement or in conjunction with other debridement techniques. Enzymatic debridement can be slow to establish a clean wound bed and should be discontinued after removal of devitalized tissues in order to avoid damage.

Autolytic Debridement

Autolytic debridement refers to using the body's own mechanisms to remove nonviable tissue. Common methods of autolytic debridement include transparent films, hydrocolloids, hydrogels, and alginates. Autolytic debridement results in a moist wound environment that permits rehydration of the necrotic tissue and eschar and allows enzymes to digest the nonviable tissue. Autolytic debridement can be used with any amount of necrotic tissue and is non-invasive and pain free. Patients and caregivers can be instructed to perform autolytic debridement with relative ease; however, this type of debridement requires a longer period of time for overall wound healing to occur. Autolytic debridement should not be performed on infected wounds.

Non-selective Debridement

Non-selective debridement involves removing both viable and nonviable tissues from a wound. Non-selective debridement is often termed "mechanical" and is most commonly performed by wet-to-dry dressings, wound irrigation, and hydrotherapy (whirlpool).

Wet-to-dry Dressings

Wet-to-dry dressings refer to the application of a moistened gauze dressing placed in an area of necrotic tissue. The dressing is then allowed to dry completely and is later removed along with the necrotic tissue that has adhered to the gauze. Wet-to-dry dressings are most often used to debride wounds with moderate amounts of exudate and necrotic tissue. This type of debridement should be used sparingly on wounds with both necrotic tissue and viable tissue since granulation tissue will be traumatized in the process. Removal of dry dressings from granulation tissue may cause bleeding and be extremely painful.

Wound Irrigation

Wound irrigation removes necrotic tissue from the wound bed using pressurized fluid. Pulsatile lavage is an example of wound irrigation that uses a pressured stream of irrigation solution. This type of debridement is most desirable for wounds that are infected or have loose debris. Most devices permit varying pressure settings and provide suction for removal of the exudate and debris.

Hydrotherapy

Hydrotherapy is most commonly employed using a whirlpool tank with agitation directed toward a wound that requires debridement. This process results in the softening and loosening of adherent necrotic tissue. Physical therapists must be aware of the side effects of hydrotherapy such as dependent positioning of the lower extremities, systemic effects such as a drop in blood pressure, and maceration of surrounding skin.

Wound Terminology

Abrasion

An abrasion is a wound that occurs from the scraping away of the surface layers of the skin, often as a result of trauma.

Contusion

A contusion is an injury in which the skin is not broken. The injury is characterized by pain, swelling, and discoloration.

Hematoma

A hematoma is a swelling or mass of blood localized in an organ, space or tissue, usually caused by a break in a blood vessel.

Laceration

A laceration is a wound or irregular tear of tissues that is often associated with trauma.

Penetrating wound

A penetrating wound is a wound that enters into the interior of an organ or cavity.

Puncture

A puncture is a wound that is made by a sharp pointed instrument or object by penetrating through the skin into underlying tissues.

Ulcer

An ulcer is a lesion on the surface of the skin or the surface of a mucous membrane, produced by the sloughing of inflammatory, necrotic tissue.

Factors Influencing Wound Healing

There are a variety of factors that are not inherent to the actual wound that can significantly impact the rate and degree of wound healing.

Age: A decreased metabolism in older adults tends to decrease the overall rate of wound healing.

Illness: Compromised medical status such as cardiovascular disease may significantly delay healing. This often results secondary to diminished oxygen and nutrients at the cellular level.

Infection: An infected wound will impact essential activity associated with wound healing including fibroblast activity, collagen synthesis, and phagocytosis.

Lifestyle: Regular physical activity results in increased circulation that enhances wound healing. Lifestyle choices such as smoking negatively impacts wound healing by limiting the blood's oxygen carrying capacity.

Medication: There are a variety of pharmacological agents that can negatively impact wound healing. Medications falling into this category include steroids, anti-inflammatory drugs, heparin, antineoplastic agents, and oral contraceptives. Undesirable physiologic effects include delayed collagen synthesis, reduced blood supply, and decreased tensile strength of connective tissues.

Scar Management

Immediately after an injury, homeostasis attempts to occur and the acute inflammatory response is triggered. The proliferative or fibroplastic phase of wound repair includes granulation tissue formation and re-epithelialization. The maturation or remodeling phase includes the remodeling of the tissue and scar formation. Scars can form in an organized manner termed normotrophic scarring or in a disorganized manner such as seen with hypertrophic or keloid scars.

General Treatment Guidelines
✓ Massage using cream twice per day (once the wound is completely healed)
✓ Use of sun block and vitamin E over the scar
✓ Use of silicone gel (softens scar)
✓ Pressure garments
✓ Consider ultrasound treatment
✓ Consider electrical stimulation treatment

Exudate Classifications

Serous: Presents as clear, light color with a thin, watery consistency. Serous exudate is considered to be normal in a healthy healing wound.

Sanguineous: Presents as red with a thin, watery consistency. Sanguineous exudate appears to be red due to the presence of blood or may be brown if allowed to dehydrate. This type of exudate may be indicative of new blood vessel growth or the disruption of blood vessels.

Serosanguineous: Presents as light red or pink color with a thin, watery consistency. Serosanguineous exudate can be normal in a healthy healing wound.

Seropurulent: Presents as opaque, yellow or tan color with a thin, watery consistency. Seropurulent exudate may be an early warning sign of an impending infection.

Purulent: Presents as yellow or green color with a thick, viscous consistency. Purulent exudate is generally an indicator of wound infection.

Pressure Ulcer Staging*

Stage I
An observable pressure related alteration of intact skin whose indicators as compared to an adjacent or opposite area on the body may include changes in skin color, skin temperature, skin stiffness or sensation.

Stage II
A partial-thickness skin loss that involves the epidermis and/or dermis. The ulcer is superficial and presents clinically as an abrasion, a blister or a shallow crater.

Stage III
A full-thickness skin loss that involves damage or necrosis of subcutaneous tissue that may extend down to, but not through, underlying fascia. The ulcer presents clinically as a deep crater with or without undermining adjacent tissue.

Stage IV
A full-thickness skin loss with extensive destruction, tissue necrosis or damage to muscle, bone or supporting structures (e.g., tendon, joint capsule).

*Resource: NPAUP The Pressure Ulcer Staging System

The Wagner Ulcer Grade Classification Scale

The Wagner Ulcer Grade Classification Scale is commonly used as an assessment instrument for the evaluation of diabetic foot ulcers.

Grade	
0	No open lesion but may possess pre-ulcerative lesions; healed ulcers; presence of bony deformity
1	Superficial ulcer not involving subcutaneous tissue
2	Deep ulcer with penetration through the subcutaneous tissue; potentially exposing bone, tendon, ligament or joint capsule
3	Deep ulcer with osteitis, abscess or osteomyelitis
4	Gangrene of digit
5	Gangrene of foot requiring disarticulation

Bony Prominences Associated with Pressure Injuries

Supine	Prone	Sidelying	Sitting (Chair)
Occiput	Forehead	Ears	Spine of the scapula
Spine of scapula	Anterior portion of acromion process	Lateral portion of acromion process	Vertebral spinous processes
Inferior angle of scapula	Anterior head of humerus	Lateral head of humerus	Ischial tuberosities
Vertebral spinous processes	Sternum	Lateral epicondyle of humerus	
Medial epicondyle of humerus	Anterior superior iliac spine	Greater trochanter	
Posterior iliac crest	Patella	Head of fibula	
Sacrum	Dorsum of foot	Lateral malleolus	
Coccyx		Medial malleolus	

Burns

Types of Burns

Thermal burn: Caused by conduction or convection. Examples include hot liquid, fire or steam.

Electrical burn: Caused by the passage of electrical current through the body. Typically there is an entrance and an exit wound. Complications can include cardiac arrhythmias, respiratory arrest, renal failure, neurological damage, and fractures. Lightning is an example of an electrical burn.

Chemical burn: Occurs when certain chemical compounds come in contact with the body. The reaction will continue until the chemical compound is diluted from the site. Compounds that cause chemical burns include sulfuric acid, lye, hydroflouric acid, and gasoline.

Burn Classification

The extent and severity of a burn is dependent on gender, age, duration of burn, type of burn, and affected area. Burns are most appropriately classified according to the depth of tissue destruction.

Superficial Burn: A superficial burn involves only the outer epidermis. The involved area may be red with slight edema. Healing occurs without evidence of scarring.

Superficial Partial-Thickness Burn: A superficial partial-thickness burn involves the epidermis and the upper portion of the dermis. The involved area may be extremely painful and exhibit blisters. Healing occurs with minimal to no scarring.

Deep Partial-Thickness Burn: A deep partial-thickness burn involves complete destruction of the epidermis and the majority of the dermis. The involved area may appear to be discolored with broken blisters and edema. Damage to nerve endings may result in only moderate levels of pain. Healing occurs with hypertrophic scars and keloids.

Full-Thickness Burn: A full-thickness burn involves complete destruction of the epidermis and dermis along with partial damage of the subcutaneous fat layer. The involved area often presents with eschar formation and minimal pain. Patients with full-thickness burns require grafts and may be susceptible to infection.

Subdermal Burn: A subdermal burn involves the complete destruction of the epidermis, dermis, and subcutaneous tissue. Subdermal burns may involve muscle and bone and as a result often require surgical intervention.

Zones of Injury

Zone of coagulation: The area of the burn that received the most severe injury along with irreversible cell damage.

Zone of stasis: The area of less severe injury that possesses reversible damage and surrounds the zone of coagulation.

Zone of hyperemia: The area surrounding the zone of stasis that presents with inflammation, but will fully recover without any intervention or permanent damage.

Rule of Nines

Allows for a gross approximation of the percentage of the body affected by a burn.

Adult Values

Head and neck	9%
Anterior trunk	18%
Posterior trunk	18%
Bilateral anterior arm, forearm, and hand	9%
Bilateral posterior arm, forearm, and hand	9%
Genital region	1%
Bilateral anterior leg and foot	18%
Bilateral posterior leg and foot	18%
Total	**100%**

Children Values
A child under one year has 9% taken from the lower extremities and added to the head region. Each year of life, 1% is distributed back to the lower extremities until age nine when the head region is considered to be the same as an adult.

Positioning and Splinting

Effective management of burns includes proper positioning and splinting. A patient that sustains a burn is prone to develop contractures due to hypertrophic scarring and overall lack of motion. A general rule is to position the affected joint in the opposite direction from which it will contract. The identified position should, if at all possible, be a position of function. Splints are usually left on overnight, worn intermittently during the day, and require frequent observation to ensure proper fit.

Ideal positioning includes placing the neck in extension, upper extremities abducted to 90 degrees, shoulder lateral

rotation, and supination of the forearm. The lower extremities should align in neutral hip extension, 20 degrees abduction, full extension of the knee, and ankle dorsiflexion.

Topical Agents Used in Burn Care

Topical Agent	Advantages	Disadvantages
Silver Sulfadiazine	Can be used with or without dressings Is painless Can be applied to wound directly Broad-spectrum Effective against yeast	Does not penetrate into eschar
Silver Nitrate	Broad-spectrum Non-allergenic Dressing application is painless	Poor penetration Discolors, making assessment difficult Can cause severe electrolyte imbalances Removal of dressings is painful
Povidone-iodine	Broad-spectrum Antifungal Easily removed with water	Not effective against Pseudomonas May impair thyroid function Painful application
Mafenide Acetate	Broad-spectrum Penetrates burn eschar May be used with or without occlusive dressings	May cause metabolic acidosis May compromise respiratory function May inhibit epithelialization Painful application
Gentamicin	Broad-spectrum May be covered or left open to air	Has caused resistant strains Ototoxic Nephrotoxic
Nitrofurazone	Bacteriocidal Broad-spectrum	May lead to overgrowth of fungus and Pseudomonas Painful application

From Trofino, RB: Nursing Care of the Burn-Injured Patient. F.A. Davis Company, Philadelphia 1991, p.46, with permission.

Skin Graft Procedures

Allograft (homograft): A temporary skin graft taken from another human, usually a cadaver, in order to cover a large burned area.

Autograft: A permanent skin graft taken from a donor site on the patient's own body.

Heterograft (xenograft): A temporary skin graft taken from another species.

Mesh graft: A skin graft that is altered to create a mesh-like pattern in order to cover a larger surface area.

Sheet graft: A skin graft that is transferred directly from the donor site to the recipient site.

Split-thickness skin graft: A skin graft that contains only a superficial layer of the dermis in addition to the epidermis.

Full-thickness skin graft: A skin graft that contains the dermis and the epidermis.

Anticipated Deformities Based on Burn Location		
Area	**Anticipated deformity**	**Splinting type**
Anterior neck	Flexion with possible lateral flexion	Soft collar, molded collar, Philadelphia collar
Anterior chest and axilla	Shoulder adduction, extension, and medial rotation	Axillary or airplane splint, shoulder abduction brace
Elbow	Flexion and pronation	Gutter splint, conforming splint, three-point splint, air splint
Hand and wrist	Extension or hyperextension of the MCP joints; flexion of the IP joints; adduction and flexion of the thumb; flexion of the wrist	Wrist splint, thumb spica splint, palmar or dorsal extension splint
Hip	Flexion and adduction	Anterior hip spica, abduction splint
Knee	Flexion	Conforming splint, three-point splint, air splint
Ankle	Plantar flexion	Posterior foot drop splint, posterior ankle conforming splint, anterior ankle conforming splint

Burn Profile

Examination

- Past medical history
- History of current condition
- Social history (caregiver support)
- Medications
- Living environment
- Systems review
- Respiratory assessment
- Neurological assessment
- Edema/girth measurements
- Sensation
- Range of motion
- Flexibility
- Strength
- Pain
- Mobility skills

Intervention

- Positioning
- Splinting
- Edema control
- Scar management
- Passive range of motion
- Massage
- Conditioning exercises
- Endurance training
- Joint mobilization
- Electrotherapeutic modalities
- Compression devices
- Hydrotherapy
- Physical agents
- Mobility training

Goals

- Maximize functional mobility
- Maintain range of motion to all affected joints
- Maximize strength and endurance
- Reduce edema to the affected areas
- Maximize proper positioning and reduce scar contracture
- Maximize patient/caregiver competence with:
    - --Positioning of joints
    - --Use of splinting
    - --Pressure garments
    - --Stretching and strengthening programs

Burn Terminology

Dermis: The vascular layer of skin below the epidermis that contains hair follicles, sebaceous glands, and sweat glands.

Donor site: A site where healthy skin is taken and used as a graft.

Epidermis: The superficial avascular layer of skin that allows for hair follicles, sebaceous glands, and sweat glands.

Eschar: The necrotic and nonviable tissue resulting from a deep burn. This skin is hard, dry, and does not possess qualities of normal skin.

Escharotomy: A surgical procedure that removes eschar from a burn site and subsequently enhances circulation.

Hypertrophic scarring: An abnormal and disorganized scar formation characterized by a raised, firm scar with collagen fibers that do not follow any pattern.

Normotrophic scarring: A scar with organized formation of collagen fibers that align in a parallel fashion.

Pressure garments: A custom-made garment that applies sustained pressure in order to improve the structure of a scar. Pressure garments are worn 22-23 hours per day and may be required for up to two years.

Recipient site: A site that has been burned and requires a graft.

Z-plasty: A surgical procedure to eliminate a scar contracture. An incision in the shape of a "z" allows the contracture to change configuration and lengthen the scar.

Chapter Six
Patient Care Skills

Patient Management

Patient Communication

✓ Verbal commands should focus the patient's attention on specifically desired actions.
✓ Instruction should remain as simplistic as possible and should not incorporate confusing medical terminology.
✓ The therapist should describe to the patient the general sequence of events that will occur prior to initiating treatment.
✓ The therapist should ask the patient questions during treatment in order to establish a rapport with the patient and to provide feedback as to the status of the current treatment.
✓ The therapist should speak clearly and vary their tone of voice as required by the situation.

Ergonomic Guidelines

Workstation Recommendations
✓ 18-20 inch monitor
✓ Easily adjustable monitor to angle or tilt
✓ Split keyboard preferred
✓ Adjustable feet for the keyboard
✓ Minimum of six feet length for keyboard cord
✓ Monitor display should be directed ten degrees below the horizontal
✓ Monitor should be placed at least twenty inches away from the eyes
✓ Minimum of 30 inches depth for desk surface to accommodate monitor and keyboard
✓ Chair should swivel 360 degrees for easy access
✓ Wrist rests should match the front edge of the keyboard in order to maximize comfort
✓ Hands-free telephone set preferred
✓ Use a mouse that contours to the hand and has sufficient cord length
✓ 30-second exercise break every hour while sitting at the desk
✓ Space under the desk should be at least 30 inches wide, 19 inches deep, and 27 inches in height; there should be 2-3 inches between the top of the thighs and the desk

Workstation Posture

Head: level, facing forward, inline with trunk

Shoulders: relaxed, arms at side

Elbows: remain close to trunk, bent 90-120 degrees

Forearms, wrists, hands: parallel to the floor, straight

Trunk: maintain normal curves of the spine with appropriate lumbar support, shoulders and pelvis are level

Hips, thighs: well supported with contoured seat, parallel to the floor

Knees: maintain a level position with a 90 degree angle of flexion, knees generally at the same height as the hips

Feet: place feet flat on the floor or supported in a slight incline

Body Mechanics

A therapist must consistently use proper body mechanics when treating patients and avoid unnecessary stress and strain by maintaining proper alignment within the musculoskeletal system.

Principles of Proper Body Mechanics
- Use the shortest lever arm possible
- Stay close to the patient when possible
- Use larger muscles to perform heavy work
- Maintain a wide base of support
- Avoid any rotary movement when lifting
- Attempt to maintain the center of gravity of the therapist and patient within the base of support

Lifting Guidelines

✓ Always attempt to increase your base of support
✓ Maintain a proper lumbar curve as you lift
✓ Pivot your feet when lifting; do not twist your back to turn
✓ Maintain a slow and consistent speed while lifting
✓ Only lift an object as a last resort

Deep Squat Lift
1. Begin with hips below the level of the knees
2. Assume a wide base of support
3. Straddle the object
4. Grasp the object from each side or from beneath
5. The trunk should remain vertical
6. Maintain a lumbar lordosis and anterior pelvic tilt

Half-Kneeling Lift
1. Begin in a half-kneel position
2. The bottom leg should be positioned behind and to the side of the object
3. Maintain a normal lumbar lordosis
4. Lift the object onto the knee and draw it closer to the trunk
5. Continue the lift by holding the object close as you assume a standing position

One Leg Stance Lift
1. Used for lifting light objects that can be lifted with one extremity
2. Face the object in a lunge position
3. Shift weight onto the forward extremity
4. Flex the forward extremity and lower to reach the object
5. The hind leg rises off the ground to counterbalance the shift in weight
6. Maintain a neutral spine throughout the lift

Power Lift
1. Begin with the hips above the level of the knees
2. Assume a wide base of support behind the object with the feet parallel to each other
3. Grasp the object from each side or from underneath
4. The trunk should remain in a vertical position
5. Maintain a lumbar lordosis and anterior tilt

Traditional Lift
1. Begin with the lower extremities in a full squat facing the object
2. The feet should be positioned in an anterior-posterior manner on each side of the object
3. Grasp the object and flex the upper extremities to initiate the lift
4. Use bilateral lower extremities to provide the work of the lift
5. Keep the object close to the trunk during the lift
6. Maintain normal lumbar lordosis
7. Do not lift with the back

Pushing or Pulling an Object

- ✓ Use a semi-squat position to push or pull
- ✓ Apply the force parallel to the surface that the object should be moved upon

- ✓ Exert an initial force that is adequate to overcome the counter force of inertia and friction
- ✓ Attempt to push, pull, slide or roll the object prior to lifting or carrying an object

Mobility

Preparation for Treatment

In order to create an effective and successful treatment environment the patient must be informed regarding all expectations of the upcoming treatment as well as have all questions answered prior to initiating the actual hands-on intervention. The therapist must obtain informed consent from the patient and document consent in the patient's chart. The therapist must also determine if there are any potential limitations to treatment due to a patient's religious or cultural beliefs. The patient must be notified as to appropriate clothing for therapy, and areas such as draping must also be discussed prior to initiation of therapy in order to ensure a patient's comfort during treatment.

Draping
Draping is a technique utilized by health care providers to ensure the patient's privacy and modesty when treating particular areas of the body. Draping assists to keep the patient warm during treatment, adequately expose the area of treatment, and protect open areas, wounds, scars, and the patient's personal belongings from being soiled or injured during treatment. Draping materials may include gowns, towels, and sheets that must be secured in a manner that will properly expose the area of the body that requires treatment, while maintaining a patient's modesty and overall level of comfort during treatment.

Bed Mobility Guidelines

- ✓ A patient that is dependent must be repositioned in bed at least every two hours
- ✓ Skin should be inspected for redness or breakdown with each position change
- ✓ A dependent patient must be lifted when changing positions in order to avoid shearing across the bed
- ✓ Use pillows, towels or blankets when positioning a patient in order to support and maintain a particular position
- ✓ A patient should always be encouraged to participate in all mobility and positioning
- ✓ Practice moving segmentally from one side of the bed to the other

✓ Utilize the "bridging" position of hip flexion and knee flexion with feet flat on the surface to assist with movement and rolling

✓ Move from a supine to sitting position by rolling into sidelying and placing the feet over the edge; assist as needed to obtain a sitting position

✓ All components of bed mobility are complete only when the patient ends in a comfortable and safe position

Transfers

Communication During Transfers

The patient should be informed about the transfer itself and their responsibility during the transfer. The explanation should be understood by the patient and should occur prior to performing the transfer.

Commands and counts are used to synchronize the actions of the participants involved in the transfer. The therapist at the head of the patient should give the commands during the transfer when more than one person is involved.

Levels of Physical Assistance

Independent: The patient does not require any assistance to complete the task.

Supervision: The patient requires a therapist to observe throughout completion of the task.

Contact Guard: The patient requires the therapist to maintain contact with the patient to complete the task. Contact guard is usually needed to assist if there is a loss of balance.

Minimal Assist: The patient requires 25% assist from the therapist to complete the task.

Moderate Assist: The patient requires 50% assist from the therapist to complete the task.

Maximal Assist: The patient requires 75% assist from the therapist to complete the task.

Dependent: The patient is unable to participate and the therapist must provide all of the effort to perform the task.

Transfer Guidelines

✓ Evaluate the patient's level of cognition and mobility

✓ When in doubt, utilize a second person to maintain patient/therapist safety

✓ Obtain all appropriate equipment prior to initiating the transfer

✓ Utilize a transfer belt

✓ Educate the patient regarding the expectations and transfer sequence through verbal explanation and demonstration

✓ Instruct the patient in smaller segments of the transfer if necessary prior to performing the entire transfer all at once

✓ Position yourself correctly around the patient and maintain a large base of support; use proper body mechanics throughout the transfer

✓ Vary the amount of assistance as needed

✓ Utilize manual contacts with the patient to direct their participation during the transfer

✓ Complete the transfer with the patient positioned comfortably and safely

Types of Transfers

Dependent Transfers

Three-person carry/lift

The three-person carry or lift is used to transfer a patient from a stretcher to a bed or treatment plinth. Three therapists carry the patient in a supine position; one therapist supports the head and upper trunk, the second therapist supports the trunk, and the third supports the lower extremities. The therapist at the head is usually the one to initiate commands. The therapists flex their elbows that are positioned under the patient and roll the patient on their side towards them. The therapists then lift on command and move in a line to the destination surface, lower, and position the patient properly.

Two-person lift

The two-person lift is used to transfer a patient between two surfaces of different heights or when transferring a patient to the floor. Standing behind the patient, the first therapist should place their arms underneath the patient's axilla. The therapist should grasp the patient's left forearm with their right hand and grasp the patient's right forearm with their left hand. The second therapist places one arm under the mid to distal thighs and the other arm is used to support the lower legs. The therapist at the head usually initiates the command to lift and transfer the patient out of the chair to the destination surface.

Dependent squat pivot transfer

The dependent squat pivot transfer is used to transfer a patient who cannot stand independently, but can bear some weight through the trunk and lower extremities. The therapist should position the patient at a 45-degree angle to the destination surface. The patient places their upper extremities on the therapist's shoulders, but should not be allowed to pull on the therapist's neck. The therapist should position the patient at the edge of the surface, hold the patient around the hips and under the buttocks, and block the patient's knees in order to avoid buckling while standing. The therapist should utilize momentum, straighten his or her legs, and raise the patient or allow the patient to remain in a squatting position. The therapist should then pivot and slowly lower the patient to the destination surface.

Hydraulic lift
The hydraulic lift is a device required for dependent transfers when a patient is obese, there is only one therapist available to assist with the transfer or the patient is totally dependent. The hydraulic lift needs to be locked in position before the transfer. The therapist positions a webbed sling under the patient and attaches the S-ring to the bars on the lift. Once all attachments are checked, the therapist should pump the handle on the device in order to elevate the patient. Once the patient is elevated, the therapist can navigate the lift with the patient to the destination surface. Once transferred, the chains should be removed, however, the webbed sling should remain in place in preparation for the return transfer.

Assisted Transfers
Sliding board transfer
The sliding board transfer is used for a patient who has some sitting balance, some upper extremity strength, and can adequately follow directions. The patient should be positioned at the edge of the wheelchair or bed and should lean to one side while placing one end of the sliding board sufficiently under the proximal thigh. The other end of the sliding board should be positioned on the destination surface. The patient should not hold onto the end of the sliding board in order to avoid pinching the fingers. The patient should place the lead hand four to six inches away from the sliding board and use both arms to initiate a push-up and scoot across the board. The therapist should guard in front of the patient and assist as needed as the patient performs a series of push-ups across the board.

Stand pivot transfer
The stand pivot transfer is used when a patient is able to stand and bear weight through one or both of the lower extremities. The patient must possess functional balance and the ability to pivot. Patients with unilateral weight bearing restrictions or hemiplegia may utilize this transfer and lead with the uninvolved side. The transfer may also be used therapeutically, leading with the involved side for a patient post CVA. A patient should be positioned at the edge of the wheelchair or bed to initiate the transfer.

The therapist can assist the patient to keep their feet flat on the floor while bringing the head and trunk forward. The therapist should assist the patient as needed with their feet. The therapist must guard or assist the patient through the transfer and instruct the patient to reach back for the surface before they begin to sit down. Once the stand pivot is performed, the therapist should assist as needed to ensure control with lowering the patient to the destination surface.

Stand step transfer
The stand step transfer is used with a patient who has the necessary strength and balance to weight shift and step during the transfer. The patient requires guarding or supervision from the therapist and performs the transfer as a stand pivot transfer except the patient actually takes a step to maneuver and reposition his or her feet instead of a pivot.

Wheelchairs

Wheelchair Facts

- Adult standard wheelchair specifications include seat width - 18 inches, seat depth - 16 inches and seat height - 20 inches.
- Hemi-height wheelchairs have decreased seat height (17.5 inches) to allow for propulsion using the unaffected foot.
- Rear wheel axles can be positioned two inches posteriorly from normal for patients with amputations to increase the base of support and to compensate for diminished weight in front of the wheelchair.
- Reclining wheelchairs allow intermittent or constant reclined positioning.
- Tilt-in-space wheelchairs allow for a reclined position without losing the required 90 degrees of hip flexion and 90 degrees of knee flexion. The entire chair reclines without any anatomical changes in positioning.

Patient Considerations
- Physical needs
- Rental versus purchase
- Manual versus power
- Physical abilities
- Cognition
- Coordination
- Level of endurance
- Functional mobility
- Seating systems (support, comfort, pressure relief)

Standard Wheelchair Measurements for Proper Fit

Measurement	Instructions	Average Adult Size
Seat height/leg length	Measure from the user's heel to the popliteal fold and add 2 inches to allow clearance of the footrest.	19.5 to 20.5 inches
Seat depth	Measure from the user's posterior buttock, along the lateral thigh to the popliteal fold; then subtract approximately 2 inches to avoid pressure from the front edge of the seat against the popliteal space.	16 inches
Seat width	Measure the widest aspect of the user's buttocks, hips or thighs and add approximately 2 inches. This will provide space for bulky clothing, orthoses, or clearance of the trochanters from the armrest side panel.	18 inches
Back height	Measure from the seat of the chair to the floor of the axilla with the user's shoulder flexed to 90 degrees and then subtract approximately 4 inches. This will allow the final back height to be below the inferior angles of the scapulae. (Note: This measurement will be affected if a seat cushion is to be used. The person should be measured while seated on the cushion or the thickness of the cushion must be considered by adding that value to the actual measurement.)	16 to 16.5 inches
Armrest height	Measure from the seat of the chair to the olecranon process with the user's elbow flexed to 90 degrees and then add approximately 1 inch. (Note: This measurement will be affected if a seat cushion is to be used. The person should be measured while seated on the cushion or the thickness of the cushion must be considered by adding that value to the actual measurement.)	9 inches above the chair seat

From Pierson, FM: Principles and Techniques of Patient Care. W.B. Saunders Company, Philadelphia 2002, p.168, with permission.

Components of a Wheelchair

Footplates/Footrests:	Foot loops Heel loops
Legrests:	Stationary Adjustable/removable Swing away Elevating
Seat:	Sling versus solid Gel cushion Air cushion Foam cushion

Armrests:	Fixed versus adjustable Stationary versus removable Full-length versus partial Desk top
Wheelchair Back:	Fixed versus removable Sling versus contoured: • Gel • Foam Tall versus low back
Brake options:	Pull-to-lock versus push-to-lock Brake extensions
Wheel options:	Quick release Axle placement Type of casters Type of tires Rim projections
Restraints:	Velcro lap belts and chest belts Airplane seat belts Automobile seat belts

Components of a Wheelchair (continued)	
Power control options:	Head control Tongue control Puff-n-sip Joystick control Power scanning Microswitching system
Wheelchair Frame:	Rigid versus folding Narrow versus standard versus large Power versus manual
Other considerations:	Lap tray Tilt versus reclining system Anti-tippers Seat belts/lap restraints Allowance for growth in the system

Ambulation

Assistive Devices

Primary indications for using an assistive device during ambulation include:

- Decreased weight bearing on the lower extremities
- Muscle weakness of the trunk or lower extremities
- Decreased balance or impaired kinesthetic awareness
- Pain

Assistive Device Selection

Parallel Bars

Parallel bars provide maximum stability and security for a patient during the beginning stages of ambulation or standing. Proper fit includes bar height that allows for 20–25 degrees of elbow flexion while grasping on the bars approximately four to six inches in front of the body. A patient must progress out of the parallel bars as quickly as possible to increase overall mobility and decrease dependence using the parallel bars.

Walker

A walker can be used with all levels of weight bearing. The walker has a significant base of support and offers good stability. The walker should allow for 20–25 degrees of elbow flexion to ensure proper fit. The standard walker has many

variations including the rolling, hemi, reciprocal, folding, or adjustable walker with brakes, upper extremity attachments and/or a seat platform. The walker is used with a three-point gait pattern.

Axillary Crutches

Axillary crutches can be used with all levels of weight bearing, however, require higher coordination for proper use. Proper fit includes positioning with the crutches six inches in front and two inches lateral to the patient. The crutch height should be adjusted no greater than three finger widths from the axilla. The handgrip height should be adjusted to the ulnar styloid process and allow for 20–25 degrees of elbow flexion while grasping the handgrip. A platform attachment can be utilized with this device. The axillary crutches can be used with two-point, three-point, four-point, swing-to, and swing-through gait patterns.

Lofstrand (forearm) Crutches

Lofstrand crutches can be used with all levels of weight bearing, however, require the highest level of coordination for proper use. Proper fit includes 20–25 degrees of elbow flexion while holding the handgrip with the crutches positioned six inches in front and two inches lateral to the patient. The arm cuff should be positioned one to one and one half inches below the olecranon process so it does not interfere with elbow flexion. A platform attachment can be utilized with this device if necessary. The Lofstrand crutches can be used with two-point, three-point, four-point, swing-to, and swing-through gait patterns.

Cane

A cane provides minimal stability and support for patients during ambulation activities. The straight cane provides the least support and is used primarily for assisting with balance. A straight cane should not be utilized for patients that are partial weight bearing. The small base and large base quad canes provide a larger base of support and can better assist with limiting weight bearing on an involved lower extremity and improving balance on unlevel surfaces, curbs, and stairs. Proper fit includes standing the cane at the patient's side and adjusting the handle to the level of the wrist crease at the ulnar styloid. The patient should have 20–25 degrees of elbow flexion while grasping the handgrip. The straight cane can be used with the two-point, four-point, modified two-point, and modified four-point gait patterns.

Levels of Weight Bearing

Non-weight bearing (NWB): A patient is unable to place any weight through the involved extremity and is not permitted to touch the ground or any surface. An assistive device is required.

Toe touch weight bearing (TTWB): A patient is unable to place any weight through the involved extremity, however, may place the toes on the ground to assist with balance. An assistive device is required.

Partial weight bearing (PWB): A patient is allowed to put a particular amount of weight through the involved extremity. The amount of weight bearing is expressed as allowable pounds of pressure or as a percentage of total weight. A therapist must monitor the amount of actual weight transferred through the involved foot during partial weight bearing. An assistive device is required.

Weight bearing as tolerated (WBAT): A patient determines the proper amount of weight bearing based on comfort. The amount of weight bearing can range from minimal to full. An assistive device may or may not be required.

Full weight bearing (FWB): A patient is able to place full weight on the involved extremity. An assistive device is not required at this level, but may be used to assist with balance.

Guidelines for Guarding during Ambulation**

✓ A gait belt is recommended
✓ Stand to the side (usually the affected side) and slightly behind the patient
✓ Grasp the gait belt with one hand; place the other hand on the patient's shoulder
✓ Do not grasp the arm, as it will interfere
✓ Move your lead foot forward when the patient moves; the assistive device and your back leg should advance as the patient ambulates

**A therapist must always consider the size, weight, and level of impairment of the patient prior to initiating ambulation activities. Guarding guidelines may require modification and/or a second therapist may be required.

Gait Patterns

An appropriate gait pattern is determined by the amount of weight bearing permitted and the severity of the patient's overall condition. Commonly used gait patterns include two-point, three-point, four-point, swing-to, and swing-through.

Two-Point Gait
This is a pattern in which a patient uses two crutches or canes. The patient ambulates moving the left crutch forward while simultaneously advancing the right lower extremity and vice versa. Each step is one-point and a complete cycle is two-points.

Three-Point Gait
This pattern can be seen with a walker or crutches. It involves one injured lower extremity that may have decreased weight bearing. The assistive device is advanced followed by the injured lower extremity and then the uninjured lower extremity. The assistive device and each lower extremity are considered separate points.

Four-Point Gait
This pattern is very similar to the two-point pattern. The primary difference is that the patient does not move the lower extremities simultaneously with the device, but rather waits and advances the opposite leg once the crutch/cane has been advanced. This gait pattern may be prescribed when a patient exhibits impaired coordination, balance or significant strength deficits. Each advancement of the crutch or cane as well as the bilateral lower extremities indicates a single point, thus allowing for a four-point gait pattern.

Swing-to Gait
A gait pattern where a patient with bilateral trunk and/or lower extremity weakness, paresis or paralysis, uses crutches or a walker and advances the lower extremities simultaneously only to the point of the assistive device.

Swing-through Gait
A gait pattern where the patient performs the same sequence as a swing-to gait pattern, however, advances the lower extremities beyond the point of the assistive device.

Guidelines for Guarding during Stair and Curb Training

✓ A gait belt is recommended
✓ When ascending stairs or curbs, remain behind the patient (usually towards the weaker side). Place the lead foot on the same step as the patient and the

other foot one step lower. Hold the gait belt in one hand and position the other hand on the patient's shoulder. Remain static when the patient is moving, then advance keeping your feet in stride position.

✓ When descending stairs or curbs, remain in front of the patient and usually towards the weaker side. Place the lead foot on the step that the patient will step on and the other foot one step lower. Hold the gait belt in one hand and position the other hand on the front of the patient's shoulder. Remain static when the patient is moving, then advance keeping your feet in stride position.

Infection Control

Infection Control Terminology

Asepsis: The elimination of the microorganisms that cause infection and the creation of a sterile field.

Contamination: A term used to describe an area, surface, or item coming in contact with something that is not sterile. Contamination assumes an environment that contains microorganisms.

Hand washing: Hand washing is an important technique for asepsis. Guidelines for acceptable hand washing are as follows:

✓ Use warm water
✓ Remove all jewelry
✓ Wash hands with soap for at least 30 seconds (the time it takes to sing "Happy Birthday" twice)
✓ Avoid touching any contaminated surface
✓ Rinse thoroughly
✓ Use a paper towel barrier when turning off the water

Medical asepsis: A technique that attempts to contain pathogens to a specific area, object, or person. A primary goal is to reduce the spread of pathogens. Example: A patient with tuberculosis is hospitalized and kept in isolation.

Personal protective equipment (PPE): Items that are worn and used as barriers to protect someone who is assisting a patient with a potentially infectious disease. Personal protective equipment includes gowns, lab coats, masks, gloves, goggles, spill kits, and mouthpieces.

Sterile field: A sterile field is used to maintain surgical asepsis. A sterile field is a designated area that is considered void of all contaminants and microorganisms. There are standard and required protocols that must be followed in order to develop and maintain a sterile field.

Surgical asepsis: A state in which an area or object is without any microorganisms. Example: A sterile field.

Infectious Disease

Infectious disease is defined as a condition where an organism invades a host and develops a parasitic relationship with the host. The invasion and multiplication of the microorganisms produces an immune response with subsequent signs and symptoms.

Potential Symptoms of Infectious Disease

• Fever, chill, malaise	• Headache
• Rash, skin lesion	• Stiff neck
• Bleeding from gums	• Myalgia
• Joint effusion	• Convulsions
• Diarrhea	• Confusion
• Frequency, urgency	• Tachycardia
• Cough, sore throat	• Hypotension
• Nausea, vomiting	

Chain of Transmission for Infection

1. Causative agent, bacteria, pathogen, virus

2. Reservoir of humans, animals, inanimate objects

3. Portal of exit through blood, intestinal tract, respiratory tract, skin/mucous membrane, open lesion, excretions, tears or semen

4. Transmission through airborne, contact, vector, vehicle or droplet modes

5. Portal of entry through non-intact skin, blood, mucous membrane, inhalation, ingestion or percutaneous injection

6. Susceptible host regarding age, health status, nutrition, and environmental status

Precautions

Universal Precautions

Universal precautions are guidelines created in 1987 and recommended by the Centers for Disease Control to protect against bloodborne pathogens such as HIV and Hepatitis B. A health care provider must treat all patients as if they are infected with a bloodborne disease. The protocol requires gloves, mask, and gown when there is contact or potential contact with blood or body fluids.

Universal Precautions require:
✓ Wash hands before and after each patient contact
✓ Clean treatment area

✓ Use of personal protective equipment as needed
✓ A therapist should cover any open area on themselves prior to contact
✓ Use of medical asepsis
✓ Place biohazard materials in the appropriate receptacle

Standard Precautions

Standard precautions are revised guidelines that update Universal precautions and are designed for the care of all patients in hospitals regardless of infection or diagnosis. These precautions combine Universal and body substance isolation precautions and apply to all blood/body fluids, secretions, and excretions.

Standard Precautions
Hand washing
✓ Use plain soap for routine hand washing; use an antimicrobial agent for specific incidences based on the infection control policy.

Gloves
✓ Wear gloves when touching all body fluids, blood secretions, excretions, and contaminated items.
✓ Change gloves between tasks with a patient after coming in contact with infectious material. Remove gloves immediately, avoid touching non-contaminated items, and wash hands at that time.

Mask
✓ Wear a mask/eye protection/face shield for protection during activities that are at risk for splashing of any body fluids.

Gown
✓ Wear a gown for protection during activities that are at risk for splashing of any body fluids. Remove gown immediately and wash hands.

Patient Care Equipment
✓ Handle all patient equipment in a manner that prevents transfer of microorganisms.
✓ Ensure that all reusable equipment is properly sanitized prior to reuse.

Occupational Health and Bloodborne Pathogens
✓ Vigilance is required when handling/disposing of sharp instruments. Never recap needles or remove syringes by hand. All sharps disposal should use puncture-resistant containers.
✓ Mouthpieces, resuscitation bags, and ventilation devices should be used as an alternative to mouth-to-mouth resuscitation.

Transmission-based Precautions

Transmission-based precautions are updated guidelines for the particular care of specified patients infected with epidemiologically important pathogens transmitted by airborne, droplet or contact modes. These are additional precautions that should be implemented in addition to standard precautions.

Airborne Precautions
▪ Airborne precautions reduce risk of airborne transmission of infectious agents through evaporated droplets in air or dust particles containing infectious agents
▪ Private room with monitored air pressure
▪ Six to twelve air changes within the room per hour
▪ Room door should remain closed with patient remaining within the room
▪ Respiratory protection worn when entering room
▪ Limit patient's transport outside of the room for only essential purposes; patient should wear a mask during transport

Examples:
measles, varicella, tuberculosis

Droplet Precautions
Droplet precautions reduce the risk of droplet transmission of infectious agents through contact of the mucous membranes of the mouth and nose; contact with the conjunctivae, through coughing, sneezing, talking or suctioning. This transmission requires close contact, as the infectious agents do not suspend in the air and travel only three feet or less.
▪ Private room
▪ May share a room with a patient that has active infection of the same microorganism
▪ Maintain at least three feet between the patient and any contact (patient, staff, visitor)
▪ Room door may remain open
▪ Wear a mask when working within three feet of the patient
▪ Limit the patient's transport outside of room for only essential purposes; patient should wear a mask during transport

Examples:
Bacterial include: Haemophilus influenzae (including meningitis, pneumonia, epiglottis, sepsis), Neissena meningitidis (including meningitis, pneumonia, epiglottis, sepsis), Diphtheria, Mycoplasma pneumonia, Pertussis, Streptococcal (group A)
Viral include: Adenovirus, Influenza, Mumps, Parovirus B19, Rubella

Contact Precautions
Contact precautions reduce the risk of transmission of infectious agents through direct or indirect contact. Direct contact involves skin-to-skin transmission; indirect contact involves a contaminated intermediate object, usually within the patient's environment.

- Private room
- May share a room with a patient that has active infection of the same microorganism
- Use of gloves when entering the room
- Change of gloves after direct contact with infectious material
- Take gloves off prior to leaving the room and perform proper hand washing technique
- Wear a gown if you will have substantial close contact with the patient and remove the gown prior to leaving the room
- Limit patient's transport outside of the room for essential purposes only
- Dedicate non-critical patient care equipment to one patient, do not share between patients or disinfect properly prior to using the equipment again

Examples:

Gastrointestinal, respiratory, skin or wound infections, multi-drug resistant bacteria, Clostridium difficile, Enterohemorrhagic escherichia coli, Shigella, Hepatitis A (for incontinence/diapered), Parainfluenza virus or enteroviral infection (infants/young children), Diphtheria, Herpes simplex virus, Impetigo, Pediculosis, Scabies, Zoster, Viral hemorrhagic infections (Ebola)

Nosocomial Infections

A term used to describe an infection that is acquired during a hospitalization. The primary factor in the prevention of nosocomial infection is proper hand washing. Staff must also follow standard precautions and all infection control procedures at all times.

"The CDC Guidelines for Isolation Precautions in Hospitals" is a document that outlines the guidelines from collaboration between the Centers for Disease Control and Prevention (CDC) and the Hospital Infection Control Practices Advisory Committee (HICPAC). This document describes infection control within the hospital setting and provides strategies for surveillance, prevention, and control of nosocomial infections within the hospital setting.

Application of Sterile Protective Garments

Gowns

- ✓ Hold gown firmly away from the sterile field
- ✓ Shake gown open so it unfolds and keep hands above waist level
- ✓ Touch only the inside of the gown as you place both arms into the sleeves
- ✓ Stop when hands reach the sleeve cuff
- ✓ The gown is tied in back

Sterile Gloves

- ✓ Use the gown's sleeve cuffs as mittens and open the glove pack
- ✓ The sterile glove has a fold at the wrist where the inside (exposed) of the glove is not sterile
- ✓ Grasp the right glove with the left hand (still using the sleeve cuff as a mitten) and pull it on over the open end of the gown sleeve
- ✓ The first three fingers of the right hand should reach under the fold (touching the sterile portion of the left glove) and hold the glove while the left hand positions inside the glove
- ✓ Once both gloves are donned the left glove can unfold the right glove's cuff

Cap and Mask

- ✓ Wash hands
- ✓ Avoid contact with the hair while applying the cap
- ✓ All hair must be contained within the cap
- ✓ Apply a mask, if necessary, by first positioning the mask over the bridge of the nose
- ✓ The mask should form to fit securely over the nose and mouth
- ✓ Secure the upper ties behind the head and the lower ties behind the neck

Sterile Field Guidelines

- ✓ All items on a sterile field must be (and remain) sterile
- ✓ The edges of all packaging of sterile items become non-sterile once the package is opened
- ✓ Sterile gowns are only considered sterile in the front from the waist level upwards, including the sleeves
- ✓ Only the top surface of the table or sterile drape is considered sterile, with the outer one-inch of the field considered non-sterile
- ✓ Avoid all unnecessary activity around the sterile field
- ✓ Any item that positions or falls below waist-level is considered contaminated
- ✓ Do not talk, sneeze or cough, as it will contaminate the sterile field
- ✓ Do not turn your back to a sterile field as the back of the gown is not sterile; constant observation of the sterile field is required
- ✓ If an object on the sterile field becomes contaminated, the field is considered non-sterile and should be discarded
- ✓ Sterile fields should never be left unattended and should be prepared as close to the treatment time as possible in order to further avoid contamination

Accessibility

Americans with Disabilities Act

The Americans with Disabilities Act is designed to provide a clear and comprehensive national mandate for the elimination of discrimination. The Americans with Disabilities Act (PL101-336) is federal legislation that was signed into law on July 26, 1990.

The Americans with Disabilities Act is divided into five titles:

Title I:	Employment
Title II:	Public Services
Title III:	Public Accommodations
Title IV:	Telecommunications
Title V:	Miscellaneous

The Americans with Disabilities Act applies primarily, but not exclusively, to "disabled" individuals. An individual is "disabled" if they meet at least one of the following criteria:
- They have a physical or mental impairment that substantially limits one or more of their major life activities.
- They have a record of such an impairment.
- They are regarded as having such an impairment.

The Employment provisions (Title I) apply to employers of fifteen employees or more. The Public Accommodations provisions (Title III) apply to all businesses, regardless of the number of employees.

Employers are required to make reasonable accommodation for qualified individuals with a disability, who are defined by the Americans with Disabilities Act as individuals who satisfy the job-related requirements of a position held or desired, and who can perform the "essential functions" of such position with or without reasonable accommodation. The Americans with Disabilities Act does not require employers to make accommodations that pose an "undue hardship." "Undue hardship" is defined as significantly difficult or expensive accommodations.

Sources of additional information on the Americans with Disabilities Act:

Employment
Equal Opportunity Commission
1801 L Street, NW
Washington, DC 20507
(800) 669-4000
(202) 663-4900
http://www.eeoc.gov

Public Accommodations
Department of Justice
Office on the Americans with Disabilities Act
Civil Rights Division
P.O. Box 66118
Washington, DC 20035-6118
(202) 514-0301
http://www.usdoj.gov
www.ada.gov

Accessible Design in New Construction and Alterations
Architectural and Transportation Barriers and Compliance Board
1331 F Street, NW
Suite 1000
Washington, DC 20004-1111
(800) 872-2253
http://www.access-board.gov

Transportation
Department of Transportation
400 Seventh Street, SW
Room 10424
Washington, DC 20590
(202) 366-4000
http://www.fta.dot.gov

Telecommunications
Federal Communications Commission
445 12th Street SW
Washington, DC 20554
(888) 225-5322
http://www.fcc.gov

Accessibility Requirements

Ramps:	Grade $\leq 8.3\%$ At least 36 inches width Must have handrails on both sides Twelve inches of length for each inch of vertical rise Handrails required for a rise of six inches or more or for a horizontal run of 72 inches or more
Doorways:	Minimum 32 inch width Maximum 24 inch depth
Thresholds:	Less than ¾ inch for sliding doors Less than ½ inch for other doors
Carpet:	Requires ½ inch pile or less
Hallway clearance:	36 inch width

Accessibility Requirements (continued)	
Wheelchair turning radius (U-turn):	60 inch width 78 inch length
Forward reach in wheelchair:	Low reach 15 inches High reach 48 inches
Side reach in wheelchair:	Reach over obstruction to 24 inches
Bathroom sink:	Not less than 29 inch height Not greater than 40 inches from floor to bottom of mirror or paper dispenser 17 inches minimum depth under sink to back wall
Bathroom toilet:	17-19 inches from floor to top of toilet Not less than 36 inch grab bars Grab bars should be 1¼ - 1½ inches in diameter 1½ inch spacing between grab bars and wall Grab bar placement 33–36 inches up from floor level
Hotels:	Approximately 2% total rooms must be accessible
Parking spaces:	96 inches wide 240 inches in length Adjacent aisle must be 60 inches by 240 inches Approximately 2% of the total spaces must be accessible

Laboratory/Diagnostic Testing

Laboratory Testing

Hematocrit
Hematocrit is the percentage of packed red blood cells in total blood volume. Hematocrit is commonly used in the identification of abnormal states of hydration, polycythemia, and anemia. A low hematocrit may result in a feeling of weakness, chills or dyspnea. A high hematocrit may result in an increased risk of thrombus formation.

Hemoglobin
Hemoglobin is the iron containing pigment of the red blood cells. Hemoglobin's function is to carry oxygen from the lungs to the tissues. The laboratory test is commonly used to assess blood loss, anemia, and bone marrow suppression. Low hemoglobin may indicate anemia or recent hemorrhage, while elevated hemoglobin suggests hemoconcentration caused by polycythemia or dehydration.

Partial thromboplastin time
Partial thromboplastin time is most commonly used to monitor oral anticoagulant therapy or to screen for selected bleeding disorders. The test examines all of the clotting factors of the intrinsic pathway with the exception of platelets. Partial thromboplastin time is more sensitive than prothrombin time in detecting minor deficiencies.

Platelet count
Platelet count refers to the number of platelets per milliliter of blood. Platelets play an important role in blood coagulation, homeostasis, and blood thrombus formation. Low platelet counts increase the risk of bruising and bleeding. High platelet counts increase the risk of thrombosis.

Prothrombin time
Prothrombin time is most commonly used to monitor oral anticoagulant therapy or to screen for selected bleeding disorders. The test examines extrinsic coagulation factors V, VII, X, prothrombin, and fibrinogen.

White blood cell count
White blood cell count refers to the number of white blood cells per milliliter of blood. White blood cell count is commonly used to identify the presence of infection, allergens, bone marrow integrity, or the degree of immunosuppression. An increase in white blood cell count can occur after hemorrhage, surgery, coronary occlusion or malignant growth.

Reference Values for Clinical Chemistry - (Blood, Serum, Plasma)

		Conventional Units	SI Units
Cholesterol, serum or EDTA plasma	Desirable range	< 200 mg/dL	< 5.18 mmol/L
	LDL cholesterol	60 - 180 mg/dL	600 - 1800 mg/L
	HDL cholesterol	30 - 80 mg/dL	300 - 800 mg/L
Oxygen, blood, arterial, room air	Partial pressure (PaO_2)	80 - 100 mm Hg	80 - 100 mm Hg
	Saturation (SaO_2)	95 - 98%	95 - 98%
pH, arterial blood		7.35 - 7.45	7.35 - 7.45

From Miller-Keane: Encyclopedia and Dictionary of Medicine, Nursing, and Allied Health. W.B. Saunders Company, Philadelphia 1997, p.1844, with permission.

Reference Values in Hematology

		Conventional Units	SI Units
Cell Counts			
Erythrocytes			
Males		4.6 - 6.2 million/mm^3	4.6 - 6.2 X 10^{12}/L
Females		4.2 - 5.4 million/mm^3	4.2 - 5.4 X 10^{12}/L
Children (varies with age)		4.5 - 5.1 million/mm^3	4.5 - 5.1 X 10^{12}/L
Leukocytes			
Total		4500 - 11,000 mm^3	4.5 - 11.0 X 10^9/L

Differential	**Percentage**	**Absolute**	**Absolute**
Myelocytes	0	0/mm^3	0/L
Band neutrophils	3 - 5	150 - 400/mm^3	150 - 400 X 10^6/L
Segmented neutrophils	54 - 62	3000 - 5800/mm^3	3000 - 5800 X 10^6/L
Lymphocytes	25 - 33	1500 - 3000/mm^3	1500 - 3000 X 10^6/L
Monocytes	3 - 7	300 - 500/mm^3	300 - 500 X 10^6/L
Eosinophils	1 - 3	50 - 250/mm^3	50 - 250 X 10^6/L
Basophils	0 - 1	15 - 50/mm^3	15 - 50 X 10^6/L

		Conventional Units	SI Units
Platelets		150,000 - 400,000/mm^3	150 - 400 X 10^9/L
Reticulocytes		25,000 - 75,000/mm^3 (0.5 - 1.5% of erythrocytes) 20 - 165 mg/dL	25 - 75 X10^9/L 0.20 - 1.65 g/L
Hematocrit			
Males		40 - 54 mL/dL	0.40 - 0.54 volume fraction
Females		37 - 47 mL/dL	0.37 - 0.47 volume fraction
Newborns		49 - 54 mL/dL	0.49 - 0.54 volume fraction
Children (varies with age)		35 - 49 mL/dL	0.35 - 0.49 volume fraction
Hemoglobin			
Males		14.0 - 18.0 gm/dL	2.17 - 2.79 mmol/L
Females		12.0 - 16.0 gm/dL	1.86 - 2.48 mmol/L
Newborns		16.5 - 19.5 gm/dL	2.56 - 3.02 mmol/L
Children (varies with age)		11.2 - 16.5 gm/dL	1.74 - 2.56 mmol/L

From Miller-Keane: Encyclopedia and Dictionary of Medicine, Nursing, and Allied Health. W.B. Saunders Company, Philadelphia 1997, p.1843, with permission.

Diagnostic Tests

Arteriography
Arteriography refers to a radiograph that visualizes injected radiopaque dye in an artery. The test can be used to identify arteriosclerosis, tumors or blockages.

Arthrography
Arthrography is an invasive test utilizing a contrast medium to provide visualization of joint structures through radiographs. Soft tissue disruption can be identified by leakage from the joint cavity and capsule. The test is commonly used at peripheral joints such as the hip, knee, ankle, elbow, and wrist.

Bone Scan
A bone scan is an invasive test that utilizes isotopes to identify stress fractures, infection, and tumors. Bone scans can identify bone disease or stress fractures with as little as 4-7% bone loss.

Computed Tomography
Computed tomography produces cross-sectional images based on x-ray attenuation. A computerized analysis of the changes in absorption produces a detailed reconstructed image. The test is commonly used to diagnose spinal lesions and in diagnostic studies of the brain.

Doppler Ultrasonography
Doppler ultrasonography is a non-invasive test that evaluates blood flow in the major veins, arteries, and cerebrovascular system. The test relies on the transmission and reflection of high frequency sound waves to produce cross-sectional images in a variety of planes. Doppler ultrasonography is safer, less expensive, and requires a shorter time period than more invasive tests such as arteriography and venography.

Electrocardiography
Electrocardiography is the recording of the electrical activity of the heart. The test identifies three distinct waveforms: P wave (atrial depolarization), QRS complex (ventricular depolarization), and the T wave (ventricular repolarization). Electrocardiography is used to help identify conduction abnormalities, cardiac arrhythmias, and myocardial ischemia.

Electroencephalography
Electroencephalography is the recording of the electrical activity of the brain. The electrical activity is collected by examining the difference between the electrical potential of two electrodes placed at different locations on the scalp. Electroencephalography is used to assess seizure activity, metabolic disorders, and cerebellar lesions.

Electromyography
Electromyography is the recording of the electrical activity of a selected muscle or muscle groups at rest and during voluntary contraction. Electromyography is performed by inserting a needle electrode percutaneously into a muscle or through the use of surface electrodes. The test is commonly used to assess peripheral nerve injuries and to differentiate between various neuromuscular disorders.

Fluoroscopy
Fluoroscopy is designed to show motion in joints through x-ray imaging. The technique permits objects placed between a fluorescent screen and a roentgen tube to become visible. Fluoroscopy is not used commonly due to excessive radiation exposure.

Magnetic Resonance Imaging
Magnetic resonance imaging is a non-invasive technique that utilizes magnetic fields to produce an image of bone and soft tissue. The test is valuable in providing images of soft tissue structures such as muscles, menisci, ligaments, tumors, and internal organs. Magnetic resonance imaging requires the patient to remain still for prolonged periods of time and is extremely expensive.

Myelography
Myelography is an invasive test that combines fluoroscopy and radiography to evaluate the spinal subarachnoid space. The test utilizes a contrast medium that is injected into the epidural space by spinal puncture. Myelography is used to identify bone displacement, disk herniation, spinal cord compression or tumors.

Venography
Venography refers to a radiograph that visualizes injected radiopaque dye in a vein. The test can be used to identify tumors or blockages in the venous network.

X-ray
X-ray is a radiographic photograph commonly used to assist with the diagnosis of musculoskeletal problems such as fractures, dislocations, and bone loss. X-ray produces planar images and as a result often requires images to be taken in multiple planes in order to visualize a lesion's location and size.

Medical Equipment

Tubes, Lines, and Equipment

Arterial Line
An arterial line is a monitoring device consisting of a catheter that is inserted into an artery and attached to an electronic monitoring system. An arterial line is used to measure blood pressure or to obtain blood samples. The device is considered to be more accurate than traditional measures of blood pressure and does not require repeated needle punctures.

External Catheter
An external catheter is applied over the shaft of the penis and is held in place by a padded strap or adhesive tape.

Foley Catheter
A Foley catheter is an indwelling urinary tract catheter that has a balloon attachment at one end. The balloon which is filled with air or sterile water must be deflated before the catheter can be removed.

Intravenous System
An intravenous system consists of a sterile fluid source, a pump, a clamp, and a catheter to insert into a vein. An intravenous system can be used to infuse fluids, electrolytes, nutrients, and medication. Intravenous lines are most commonly inserted into superficial veins such as the basilic, cephalic or antecubital.

Nasal Cannula
A nasal cannula consists of tubing extending approximately one centimeter into each of the patient's nostrils. The tubing is connected to a common tube that is attached to an oxygen source. This method of oxygen therapy is capable of delivering up to 6 liters of oxygen per minute.

Nasogastric Tube
A nasogastric tube is a plastic tube inserted through a nostril and extending into the stomach. The device is commonly used for liquid feeding, medication administration or to remove gas from the stomach.

Oximeter
An oximeter is a photoelectric device used to determine the oxygen saturation of blood. The device is most commonly applied to the finger or the ear. Oximetry is often used by therapists to assess activity tolerance.

Suprapubic Catheter
A suprapubic catheter is an indwelling urinary catheter that is surgically inserted directly into the patient's bladder. Insertion of a suprapubic catheter is performed under general anesthesia.

Swan-Ganz Catheter
A Swan-Ganz catheter is a soft, flexible catheter that is inserted through a vein into the pulmonary artery. The device is used to provide continuous measurements of pulmonary artery pressure. Patients utilizing a Swan-Ganz catheter can exercise with the device in place, however, the patient should avoid activities that increase pressure on the catheter's insertion site.

Chapter Seven
Physical Agents

Therapeutic Modalities

Indications for Therapeutic Modalities

Inflammation and Repair: Modalities can alter circulation, chemical reactions, flow of body fluids, and cell function throughout all phases of healing. Modalities enhance and accelerate the healing process and reduce the risk of adverse effects associated with inflammation.

Pain: Modalities can control pain by altering the cause of the pain or altering the process of pain perception.

Restriction in Motion: Thermal agents are used to enhance extensibility of collagen to allow for greater range of motion and tolerance to stretch.

Abnormal Tone: Modalities can influence tonal abnormalities from pain, musculoskeletal or neurological pathology. Alteration in nerve conduction, reduction of pain, and change in muscle biomechanical properties can normalize tone and enhance functional outcome.

Phases of Tissue Healing*

Inflammation Phase
- Lasts one to six days
- Occurs secondary to trauma or disease
- Required for healing to occur
- Presents with calor, rubor, tumor, dolor
- Clot formation and phagocytosis occur

Proliferative Phase
- Lasts from day three through day 20
- Involves connective tissues and epithelial cells
- Epithelialization, collagen production, wound contracture, and neurovascularization occur

Maturation Phase
- Begins at approximately day nine and is ongoing
- This phase is the longest in duration; can last over one year
- Progression towards restoration of the prior function of the injured tissues
- Collagen synthesis and lysis balance
- Collagen fiber orientation

*****Phases of tissue healing can overlap**

Keloid Scar
A keloid scar can occur during the healing process when collagen production greatly exceeds collagen lysis. A keloid scar extends beyond the original boundaries of an injury and damages healthy tissues.

Hypertrophic Scar
A hypertrophic scar can occur during the healing process when collagen production greatly exceeds collagen lysis. A hypertrophic scar will be raised, but remain within the borders of the original injury.

Principles of Heat Transfer

Conduction: The gain or loss of heat as a result of direct contact between two materials at different temperatures. Examples include hot pack, paraffin, ice massage, and ice pack.

Convection: The gain or loss of heat as a result of air or water moving in a constant motion across the body. Examples include fluidotherapy and whirlpool.

Conversion: The transfer of heat when nonthermal energy (mechanical, electrical) is absorbed into tissue and transformed into heat. Examples include diathermy and ultrasound.

Evaporation: The transfer of heat as a liquid absorbs energy and changes form to a vapor. An example is a vapocoolant spray.

Radiation: The direct transfer of heat from a radiation energy source of higher temperature to one of cooler temperature. Heat energy is directly absorbed without the need for a medium. An example is an infrared lamp.

Types of Pain		
ACUTE	**CHRONIC**	**REFERRED**
- Pain that lasts during the time of healing	- Pain that lasts beyond the time of healing	- Experience pain in one area with the injury in another area

Types of Pain (continued)		
ACUTE	**CHRONIC**	**REFERRED**
• There is a known causative factor or etiology	• Activation of abnormal neurological responses	• Can refer joint to joint
• Well-localized and defined	• Pain continues after noxious stimuli ceases	• Can refer from a peripheral nerve to its distal innervation
• Pain will last as long as the noxious stimuli persists	• Associated with physical, psychological, social dysfunction	• Can refer from an organ to outside tissues

Cryotherapy

Therapeutic Effects:

- Initial decrease in blood flow to the treated area
- Initial vasoconstriction
- Decrease temperature
- Decrease nerve conduction velocity
- Increase pain threshold
- Reduce spasticity of muscle
- Decrease metabolism
- Produce analgesic effects
- Decrease edema

Indications:

- Acute or chronic pain
- Acute or subacute inflammation
- Myofascial pain syndrome
- Musculoskeletal trauma
- Muscle spasm
- Reduction of spasticity
- Bursitis
- Tendonitis

Contraindications:

- Area of compromised circulation
- Raynaud's phenomenon
- Peripheral vascular disease
- Cold urticaria
- Ischemic tissue
- Hypertension
- Cold hypersensitivity
- Cryoglobinemia
- Infection

Stages of Perceived Sensations during Cryotherapy

1. Intense cold within three minutes
2. Aching and/or burning sensation from four to seven minutes
3. Anesthesia to analgesia from eight to 15 minutes
4. Numbness from 15 to 30 minutes

Ice Massage

Ice massage is typically performed by freezing water in paper cups and applying the ice directly to the treatment area. Ice massage is ideal for small or contoured areas, allows for observation, and is inexpensive to use.

Treatment Parameters: Ice massage can be administered using a frozen water popsicle or frozen water in a paper cup. Directly apply ice massage to the area for five to ten minutes.

Cold Pack

A cold pack typically contains silica gel and is available in a variety of shapes and sizes. The cold pack is stored in a refrigeration unit and is usually applied with a moist towel. Cold packs are easy to use, require minimal clinician time, and can cover a large area. Cold packs may not maintain uniform contact with the body and require frequent observation of the skin.

Treatment Parameters: A cold pack requires a temperature of 23 degrees Fahrenheit (−5 degrees Celsius). Apply the cold pack wrapped in a moistened towel to the area for 15 minutes. Application may extend to 30 minutes for reduction in spasticity, however, the skin requires observation every ten minutes. Cold packs can be applied every one to two hours for reduction of inflammation and pain control.

Cold Bath

A cold bath is commonly used for immersion of the distal extremities. A basin or whirlpool is most often used to hold the cold water.

Treatment Parameters: A cold bath requires water temperature ranging from 55 to 64 degrees Fahrenheit (13 to 18 degrees Celsius). A whirlpool or container of water with crushed ice can be used. The body part should be immersed for 5 to 15 minutes to attain the desired therapeutic effects.

Vapocoolant Spray

Vapocoolant sprays are often used in conjunction with passive stretching. Fluori-Methane is a commonly used vapocoolant spray that is typically applied from the proximal to distal muscle attachments. Vapocoolant sprays allow for a short duration of cooling to a very localized area of application, however, may be harmful to the environment and dangerous if inhaled.

Treatment Parameters: Identify the trigger point and make two to five sweeps with the spray in the direction of the muscle fibers. Keep the spray 12 to 18 inches from the skin and apply at a 30-degree angle. Stretching should begin while applying the spray and continue with steady tension and stretch. Repeated applications during the same treatment are safe if the skin is rewarmed between applications. Chlorofluorocarbons are exempt from the Clean Air Act when used for medical purposes, however, may cause environmental and ozone damage.

Superficial Heating Agents

Therapeutic Effects:

Increase temperature	Vasodilation
Increase blood flow to the treated area	Increase nerve conduction velocity
Decrease nerve conduction latency	Increase metabolic rate
Temporarily decrease muscle strength	Increase muscle elasticity
Increase pain threshold	Increase collagen extensibility
Increase edema	Decrease muscle tone

Indications:

Pain control	Muscle spasm
Chronic inflammatory conditions	Decreased range of motion
Trigger point	Desensitization
Tissue healing	

Contraindications:

Circulatory impairment	Bleeding or hemorrhage
Area of malignancy	Sensory impairment
Acute musculoskeletal trauma	Thrombophlebitis
	Arterial disease

Fluidotherapy

Fluidotherapy consists of a container that circulates warm air and small cellulose particles. The extremity is placed into the container and dry heat is generated through the energy transferred by forced convection. The therapeutic effects include the promotion of tissue healing, skin desensitization, and prevention of edema. Fluidotherapy allows for active movement during treatment and constant treatment temperature, however, it is expensive and may require the extremity to be placed in a dependent position.

Treatment Parameters: The body part to be treated should be placed into the fluidotherapy unit prior to turning the machine on. The temperature should be set between 111 to 125 degrees Fahrenheit (44 to 52 degrees Celsius) and the degree of agitation should be adjusted to patient comfort. Treatment time is usually 20 minutes. A protective covering is required for any open area.

Hot Pack

A hot pack consists of a canvas or nylon covered pack filled with a hydrophilic silicate gel that provides a moist heat. The size and shape of the hot pack varies depending on the size and contour of the treatment area. A hot pack is easy to use, inexpensive, and can cover large areas. The main therapeutic effects include soft tissue healing, promoting relaxation, and decreasing pain and stiffness. Disadvantages of a hot pack include the need for close monitoring of the skin, the inability to maintain total contact, and the inability to move during treatment.

Treatment Parameters: A hot pack must be stored in hot water between 158 to 167 degrees Fahrenheit (77 to 75 degrees Celsius). Application requires six to eight layers of towels around the hot pack. The hot pack should be applied on top of the patient. If the patient lies on top of the hot pack additional towels are required. Skin checks are required after five minutes for excess redness or signs of a burn. A patient must have a call device to notify the therapist of discomfort. Hot packs require approximately 20 minutes to achieve the desired effects.

Infrared Lamp (IR)

An infrared lamp produces superficial heating of tissue through radiant heat. This form of heating is usually limited to penetration of less than one to three millimeters. Infrared does not require contact with the area to be treated and allows for constant observation, however, it requires skill to localize a treatment site. The main therapeutic effect is the enhancement of soft tissue healing. The use of infrared is declining due to the limited depth of penetration, dehydrating effects on wounds, and the risk of burns during treatment.

Treatment Parameters: The patient should be positioned approximately 20 inches from the source. A moist towel should be placed over the treatment area and the skin should be monitored intermittently throughout treatment. The standard formula indicates 20 inches in distance should equal 20 minutes of treatment. As the distance decreases, the intensity will increase, and the time of total treatment should decrease.

Paraffin

Paraffin wax is the most commonly used superficial heating agent of the distal extremities. It has the ability to maintain contact over all contoured areas and due to the low specific heat and slower conduction it does not feel as hot as water at the same temperature. Paraffin is easy to use, inexpensive, and can be used at home, however, it cannot be used over open areas.

Treatment Parameters: Temperature of the paraffin mixture should be maintained between 113 and 126 degrees Fahrenheit (45 to 52 degrees Celsius). There are three methods of paraffin application: dip-wrap, dip-reimmersion or paint application. The distal extremities utilize the dip-wrap or dip-reimmersion methods. The patient's skin should be dry and clean prior to treatment. The patient is required to maintain a static position as the distal extremity dips into the paraffin bath and is removed. Wait a few seconds for the paraffin to harden and redip six to ten times using the dip-wrap method. Next, place a plastic bag over the extremity with a towel around it to insulate and maintain heating for approximately 15 to 20 minutes. Using the dip-reimmersion method place the distal extremity back into the paraffin bath after the initial six to ten dips and allow it to remain for the duration of treatment, up to 20 minutes. The paint method is used for body parts that cannot be immersed into the paraffin bath. A layer of paraffin is painted on the body with a brush. After a few seconds, six to ten additional layers are applied and a plastic wrap is placed over the paraffin with a towel on top to insulate the treatment area. Removal of the paraffin is the same for all forms of application. Paraffin should be peeled off after treatment and placed back into the container to melt or simply be discarded.

Deep Heating Agents

Diathermy

Diathermy is a deep heating agent that converts high frequency electromagnetic energy into therapeutic heat. Electrical energy produces vibration of molecules within a specific tissue, generates heat, and elevates tissue temperature. The main therapeutic effect of diathermy is the enhancement of soft tissue healing. Shortwave diathermy can be delivered in a continuous or pulsed mode. A pulsed mode is typically utilized to attain nonthermal effects while a continuous mode is used for thermal effects. The most common frequency used for shortwave diathermy is 27.12 MHz. Shortwave diathermy can utilize a capacitance technique or inductance technique. Capacitive plate applicators produce a high frequency electrical current that alternates between the plates. The patient becomes part of the electrical circuit and the oscillation of ions increases tissue temperature. Inductive coil applicators utilize a coil that generates alternating electric current, creates a magnetic field perpendicular to the coil, and produces eddy currents within the tissues. Eddy currents cause the oscillation of ions that increases tissue temperature. Inductive coil applicators are bundled as cables that wrap around an extremity or as a drum applicator.

Therapeutic Effects:

• Increase temperature	• Vasodilation
• Altered cell membrane function	• Increase nerve conduction velocity
• Decrease nerve conduction latency	• Increase metabolic rate
• Increase pain threshold	• Increase collagen extensibility
• Increase muscle elasticity	• Alteration of muscle strength
• Increase edema	

Indications:

• Decreased collagen extensibility	• Degenerative joint disease
• Pain	• Joint stiffness
• Tissue healing	• Bursitis
• Chronic inflammatory pelvic disease	• Peripheral nerve regeneration
• Muscle guarding	• Chronic inflammation

Contraindications:

• Low back, abdomen, pelvis of a pregnant woman	• Pain and temperature sensory deficits
• Internal and external metal objects	• Moist wound dressing
• Eyes	• Over hemorrhagic region
• Malignant area	• Testes
• Intrauterine device	• Acute inflammation
• Cardiac pacemaker	• Ischemic tissue

Capacitive Plate Method
- Metal plates encased in a plastic housing
- Field radiation is a strong electrical field and a weaker magnetic field
- Energy is absorbed most within the skin and less into deeper structures
- The heating pattern is superficial
- Application is generally over areas of low-fat content

Inductive Coil Method
- Rigid metal coils encased
- Field radiation is a strong magnetic field and a weaker electrical field
- Energy is absorbed most within the deeper structures; tissues with the highest electrical conductivity such as muscle and synovial fluid
- The heating pattern is deeper
- Application is generally over areas of high water content

Treatment Parameters: A therapist should first select the most appropriate diathermy technique and device based on patient examination. The patient must remove all metal and jewelry in the area surrounding the treatment site. Position the patient and check for clean and dry skin. When using an inductive applicator the therapist must wrap the coils around the extremity that has been covered by a towel. When using a drum the therapist should place the drum directly over the treatment area. When using a capacitive applicator place the two plates over both sides of the treatment area ensuring equal distance from the plates to the skin (two to ten centimeters). The patient must remain in the same position throughout treatment for complete and consistent heating. The patient should have a call bell and should be checked within the first few minutes of treatment. Treatment time varies from 15 to 30 minutes based on diagnosis and desired effects.

Ultrasound

Ultrasound is a common deep heating agent that transfers heat through conversion, elevates tissue temperature to depths up to five centimeters, and uses inaudible acoustic mechanical vibrations of high frequency to produce thermal and nonthermal effects. The piezoelectric crystal transducer converts electrical energy into sound. The main therapeutic effects of ultrasound include enhanced soft tissue healing, decreased inflammatory response, and decreased pain. Therapeutic ultrasound has a frequency between .75 and 3 MHz. Ultrasound requires the use of a coupling agent and can be applied using the stationary or moving technique. Ultrasound can be administered using a pulsed or continuous mode. Continuous mode ultrasound is more effective in elevating tissue temperature where pulsed mode ultrasound conversely minimizes the thermal effects. Duty cycle indicates the portion of treatment time that ultrasound is generated during the entire treatment. For example, continuous ultrasound generates constant ultrasound waves that correlates to a 100% duty cycle and produces thermal effects at a higher intensity and nonthermal effects at a lower intensity. Pulsed ultrasound that generates ultrasound 20% of the treatment time correlates to a 20% duty cycle and will produce nonthermal effects. A frequency setting of 1 MHz is used for heating of deeper tissues (up to five centimeters) where a setting of 3 MHz produces a higher temperature with a depth of penetration of less than two centimeters.

Therapeutic Effects:

Thermal	*Nonthermal*
• Increase extensibility of collagen structures	• Stimulation of tissue regeneration
• Decrease joint stiffness	• Increase macrophage responsiveness
• Pain relief	• Pain relief
• Increase blood flow	• Soft tissue repair
• Decrease muscle spasm	• Increase blood flow
	• Increase skin and cell membrane permeability

Indications:

• Soft tissue repair	• Scar tissue
• Contracture	• Pain
• Bone fracture	• Plantar wart
• Trigger point	• Muscle spasm
• Dermal ulcer	

Contraindications:

• Over eyes	• Over heart
• Over pregnant uterus	• Over testes
• Over cemented prosthetic joint	• Over epiphyseal areas in children
• Impaired circulation	• Infection
• Thrombophlebitis	• Over malignancy
• Impaired pain or temperature sensory deficits	

Treatment Parameters: Ultrasound can be administered using a stationary or moving technique. For all techniques the therapist should decide the duration, frequency, duty cycle, and intensity of treatment based on diagnosis and desired effects. Apply the coupling medium to the treatment area or place the area to be treated under water if using the immersion technique. Place the transducer on the treatment area or one half-inch parallel to the treatment area under water and then turn on the machine. During the moving technique the transducer should continuously move in a small circular pattern over the treatment area. Maintain contact with the skin and stay within the treatment area. An area two to three times the size of the transducer typically requires a duration of five minutes of treatment. Intensity for continuous ultrasound is normally set between .5 to 2 W/cm^2 for thermal effects. Pulsed ultrasound is normally set between .5 to .75 W/cm^2 with a 20% duty cycle for nonthermal effects.

Beam Nonuniformity Ratio (BNR)

- BNR is the ratio of intensity of the highest peak to the average intensity of all peaks.
- The lower the BNR, the more favorable, since patients will be less likely to experience hot spots and/or discomfort during treatment.
- The BNR of a particular unit is required to be listed on the device for consumer education and awareness.
- The BNR is derived from the intrinsic factors and quality of the piezoelectric transducer. The higher the quality of the transducer, the lower the BNR. BNR values should range between 2:1 and 6:1; most devices often fall in the 5:1 or 6:1 range.

Effective Radiating Area (ERA)

The ERA is the area of the transducer that transmits ultrasound energy. The ERA is always smaller than the total size of the transducer head.

Acoustic Cavitation

Acoustic cavitation occurs as a result of the acoustic energy generated by ultrasound that develops into microscopic bubbles causing cavities that surround soft tissues. The microscopic, vapor-filled bubbles expand and contract. There are two types of cavitation that occur:

- *Stable cavitation:* The microscopic bubbles increase and decrease in size, but do no burst. Stable cavitation triggers microstreaming.

- *Transient (unstable) cavitation:* The microscopic bubbles increase in size over multiple cycles and implode. This causes brief moments of local temperature and pressure increases in the area surrounding these bubbles. This process should not

occur during therapeutic ultrasound since the intensities required are much higher than 3 W/cm^2.

Microstreaming

Microstreaming is the minute flow of fluid that takes place around the vapor-filled bubbles that oscillate and pulsate.

Acoustic Streaming

Acoustic streaming is the term for the consistent and circular flow of cellular fluids that results from ultrasound. Acoustic streaming is responsible for altering cellular activity and the transport of fluids to different portions of the field.

Phonophoresis describes the use of ultrasound for transdermal delivery of medication. Ultrasound enhances the distribution of the medication through the skin, provides a high concentration of the drug directly to the treatment site, and avoids risks that may be involved with injection of medication. Medications regularly used in phonophoresis include anti-inflammatory agents or analgesics. Phonophoresis is effective with both continuous and pulsed techniques.

Hydrotherapy

Hydrotherapy transfers heat through conduction or convection and is administered in tanks of varying size ranging from extremity whirlpool to Olympic size pools. The main therapeutic effects of hydrotherapy include wound care, unloading of weight, and reduction of edema. The specific instrument to be used depends on the treatment objectives and site of the pathology.

Properties of Water

Buoyancy
Archimedes' principle of buoyancy states that there is an upward force on the body when immersed in water equal to the amount of water that has been displaced by the body. The ability to float in water results from the body possessing a specific gravity less than that of water.

Hydrostatic pressure
Water exerts pressure that is perpendicular to the body and increases in proportion with the depth of immersion.

Resistance
Water molecules tend to attract to each other and provide resistance to movement of the body in the water. Resistance by water increases in proportion to speed of motion.

Specific Gravity

The computation for the specific gravity of water is equal to 1. The human body varies based on size and somatotype but typically has a specific gravity of less than 1 (average .974). Therefore, a person will generally float when fully submerged in water.

Specific Heat

The specific heat is the measure of the ability of a fluid to store heat. This is calculated as the amount of thermal energy required to increase the fluid's temperature by one unit. Water can store four times the heat as compared to air. Water's thermal conductivity is approximately 25 times faster then air at the same temperature.

Total Drag Force

The total drag force is comprised of profile drag, wave drag, and surface drag forces. This is a hydromechanic force exerted on a person submerged in water that normally opposes the direction of the body's motion.

Therapeutic Effects:

- Increase blood flow
- Increase core temperature
- Relaxation
- Pain relief
- Vasodilation
- Decrease abnormal tone
- Wound/debridement

Indications:

- Burn care
- Superficial heating or cooling
- Edema control
- Muscle strain
- Arthritis
- Desensitization of residual limb with contrast bath
- Pain management
- Wound care
- Decreased range of motion
- Pool therapy/exercise
- Sprain
- Joint stiffness
- Muscle spasm/spasticity

Contraindications:

- Peripheral vascular disease
- Gangrene
- Severe infection
- Urinary/fecal incontinence
- Advanced cardiovascular or pulmonary disease
- Buerger's disease with contrast bath
- Impaired circulation
- Renal infection
- Bleeding surface area
- Diminished sensation

Types of Hydrotherapy

Extremity Tank

An extremity tank is used for the distal upper or lower extremity. Approximate dimensions for the extremity tank are a depth of 18 to 24 inches, a length of 28 to 32 inches, and a width of 15 inches. (10-45 gallons)

Lowboy Tank

A lowboy tank is used for larger parts of the extremities and permits long sitting with water up to the midthoracic level. Approximate dimensions for the lowboy tank are a depth of 18 inches, a length of 52 to 65 inches, and a width of 24 inches. (90-105 gallons)

Highboy Tank

A highboy tank is used for larger parts of the extremities and the trunk and permits sitting in chest-high water with hips and knees flexed. Approximate dimensions for the highboy tank are a depth of 28 inches, a length of 36 to 48 inches, and a width of 20 to 24 inches. (60-105 gallons)

Hubbard Tank

The Hubbard tank is used for full-body immersion. Approximate dimensions for the Hubbard tank are a depth of four feet, a length of eight feet, and a width of six feet. Contraindications specific to full-body immersion include unstable blood pressure and incontinence. Treatment time ranges between 10 to 20 minutes. Temperature should not exceed 100 degrees Fahrenheit (39 degrees Celsius). (425 gallons)

Therapeutic Pool

A therapeutic pool is used for exercising in a water medium. Temperature should range between 79 to 98 degrees Fahrenheit (26 to 37 degrees Celsius) depending on patient age, health status, and goals.

Treatment Temperature Guidelines

Degrees F	Degrees C	Purpose
32 - 79 °F	(0 - 26 °C)	Acute inflammation of distal extremities
79 - 92 °F	(26 - 33 °C)	Exercise
92 - 96 °F	(33 - 36 °C)	Wound care, spasticity
96 - 98 °F	(36 - 37 °C)	Cardiopulmonary compromise, treatment of burns
99 - 104 °F	(37 - 40 °C)	Pain management
104 - 110 °F	(40 - 44 °C)	Chronic rheumatoid or osteoarthritis, increased range of motion

Treatment Parameters for whirlpool: Prior to treatment the therapist should explain the sensations the patient will experience during treatment. Select the water temperature based on diagnosis and goals and assist the patient into a comfortable position. Adjust and turn on the turbine. Monitor the patient's vital signs and level of comfort. Treatment time ranges between 10 and 30 minutes. Exercise can be performed during whirlpool as indicated. After treatment dry and inspect the treated area.

Treatment Parameters for pool therapy: In addition to general contraindications for superficial or deep heating, specific contraindications include incontinence, open areas, fear of water, confusion, and significant respiratory pathology. The therapist should assist the patient as needed into the pool and throughout treatment. The therapist must stay with the patient and monitor vital signs and tolerance to activity. Advantages of pool therapy include decreased weight bearing with the assistance of buoyancy, easier handling by the therapist, control over the amount of resistance during exercise, and diminished risk of falling with activity. Recommended populations for pool therapy include patients with arthritis, musculoskeletal injuries, neurological deficits, spinal cord injury, CVA, multiple sclerosis, and selected cardiopulmonary diagnoses. The tank must be thoroughly cleaned after each use with a disinfectant and antibacterial agent.

Contrast Bath

A contrast bath utilizes alternating heat and cold in order to decrease edema in a distal extremity. The alternating vasodilation and vasoconstriction is theorized to stimulate local circulation and systemic circulation to a lesser degree. The technique provides good contact over irregularly shaped areas, allows for movement during treatment, and assists with pain management. Disadvantages include potential intolerance to cold, dependent positioning, and lack of credible research to support the theory of contrast baths and its effect on edema.

Treatment Parameters: The therapist should position the patient so that both baths are accessible to the patient. The treatment should begin with the patient's distal extremity immersed in the hot whirlpool with a temperature between 100 to 110 degrees Fahrenheit (27 to 40 degrees Celsius) for three to four minutes. The patient should then place the distal extremity into the cold bath with a temperature between 55 to 67 degrees Fahrenheit (13 to 20 degrees Celsius) for one minute. The patient should repeat this hot/cold sequence for 20-30 minutes. The patient should end the treatment in the hot whirlpool and then dry off immediately. Contrast baths are utilized

primarily with arthritis of the smaller joints, musculoskeletal sprains and strains, RSD, and to desensitize the residual limb of a patient status post amputation.

Mechanical Agents

Traction

Traction is a modality that applies mechanical forces to the body to separate joint surfaces and decrease pressure. The force can be applied manually by the therapist or mechanically by a machine. Traction is indicated for many diagnoses and allows for variation and adjustment of the established protocol based on individual patient need. Traction affects many of the body's systems and requires ongoing monitoring and reassessment of treatment parameters. Mechanical traction, self-traction, manual traction, and positional traction are commonly utilized techniques.

Therapeutic Effects:

• Joint distraction	• Muscle relaxation
• Soft tissue stretching	• Joint mobility
• Reduction of disk protrusion	

Indications:

• Nerve impingement	• Joint hypomobility
• Herniated or protruding disc	• Paraspinal muscle spasm
• Subacute joint inflammation	• Degenerative joint disease
• Spondylolisthesis	• Osteophyte formation

Contraindications:

• When motion is contraindicated	• Acute inflammatory response
• Joint instability	• Acute sprain
• Tumor	• Osteoporosis
• Pregnancy	• Fracture

Treatment Parameters: Mechanical traction can be performed to the cervical or lumbar spine. All halters and belts should be secured and the patient instructed in what to expect from treatment. The therapist should then set the time of treatment, force of pull, and determine static or intermittent control with hold and relax ratio settings. During treatment the patient should have the ability to stop the machine and call for help. Treatment time varies based on diagnosis and therapeutic goals and falls between five and 20 minutes. To initiate cervical traction the therapist should position the patient in supine with approximately 25-35 degrees of neck flexion or in a sitting position. Cervical traction should start with a force between 10-15 pounds and progress to 7% of the patient's body weight as tolerated for separation of the vertebrae. Application of lumbar traction should be performed in supine or prone. The force of lumbar traction is dependent on the goals of treatment and should be set with a force of less than half of the body weight for the initial treatment. Traction force of 25 – 50 pounds is recommended when initiating mechanical lumber traction. Force of up to 50% of the body weight is required for actual separation of the vertebrae.

Compression

Compression is a physical agent that applies a mechanical force that increases pressure on the treated body part. Compression works to keep venous and lymphatic flow from pooling into the interstitial space. Static compression utilizes bandaging and compression garments to shape residual limbs, control edema, prevent abnormal scar formation, and reduce the risk of deep vein thrombosis. Intermittent compression with a pneumatic device is primarily used to reduce chronic or post-traumatic edema and requires adjusting the parameters of inflation pressure, on/off ratio, and total treatment time. Compression appliances have coupled compression with therapeutic cold and electrical stimulation.

Therapeutic Effects:
• Control of peripheral edema	• Improve lymphatic and venous return
• Shaping of residual limb	• Prevention of deep vein thrombosis
• Management of scar formation	

Indications:
• Lymphedema	• Edema
• New residual limb	• Stasis ulcers
• Risk for deep vein thrombosis	• Hypertrophic scarring

Contraindications:
• Malignancy of treated area	• Infection of treated area
• Deep vein thrombosis	• Pulmonary edema
• Unstable or acute fracture	• Circulatory obstruction
• Heart failure	

Treatment Parameters: The therapist must ask the patient to remove all jewelry and ensure appropriate fit of the compression sleeve prior to treatment. The patient should be placed in a comfortable position with the extremity elevated. Blood pressure and girth measurements should be recorded. The therapist should apply the stockinette over the extremity and adjust the compression sleeve. The therapist should set parameters based on desired effect. A 3:1 ratio is generally used for on/off time with inflation between 40 to 100 seconds and deflation between 10 to 35 seconds. Inflation pressure generally ranges from 30 to 80 mm Hg and should not exceed the patient's diastolic blood pressure. Treatment of the upper extremities generally requires between 30 and 60 mm Hg of inflation pressure while treatment of the lower extremities generally requires between 40 and 80 mm Hg of inflation pressure. Treatment time varies based on diagnosis from two to four hours and is utilized from three times per week to three times per day. The patient should have a call bell and should be monitored for comfort and blood pressure readings throughout treatment. When treatment time is complete the therapist should reassess the extremity, girth measurements, and blood pressure readings.

Additional Physical Agents

Ultraviolet (UV)

Ultraviolet light is a form of energy that is used therapeutically and absorbed one to two millimeters into the skin. Ultraviolet is divided into UV-A, UV-B, and UV-C according to wavelength and place on the electromagnetic spectrum. Treatment parameters and application are based on diagnosis, desired effects, and minimal erythemal dose. The most effective use of UV is to treat skin disorders.

Therapeutic Effects:
• Facilitate healing	• Tanning
• Exfoliation	• Bacteriocidal effects
• Vitamin D production	• Thickening of epidermis
• Increase pigmentation	

Indications:
• Acne	• Chronic ulcer/wound
• Psoriasis	• Osteomalacia/rickets
• Tetany	• Sinusitis
• Vitamin D deficiency	

Contraindications:
• Photosensitive medication	• Renal or hepatic pathology
• Lupus erythematosus	• Diabetes mellitus
• Tuberculosis	• Pellagra
• Herpes simplex	

Treatment Parameters: Prior to treatment with UV a therapist must obtain a minimal erythemal dose (MED). This is the time of exposure needed to produce an area of mild redness between eight and 24 hours after treatment. The MED is tested by placing a piece of paper with five one-inch cut outs over a patient's anterior forearm. The patient should have all other non-treatment areas covered as well as wear protective goggles. Once the lamp is warmed up it should be positioned at a 90-degree angle to the area of treatment (for maximum absorption) and at a distance between 24 to 40 inches from the forearm. The squares should be exposed sequentially in 15 second increments for 15, 30, 45, 60, and 75 seconds. Visual inspection after an 8-hour period will determine the MED. Parameters including distance from the lamp, position of the lamp at a 90-degree angle to the treatment site, and MED must remain consistent over the course of treatment. The treatment time should increase each consecutive treatment day since the skin adapts to UV exposure. The therapist should utilize a stopwatch and continue with ongoing visual inspection during all treatment sessions.

Massage

Massage is a manual therapeutic modality that produces physiologic effects through different types of stroking, rubbing, and pressure. Massage is capable of producing mechanical and reflexive effects.

Massage Techniques

Effleurage: Effleurage is a massage technique that is usually light in stroke and produces a reflexive response. The technique is performed at the beginning and at the end of a massage to allow the patient to relax and should be directed towards the heart. Effleurage can be applied as a deep stroke to produce both a mechanical and a reflexive response.

Friction: Friction is a massage technique that incorporates small circular motions over a trigger point or muscle spasm. This is a deep massage technique that penetrates into the depth of a muscle and attempts to reduce edema, loosen adhesions, and relieve muscle spasm. Friction massage is used quite frequently with chronic inflammation or with overuse injuries.

Petrissage: Petrissage is a massage technique described as kneading where the muscle is squeezed and rolled under the therapist's hands. The goal of petrissage is to loosen adhesions, improve lymphatic return, and facilitate removal of metabolic waste from the treatment area. Petrissage must provide a distal to proximal sequence of kneading over the muscle.

Petrissage can be performed with two hands over larger muscle groups or with as few as two fingers over smaller muscles.

Tapotement: Tapotement is a massage technique that provides stimulation through rapid and alternating movements such as tapping, hacking, cupping, and slapping. The primary purpose of tapotement is to enhance circulation and stimulate peripheral nerve endings.

Vibration: Vibration is a massage technique that places the therapist's hands or fingers firmly over an area and utilizes a rapid shaking motion that causes vibration to the treatment area. The therapist initiates this motion from the forearm while maintaining firm contact on the treatment area. Vibration is used primarily for relaxation.

Therapeutic Effects:

Increase lymphatic circulation	Stimulate reflexive effects
Improve circulation	Reduction of edema
Removal of metabolic waste	Alters pain transmission
Decrease muscle atrophy	Decrease muscle spasm
Decrease anxiety and tension	Loosen adhesions
Facilitate healing	Relaxation

Indications:

Pain	Trigger point
Decreased range of motion	Muscle spasm and cramping
Edema	Scar tissue
Adhesions	Bursitis
Myositis	Tendonitis
Lactic acid accumulation	Intermittent claudication
Migraine or general headache	Raynaud's syndrome

Contraindications:

Infection	Acute injury
Arteriosclerosis	Embolus
Thrombus	Cancer
Cellulitis	

Treatment Parameters: The patient should be comfortable and properly draped prior to the initiation of treatment. The therapist's hands must be clean, dry, and warm. The therapist must be positioned in an efficient posture during treatment and maintain the required pressure and rhythm based on the goals of treatment. The massage should start using the effleurage technique. The amount of time required for each treatment is dependent on the body part and therapeutic goal. Generally, the back requires 15 minutes as opposed to a smaller area or joint that requires eight to ten minutes. The intensity should progressively increase and then decrease, using effleurage again to end the treatment session. Lubricant is indicated with all strokes except friction massage.

Electrotherapy

Electrotherapy is utilized in physical therapy for various reasons including facilitation of skeletal muscle contraction, stimulation of denervated muscle, pain management, to retard muscle atrophy, osteogenesis, driving medications through the skin, and wound management.

Therapeutic Effects:

- Relaxation of muscle spasm
- Muscle strengthening
- Improve range of motion
- Facilitate wound healing
- Decrease edema
- Eliminate disuse atrophy
- Muscle re-education
- Increase local circulation
- Facilitate bone repair
- Decrease pain

Indications:

- Muscle spasms
- Muscle weakness
- Pain
- Decreased range of motion
- Idiopathic scoliosis
- Fracture
- Joint effusion
- Facial neuropathy
- Muscle atrophy
- Open wound/ulcer
- Bell's palsy
- Use with labor and delivery
- Stress incontinence
- Shoulder subluxation

Contraindications:

- Cardiac pacemaker
- Patient with a bladder stimulator
- Use over carotid sinus
- Seizure disorders
- Phlebitis
- Malignancy
- Use over a pregnant uterus
- Cardiac arrhythmia
- Osteomyelitis

Electrode Configuration

Monopolar Technique: The stimulating or active electrode is placed over the target area. A second dispersive electrode is placed at another site away from the target area. Typically the active electrode is smaller than the dispersive electrode. This technique is used with wounds, ionotophoresis, and in the treatment of edema.

Bipolar Technique: Two active electrodes are placed over the target area. Typically the electrodes are equal in size. This technique is used for muscle weakness, neuromuscular facilitation, spasms, and range of motion.

Quadripolar Technique: Two electrodes from two separate stimulating circuits are positioned so that the individual currents intersect with each other. This technique is utilized with interferential current.

Electrode Size

When using a smaller electrode it is particularly important to understand that since the current density is quite high compared to a larger electrode, the patient will be more susceptible to pain and potential tissue damage.

Small Electrodes	Large Electrodes
- Increased current density - Increased impedance - Decreased current flow	- Decreased current density - Decreased impedance - Increased current flow

Treatment Parameters

Direct Current

Direct current, also referred to as Galvanic current, is characterized by a constant flow of electrons from the anode to the cathode (for a period of greater than one second) without interruption. Polarity remains constant and is determined by the therapist based on treatment goals. Iontophoresis uses direct current.

Alternating Current

Alternating current is characterized by polarity that continuously changes from positive to negative with the change in direction of current flow. Alternating current is biphasic, symmetrical or asymmetrical, and is characterized by a waveform that is sinusoidal in shape. Alternating current is used in muscle retraining, spasticity, and stimulation of denervated muscle.

Interferential Current

Interferential current combines two high frequency alternating waveforms that are biphasic. This type of current is used for deep muscle stimulation. Interferential current attempts to reach deeper tissues using the higher frequencies of each waveform along with the overall shorter pulse widths. Interferential uses a frequency of 50-120 pulses per second and a pulse width of 50-150 microseconds for pain management; and a frequency of

20-50 pulses per second and a pulse width of 100-200 microseconds for muscle contraction.

Indications:

- Pain management
- Urinary incontinence
- Edema management
- Osteoarthritic pain
- Migraines

Contraindications:

- Malignancy
- With all types of electronic implants
- During the first trimester of pregnancy
- Over lower abdomen/uterus during pregnancy
- Over the anterior transcervical area

Common Methods of Delivery

- Bipolar
- Quadripolar
- Quadripolar with automatic vector scan

Bipolar Delivery

Bipolar delivery utilizes two electrodes connected to a single channel with two medium sinusoidal currents. For example, one medium-frequency sinusoidal current produces 3,000 Hz and another medium-frequency sinusoidal current produces 3,050 Hz. The interference between the two currents creates an amplitude modulated interferential current with a beat frequency of 50 bps (beats per second). This is the net difference between the two currents. The bipolar method allows for the interferential current to be modulated prior to delivery of the current to the electrodes.

Quadripolar Delivery

Quadripolar delivery utilizes four electrodes with each pair connected to a single channel. The interference between the currents using this method occurs at the level of the treatment area within the targeted tissues (as opposed to the previous method where it occurs prior to the electrode level). When the currents intersect at a 90 degree angle the maximum resultant amplitude occurs halfway between the two lines of current. The current treatment area creates a four-leaf clover shaped treatment field within the area between all four electrodes.

Quadripolar with Automatic Vector Scan

The quadripolar method with automatic vector scan is used when there is a need to increase the size of the field of current that is created by the quadripolar method. One of the circuits is allowed to vary in amplitude and this allows the field pattern to automatically rotate between the two lines of current. The field is circular in shape as opposed to the cloverleaf and allows for the overall larger field of current.

Russian Current

Russian current is a medium frequency polyphasic waveform. The intensity of this form of alternating current is produced in a 50 burst per second interval with a pulse width range of 50-200 microseconds, and an interburst interval of 10 milliseconds. Russian current is a type of NMES or FES and is believed to augment muscle strengthening by depolarizing both sensory and motor nerve fibers resulting in tetanic contractions that are painless and stronger than those made voluntarily by the patient. Since the mode of delivery is theoretically painless, the increased current amplitude allows the deeper motor nerve fibers to depolarize concomitantly.

Indications:

- The primary indication is to strengthen the muscle groups of otherwise healthy individuals and athletes

Contraindications:

- Over the abdominal and pelvic area of a pregnant woman
- Over hemorrhage area
- Malignancy
- Over the anterior cervical area
- Over electronic implants

Treatment Parameters: Prior to treatment the therapist should ensure that the patient's skin is clean and dry. The electrode orientation should be placed parallel to the muscle fibers along the line of pull of the muscle group. The electrode placement can be monopolar, bipolar, quadripolar, or multipolar in arrangement. Current transmission relies on a coupling gel that is applied to the entire treatment surface area of each electrode. Russian stimulation has an average peak current amplitude of 100 mA, 50 bursts per second, with an on/off time ratio of 10/50. A popular training protocol with Russian current suggests a treatment of 10 evoked contractions with a 10 second contraction and a 50 second rest period between each of the ten contractions.

Neuromuscular Electrical Stimulation (NMES)

Neuromuscular electrical stimulation (NMES) or functional electrical stimulation (FES) is a technique used to facilitate skeletal muscle activity. Stimulation of an innervated muscle occurs when an electrical stimulus of appropriate intensity and duration is administered to the corresponding peripheral nerve. Electrical stimulation of a denervated muscle has been used in an attempt to maintain the muscle, however, there is little documented evidence that supports this treatment option. Neuromuscular electrical stimulation is a commonly used therapeutic technique to facilitate the return of controlled functional muscular activity or to maintain postural alignment until recovery occurs.

***Treatment Parameters*:** The patient should be positioned comfortably. The therapist uses a bipolar electrode placement over the target muscle. An interrupted or surged current is utilized with a range of 20 – 40 pulses per second and an on time of six to ten seconds followed by an off time of approximately 50 – 60 seconds in order to avoid immediate motor fatigue. Treatment time ranges from 15 to 20 minutes and can be repeated several times each day.

Transcutaneous Electrical Nerve Stimulation (TENS)

Transcutaneous electrical nerve stimulation is widely used for acute and chronic pain management. Areas of use include obstetrics, temporomandibular joint pain, and post-operative pain. The main therapeutic effects of TENS include pain relief through the gate control theory of Wall and Melzak or the endogenous opiate pain control theory. TENS units are portable and indicated for home use.

Indications:
- Post-operative pain
- During labor and delivery
- Bone fractures
- Chronic pain
- Trigeminal neuralgia
- Phantom pain
- For antiemetic effects
- Improved blood blow

Contraindications:
- Cardiac pacemakers (relative contraindication)
- Epilepsy
- During the first trimester of pregnancy
- Over lower abdomen/uterus during pregnancy
- Over the anterior transcervical area

***Treatment Parameters*:** The waveforms used are monophasic pulsatile current or biphasic pulsatile current with a spiked square, rectangular or sinewave form. Electrode placement may be based on sites of nerve roots, trigger points, acupuncture sites or key points of pain and

sensitivity. Net polarity is normally equal to zero. If the waveform is unbalanced there will be an accumulation of charges that will lead to skin irritation under the electrodes. Generally, the parameters when using TENS include a pulse duration that can vary from 20 – 400 microseconds; pulse frequency that varies in range from 1 – 200 Hz; and current amplitude from .1 – 120 mA. Sensory level stimulation requires the patient to experience perceptible tingling.

**TENS	Frequency	Duration	Amplitude
Conventional	50–50HZ	20–100 microseconds	10–30mA
Acupuncture-like (AL)	1–4 HZ	100–200 microseconds	30–80mA
Pulse burst	70–100 Hz/burst	40–75 microseconds	30–60mA
Brief intense (high-intensity)	70–100 Hz/burst	150–200 microseconds	30–60mA

**This chart demonstrates a typical range for each type of TENS, however, there are discrepancies that exist from author to author regarding the appropriate settings for TENS as well as each diagnoses' parameters. Thus, this chart is to be used as a guideline for overall understanding of the mechanism of action behind each type of TENS and its outcome based on those settings.

Iontophoresis

Iontophoresis is the process by which medications are induced through the skin into the body by means of continuous direct current electrical stimulation. The medication is separated into ions based on the polarity of the current.

Acidic Reaction: A patient may have an acidic reaction from the iontophoresis treatment that is sclerotic in nature and can cause hardening of the skin over time.

Alkaline Reaction: A patient may have an alkaline reaction from the iontophoresis treatment that is sclerolytic in nature and can soften the skin over time, exposing it to the risk of irritation and burn during further treatment.

Buffering: Buffering is a technique used to stabilize the pH of the skin during iontophoresis by placing buffering agents into the electrode pads that cover the designated drug reservoir area within the electrode. This maintains the hydrogen concentration and avoids any significant pH change during treatment.

Electrolysis: Electrolysis is a term used to describe the decomposition of a compound that results from passing an electrical current through it.

Electron Exchange: Electron exchange occurs during iontophoresis where there is an exchange between the ions within the solutions and the electrodes.

Redox Reaction: A redox reaction is the decomposition of water when an electrical current is passed through it. Water will be reduced to a net accumulation of hydrogen ions (H+) under the anode and hydroxyl ions (OH-) under the cathode.

Treatment Parameters: The patient should be positioned comfortably, but should never lie on top of the electrodes. The unit should be set to continuous direct current. Polarity must be set to the same polarity as the ion solution. The ion solution should be massaged into the treatment site or placed into the designated space within the electrode. The therapist must ensure that the conductive surface area of the negative electrode (cathode) is twice the size of the conductive surface area of the positive electrode (anode) regardless of which one is the active electrode. The active electrode should be placed over the target area and the dispersive electrode should be placed as far as possible from the active electrode. The therapist should secure the electrodes and slowly increase the intensity towards a maximum of five milliamperes. Treatment should last 15 to 20 minutes. Additional time is required for treatment at an intensity of less than five milliamperes. The therapist must monitor the patient during treatment to ensure that the skin is not burned under the electrode. Upon completion of treatment the therapist must slowly decrease the intensity, remove the electrodes, and provide the area of skin under the negative electrode with a thorough cleaning followed by the application of lotion to minimize irritation.

| Therapeutic Ions and Charge ||
+ (Positive charge)	– (Negative charge)
Lidocaine	Acetate
Hydrocortisone	Dexamethasone
Histamine	Salicylate
Lithium	Iodine
Magnesium	Chlorine
Zinc	Tap water (+ and –)

High-Voltage Pulsed Current (HVPC)

High-volt pulsed current, also known as high-volt or high-voltage pulsed galvanic current, is a twin-peak (pair of monophasic spike waveforms) monophasic, pulsed current. It is differentiated from other stimulators by the high electromotive forces produced. HVPC has a phase duration of 5-20 microseconds (fixed in most machines), a short pulse duration (includes both spikes and the interspike interval) that ranges between 100-200

microseconds, and voltage greater than 150V to a maximum of 500V. There is one large dispersive pad along with one, two, or four active electrodes. The active electrodes can be positive or negative in polarity based on the treatment goals.

Indications:
- Wound management
- Pain management
- Soft tissue edema
- Levator ani syndrome
- Muscle spasm
- Muscle weakness
- Bell's palsy

Contraindications:
- Cardiac pacemakers (relative contraindication)
- Over heavy scarring tissues
- Malignancy
- Over lower abdomen/uterus during pregnancy
- Over the anterior transcervical area
- Over osteomyelitis
- Anterior cervical region

Treatment Parameters: General treatment parameters are found above. An example of using HVPS for wound healing is as follows: Prepare the patient so the patient is comfortable and the wound is clean from any exudate or foreign materials. The therapist must wash the hands and apply proper protective garments. Secure one electrode over the wound (using a warm sterile gauze and sponge) and the other over healthy skin a minimum of 5 cm from the wound itself. The polarity should be in reversal mode so that it allows for 50% of treatment with negative polarity and 50% of treatment with positive polarity. The frequency is generally 30-200 pps, amplitude 1-500V and duration of treatment from 10-60 minutes per session. Dermal wounds should be treated five to seven days per week for best results.

Electromyography

Electromyography is the science of evaluating motor units (the anterior horn cell, its axon, neuromuscular junctions and muscle fibers innervated by the unit) through the use of intramuscular needle electrodes or surface electrodes. Surface electrodes are used to monitor larger muscle groups while indwelling electrodes are used for small or deep muscles or when there is a need to record a single motor unit potential.

Muscles at rest: A normal relaxed muscle should exhibit electrical silence (no electrical potentials). Spontaneous potentials during rest are significant abnormal findings.

Abnormal Potentials

Spontaneous

Fibrillation potentials: indicative of lower motor neuron disease

Positive sharp wave: denervated muscle disorders at rest, primary muscle disease such as muscular dystrophy

Fasciculations: irritation/degeneration of anterior horn cell, nerve root compression or muscle spasms

Repetitive discharges: lesions of anterior horn cell and peripheral nerves; and myopathies

Voluntary

Polyphasic potentials: myopathies; muscle or peripheral nerve involvement

Common Muscles used for Insertion of Needle Electrodes			
Upper Extremity		**Lower Extremity**	
C5-6	Lateral deltoid	L4-5	Tibialis anterior
C5-6	Biceps brachii	L5-S1	Peroneus longus
C6-7	Triceps brachii	S1-2	Gastrocnemius
C6-7	Flexor carpi radialis	L2, 3, 4	Vastus medialis
C8-T1	Abductor pollicis brevis	L4-5, S1	Tensor fasciae latae
C8-T1	First dorsal interossei	L5, S1-2	Gluteus maximus
C7-8	Extensor indicis propius	L5, S1-2	Hamstrings

Biofeedback

Biofeedback is a modality that uses an electromechanical device to provide visual and/or auditory feedback. Biofeedback can be utilized to receive information related to motor performance, kinesthetic performance or physiological response. Biofeedback can measure peripheral skin temperature, changes in blood volume through vasodilation and vasoconstriction using finger phototransmission, sweat gland activity, and electrical activity during muscle contraction. Electromyographic biofeedback is the most commonly used biofeedback modality in the clinical setting.

Biofeedback Measures:

- Muscle activity
- Heart rate
- Balance
- Abnormal/normal movement
- Skin temperature
- Blood pressure
- Posture

Types of Biofeedback:

- Myoelectric/electromyographic biofeedback (EMG-BF)
- Position biofeedback
- Blood pressure biofeedback
- Respiratory biofeedback
- Sphincter control biofeedback
- Temperature and blood flow biofeedback
- Electroencephalographic biofeedback

Therapeutic Effects:

- Muscle relaxation
- Improve muscle strength
- Decrease muscle spasm
- Neuromuscular control
- Decrease accessory muscle use
- Decrease pain

Indications:

- Muscle spasm
- Pain
- Spinal cord injury
- Urinary incontinence
- Improve neuromuscular control
- Muscle weakness
- Hemiplegia
- Cerebral palsy
- Bowel incontinence
- Promote relaxation

Contraindications:

- Any condition where muscle contraction is detrimental
- Skin irritation at electrode site

Treatment Guidelines

- ✓ Biofeedback normally uses visual and/or auditory feedback related to the amount of electrical activity detected
- ✓ Biofeedback does not measure muscle contraction but rather the electrical activity associated with muscle contraction
- ✓ Noise is any extraneous electrical activity not produced by the contraction of the muscle
- ✓ Two active electrodes and one ground electrode in a bipolar arrangement best deletes "noise"

✓ Surface electrodes with some form of conduction gel are required to adhere to prepared, clean skin
✓ The electrodes should be placed parallel to the direction of the muscle fibers
✓ Set the level of sensitivity on the device relative to the treatment goals (use low-level sensitivity settings for muscle re-education, use a high-level sensitivity settings for relaxation).

Treatment Parameters: Prior to treatment the therapist should ensure that the patient's skin is clean and dry. The two active electrodes should be placed parallel to the muscle fibers and close to each other. The reference or ground electrode can be placed anywhere on the body, but is often secured between the two active electrodes. The signals are transmitted to a differential amplifier and information is conveyed through visual and audio feedback.

The treatment for muscle re-education should begin with the patient performing a maximal muscle contraction. The sensitivity of the biofeedback unit should be set at a low sensitivity setting and adjusted so that the patient can perform the repetitions at a ratio of two-thirds of the maximal muscle contraction. Isometric contractions should continue for six to ten seconds with relaxation in between each contraction. Treatment duration for a single muscle group is five to ten minutes. The treatment for muscle relaxation requires a high sensitivity setting and a similar electrode placement with active electrodes initially positioned close to each other. As the patient improves with relaxation, the electrodes should be placed further apart and the sensitivity setting increased. During this treatment, the patient may also benefit from adjunct relaxation techniques such as imagery. Treatment duration of 10 to 15 minutes is usually adequate to attain relaxation.

Electrical Equipment Care and Maintenance

The use of electrical equipment can be a potential hazard to both the therapist and the patient. The following is a very abbreviated list of techniques that can minimize the risks of electrical equipment danger.

- Utilize experts to conduct routine inspections to ensure that you meet or exceed all local, state, and federal operation standards.
- Never use a piece of electrical equipment until you have a complete understanding of all aspects of its operation.

- Have routine scheduled service on all electrical equipment at or before the manufacturer's suggested service dates.
- Have repairs performed immediately after the identification of a potential problem.
- Conduct routine inspections of all electrical equipment to identify potential problems.
- Display electrical equipment operation manuals in an accessible location for staff members to use as a resource.

Ground-Fault Circuit Interrupter (GFCI)

A GFCI is a device designed to cut off electrical supply to a piece of equipment if it detects any form of leakage or ground-fault. This prevents a staff member or patient from becoming a ground-fault for electrical current resulting in harmful or deadly injuries.

- All electrical outlets should have the three-prong GFCI outlets
- Ensure all line-powered equipment has a testing seal (maximum leakage of a current < 1 mA)
- Never use extension cords
- Unplug all line-powered equipment at the end of each day
- A sticker should be placed on equipment noting the last inspection/maintenance
- Keep an updated log for all equipment used in the physical therapy department

Electrotherapy Terminology

Accommodation: Accommodation is an occurrence whereby a nerve and muscle membrane's threshold for excitability increases secondary to a stimulation by a pulse that has a slow phase rise time. The quicker the rise time, the less the nerve can accommodate to the impulse.

Alternating current (biphasic): Alternating current allows for the constant change in flow of ions.

Ampere: An ampere is a unit of measure used to describe the rate of current.

Amplitude: Amplitude refers to the magnitude of current. Amplitude controls are often labeled intensity or voltage.

Anode: The anode used during direct current electrotherapy is the positively charged electrode that attracts negative ions.

Biphasic: Biphasic describes a pulse that moves in one direction, returns to baseline, then in the other direction and back to baseline again within a predetermined amount of time.

- ### Types of Biphasic Pulse
  Symmetrical: the positive phase is identical to the negative phase
  Asymmetrical: the positive phase and the negative phase are not identical in shape
  Balanced: the positive phase's electrical charge is equal to the negative phase's electrical charge
  Unbalanced: the positive phase and negative phase do not have identical electrical charges

Burst: A burst is an interrupted group of pulses that are delivered in a finite series and a predetermined frequency.

Capacitance: Capacitance is a property of an insulator that allows for the storage of energy when the opposing surfaces of the insulator have an electrical potential difference.

Cathode: The cathode used during direct current electrotherapy is the negatively charged electrode that attracts positive ions.

Chronaxie: Chronaxie is a testing procedure used to measure the amount of time required to produce a small muscle contraction at a particular intensity.

Conductance: Conductance describes the ease at which a particular material will allow current flow (mho).

Current: Current describes the flow of electrons from one place to another.

Direct current (monophasic or Galvanic): Direct current refers to the constant unidirectional flow of ions. The direction of the current is dependent on polarity.

Duration of stimulus/Duration of rest: Duration of stimulus/duration of rest refers to the time period of stimulation and the time period of rest between periods of stimulation. The controls that correspond to the periods of stimulation and rest are labeled on time and off time.

Duty cycle: Duty cycle refers to the percentage of time that electrical current is on in relation to the entire treatment time.

Electrical impedance: Electrical impedance is the resistance of a tissue to electrical current.

Frequency: Frequency determines the number of pulses delivered through each channel per second. Frequency controls are often labeled rate.

High-volt current: High-volt current is characterized by a waveform greater than 150 volts with a short pulse duration. High-volt is intermittent and is used for deeper tissue penetration.

Impedance: Impedance is the property of a substance that provides resistance to the flow of current by offering an alternate current.

Inductance: Inductance describes how easily a certain material will induce an electromotive force (emf) within a circuit.

Interpulse interval: The interpulse interval is the period of time of electrical inactivity between each pulse, usually expressed in microseconds or milliseconds.

Ion: An ion is a positively or negatively charged atom.

Low-volt current: Low-volt current is characterized by a waveform of less than 150 volts and is used for neuromuscular stimulation.

Monophasic: Monophasic describes a pulse that has either a positive or negative polarity and moves in only one direction from a zero baseline and returns to the baseline within a predetermined amount of time.

Negative ion: A negative ion has gained one or more electrons and possesses a negative charge.

Ohm's law: Ohm's law describes the current of an electrical circuit. There is a direct proportional relationship between current and voltage and an indirect proportional relationship between current and resistance.

Positive ion: A positive ion has lost one or more electrons and possesses a positive charge.

Pulse: A pulse is one individual waveform.

Pulse duration: The pulse duration is the amount of time that it takes to complete all phases of a single pulse (which is also termed the positive phase of the waveform). Pulse duration controls are often labeled pulse width.

Pulsed current (interrupted): Pulsed current allows for a non-continuous flow of either alternating or direct current with periods of no electrical activity.

Ramp: Ramp refers to the number of seconds it takes for the amplitude to gradually increase or decrease to the maximum value set by the amplitude control.

Resistance: Resistance describes the ability of a material to oppose the flow of ions through it.

Rheobase: Rheobase is the minimal intensity used with a long current duration that produces a small muscle contraction.

Volt: A volt is a unit of measure of electrical power or electromotive force.

Waveform: A waveform is the consistent pattern of a current measured on an oscilloscope.

Chapter Eight
Education

Psychology

Maslow's Hierarchy of Needs

Maslow's hierarchy of needs hypothesizes that there is a hierarchy of biogenic and psychogenic needs that individuals must progress through. In order to move to a higher level of needs an individual must attain the objectives associated with the previous level. In essence an individual must achieve basic or fundamental needs before moving to upper level needs.

Self-actualization needs: The need to realize one's full potential as a human being.

Esteem needs: The need to feel good about oneself and one's capabilities; to be respected by others, and to receive recognition and appreciation.

Affiliative needs: The need for security, stability, and a safe environment.

Physiological needs: The need for basic things necessary in order to survive such as food, water, and shelter.

Classical Conditioning (Pavlov)

Classical conditioning is a process where learning occurs when an unconditioned stimulus (food) is repeatedly preceded by a neutral stimulus (bell), the neutral stimulus serves as a conditioned stimulus and the learned reaction that results is termed the conditioned response. In order to maintain a conditioned response the conditioned and unconditioned stimuli must occasionally be paired.

Operant Conditioning (B.F. Skinner)

Operant conditioning is a process where learning occurs when an individual engages in specific behaviors in order to receive certain consequences.

Positive reinforcement: Administering desirable consequences to individuals who perform a specific behavior.

Negative reinforcement: Removing undesirable consequences from individuals who perform a specific behavior.

Extinction: Removing selected variables that reinforce a specific behavior.

Punishment: Administering negative consequences to individuals who perform undesirable behaviors.

Reinforcement Frequency and Schedules:

Continuous reinforcement
   A behavior is reinforced every time it occurs.

Partial reinforcement
   A behavior is reinforced intermittently.

Fixed-interval schedule
   The period of time between the occurrences of each instance of reinforcement is fixed or set.

Variable-interval schedule
   The amount of time between reinforcements varies around a constant average.

Social Learning Theory

Social learning theory is a theory that takes into account the influence of thoughts and feelings in learning.

Vicarious learning: Learning that occurs when one person learns a behavior by observing another person perform the behavior.

Self-control: Self-discipline that allows a person to learn to perform a behavior even though there is no external pressure to do so.

Self-reinforcers: Consequences or rewards that individuals can supply to themselves.

Patient Education

Adult Learning

- Therapists must strive to make patient education sessions practical and useful for the patient.
- Failure to identify the relevance of the presented information will promote disinterest and decrease compliance.

Guidelines to Promote Adult Learning

- Design learning activities that will incorporate the patient's past experiences.
- Encourage the learner to play an active role in their educational program.
- Attempt to demonstrate the relevance of selected learning activities.
- Provide ample opportunities for practice and feedback.
- Recognize skill acquisition or objective improvement in patient performance.

Domains of Learning

Domains of learning are educational terms that describe various aspects of human behavior. The three most commonly recognized domains of learning are the cognitive, psychomotor, and affective domains. Recognizing the various levels of each of the domains can assist therapists to plan appropriate patient learning activities.

Affective domain: The affective domain is primarily concerned with attitudes, values, and emotions.
The domain consists of five specific levels: receiving, responding, valuing, organization, and characterization.

Cognitive domain: The cognitive domain is primarily concerned with knowledge and understanding.
The domain consists of six specific levels: knowledge, comprehension, application, analysis, synthesis, and evaluation.

Psychomotor domain: The psychomotor domain is primarily concerned with physical action or motor skill.
The domain consists of seven specific levels: perception, set, guided response, mechanism, complex overt response, adaptation, and origination.

Learning Style

Therapists can often obtain information related to a patient's preferred learning style by asking a few basic questions.

- ✓ Do you prefer to learn new information by observing, reading, listening or experiencing?
- ✓ Are you more comfortable learning in an active or passive manner?
- ✓ What increases your motivation to learn?

Teaching Methods

Individual

- Therapists most commonly instruct patients on an individual basis.
- The individual approach allows the therapist to focus on the needs of the learner and is the model of choice when the objectives of the session are unique to an individual patient.
- The individual approach allows the therapist to strengthen the patient/therapist bond and provides additional opportunities for specific feedback.

Group

- Therapists often instruct patients in a group.
- Group teaching may occur with patients, family members, staff, and support persons.
- Group teaching can be difficult if patients are not supportive of each other or if the learning needs of the group are diverse.
- Some patients may be intimidated by selected group members and tend to withdraw, while others may attempt to take control of the group.
- Since individuals typically receive less individual attention in a group it is critical for the therapist to regularly assess individual patient progress.
- Group teaching allows participants to support each other in the educational process and permits therapists to effectively use scarce resources such as time or money.
- Patients participating in group activities often feel a sense of camaraderie interacting with others who have similar personal experiences.

Guidelines for Effective Patient Education

- Attempt to establish a positive rapport with the patient.
- Assess the patient's readiness and motivation to learn.
- Attempt to identify the patient's preferred learning style and available resources.
- Identify potential barriers to patient progress.

- Design an individualized education program for the patient based on his/her medical condition and personal goals.
- Coordinate education with the other members of the health care team.
- Focus the majority of available time on the most important concepts.
- Provide clear and succinct communication to the patient.
- Use repetition to improve patient learning.
- Provide frequent feedback to the patient.
- Utilize appropriate teaching resources to facilitate patient learning.
- Assess the effectiveness of patient education.
- Modify the patient education program based on the assessment results.

Principles of Motivation

- Readiness to learn significantly influences motivation.
- Individuals respond differently to selected motivational strategies.
- Success is more motivating than failure.
- Internal motivation has a greater potential to contribute to meaningful and lasting change than external motivation.
- Positive patient/therapist relationship enhances motivation.
- Limited anxiety may serve to motivate, while excessive anxiety may debilitate.
- Affiliation and approval can be motivating.

Cultural Influences

- Understanding cultural differences in patients can assist therapists to function as more effective educators.
- Patient culture is influenced and shaped by society, community, family, personal values, and attitudes.
- Language barriers, nonverbal communication, and limited personal experience can serve as obstacles when educating patients with significant cultural differences.
- Therapists should embrace cultural diversity and avoid efforts to make patients conform to any particular norm or standard.
- Therapists must be cautious when interpreting specific language or behavior and avoid labeling patients as unmotivated or disinterested.
- Therapists should use available resources such as experienced staff members, interpreters or consultants as necessary to achieve desired outcomes.

Designing Effective Patient Education Materials

- Design the materials to convey only the necessary information.
- Emphasize essential information.
- Utilize active instructions such as "you" and avoid passive terms such as "patient."
- Larger print may be more desirable than smaller print.
- Avoid long sentences or complex medical terminology.
- Pictures or graphics should be used where appropriate to complement written information.
- Incorporate answers to frequently asked questions.
- Written materials should flow in a logical sequence.
- Written materials should utilize a reading level appropriate for the target audience.

Teaching Guidelines for Specific Patient Categories

Therapists often vary their approach when educating patients of various ages and ability. It is difficult to develop recommendations that apply to all patients in a given category, however, the following represent general guidelines for therapists to consider when treating selected patient categories.

Infants/Children

- Therapists should try to make therapy sessions with infants/children interactive.
- Sessions should include structured play and should be of relatively short duration.
- Frequent breaks and positive reinforcement will serve to increase the patient's level of participation.

Adolescents

- Therapists should try to assume the role of an advocate when working with adolescents.
- It is important for therapists to establish patients' trust and incorporate patient goals into the plan of care.
- Adolescents prefer to be treated like adults and may resent the presence of parents during therapy sessions.
- Therapists should provide patients with clear and concise instructions and offer frequent positive reinforcement.

Adults

- Therapists should involve adults in determining education outcomes.
- The education program should be compatible with the patient's daily routine and goals.

- Emphasizing the relevance of educational activities will serve to increase patient compliance.
- Therapists should be aware of the available patient support system and identify any barriers to progress.

Elderly

- Therapists may find it necessary to introduce new information gradually when working with the elderly.
- Special attention should be paid to identify signs of hearing loss or visual impairments.
- The elderly population often benefits from the social benefits of group activities.
- Education sessions for the elderly should not be longer in duration, however, the achievement of selected outcomes may require additional sessions.

Terminally Ill

- Therapists should incorporate patient goals as an integral component of any educational session for patients with terminal illness.
- Family members and other support personnel should be encouraged to participate in the educational session, however, it is important to provide the patient with the opportunity to make independent decisions whenever possible.
- Goals for the terminally ill patient often include maximizing function, safety, and comfort.
- Therapists may alter their teaching methods based on the current mental and physical well-being of the patient.

Cognitively Impaired

- The therapist should focus on the education of the caregiver and incorporate the patient whenever possible.
- When incorporating the patient in the session, instructions should be clear and concise and should be summarized though demonstration and pictures.
- Therapists should encourage the patient to compensate for any memory deficit.

Illiteracy

- Therapists should attempt to determine the literacy level of their patients.
- If a patient is determined to be illiterate the therapist may elect to modify language to use basic wording and short sentences.
- Demonstration, repetition, and pictures should be incorporated into educational sessions.
- Therapists may include more detailed written information in educational sessions if the patient has adequate support at home.

Stages of Dying

Elizabeth Kubler-Ross identified five stages in coming to terms with death after interviewing 500 terminally ill patients. The stages Kubler-Ross identified were denial, anger, bargaining, depression, and acceptance.

Denial

The denial stage is characterized by a failure of the individual to believe that his/her condition is terminal. Therapists should attempt to establish trust with a patient in this stage and avoid trying to make the patient accept their condition.

Anger

The anger stage is characterized by frustration and negative emotional feelings often directed at anyone the individual comes in contact with. Individuals often ask "Why me?" Therapists should avoid taking the anger personally and recognize that expressing anger is often a useful step for the individual to move beyond this stage.

Bargaining

The bargaining stage is characterized by the individual trying to negotiate with fate. The individual may try to make a deal with a higher being based on good behavior, compliance with an exercise program or dedication of their life to a specific cause. Therapists should facilitate discussion with the patient and serve as a good listener.

Depression

The depression stage is characterized by the individual expressing the depths of his/her anguish. The individual is often deeply depressed and may show little interest in any form of medical intervention. Therapists should listen to the individual and exhibit a great deal of patience during this stage.

Acceptance

The acceptance stage is characterized by the individual coming to terms with their fate. The individual may attempt to resolve any unfinished business and may experience a sense of inner peace. Therapists should encourage the individual and family to ask questions and attempt to spend meaningful time with the individual.

Education Concepts

Practice

Practice refers to repeated performance of an activity in order to learn or perfect a skill. There are several commonly used terms that describe various types of practice.

Massed practice: The practice time in a trial is greater than the amount of rest between trials.

Distributed practice: The amount of rest time between trials is equal to or is greater than the amount of practice time for each trial.

Constant practice: Practice of a given task under a uniform condition.

Variable practice: Practice of a given task under differing conditions.

Random practice: Varying practice amongst different tasks.

Blocked practice: Consistent practice of a single task.

Whole training: Practice of an entire task.

Part training: Practice of an individual component or selected components of a task.

Feedback

Therapists should provide patients with specific and timely feedback in a manner that will promote attainment of the learning objective.

Summary feedback: Provided at the end of a defined number of activities or at the conclusion of the entire session.

Immediate feedback: Provided at the conclusion of a given activity.

Intrinsic feedback: Provided by the individual's internal sensory system.

Extrinsic feedback: Provided by an external source such as a therapist, spouse or physician.

Team Models

Unidisciplinary: A single discipline provides patient care services.

Multidisciplinary: Several different disciplines are involved in providing patient care, however, the disciplines tend to function independently and communication occurs primarily through the medical record.

Interdisciplinary: Several different disciplines are involved in providing patient care. The disciplines function independently, however, routinely report to each other and may coordinate patient care.

Transdisciplinary: Numerous disciplines function as a collective unit to provide patient care services. Team goals are established rather than individual discipline goals and as a result, discipline specific boundaries tend to erode.

Chapter Nine
Research

Research Basics

Types of Research

Historical Research
Investigating, recording, analyzing, and interpreting the events of the past for the purpose of discovering generalizations that are helpful in understanding the past, the present, and to a limited extent, anticipating the future.

Descriptive Research
Recording, analyzing, and interpreting conditions that exist. Descriptive research involves some type of comparison or contrast and attempts to discover relationships between existing and non-manipulated variables.

Experimental Research
A description of what will result when certain variables are carefully controlled or manipulated. The focus is on variable relationships.

Ethical Considerations

Informed Consent
Recruitment of volunteers for experimentation must involve the subject's complete understanding of the procedures, risks, and demands that may be made.

Confidentiality
The researcher must hold all information gathered in an experiment in strict confidence, maintaining the subject's anonymity at all times.

Protection from Harm or Danger
When using treatments that may have a temporary or permanent effect on a subject, the researcher must take all precautions to preserve the subject's well-being.

Knowledge of Outcome
Subjects have a right to receive an explanation for the experimental procedures and the results of the investigation.

Reliability

The degree of consistency that a measuring method or device produces.

Intrarater Reliability: The consistency of repeated measurements of the same observation by the same rater.

Interrater Reliability: The consistency of repeated measurements of the same observation by different raters.

Validity

Validity is the degree to which data or results of a study are correct or true.

Concurrent Validity: The degree to which the measurement being validated agrees with an established measurement standard administered at approximately the same time. Concurrent validity is a form of criterion validity.

Construct Validity: The relationship between an instrument and an established theoretical framework. Construct validity is based on theory and not statistical analysis.

Content Validity: The degree to which the indicator provides a complete representation of the domain of interest.

Criterion Validity: The degree to which a relationship exists between a measurement being validated and other measures.

External Validity: The degree to which results of the research study are generalizable.

Internal Validity: The degree to which the reported outcomes of the research study are a consequence of the relationship between the independent and dependent variables and not the result of extraneous factors.

Predictive Validity: The ability of an instrument to predict the occurrence of a future behavior or event. Predictive validity is a form of criterion validity.

Variables

Independent Variable: The factors in a research study that are manipulated by the researcher.

Dependent Variable: The factors in a research study used to measure the effect of the independent variable.

Discrete Variable: A variable whose measurements are expressed as integers.

Continuous Variable: A variable whose measurements can assume any value along a continuum. Values are not limited to integers and instead are only limited by the degree of accuracy of the measuring instrument.

Levels of Measurement

Nominal
This is the weakest level of measurement. Categories are very broad and each participant of the study will fit into only one of the categories. Each category is independent of the other.

> **Example:** male vs. female, yes vs. no

Ordinal
This level of measurement is also known as a ranking scale. Data that is collected will be placed into independent categories, however, the categories have a qualitative relationship regarding the order of ranking. There is not equality between each category.

> **Example:** Manual muscle testing, levels of assistance

Interval
A metric measurement scale where the distance between any two numbers is of equal amounts. In this scale the unit of measure and zero are both arbitrary.

> **Example:** Celsius temperature scale, calendar time

Ratio
A metric measurement scale where the unit of measurement is arbitrary, however, there is an absolute zero.

> **Example:** weight and length scales

Research Design

Controlled Trials: Controlled trials require the experimental procedure to be compared with a placebo or another previously accepted procedure. Controlled studies are more likely than uncontrolled studies to determine whether differences are due to the experimental treatment or to some other extraneous factor.

Uncontrolled Trials: Uncontrolled trials involve the investigators describing their experience with an experimental procedure, however, the experimental procedure is not formally compared with a placebo or another previously accepted procedure.

Quantitative Observations: Quantitative observations have characteristics measured on a numerical scale.

Qualitative Observations: Qualitative observations have characteristics measured on a nominal scale.

Single-blind Study: A single-blind study is a study in which the investigator does not know if the subject is in the treatment or the control group.

Double-blind Study: A double-blind study is a study in which neither the investigator nor the subject knows if the subject is in the treatment or the control group.

Sampling

Probability Sampling
Probability sampling requires an investigator to identify the parameters of a population. Every member of the population must have the same probability of being selected for the sample. Probability sampling generates smaller sampling error and therefore is often more desirable when an investigator would like to generalize from a specific population to a larger population.

Probability Sampling Methods:
- *Simple random sampling*
  Subjects have an equal chance of being selected for the sample. The sampling method often relies on a table of random numbers to determine the sample. Sampling can be performed with or without replacement.

- *Systematic sampling*
  Subjects are selected by taking every n[th] subject from the population. The size of the interval is based on the desired sample size. Systematic sampling is more efficient than simple random sampling and is most commonly employed when a researcher is drawing from a very large sample.

- *Stratified random sampling*
  Subjects are randomly selected from predetermined characteristics related to a particular study. Stratified random sampling enhances the sample representation and lowers sampling error by allowing subgroups to remain homogenous.

- *Cluster sampling*
  Subjects are selected based on a random sample of naturally occurring groups. Cluster sampling allows a random sample without a complete listing of each unit. The sampling technique is less costly and more efficient than simple random sampling.

Non-probability Sampling

Non-probability sampling does not require the parameters of a population to be identified and there is an absence of randomization. This type of sampling is often utilized in physical therapy due to the increased difficulty of meeting the more rigid requirements of probability sampling.

Non-probability Sampling Methods:

- *Convenience sampling*
  Subjects are selected as they become available until the desired sample is reached.

- *Purposive sampling*
  Subjects are deliberately selected based on predefined criteria chosen by the investigators.

- *Snowball sampling*
  Subjects are identified by asking existing subjects to identify the names of other potential participants. Snowball sampling is often used when members of a given sample are difficult to identify.

Research Terminology

Hawthorne effect (placebo effect): An untreated subject experiences a change simply from participating in a research study.

Hypothesis: A statement of belief about population parameters.

Level of significance (alpha): Expresses the probability of rejecting the null hypothesis when it is true. Since it is desirable to limit this probability, traditional values for alpha are .05 and .01. Alpha is synonymous with the probability of a type I error.

Null hypothesis: A statement indicating there is no difference between the population mean and the hypothesized value.

One-tailed test: Used when investigators have a prior expectation about the size of a sample mean and want to test whether it is larger or smaller than the population mean.

Parameter: Numerical measurement describing some characteristic of a population.

Population: Group of all elements to be studied.

Sample: Subgroup of elements drawn from a population.

Sensitivity: The percentage of individuals with a particular diagnosis that are correctly identified as positive.

Specificity: The percentage of individuals without a particular diagnosis that are correctly identified as negative.

Statistic: Numerical measurement describing some characteristic of a sample.

Two-tailed test: Used when investigators do not have a prior expectation about the size of a sample mean and want to test whether it is different from the population mean in either direction.

Type I error (alpha error): Rejecting the null hypothesis when it is in fact true. If the level of significance was set at .01, there would be a 1% chance of a type I error occurring.

Type II error (beta error): Accepting the null hypothesis when it is in fact false. An example of a type II error occurs when a researcher concludes that a given intervention did not have a positive outcome on a dependent variable when it actually did. Type I and Type II errors vary inversely.

Statistics

Types of Statistics

Descriptive Statistics: Descriptive statistics summarize or describe important characteristics of a known set of population data. Conditions cannot be extended beyond the known set of population data and any similarity to data outside the known set cannot be assumed.

Inferential Statistics: Inferential statistics use sample data to make inferences about a population. This form of statistics is often utilized to determine whether there are significant differences between groups.

Measures of Central Tendency

Mean: The results obtained by adding all of the values and dividing by the total number of values that were added.

Median: The point on a distribution at which 50% of the values fell above and below. The median is identified by first rank ordering the values. If the number of values is odd, the median is the middle value. If the number of values is even, the median is found by determining the mean of the two middle values.

Mode: The value that occurs most frequently. A distribution with two modes is termed bimodal. A distribution with more than two modes is termed multimodal.

Measures of Variation

Range: The difference between the highest and lowest value.

Variance: The sum of the squared deviation from the mean divided by the total number of values.

Standard Deviation: The average deviation of values around the mean. Standard deviation is based on the distance of sample values from the mean and equals the square root of the mean of the squared deviation. Expressed differently, the standard deviation is the square root of the variance.

Normal Distribution

A bell shaped curve that is symmetrical around its vertical axis with the values tending to cluster around the mean. The mean, median, and mode have the same value. The curve has no boundaries and only a small fraction of the values fall outside of three standard deviations above or below the mean.

- Approximately 68% of all values fall within one standard deviation above or below the mean.

- Approximately 95% of all values fall within two standard deviations above or below the mean.

- Approximately 99% of all values fall within three standard deviations above or below the mean.

Skewness: Refers to the symmetry or lack of symmetry in the shape of a frequency distribution. Negatively skewed or left skewed data is characterized by the mean and median being to the left of the mode. Positively skewed or right skewed data is characterized by the mean and median being to the right of the mode.

Steps in Testing a Statistical Hypothesis

1. State the research question in terms of statistical hypothesis
   a. null hypothesis
   b. alternative hypothesis
2. Decide on the appropriate test statistic
3. Select the level of significance for the statistical test
4. Determine the value the test statistic must attain to be declared significant
5. Perform the calculations
6. State the conclusion

Parametric Statistics

Parametric statistics assume that samples come from populations that are normally distributed and there is homogeneity of variance. Parametric statistical tests are applied to both interval and ratio level data.

Parametric Statistical Tests

- *t-test*
  A statistical procedure for comparing a mean with a norm or comparing two means with sample sizes less than or equal to 30.

z-test
A statistical procedure for comparing a mean with a norm or comparing two means for larger sample sizes greater than 30.

Independent t-test
A statistical procedure used to compare two independent samples. A sample is independent if the sample selected from one population is not related to the sample selected from the other population.

Dependent t-test
A statistical procedure used to compare the difference in a numerical variable observed for two paired groups. The test is also used when the same group is subjected to pre-test and post-test measurements.

Analysis of variance
A statistical procedure used to compare differences between two or more population means by analyzing sample variances.

One-way analysis of variance
A statistical procedure similar to the independent t-test, however, the test is designed to accommodate two or more population means. One-way refers to the fact that only one independent variable is examined.

Two-way analysis of variance
A statistical procedure used to compare two or more population means with two or more independent variables.

Nonparametric Statistics

Nonparametric statistics do not assume that samples come from populations that are normally distributed and do not assume homogeneity of variance. Nonparametric statistical tests are most commonly applied to nominal or ordinal level data.

Nonparametric Statistical Tests

- **Chi Square**
  A statistical procedure used to determine the probability that group differences result from chance. The nonparametric test uses nominal level data.

- **Kruskal-Wallis test**
  A statistical procedure used to determine if two or more samples come from the same population. The test is the nonparametric version of the one-way analysis of variance.

- **Mann-Whitney test**
  A statistical procedure used to compare two independent samples with ordinal level data. The test is the nonparametric alternative of the independent t-test.

- **Wilcoxon Signed Rank test**
  A statistical procedure used to compare two dependent samples with ordinal level data. The test is the nonparametric alternative of the dependent t-test.

Correlation

The relationship between two variables when one is related to the other.

Correlation coefficient:
The correlation coefficient is the measure of the linear relationship between paired variables in a sample.
- A perfect positive correlation indicates that for every unit increase in one variable there is a proportionate unit increase in the other variable. A perfect positive correlation is indicated by +1.0.
- A perfect negative correlation indicates that for every unit increase in one variable there is a proportionate unit decrease in the other variable. A perfect negative correlation is indicated by –1.0.

Pearson Product Moment Correlation (r):
The Pearson product moment correlation is a type of correlation statistic that requires interval level data. The test yields a value between –1.0 and +1.0.

Spearman rho:
The Spearman rho is a type of correlation statistic that requires ordinal level data. The test yields a value between –1.0 and +1.0. When interpreting a correlation coefficient it is important to remember that the coefficient does not imply a cause and effect relationship between variables. Attempt to avoid using rates or averages since this type of data reduces variation and may result in an inflated correlation coefficient.

Graphs

Histogram: A graphical display of a frequency distribution. A histogram typically includes the measurement of interest along the x-axis and the number or percentage of observations along the y-axis.

Dotplots: A graphical display in which each piece of data is plotted as a dot along a horizontal scale. When values occur more than once at a given point on the horizontal scale the dots are stacked vertically.

Stem and leaf plots: A graphical display which enables the reader to observe the entire distribution of data without losing any information. Most commonly this is done by organizing data into categories (e.g., 20-29, 30-39), and then dividing a number into two digits. The first digit is placed to the left side of a vertical line (stem) and the second digit is placed on the right side of the vertical line (leaves). The first digit within a category (stem) does not need to be repeated, however, the second digit (leaves) should be repeated.

Scatterplot: A graphical display that illustrates the relationship between two measures or variables measured on a numeric scale. Each value is represented by a point or dot on the scatterplot. A scatterplot should not be used to determine if a relationship is significant or occurs due to chance.

Box and whisker plot: A graphical display constructed based on the information in a stem and leaf plot. The graph illustrates both the frequencies and the distribution of the data and is commonly used to illustrate certain locations in the distribution.

Chapter Ten
Administration

Documentation

Purpose of Documentation

- Communicate with other treating professionals
- Assistance with discharge planning
- Reimbursement
- Assistance with utilization review
- A legal document regarding the course of therapy

Types of Documentation

Record

- An increase in specialization of care and multidisciplinary treatment increases the need for medical records to serve as a means of communication among clinicians.
- Progress notes and referrals related directly to patient care are examples of clinical records.
- Departmental statistics and records are examples of administrative records.

Referral

- Acceptable forms of referral range from a signed prescription form to a highly structured checklist. The referral must include the name of the patient and be signed and dated by the referring physician.
- Referrals commonly include some indication as to the number and frequency of treatments desired and any special precautions or instructions.

Progress Note

- Improvement of patient care is the most important function of progress notes.
- Progress notes allow members of all health services to know what the patient is accomplishing in each given area.
- Progress notes should contain patient identification, the date, and the signature of the therapist.

- Progress notes should be written when the patient's condition changes during the course of treatment. Specific frequency of progress notes is usually dictated by department policy.
- Appropriate forms of documentation include diagrams, videotapes, and flow sheets as well as many other less frequently used media.

S.O.A.P. Note

A commonly used record to write daily notes is the S.O.A.P. note. S.O.A.P. stands for:

S: Subjective
O: Objective
A: Assessment
P: Plan

Subjective
Refers to information the patient communicates to the therapist. This could include social or medical history not previously recorded. It could also include the patient's statements or complaints.

Objective
Refers to information the therapist observes. Common examples include range of motion measurements, muscle strength, and functional abilities. It also includes manual techniques and equipment used during treatment.

Assessment
Allows the therapist to express their professional opinion. Short and long-term goals are often expressed in this section as well as changes in the treatment program.

Plan
Includes ideas for future physical therapy sessions. Frequency and expected duration of physical therapy services can also be incorporated into this section.

Discharge Summary

A discharge summary should provide a capsule view of the patient's progress during therapy. The discharge summary is usually conducted on the day of the patient's last therapy session.

Guidelines for Physical Therapy Documentation

Preamble

The American Physical Therapy Association (APTA) is committed to meeting the physical therapy needs of society, to meeting the needs and interests of its members and to developing and improving the art and science of physical therapy, including practice, education, and research. To help meet these responsibilities, the APTA Board of Directors has approved the following guidelines for physical therapy documentation. It is recognized that these guidelines do not reflect all of the unique documentation requirements associated with the many specialty areas within the physical therapy profession. Applicable for both handwritten and electronic documentation systems, these guidelines are intended to be used as a foundation for the development of more specific documentation guidelines in specialty areas, while at the same time providing guidance for the physical therapy profession across all practice settings.

It is the position of APTA that physical therapy examination, evaluation, diagnosis, and prognosis shall be documented, dated, and authenticated by the physical therapist that performs the service. Intervention provided by the physical therapist or physical therapist assistant is documented, dated, and authenticated by the physical therapist or, when permissible by law, the physical therapist assistant, or both.

Other notations or flow charts are considered a component of the documented record but do not meet the requirements of documentation in, or of, themselves (Position on Authority for Physical Therapy Documentation, HOD 06-98-11-11).

Operational Definitions

Guidelines: APTA defines "guidelines" as approved non-binding statements of advice.

Documentation: Any entry into the client record, such as consultation report, initial examination report, progress note, flow sheet/checklist that identifies the care/service provided, re-examination or summation of care.

Authentication: The process used to verify that an entry is complete, accurate, and final. Indications of authentication can include original written signatures and computer "signatures" on secured electronic record systems only.

I. General Guidelines
  A. All documentation must comply with the applicable jurisdictional/regulatory requirements.

1. All handwritten entries shall be made in ink and will include original signatures. Electronic entries are made with appropriate security and confidentiality provisions.
2. Charting errors should be corrected by drawing a single line through the error and initializing and dating the chart or through the appropriate mechanism for electronic documentation that clearly indicates that a change was made without deletion of the original record.
3. Identification
    3.1 Include patient's/client's full name and identification number, if applicable, on all official documents.
    3.2 All entries must be dated and authenticated with the provider's full name and appropriate designation (i.e., PT or PTA).
    3.3 Documentation by graduates or others pending receipt of an unrestricted license shall be authenticated by a licensed physical therapist.
    3.4 Documentation by students (SPT/SPTA) in physical therapist or physical therapist assistant programs must be additionally authenticated by the physical therapist or, when permissible by law, documentation by physical therapist assistant students may be authenticated by a physical therapist assistant.
4. Documentation should include the referral mechanism by which physical therapy services are initiated.
    Examples include:
      Ex 4.1 Self-referral/direct access
      Ex 4.2 Request for consultation from another practitioner

II. Initial Patient/Client Management
  A. Documentation is required at the onset of each episode of physical therapy care and shall include the elements of examination, evaluation, diagnosis, and prognosis.
  B. Documentation of the initial episode of physical therapy care shall include the elements of examination, a comprehensive screening and specific testing process leading to diagnostic classification, or, as appropriate, to a referral to another practitioner. The examination has three components: the patient/client history, the systems review, and tests and measures.
  1. Documentation of appropriate history:
      1.1 General demographics
          Social history
          Employment/work (Job/School/Play)

Growth and development
Living environment
General health status (self-report, family report, caregiver report)
Social/health habits (past and current)
Family history
Medical/surgical history
Current condition(s)/Chief complaint(s)
Functional status and activity level
Medications
Other clinical tests

2. Documentation of systems review
   2.1 Documentation of physiologic and anatomical status to include the following systems:
   Cardiovascular/pulmonary
   Blood pressure
   Edema
   Heart rate
   Respiratory rate
   Integumentary
   Presence of scar formation
   Skin color
   Skin integrity
   Musculoskeletal
   Gross range of motion
   Gross strength
   Gross asymmetry
   Height
   Weight
   Neuromuscular
   Gross coordinated movement (e.g., balance, locomotion, transfers, and transitions)

   2.2 A review of communication, affect, cognition, language, and learning style
   Ability to make needs known
   Consciousness
   Orientation
   Expected emotional/behavioral responses
   Learning preferences

   2.3 Documentation of selection and administration of appropriate tests and measures to determine patient/client status in a number of areas and documentation of findings. The following is a partial list of these areas to be addressed in the documented examination and evaluation, including categories of tests and measures for each area:

Aerobic Capacity/Endurance

Examples of examination findings include:
   3.1.1 Aerobic capacity during functional activities
   3.1.2 Aerobic capacity during standardized exercise test protocols
   3.1.3 Cardiovascular signs and symptoms in response to increased oxygen demand with exercise or activity
   3.1.4 Pulmonary signs and symptoms in response to increased oxygen demand with exercise or activity

Anthropometric Characteristics

Examples of examination findings include:
   3.2.1 Body composition
   3.2.2 Body dimensions
   3.2.3 Edema

Arousal, Attention, and Cognition

Examples of examination findings include:
   3.3.1 Arousal and attention
   3.3.2 Cognition
   3.3.3 Communication
   3.3.4 Consciousness
   3.3.5 Motivation
   3.3.6 Orientation to time, person, place, and situation
   3.3.7 Recall

Assistive and Adaptive Devices

Examples of examination findings include:
   3.4.1 Assistive or adaptive devices and equipment use during functional activities
   3.4.2 Components, alignment, fit, and ability to care for the assistive or adaptive devices and equipment
   3.4.3 Remediation of impairments, functional limitations, or disabilities with use of assistive or adaptive devices and equipment
   3.4.4 Safety during use of assistive or adaptive devices and equipment

Circulation (Arterial, Venous, Lymphatic)

Examples of examination findings include:
   3.5.2 Cardiovascular symptoms
   3.5.3 Physiological responses to position change

Cranial and Peripheral Nerve Integrity

Examples of examination findings include:
- 3.6.1   Electrophysiological integrity
- 3.6.2   Motor distribution of the cranial nerves
- 3.6.3   Motor distribution of the peripheral nerves
- 3.6.4   Response to neural provocation
- 3.6.5   Response to stimuli, including auditory, gustatory, olfactory, pharyngeal, vestibular, and visual
- 3.6.6   Sensory distribution of the cranial nerves
- 3.6.7   Sensory distribution of the peripheral nerves

Environmental, Home, Work (Job/School/Play) Barriers

Examples of examination findings include:
- 3.7.1   Current and potential barriers
- 3.7.2   Physical space and environment

Ergonomics and Body Mechanics

Examples of examination findings for ergonomics include:
- 3.8.1   Dexterity and coordination during work
- 3.8.2   Functional capacity and performance during work actions, tasks, or activities
- 3.8.3   Safety in work environments
- 3.8.4   Specific work conditions or activities
- 3.8.5   Tools, devices, equipment, and workstations related to work actions, tasks, or activities

Examples of examination findings for ergonomics include:
- 3.8.6   Body mechanics during self-care, home management, work, community, or leisure actions, tasks, or activities

Gait, Locomotion, and Balance

Examples of examination findings include:
- 3.9.1   Balance during functional activities with or without the use of assistive, adaptive, orthotic, protection, supportive, or prosthetic devices or equipment
- 3.9.2   Balance (dynamic and static) with or without the use of assistive, adaptive, orthotic, protective, supportive, or prosthetic devices or equipment
- 3.9.3   Gait and locomotion during functional activities with or without the use of assistive, adaptive, orthotic, protective, supportive, or prosthetic devices or equipment
- 3.9.4   Gait and locomotion with or without the use of assistive, adaptive, orthotic, protective, supportive, or prosthetic devices or equipment
- 3.9.5   Safety during gait, locomotion, and balance

Integumentary Integrity

Examples of examination findings include:
- 3.10.1.1   Associated with skin:
- 3.10.1.2   Activities, positioning, and postures that produce or relieve trauma to the skin
- 3.10.1.3   Assistive, adaptive, orthotic, protective, supportive, or prosthetic devices and equipment that may produce or relieve trauma to the skin
- 3.10.1.4   Skin characteristics
- 3.10.1.5   Wound
- 3.10.1.6   Postures that aggravate the wound or scar or that produce or relieve trauma
- 3.10.1.7   Burn
- 3.10.1.8   Signs of infection
- 3.10.1.9   Wound characteristics
- 3.10.1.10   Wound scar tissue characteristics

Joint Integrity

Examples of examination findings include:
- 3.11   Joint integrity and mobility
- 3.11.1   Joint play movements
- 3.11.2   Specific body parts

Motor Function

Examples of examination findings include:
- 3.12.1   Dexterity, coordination, and agility
- 3.12.2   Electrophysiological integrity
- 3.12.3   Hand function
- 3.12.4   Initiation, modification, and control of movement patterns and voluntary postures

Muscle Performance

Examples of examination findings include:
- 3.13.1   Electrophysiological integrity
- 3.13.2   Muscle strength, power, and endurance

3.13.3   Muscle strength, power, and endurance during functional activities
3.13.4   Muscle tension

Neuromotor Development and Sensory Integration
Examples of examination findings include:
3.14.1   Acquisition and evolution of motor skills
3.14.2   Oral motor function, phonation, and speech production
3.14.3   Sensorimotor integration

Orthotic, Protective, and Supportive Devices

Examples of examination findings include:
3.15.1   Components, alignment, fit, and ability to care for the orthotic, protective, and supportive devices and equipment
3.15.2   Orthotic, protective, and supportive devices and equipment use during functional activities
3.15.3   Remediation of impairments, functional limitations, or disabilities with use of orthotic, protective, and supportive devices and equipment
3.15.4   Safety during use of orthotic, protective, and supportive devices and equipment

Pain

Examples of examination findings include:
3.16.1   Pain, soreness, and nociception
3.16.2   Pain in specific body parts

Posture

Examples of examination findings include:
3.17.1   Postural alignment and position (dynamic)
3.17.2   Postural alignment and position (static)
3.17.3   Specific body parts

Prosthetic Requirements

Examples of examination findings include:
3.18.1   Components, alignment, fit, and ability to care for prosthetic device
3.18.2   Prosthetic device use during functional activities
3.18.3   Remediation of impairments, functional limitations, or disabilities with use of the prosthetic device

3.18.4   Residual limb or adjacent segment
3.18.5   Safety during use of the prosthetic device

Range of Motion

Examples of examination findings include:
3.19.1   Functional ROM
3.19.2   Joint active and passive movement
3.19.3   Muscle length, soft tissue extensibility, and flexibility

Reflex Integrity

Examples of examination findings include:
3.20.1   Deep reflexes
3.20.2   Electrophysiological integrity
3.20.3   Postural reflexes and reactions, including righting, equilibrium, and protective reactions
3.20.4   Primitive reflexes and reactions
3.20.5   Resistance to passive stretch
3.20.6   Superficial reflexes and reactions

Self-Care and Home Management

Examples of examination findings include:
3.21.1   Ability to gain access to home environments
3.21.2   Ability to perform self-care and home management activities with or without assistive, adaptive, orthotic, protective, supportive, or prosthetic devices and equipment
3.21.3   Safety in self-care and home management activities and environments

Sensory Integrity

Examples of examination findings include:
3.22.1   Combined/cortical sensations
3.22.2   Deep sensations
3.22.3   Electrophysiological integrity

Ventilation and Respiration

Examples of examination findings include:
3.23.1   Pulmonary signs of respiration/gas exchange
3.23.2   Pulmonary signs of ventilatory function
3.23.3   Pulmonary symptoms
3.23.4   Work (job/school/play), community and leisure integration or reintegration

Vocational

Examples of examination findings include:

3.24.1 Ability to assume or resume work (job/school/play), community and leisure activities with our without assistive, adaptive, orthotic, protective, supportive, or prosthetic devices and equipment

3.24.2 Ability to gain access to work (job/school/play), community and leisure environments

3.24.3 Safety in work (job/school/play), community and leisure activities and environments

C. Documentation of evaluation (a dynamic process in which the physical therapist makes clinical judgments based on data gathered during the examination).

D. Documentation of diagnosis (a label encompassing a cluster of signs and symptoms, syndromes, or categories that reflects the information obtained from the examination).

E. Documentation of prognosis (determination of the level of optimal improvement that might be attained through intervention and the amount of time required to reach that level. Documentation shall include anticipated goals, expected outcomes, and plan of care).

1. Patient/client (and family members and significant others, if appropriate) is involved in establishing anticipated goals and expected outcomes.

2. All anticipated goals and expected outcomes are stated in measurable terms.

3. Anticipated goals and expected outcomes are related to impairments, functional limitations, and disabilities and the changes in health, wellness, and fitness needs identified in the examination.

4. The plan of care:

4.1 Is based on the examination, evaluation, diagnosis, and prognosis

4.2 Identifies anticipated goals and expected outcomes of all proposed interventions

4.3 Describes the proposed interventions taking into consideration the expectations of the patient/client and others as appropriate

4.4 Includes frequency and duration of all proposed interventions to achieve the anticipated goals and expected outcomes

4.5 Involves appropriate coordination and communication of care with other with other professionals/services

4.6 Includes plan for discharge

F. Authentication by an appropriate designation of the physical therapist.

III. Documentation of the Continuation of Care

A. Documentation of intervention or services provided and current patient/client status.

1. Documentation is required for every visit/encounter.

1.1 Authentication and appropriate designation of the physical therapist or the physical therapist assistant providing the service under the direction and supervision of a physical therapist.

2. Documentation of each visit/encounter shall include the following elements:

2.1 Patient/client self-report (as appropriate)

2.2 Identification of specific interventions provided, including frequency, intensity and duration as appropriate. Examples include:

Ex 2.2.1 Knee extension, 3 sets, 10 repetitions, 10 lb. weight.

Ex 2.2.2 Transfer training bed to chair with sliding board.

2.3 Equipment provided.

2.4 Changes in patient/client status as they relate to the plan of care.

2.5 Adverse reaction to interventions, if any.

2.6 Factors that modify frequency or intensity of intervention and progression toward anticipated goals, including patient/client adherence to patient/client related instructions.

2.7 Communication/consultation with providers/patient/client/family/ significant other.

B. Documentation of re-examination

1. Documentation of re-examination is provided as appropriate to evaluate progress and to modify or redirect intervention.

2. Documentation of re-examination shall include the following elements:

    2.1   Documentation of selected components of examination to update patient's/client's status.

    2.2   Interpretation of findings and, when indicated, revision of anticipated goals, and expected outcomes.

    2.3   When indicated, revision of plan of care as directly correlated with anticipated goals and expected outcomes as documented.

    2.4   Authentication by and appropriate designation of the physical therapist.

IV. Documentation of Summation of Episode of Care

  A. Documentation is required following conclusion of the current episode of the physical therapy intervention sequence.

  B. Documentation of the summation of the episode of care shall include the following elements:

    1. Criteria for termination of services:

      Examples of discharge include:

      Ex 1.1 Anticipated goals and expected outcomes have been achieved.

      Examples of discontinuation include:

      Ex 1.2 Patient/client, caregiver or legal guardian declines to continue intervention.

      Ex 1.3 Patient/client is unable to continue to progress toward anticipated goals due to medical or psychosocial complications or because financial/insurance resources have been expended.

      Ex 1.4 Physical therapist determines that the patient/client will no longer benefit from physical therapy.

    2. Current physical/functional status.

    3. Degree of anticipated goals and expected outcomes achieved and reasons for goals and outcomes not being achieved.

    4. Discharge or discontinuation plan that includes written and verbal communication related to the patient's/client's continuing care.

      Examples include:

      Ex 4.1 Home program.

      Ex 4.2 Referrals for additional services.

      Ex 4.3 Recommendations for follow-up physical therapy care.

      Ex 4.4 Family and caregiver training.

      Ex 4.5 Equipment provided.

    5. Authentication by and appropriate designation of the physical therapist.

Additional References:

1. *Direction and supervision of the Physical Therapist Assistant* (HOD 06-00-16-27).
2. *Comprehensive Accreditation Manual for Hospitals.* Oakbrook Terrace, Ill: Joint Commission on the Accreditation of Health care Organizations.
3. *Glossary of Terms Related to Information Security.* Schaumburg, Ill: Computer-based Patient Record Institute.
4. *Guidelines for Establishing Information Security Policies at Organizations Using Computer-based Patient Records.* Schaumburg, Ill: Computer-based Patient Record Institute.
5. *Current Procedural Terminology.* Chicago: American Medical Association (AMA); 2000.
6. *Coding and Payment Guide for the Physical Therapist 2000.* St. Anthony's Publishing and the American Physical Therapy Association.
7. Health care Financing Administration (HCFA) (www.hcfa.gov) Minimal Data Set (MDS) Regulations, HCFA/AMA documentation guidelines, Home Health Regulations.

From American Physical Therapy Association, with permission.

Military Time

The 24-hour clock (military time) is used to standardize time in the medical record.

Standard Time:	Military Time:
Noon	1200 hours
1:00 PM	1300 hours
2:00 PM	1400 hours
3:00 PM	1500 hours
4:00 PM	1600 hours
5:00 PM	1700 hours
6:00 PM	1800 hours
7:00 PM	1900 hours
8:00 PM	2000 hours
9:00 PM	2100 hours
10:00 PM	2200 hours
11:00 PM	2300 hours
Midnight	2400 hours

Symbols Commonly Used in Clinical Practice	
=	Equal
≠	Unequal
>	Greater than
<	Less than

Symbols Commonly Used in Clinical Practice (continued)

↑	Increase
↗	Increasing
↓	Decrease
↘	Decreasing
−	Negative, minus, deficiency, alkaline, reaction
±	Very slight trace or reaction, indefinite
+	Slight trace or reaction, positive, plus excess, acid reaction
++	Trace or notable reaction
+++	Moderate amount of reaction
++++	Large amount or pronounced reaction
#	Number, pound, has been given or done
→	Yields, leads to
←	Resulting from or secondary to
1°, 2°	Primary, secondary

From Miller-Keane: Encyclopedia and Dictionary of Medicine, Nursing, and Allied Health. W.B. Saunders Company, Philadelphia 1997, p.1802, with permission.

Measurement

Metric versus United States Units of Measure

1 inch = 2.54 centimeters	$°C = (°F -32) \times 1.8$
1 foot = 30.5 centimeters	$°F = (°C \times 1.8) + 32$
1 mile = 1.61 kilometers	Boiling = 212 °F
1 meter = 3.28 feet	100 °C
1 gram = .0353 ounce	Freezing = 32 °F
1 ounce = 28.35 grams	0 °C
1 pound = 454 kilograms	
1 kilogram = 2.2 pounds	
1 pound = 4.45 Newtons	
1 liter = .2642 gallons	
1 milliliter = .0338 once	
1 gallon = 3.785 liters	
1 calorie = 4.18 Joule	

Length

- 1cm = 0.3937 inch
- 1 m = 39.37 inches = 3.28 ft = 1.09 yds
- 1 km = 0.62 mile
- 1 inch = 2.54 centimeters (cm) = 25.4 millimeters (mm) = 0.0254 meters (m)
- 1 foot = 30.48 cm = 304.8 mm = 0.304 m
- 1 mile = 5280 ft = 1760 yds = 1609.35 m = 1.61 kilometers (km)

Weight

- 1 ounce (oz) = 0.0625 pounds (lb) = 28.35 grams (g) = 0.028 kilograms (kg)
- 1 pound (lb) = 16 oz = 454 g = 0.454 kg
- 1 g = 0.035 oz = 0.0022 lb = 0.001 kg
- 1 kg = 35.27 oz = 2.2 lb = 1000 g

Energy and Work

- 1 kcal = 3086 foot-pounds (ft-lbs) = 426.4 kilogram-meter (kg-m) = kilojoules (kJ)
- 1 kJ = 1000 joules (J) = 0.23892 kcal
- 1 liter O_2 consumed = 5.05 kcal = 15.575 ft-lbs = 2153 kg-m = 21.237 kJ
- 1 MET = 3.5 mL O_2/kg-min = 0.0175 kcal/kg = 0.0732 kJ/kg
- 1 ft-lb = 0.1383 kg-m
- 1kg-m = 7.23 ft-lbs

Temperature

- 0°C = 32°F = 273°K
- 100°C = 212°F
- $°C = (°F − 32) \times 5/9$
- $°F = (°C \times 9/5) + 32$

Ethics

Ethical Principles

Autonomy: Requires that the wishes of competent individuals must be honored. Autonomy is often referred to as self-determination.

Beneficence: A moral obligation of health care providers to act for the benefit of others.

Nonmaleficence: The obligation of health care providers to above all else, do no harm.

Veracity: Obligation of health care providers to tell the truth.

Management

Quality Management Process

- Review selected patient medical records
- Prioritize adverse event outcomes
- Conduct a thorough review of care
- Identify problematic areas of care
- Develop a plan to change identified aspects of care
- Implement the plan
- Monitor the plan
- Determine if the implemented change results in a measurable difference

Quality Improvement

A form of objective self-examination designed to improve the quality of services.

Agencies Responsible for Quality Improvement
- Joint Commission on Accreditation of Healthcare Organizations (JCAHO)
- Professional Standards Review Organization (PSRO)
- Commission of Accreditation of Rehabilitation Facilities (CARF)
- National Committee for Quality Assurance (NCQA)

Measures the structure, process, and outcome of physical therapy care. According to the American Physical Therapy Association structure, process, and outcome are defined as follows:

- **Structure**
  A review of structure is an assessment of organization, staffing and staff qualifications, rules and policies governing physical work, records, equipment, and physical facilities. The assessment may include a judgment of the adequacy as well as the presence of the element of structure being examined.

- **Process**
  Process assessment is based on the degree or extent to which the therapist conforms to accepted professional practices in providing services. The various approaches to care, their application, efficacy, adequacy, and timeliness are considered. A process review requires that considerable attention be given to developing and specifying the standards to be used in the assessment.

- **Outcome**
  Outcome assessment is based on the condition of the patient at the conclusion of care in relation to the goals of treatment. Assessment of outcome provides a means of reviewing the practitioner, the services, and events that led to the results of care. The results of outcome assessment ultimately may lead to the evaluation of the basic treatment procedures and modalities of physical therapy and validation of the approaches to patient care. Outcomes are the ultimate manifestations of effectiveness and quality of care.

Legal

Elements of a Risk Management Program

- Management involvement
- Risk management organization
- Incident reporting and investigation
- Inspections
- Communications

Recommendations to Avoid Litigation

- Conduct a thorough examination
- Seek consultation when in doubt
- Check the condition of your equipment
- Instruct patients thoroughly
- Keep the referring physician informed
- Obtain proper consent for treatment
- Do not delegate to unqualified individuals
- Keep accurate and timely written records

Legal Terminology

Abandonment: Unacceptable one-sided termination of services by a health care professional without patient consent or agreement.

Administrative law: Administrative agencies at the federal and state level develop rules and regulations to supplement statutes and executive orders.

Common law: Refers to court decisions in the absence of statutory law. Common law often creates legal precedent in areas where statutes have not been enacted.

Constitutional law: Involves law that is derived from the federal Constitution. The United States Supreme Court is responsible for ultimately interpreting and enforcing the Constitution.

Informed consent: The patient is required to sign a document and give permission to the health care professional to render treatment. This should be obtained from the patient in accordance with the standards of practice prior to initiation of treatment. The patient has the right to full disclosure of treatment procedures, risks, expected outcomes, and goals.

Malpractice: The failure to exercise the skills that would normally be exercised by other members of the profession with similar skills and training. This can include areas of professional negligence, breach of contract issues, and intentional conduct by a health care professional.

Negligence: The failure to do what a reasonable and prudent person would ordinarily have done under the same or similar circumstances for a given situation. In order to prove negligence, the plaintiff must prove all of the following:

- There was a duty owed to the plaintiff by the defendant.
- There was a breach of that duty under conditions that constituted negligence and the negligence was the proximate cause of the breach.
- There was damage to the plaintiff's person or property.

Risk management: The identification, analysis, and evaluation of risks and the selection of the most advantageous method for treating them.

Statutory law: Congress and state legislatures are responsible for enacting statutes. Examples of federal statutes affecting health care include the Americans with Disabilities Act and the Family and Medical Leave Act.

Tort: A private or civil wrong or injury, involving omission and/or commission.

Delegation and Supervision

American Physical Therapy Association Direction, Delegation, and Supervision in Physical Therapy Services

Delegated responsibilities must be commensurate with the qualifications, including experience, education, and training of the individuals to whom the responsibilities are being assigned. When the physical therapist of record delegates patient care responsibilities to physical therapist assistants or other supportive personnel, that physical therapist holds responsibility for supervision of the physical therapy program. Regardless of the setting in

which the service is given, the following responsibilities must be borne solely by the physical therapist:

1. Interpretation of referrals when available.
2. Initial examination, evaluation, diagnosis, and prognosis.
3. Development or modification of a plan of care that is based on the initial examination or the re-examination and that includes physical therapy anticipated goals and expected outcomes.
4. Determination of (1) when the expertise and decision-making capability of the physical therapist requires the physical therapist to personally render physical therapy interventions and (2) when it may be appropriate to utilize the physical therapist assistant. A physical therapist determines the most appropriate utilization of the physical therapist assistant that will ensure the delivery of service that is safe, effective, and efficient.
5. Re-examination of the patient/client in light of the anticipated goals, and revision of the plan of care when indicated.
6. Establishment of the discharge plan and documentation of discharge summary/status.
7. Oversight of all documentation for services rendered to each patient.

From Guide to Physical Therapist Practice. American Physical Therapy Association, Alexandria 1999, p.1-11, with permission.

Support Personnel Supervised by Physical Therapists

Physical Therapist Assistants

The physical therapist assistant is a technically educated health care provider who assists the physical therapist in the provision of physical therapy. The physical therapist assistant, under the direction and supervision of the physical therapist, is the only paraprofessional who provides physical therapy interventions. The physical therapist assistant is a graduate of a physical therapist assistant associate degree program accredited by the Commission on Accreditation in Physical Therapy Education (CAPTE).

The physical therapist of record is directly responsible for the actions of the physical therapist assistant. The physical therapist assistant may perform specific components of physical therapy interventions, where allowable by law or regulations that have been selected by the supervising physical therapist. The ability of the physical therapist assistant to perform the selected interventions should be assessed on an ongoing basis by the supervising physical therapist. The physical therapist assistant may modify an intervention only in accordance with changes in patient/client status and within the scope of the plan of care that has been established by the physical therapist.

Physical Therapy Aides

Aides are any support personnel who may be involved in the provision of physical therapist directed support services. The physical therapy aide is a non-licensed worker who is specifically trained under the direction and supervision of a physical therapist.

Physical therapist directed support services are limited to those tasks which may include methods and techniques that do not require clinical decision making by the physical therapist or clinical problem solving by the physical therapist assistant. The determination of what tasks are appropriately directed to the aide must be made by the physical therapist or, where allowable by law or regulations, the physical therapist assistant. To make this determination, the physical therapist or physical therapist assistant must have direct contact with the patient/client during each session. The aide may function only with continuous on-site supervision by the physical therapist or, when allowable by law or regulations, the physical therapist assistant.

From Guide to Physical Therapist Practice. American Physical Therapy Association, Alexandria 1999, p.1-10, with permission.

Health Care Professions

Audiologists

Audiologists assess patients with suspected hearing disorders. The audiologist can educate patients on how to make the best use of their available hearing and assist them in selecting and fitting appropriate aids. Audiologists are required to possess a master's degree or equivalent. The vast majority of states require audiologists to obtain a license to practice.

Chiropractors

Chiropractors diagnose and treat patients whose health problems are associated with the body's muscular, nervous, and skeletal systems. Patient care activities include manually adjusting the spine, ordering and interpreting X-rays, performing postural analysis, and administering various physical agents. Chiropractors are required to complete a four-year chiropractic curriculum leading to the Doctor of Chiropractic degree. All states require chiropractors to obtain a license to practice.

Home Health Aides

Home health aides provide health related services to the elderly, disabled, and ill in their homes. Patient care activities include performing housekeeping duties, assisting with ambulation or transfers, and promoting personal hygiene. A registered nurse, physical therapist, or social worker is often the health care professional that assigns specific duties and supervises the home health aide. The federal government has established guidelines for home health aides whose employers receive reimbursement from Medicare. The National Association for Home Care offers voluntary national certification for home health aides.

Licensed Practical Nurses

Licensed practical nurses care for the sick, injured, convalescent, and disabled under the direction of physicians and registered nurses. Patient care activities include taking vital signs, performing transfers, applying dressings, administering injections, and instructing patients and families. In some states licensed practical nurses can administer prescribed medications or start intravenous fluids. Experienced licensed practical nurses may supervise nursing assistants and aides. Educational programs for licensed practical nurses are approximately one year in length and include classroom study and supervised clinical practice. All states require a license to practice.

Medical Assistants

Medical assistants perform routine administrative and clinical tasks in a medical office. Administrative duties include answering telephones, updating patient files, completing insurance forms, and scheduling appointments. Clinical duties include taking medical histories, measuring vital signs, and assisting the physician during treatment. Educational programs for medical assistants are typically one to two years in length.

Occupational Therapists

Occupational therapists help people improve their ability to perform activities of daily living, work, and leisure skills. The educational preparation of occupational therapists emphasizes the social, emotional, and physiological effects of illness and injury. Occupational therapists most commonly work with individuals who have conditions that are mentally, physically, developmentally or emotionally disabling. Occupational therapists can enter the field with bachelor's, master's or doctoral degrees. All states require occupational therapists to obtain a license to practice.

Occupational Therapy Aides

Occupational therapy aides work under the direction of occupational therapists to provide rehabilitation services to persons with mental, physical, developmental or emotional impairments. Occupational therapy aides often prepare materials and assemble equipment used during treatment and may be responsible for a variety of clerical tasks. The majority of training for occupational therapy aides occurs on the job.

Occupational Therapy Assistants

Occupational therapy assistants work under the direction of occupational therapists to provide rehabilitation services to persons with mental, physical, developmental or emotional impairments. Occupational therapy assistants perform a variety of rehabilitative activities and exercises as outlined in an established treatment plan. To practice as an occupational therapy assistant individuals must complete an associate's degree or certificate program from an accredited academic institution. Occupational therapy assistants are regulated in the majority of states.

Physical Therapists

Physical therapists provide services to help restore function, improve mobility, relieve pain, and prevent or limit permanent physical disabilities of patients suffering from injuries or disease. Physical therapists engage in examination, evaluation, diagnosis, prognosis, and intervention in an effort to maximize patient outcomes. Physical therapists can enter the field with a master's or doctorate degree. As of 2002, all physical therapy programs seeking accreditation were required to offer a minimum of a master's degree. All states require physical therapists to obtain a license to practice.

Physical Therapist Aides

Physical therapy aides are considered support personnel who may be involved in support services directed by physical therapists. Physical therapy aides receive on the job training under the direction and supervision of a physical therapist and are permitted to function only with continuous on-site supervision by a physical therapist or in some cases a physical therapist assistant. Support services are limited to methods and techniques that do not require clinical decision making by the physical therapist or clinical problem solving by the physical therapist assistant.

Physical Therapist Assistants

Physical therapist assistants perform components of physical therapy procedures and related tasks selected and delegated by a supervising physical therapist. Physical therapist assistants may modify an intervention only in accordance with changes in patient status and within the established plan of care developed by the physical therapist. Physical therapist assistants are the only paraprofessionals that perform physical therapy interventions. Typically physical therapist assistants have an associate's degree from an accredited physical therapist assistant program. The majority of states require physical therapist assistants to obtain a license to practice.

Physicians

Physicians diagnose illnesses and prescribe and administer treatment for people suffering from injury or disease. The term physician encompasses both the Doctor of Medicine (M.D.) and the Doctor of Osteopathic Medicine (D.O.). The role of the M.D. and D.O. are very similar, however, the D.O. tends to place special emphasis on the body's musculoskeletal system, preventive medicine, and holistic patient care. All states require physicians to obtain a license to practice.

Physician Assistants

Physician assistants provide health care services with supervision by physicians. The supervising physician and established state law determine the specific duties of the physician assistant. In the vast majority of states physician assistants may prescribe medication. Physician assistants work with the supervision of a physician. All states with the exception of Mississippi require physician assistants to obtain a license to practice.

Psychologists

Psychologists use various techniques including interviewing and testing to advise people how to deal with problems of every day life. In the health care setting psychologists may be involved in counseling programs designed to help people achieve goals such as weight loss or smoking cessation. A doctoral degree is usually required for employment as a licensed clinical or counseling psychologist. All states require psychologists to obtain a license to practice.

Recreational Therapists

Recreational therapists provide treatment services and recreation activities to individuals with disabilities or illness. In acute care hospitals and rehabilitation hospitals recreational therapists work closely with other health care professionals to treat and rehabilitate individuals with specific medical conditions. In long-term care settings recreational therapists function primarily by offering structured group sessions emphasizing leisure activities. Recreational therapists are required to have a bachelor's degree in order to be eligible for certification as certified therapeutic recreation specialists.

Registered Nurses

Registered nurses work to promote health, prevent disease, and help patients cope with illness. Patient care activities are extremely diverse including tasks such as assisting physicians during treatments and examinations, administering medications, recording symptoms and reactions, and instructing patients and families. Registered nurse programs include associate's, bachelor's, and diploma programs. All states require registered nurses to obtain a license to practice.

Respiratory Therapists

Respiratory therapists evaluate, treat, and care for patients with breathing disorders. The vast majority of respiratory therapists are employed in hospitals. Patient care activities include performing bronchial drainage techniques, measuring lung capacities, administering oxygen and aerosols, and analyzing oxygen and carbon dioxide concentrations. Educational programs for respiratory therapists are offered by hospitals, colleges, and universities, vocational-technical institutes, and the military. The vast majority of states require respiratory therapists to obtain a license to practice.

Social Workers

Social workers help patients and their families to cope with chronic, acute or terminal illnesses and attempt to resolve problems that stand in the way of recovery or rehabilitation. A bachelor's degree is often the minimum requirement to qualify for employment as a social worker, however, in the health field the master's degree is often required. All states have licensing, certification or registration requirements for social workers.

Speech-Language Pathologists

Speech-language pathologists evaluate speech, language, cognitive-communication, and swallowing skills of children and adults. The majority of practitioners provide direct clinical services to individuals with communication disorders. Speech-language pathologists are required to possess a master's degree or equivalent. The vast majority of states require speech-language pathologists to obtain a license to practice.

Physical Therapy Practice

The Elements of Patient/Client Management Leading to Optimal Outcomes

Examination: The process of obtaining a history, performing a systems review, and selecting and administering tests and measures to gather data about the patient/client. The initial examination is a comprehensive screening and specific testing process that leads to a diagnostic classification. The examination process also may identify possible problems that require consultation with, or referral to, another provider.

Evaluation: A dynamic process in which the physical therapist makes clinical judgments based on data gathered during the examination. This process also may identify possible problems that require consultation with, or referral to, another provider.

Diagnosis: Both the process and the end result of evaluating examination data, which the physical therapist organizes into defined clusters, syndromes or categories to help determine the prognosis (including the plan of care) and the most appropriate intervention strategies.

Prognosis (Including Plan of Care): Determination of the level of optimal improvement that may be attained through intervention and the amount of time required to reach that level. The plan of care specifies the interventions to be used and their timing and frequency.

Intervention: Purposeful and skilled interaction of the physical therapist with the patient/client and, if appropriate, with other individuals involved in the care of the patient/client, using various physical therapy methods and techniques to produce changes in the condition that are consistent with the diagnosis and prognosis. The physical therapist conducts a re-examination to determine changes in patient/client status and to modify or redirect intervention. The decision to re-examine may be based on new clinical findings or on lack of patient/client progress. The process of re-examination also may identify the need for consultation with, or referral to, another provider.

Outcomes: Results of patient/client management, which include the impact of physical therapy interventions in the following domains: pathology/pathophysiology (disease, disorder, or condition); impairments, functional limitations, and disabilities, risk reduction/prevention, health, wellness, and fitness; societal resources; and patient/client satisfaction.

From Guide to Physical Therapist Practice. American Physical Therapy Association, (Phys. Ther. 2001, Vol. 81, Number 1, 43), with permission.

Standards of Practice for Physical Therapy and the Criteria

Preamble

The physical therapy profession's commitment to society is to promote optimal health and function in individuals by pursuing excellence in practice. The American Physical Therapy Association attests to this commitment by adopting and promoting the following *Standards of Practice for Physical Therapy*. These *Standards* are the profession's statement of conditions and performances that are essential for provision of high quality professional service to society, and provide a foundation for assessment of physical therapist practice.

I. Ethical/Legal Considerations

A. Ethical Considerations

The physical therapist practices according to the *Code of Ethics* of the American Physical Therapy Association.

The physical therapist assistant complies with the *Standards of Ethical Conduct for the Physical Therapist Assistant* of the American Physical Therapy Association.

B. Legal Considerations

The physical therapist complies with all the legal requirements of jurisdictions regulating the practice of physical therapy.

The physical therapist assistant complies with all the legal requirements of jurisdictions regulating the work of the assistant.

II. Administration of the Physical Therapy Service

A. Statement of Mission, Purposes, and Goals

The physical therapy service has a statement of mission, purposes, and goals that reflects the needs and interests of the patients and clients served, the physical therapy personnel affiliated with the service, and the community.

The statement of mission, purposes, and goals:
- Defines the scope and limitations of the physical therapy service.
- Identifies the goals and objectives of the service.
- Is reviewed annually.

B. Organizational Plan

The physical therapy service has a written organizational plan.

The organizational plan:
- Describes relationships among components within the physical therapy service and, where the service is part of a larger organization, between the service and other components of that organization.
- Ensures that the service is directed by a physical therapist.
- Defines supervisory structures within the service.
- Reflects current personnel functions.

C. Policies and Procedures

The physical therapy service has written policies and procedures that reflect the operation, mission, purposes, and goals of the service, and are consistent with the Association's standards, policies, positions, guidelines, and Code of Ethics.

The written policies and procedures:
- Are reviewed regularly and revised as necessary.
- Meet the requirements for federal and state law and external agencies.
- Apply to, but are not limited to:

Care of patients/clients, including guidelines
Clinical education
Clinical research
Collaboration
Competency assessment
Criteria for access to care
Criteria for initiation and continuation of care
Criteria for referral to other appropriate health care providers
Criteria for termination of care
Documentation
Environmental safety
Equipment maintenance
Fiscal management
Improvement of quality of care and performance of services
Infection control
Job/position descriptions
Medical emergencies
Care of patients/clients, including guidelines
Rights of patients/clients
Personnel-related policies
Staff orientation

D. Administration

The physical therapist is responsible for the direction of the physical therapy service:
- Ensures compliance with local, state, and federal requirements.
- Ensures compliance with current APTA documents, including Standards of Practice for Physical Therapy and the Criteria, Guide to Physical Therapist Practice, Code of Ethics, Guide for Professional Conduct, Standards of Ethical Conduct for the Physical Therapist Assistant, and Guide for Conduct of the Affiliate Member.
- Ensures that services are consistent with the mission, purposes, and goals of the physical therapy service.

- Ensures that services are provided in accordance with established policies and procedures.
- Reviews and updates policies and procedures.
- Provides training of physical therapy support personnel that ensures continued competence for their job description.
- Provides for continuous inservice training on safety issues and for periodic safety inspection of equipment by qualified individuals.

E. Fiscal Management

The director of the physical therapy service, in consultation with physical therapy staff and appropriate administrative personnel, participates in planning for, and allocation of, resources. Fiscal planning and management of the service are based on sound accounting principles.

The fiscal management plan:
- Includes a budget that provides for optimal use of resources.
- Ensures accurate recording and reporting of financial information.
- Ensures compliance with legal requirements.
- Allows for cost-effective utilization of resources.
- Uses a fee schedule that is consistent with the cost of physical therapy services and that is within customary norms of fairness and reasonableness.

F. Improvement of Quality of Care and Performance

The physical therapy service has a written plan for continuous improvement of quality of care and performance of services.
The improvement plan:
- Provides evidence of ongoing review and evaluation of the physical therapy service.
- Provides a mechanism for documenting improvement in quality of care and performance.
- Is consistent with requirements of external agencies, as applicable.

G. Staffing

The physical therapy personnel affiliated with the physical therapy service demonstrates competence and are sufficient to achieve the mission, purposes, and goals of the service.

The physical therapy service:
- Meets all legal requirements regarding licensure and certification of appropriate personnel.

- Ensures that the level of expertise within the service is appropriate to the needs of the patients/clients served.
- Provides appropriate professional and support personnel to meet the needs of the patient/client population.

H. Staff Development

The physical therapy service has a written plan that provides for appropriate and ongoing staff development.

The staff development plan:
- Includes self-assessment, individual goal setting, and organizational needs in directing continuing education and learning activities.
- Includes strategies for lifelong learning and professional career development.
- Includes mechanisms to foster mentorship activities.

I. Physical Setting

The physical setting is designed to provide a safe and accessible environment that facilitates fulfillment of the mission, purposes, and goals of the physical therapy service. The equipment is safe and sufficient to achieve the purposes and goals of the physical therapy.

The physical setting:
- Meets all applicable legal requirements for health and safety.
- Meets space needs appropriate for the number and type of patients/clients served.

The equipment:
- Meets all applicable legal requirements for health and safety.
- Is inspected routinely.

J. Collaboration

The physical therapy service collaborates with all disciplines as appropriate.

The collaboration when appropriate:
- Uses a team approach for the care of patients/clients.
- Provides instruction to patients/clients and families.
- Ensures professional development and continuing education.

III. Patient/Client Management

A. Patient/Client Collaboration

Within the patient/client management process, the physical therapist and the patient/client establish and maintain an ongoing collaborative process of decision-making that exists throughout the provision of services.

B. Initial Examination/Evaluation/ Diagnosis/Prognosis

The physical therapist performs an initial examination and evaluation to establish a diagnosis and prognosis prior to intervention.

The physical therapist examination:
- Is documented, dated, and appropriately authenticated by the physical therapist who performed it.
- Identifies the physical therapy needs of the patient/client.
- Incorporates appropriate tests and measures to facilitate outcome measurement.
- Produces data that are sufficient to allow evaluation, diagnosis, prognosis, and the establishment of a plan of care.
- May result in recommendations for additional services to meet the needs of the patient/client.

C. Plan of Care

The physical therapist establishes a plan of care and manages the needs of the patient/client based on the examination, evaluation, diagnosis, prognosis, goals, and outcomes of the planned interventions for the identified impairments, functional limitations, and disabilities.

The physical therapist involves the patient/client and appropriate others in the planning, implementation, and assessment of the plan of care.

The physical therapist, in consultation with appropriated disciplines, plans for discharge of the patient/client taking into consideration achievement of anticipated goals and expected outcomes, and provides for appropriate follow-up or referral.

The plan of care:
- Is based on the examination, evaluation, diagnosis, and prognosis.
- Identifies goals and outcomes.
- Describes the proposed intervention, including frequency and duration.
- Includes documentation that is dated and appropriately authenticated by the physical therapist who established the plan of care.

D. Intervention

The physical therapist provides, or directs and supervises, the physical therapy intervention in a manner that is consistent with the examination, evaluation, diagnosis, prognosis, and plan of care.

The intervention:
- Is based on the examination, evaluation, diagnosis, prognosis, and plan of care.
- Is provided under the ongoing direction and supervision of the physical therapist.
- Is provided in such a way that directed and supervised responsibilities are commensurate with the qualifications and the legal limitations of the physical therapist assistant.
- Is altered in accordance with changes in response or status.
- Is provided at a level that is consistent with current physical therapy practice.
- Is interdisciplinary when necessary to meet the needs of the patient or client.
- Documentation of the intervention is consistent with the Guidelines for Physical Therapy Documentation.
- Is dated and appropriately authenticated by the physical therapist or when permissible by law, by the physical therapist assistant.

E. Re-examination

The physical therapist re-examines the patient/client as necessary during an episode of care to evaluate progress or change in patient/client status and modifies the plan of care accordingly or discontinues physical therapy services.

The physical therapist re-examination:
- Is documented, dated, and appropriately authenticated by the physical therapist who performs it.
- Includes modifications to the plan of care.

F. Discharge/Discontinuation of Intervention

The physical therapist discharges the patient/client from physical therapy when the anticipated goals or expected outcomes for the patient/client have been achieved.

The physical therapist discontinues intervention when the patient/client is unable to continue to progress toward goals or when the physical therapist determines that the patient/client will no longer benefit from physical therapy.

Discharge documentation:
- Includes the status of the patient/client at discharge and the goals and functional outcomes attained.
- Is dated and appropriately authenticated by the physical therapist who performed the discharge.
- Includes, when a patient/client is discharged prior to attainment of goals and functional outcomes, the status of the patient/client and the rationale for discontinuation.

G. Communication/Coordination/ Documentation

The physical therapist communicates, coordinates and documents all aspects of patient/client management including the results of the initial examination and evaluation, diagnosis, prognosis, plan of care, interventions, response to interventions, changes in patient/client status relative to the interventions, re-examination, and discharge/discontinuation of intervention and other patient/client management activities.

Physical therapist documentation:
- Is dated and appropriately authenticated by the physical therapist who performed the examination and established the plan of care.
- Is dated and appropriately authenticated by the physical therapist who performed the intervention or, when allowable by law or regulations, by the physical therapist assistant who performed specific components of the intervention as selected by the supervising physical therapist.
- Is dated and appropriately authenticated by the physical therapist who performed the re-examination, and includes modifications to the plan of care.
- Is dated and appropriately authenticated by the physical therapist who performed the discharge, and includes the status of the patient/client and the goals and outcomes achieved.
- Includes, when a patient/client is discharged prior to achievement of goals and outcomes, the status of the patient/client and the rationale for discontinuation.

IV. Education

The physical therapist is responsible for individual professional development. The physical therapist assistant is responsible for individual career development.

The physical therapist and the physical therapist assistant under the direction and supervision of the physical therapist, participate in the education of students.

The physical therapist educates and provides consultation to consumers and the general public regarding the purposes and benefits of physical therapy.

The physical therapist educates and provides consultation to consumers and the general public regarding the roles of the physical therapist and the physical therapist assistant.

The physical therapist:
- Educates and provides consultation to consumers and the general public regarding the roles of the physical therapist, the physical therapist assistant, and other support personnel.

V. Research

The physical therapist applies research findings to practice and encourages, participates in, and promotes activities that establish the outcomes of patient/client management provided by the physical therapist.

The physical therapist:
- Ensures that his or her knowledge of research literature related to practice is current.
- Ensures that the rights of research subjects are protected and the integrity of research is maintained.
- Participates in the research process as appropriate to individual education, experience, and expertise.
- Educates physical therapists, physical therapist assistants, students, other health professionals, and the general public about the outcomes of physical therapist practice.

VI. Community Responsibility

The physical therapist demonstrates community responsibility by participating in community and community agency activities, educating the public, formulating public policy or providing pro bono physical therapy services.

The physical therapist:
- Participates in community and community agency activities.
- Educates the public, including prevention, education, and health promotion.
- Helps formulate public policy.
- Provides pro bono physical therapy services.

HOD 06-03-09-10
BOD 03-00-22-53

From Standards of Practice for Physical Therapy and Criteria. American Physical Therapy Association, with permission.

Code of Ethics

Preamble
This *Code of Ethics* of the American Physical Therapy Association sets forth principles for the ethical practice of physical therapy. All physical therapists are responsible for maintaining and promoting ethical practice. To this end, the physical therapist shall act in the best interest of the patient/client. This *Code of Ethics* shall be binding on all physical therapists.

Principle 1
A physical therapist shall respect the rights and dignity of all individuals and shall provide compassionate care.

Principle 2
A physical therapist shall act in a trustworthy manner toward patients/clients and in all other aspects of physical therapy practice.

Principle 3
A physical therapist shall comply with laws and regulations governing physical therapy and shall strive to effect changes that benefit patients/clients.

Principle 4
A physical therapist shall exercise sound professional judgment.

Principle 5
A physical therapist shall achieve and maintain professional competence.

Principle 6
A physical therapist shall maintain and promote high standards for physical therapy practice, education, and research.

Principle 7
A physical therapist shall seek only such remuneration as is deserved and reasonable for physical therapy services.

Principle 8
A physical therapist shall provide and make available accurate and relevant information to patients/clients about their care and to the public about physical therapy services.

Principle 9
A physical therapist shall protect the public and the profession from unethical, incompetent, and illegal acts.

Principle 10
A physical therapist shall endeavor to address the health needs of society.

Principle 11
A physical therapist shall respect the rights, knowledge, and skills of colleagues and other health care professionals.

HOD 06-00-12-23

From Code of Ethics, American Physical Therapy Association, 2004, with permission.

Guide for Professional Conduct

Purpose
This *Guide for Professional Conduct* (Guide) is intended to serve physical therapists in interpreting the *Code of Ethics* (Code) of the American Physical Therapy Association (Association), in matters of professional conduct. The Guide provides guidelines by which physical therapists may determine the propriety of their conduct. It is also intended to guide the professional development of physical therapist students. The Code and the Guide apply to all physical therapists. These guidelines are subject to change as the dynamics of the profession change and as new patterns of health care delivery are developed and accepted by the professional community and the public. This Guide is subject to monitoring and timely revision by the Ethics and Judicial Committee of the Association.

Interpreting Ethical Principles
The interpretations expressed in this Guide reflect the opinions, decisions, and advice of the Ethics and Judicial Committee. These interpretations are intended to assist a physical therapist in applying general ethical principles to specific situations. They should not be considered inclusive of all situations that could evolve.

Principle 1:

A physical therapist shall respect the rights and dignity of all individuals and shall provide compassionate care.

1.1   Attitudes of a Physical Therapist
A.   A physical therapist shall recognize individual differences and shall respect and be responsive to those differences.
B.   A physical therapist shall be guided by concern for the physical, psychological, and socioeconomic welfare of patients/clients.
C.   A physical therapist shall not harass, abuse or discriminate against others.

Principle 2:

A physical therapist shall act in a trustworthy manner towards patients/clients, and in all other aspects of physical therapy practice.

2.1   Patient/Physical Therapist Relationship
A.   To act in a trustworthy manner the physical therapist shall act in the patient/client's best interest. Working in the patient/client's best interest requires knowledge of the patient/client's needs from the patient/client's perspective. Patients/clients often come to the physical therapist in a vulnerable state and normally will rely on the physical therapist's advice, which they perceive to be based on superior knowledge, skill, and experience. The trustworthy physical therapist acts to ameliorate the patient's/client's vulnerability, not to exploit it.
B.   A physical therapist shall not exploit any aspect of the physical therapist/patient relationship.
C.   A physical therapist shall not engage in any sexual relationship or activity, whether consensual or nonconsensual, with any patient while a physical therapist/patient relationship exists.
D.   The physical therapist shall encourage an open and collaborative dialogue with the patient/client.
E.   In the event the physical therapist or patient terminates the physical therapist/patient relationship while the patient continues to need physical therapy services, the physical therapist should take steps to transfer the care of the patient to another provider.

2.2   Truthfulness
A physical therapist shall not make statements that he/she knows or should know are false,

deceptive, fraudulent or unfair. See Section 8.2.C and D.

2.3   Confidential Information
A.   Information relating to the physical therapist/patient relationship is confidential and may not be communicated to a third party not involved in that patient's care without the prior consent of the patient, subject to applicable law.
B.   Information derived from peer review shall be held confidential by the reviewer unless the physical therapist who was reviewed consents to the release of the information.
C.   A physical therapist may disclose information to appropriate authorities when it is necessary to protect the welfare of an individual or the community or when required by law. Such disclosure shall be in accordance with applicable law.

2.4   Patient Autonomy and Consent
A.   A physical therapist shall respect the patient's/client's right to make decisions regarding the recommended plan of care, including consent, modification, or refusal.
B.   A physical therapist shall communicate to the patient/client the findings of his/her examination, evaluation, diagnosis, and prognosis.
C.   A physical therapist shall collaborate with the patient/client to establish the goals of treatment and the plan of care.
D.   A physical therapist shall use sound professional judgment in informing the patient/client of any substantial risks of the recommended examination and intervention.
E.   A physical therapist shall not restrict patients' freedom to select their provider of physical therapy.

Principle 3:

A physical therapist shall comply with laws and regulations governing physical therapy and shall strive to effect changes that benefit patients/clients.

3.1   Professional Practice
A physical therapist shall comply with laws governing the qualifications, functions, and duties of a physical therapist.

3.2   Just Laws and Regulations
A physical therapist shall advocate the adoption of laws, regulations, and policies by providers, employers, third party payers, legislatures, and

regulatory agencies to provide and improve access to necessary health care services for all individuals.

3.3 Unjust Laws and Regulations

A physical therapist shall endeavor to change unjust laws, regulations, and policies that govern the practice of physical therapy. See Section 10.2.

Principle 4:

A physical therapist shall exercise sound professional judgment.

4.1 Professional Responsibility

A. A physical therapist shall make professional judgments that are in the patient/client's best interests.

B. Regardless of practice setting, a physical therapist has primary responsibility for the physical therapy care of a patient and shall make independent judgments regarding that care consistent with accepted professional standards. See Section 2.4.

C. A physical therapist shall not provide physical therapy services to a patient/client while his/her ability to do so safely is impaired.

D. A physical therapist shall exercise sound professional judgment based upon his/her knowledge, skill, education, training, and experience.

E. Upon accepting a patient/client for physical therapy services, a physical therapist shall be responsible for: the examination, evaluation, and diagnosis of that individual; the prognosis and intervention; re-examination and modification of the plan of care; and the maintenance of adequate records, including progress reports. A physical therapist shall establish the plan of care and shall provide and/or supervise and direct the appropriate interventions. See Section 2.4 and 6.1.

F. If the diagnostic process reveals findings that are outside the scope of the physical therapist's knowledge, experience, or expertise, the physical therapist shall so inform the patient/client and refer to an appropriate practitioner.

G. When the patient has been referred from another practitioner, the physical therapist shall communicate the findings and/or information to the referring practitioner.

H. A physical therapist shall determine when a patient/client will no longer benefit from physical therapy services. See Section 7.1.D.

4.2 Direction and Supervision

A. The supervising physical therapist has primary responsibility for the physical therapy care rendered to a patient/client.

B. A physical therapist shall not delegate to a less qualified person any activity that requires the unique skill, knowledge, and judgment of the physical therapist.

4.3 Practice Arrangements

A. Participation in a business, partnership, corporation, or other entity does not exempt physical therapists, whether employers, partners, or stockholders, either individually or collectively, from the obligation to promote, maintain and comply with the ethical principles of the Association.

B. A physical therapist shall advise his/her employer(s) of any employer practice that causes a physical therapist to be in conflict with the ethical principles of the Association. A physical therapist shall seek to eliminate aspects of his/her employment that are in conflict with the ethical principles of the Association.

4.4 Gifts and Other Considerations

A. A physical therapist shall not invite, accept, or offer gifts, monetary incentives, or other considerations that affect or give an appearance of affecting his/her professional judgment.

B. A physical therapist shall not offer or accept kickbacks in exchange for patient referrals. See Sections 7.1.F and G and 9.1.D.

Principle 5:

A physical therapist shall achieve and maintain professional competence.

5.1 Scope of Competence

A physical therapist shall practice within the scope of his/her competence and commensurate with his/her level of education, training, and experience.

5.2 Self-assessment

A physical therapist has a lifelong professional responsibility for maintaining competence through on-going self-assessment, education, and enhancement of knowledge and skills.

5.3   Professional Development

A physical therapist shall participate in educational activities that enhance his/her basic knowledge and skills. See Section 6.1.

Principle 6:

A physical therapist shall maintain and promote high standards for physical therapy practice, education and research.

6.1   Professional Standards

A physical therapist's practice shall be consistent with accepted professional standards. A physical therapist shall continuously engage in assessment activities to determine compliance with these standards.

6.2   Practice

A.   A physical therapist shall achieve and maintain professional competence. See Section 5.

B.   A physical therapist shall demonstrate his/her commitment to quality improvement by engaging in peer and utilization review and other self-assessment activities.

6.3   Professional Education

A.   A physical therapist shall support high quality education in academic and clinical settings.

B.   A physical therapist participating in the educational process is responsible to the students, the academic institutions, and the clinical settings for promoting ethical conduct. A physical therapist shall model ethical behavior and provide the student with information about the Code of Ethics, opportunities to discuss ethical conflicts, and procedures for reporting unresolved ethical conflicts. See Section 9.

6.4   Continuing Education

A.   A physical therapist providing continuing education must be competent in the content area.

B.   When a physical therapist provides continuing education, he/she shall ensure that course content, objectives, faculty credentials, and responsibilities of the instructional staff are accurately stated in the promotional and instructional course materials.

C.   A physical therapist shall evaluate the efficacy and effectiveness of information

and techniques presented in continuing education programs before integrating them into his or her practice.

6.5   Research

A.   A physical therapist participating in research shall abide by ethical standards governing protection of human subjects and dissemination of results.

B.   A physical therapist shall support research activities that contribute knowledge for improved patient care.

C.   A physical therapist shall report to appropriate authorities any acts in the conduct or presentation of research that appear unethical or illegal. See Section 9.

Principle 7:

A physical therapist shall seek only such remuneration as is deserved and reasonable for physical therapy services.

7.1   Business and Employment Practices

A.   A physical therapist's business/employment practices shall be consistent with the ethical principles of the Association.

B.   A physical therapist shall never place his/her own financial interest above the welfare of individuals under his/her care.

C.   A physical therapist shall recognize that third-party payer contracts may limit, in one form or another, the provision of physical therapy services. Third-party limitations do not absolve the physical therapist from making sound professional judgments that are in the patient's best interest. A physical therapist shall avoid under utilization of physical therapy services.

D.   When a physical therapist's judgment is that a patient will receive negligible benefit from physical therapy services, the physical therapist shall not provide or continue to provide such services if the primary reason for doing so is to further the financial self-interest of the physical therapist or his/her employer. A physical therapist shall avoid over utilization of physical therapy services. See Section 4.1.H.

E.   Fees for physical therapy services should be reasonable for the service performed, considering the setting in which it is provided, practice costs in the geographic area, judgment of other organizations, and other relevant factors.

F.   A physical therapist shall not directly or indirectly request, receive, or participate in the dividing, transferring, assigning or rebating of an unearned fee. See Sections 4.4.A and B.

G. A physical therapist shall not profit by means of credit or other valuable consideration, such as an unearned commission, discount, or gratuity, in connection with the furnishing of physical therapy services. See Sections 4.4.A and B.

H. Unless laws impose restrictions to the contrary, physical therapists who provide physical therapy services within a business entity may pool fees and monies received. Physical therapists may divide or apportion these fees and monies in accordance with the business agreement.

I. A physical therapist may enter into agreements with organizations to provide physical therapy services if such agreements do not violate the ethical principles of the Association or applicable laws.

7.2   Endorsement of Products or Services

A. A physical therapist shall not exert influence on individuals under his/her care or their families to use products or services based on the direct or indirect financial interest of the physical therapist in such products or services. Realizing that these individuals will normally rely on the physical therapist's advice, their best interest must always be maintained, as must their right of free choice relating to the use of any product or service. Although it cannot be considered unethical for physical therapists to own or have a financial interest in the production, sale or distribution of products/services, they must act in accordance with law and make full disclosure of their interest whenever individuals under their care use such products/services.

B. A physical therapist may receive remuneration for endorsement or advertisement of products or services to the public, physical therapists, or other health professionals provided he/she discloses any financial interest in the production, sale, or distribution of said products or services.

D. When endorsing or advertising products or services, a physical therapist shall use sound professional judgment and shall not give the appearance of Association endorsement unless the Association has formally endorsed the products or services.

7.3   Disclosure

A physical therapist shall disclose to the patient if the referring practitioner derives compensation from the provision of physical therapy.

Principle 8:

A physical therapist shall provide and make available accurate and relevant information to patients/clients about their care and to the public about physical therapy services.

8.1   Accurate and Relevant Information to the Patient

A. A physical therapist shall provide the patient/client information about his/her condition and plan of care. See Section 2.4

B. Upon the request of the patient, the physical therapist shall provide, or make available, the medical record to the patient or a patient-designated third party.

C. A physical therapist shall inform patients of any known financial limitations that may affect their care.

D. A physical therapist shall inform the patient when, in his/her judgment, the patient will receive negligible benefit from further care. See Section 7.1.C.

8.2   Accurate and Relevant Information to the Public

A. A physical therapist shall inform the public about the societal benefits of the profession and who is qualified to provide physical therapy services.

B. Information given to the public shall emphasize that individual problems cannot be treated without individualized examination and plans/programs of care.

C. A physical therapist may advertise his/her services to the public. See Section 2.2.

D. A physical therapist shall not use, or participate in the use of, any form of communication containing a false, plagiarized, fraudulent, deceptive, unfair, or sensational statement or claim. See section 2.2.

E. A physical therapist who places a paid advertisement shall identify it as such unless it is apparent from the context that it is a paid advertisement.

Principle 9:

A physical therapist shall protect the public and the profession from unethical, incompetent and illegal acts.

9.1 **Consumer Protection**
   A. A physical therapist shall provide care that is within the scope of practice as defined by the state practice act.
   B. A physical therapist shall not engage in any conduct that is unethical, incompetent or illegal.
   C. A physical therapist shall report any conduct that appears to be unethical, incompetent, or illegal.
   D. A physical therapist may not participate in any arrangements in which patients are exploited due to the referring sources' enhancing their personal incomes as a result of referring for, prescribing, or recommending physical therapy. See Sections 2.1.B, 4, and 7.

Principle 10:

A physical therapist shall endeavor to address the health needs of society.

10.1 **Pro Bono Services**
   A physical therapist shall render pro bono publico (reduced or no fee) services to patients lacking the ability to pay for services, as each physical therapist's practice permits.

10.2 **Individual and Community Health**
   A. A physical therapist shall be aware of the patient's health-related needs and act in a manner that facilitates meeting those needs.
   B. A physical therapist shall endeavor to support activities that benefit the health status of the community. See Section 3.

Principle 11:

A physical therapist shall respect the rights, knowledge, and skills of colleagues and other health care professionals.

11.1 **Consultation**
   A physical therapist shall seek consultation whenever the welfare of the patient will be safeguarded or advanced by consulting those who have special skills, knowledge or experience.

11.2 **Patient/Provider Relationships**
   A physical therapist shall not undermine the relationship(s) between his/her patient and other health care professionals.

11.3 **Disparagement**
   Physical therapists shall not disparage colleagues and other health care professionals. See Section 9 and Section 2.4.A.

Issued by Ethics and Judicial Committee
American Physical Therapy Association
October 1981
Last Amended January 2004

From Guide to Professional Conduct, American Physical Therapy Association, with permission.

Health Insurance

There are three major classifications of health insurance companies. They include private health insurance companies, independent health plans, and government health insurance.

Private Health Insurance Companies

Private health insurance companies include stock companies, mutual companies, and non-profit insurance plans. Reimbursement for physical therapy services is usually on a fee for service basis.

Stock Companies: Operated nationally and are owned by independent stockholders.

Mutual Companies: Operated nationally and are owned by the individual policyholders.

Non-profit Insurance Plans: Operate in a specific geographic region and are subject to specific state regulations. They are classified as tax exempt due to their nonprofit status.

Independent Health Plans

Independent health plans are organized into various groups. Health maintenance organizations and self-insurance plans are examples of independent health plans. Reimbursement is typically based on fee-for-service or a predetermined fixed fee.

Managed Care: A concept of health care delivery where subscribers utilize health care providers that are contracted by the insurance company at a lower cost. Health maintenance organizations (HMO) and preferred provider organizations (PPO) are two examples of a managed care system. This concept attempts to attain the highest quality of care at the lowest cost.

Health Maintenance Organization: Subscribers to these insurance plans agree to receive all of their health care services through the predetermined providers of the HMO. The primary physician of the subscriber controls health care access through a referral system. Cost containment is a high priority and subscribers cannot receive care from providers outside of the plan except in an emergency.

Preferred Provider Organization: Subscribers can choose their health care services from a list of providers that contract with the insurance plan. These contracts provide extreme discounts for health care. Subscribers can use a health care provider that is not associated with the PPO, however, they will absorb a greater portion of the cost.

Consolidated Omnibus Budget Reconciliation Act (COBRA): A law passed that requires an employer to allow an employee to remain under an employer's group plan for a period of time after the loss of a job, death of a spouse, a decrease in hours or a divorce. The employee may be required to pay the employer's portion of the premiums for their insurance coverage as well as their own portion.

Fee for Service versus Managed Care

Fee for Service:	Managed Care:
• Payers assume primary financial risk	• Providers share in financial risk
• Provides enrollees with freedom of choice	• Services provided by a specific pool of providers
• Unlimited access to specialty providers	• Primary care provider serves as a gatekeeper
• Co-payments often in the form of 80%/20%	• Provides services for a fixed, prepaid monthly fee
• Limited internal/external cost controls	• Formal quality assurance and utilization review
• Minimal emphasis on health promotion and education	• Health education and preventive medicine emphasized

Government Health Insurance

Government health insurance programs such as Medicare and Medicaid are administered by the federal government. The government uses private contractors to manage the payment process of each health plan.

Medicare

Medicare provides health insurance for individuals over 65 years of age and the disabled. Medicare is a nationwide program operated by the Centers for Medicare and Medicaid Services.

Established in 1966, Medicare was the second mandated health insurance program in the United State (Workers' Compensation was the first). In 1972 Medicare coverage was expanded to include certain categories of the disabled, renal dialysis, and transplant patients.

- **Medicare Part A:**
  Provides benefits for care provided in hospitals, outpatient diagnostic services, extended care facilities, hospice, and short-term care at home required by an illness for which the patient is hospitalized.

  Enrollment in Medicare Part A is automatic and funding is through payroll taxes.

- **Medicare Part B:**
  Provides benefits for outpatient care, physician services and services ordered by physicians such as diagnostic tests, medical equipment, and supplies.

  Enrollment in Medicare Part B is voluntary and funding is through premiums paid by beneficiaries and general federal tax revenues.

Cost Sharing

The Medicare program requires beneficiaries to share in the costs of health care through deductibles and coinsurance.

- **Deductibles** require beneficiaries to reach a predetermined amount of personal expenditure each 12-month period before Medicare payment is activated.

- **Coinsurance** requires that 20% of the costs for hospitalization is covered by the patient.

Medicare sets limits on the total days of hospital care that will be paid based on a lifetime pool of days limit. Medicare payments for post hospital stays in extended care facilities are limited to 100 days.

Providers are reimbursed for Medicare services through intermediaries such as Blue Cross.

Medicaid

Medicaid provides basic medical services to the economically indigent population who qualify by reason of low income or who qualify for welfare or public assistance benefits in the state of their residence. Medicaid is a jointly funded program through the federal and state governments.

Established in 1965, Medicaid is funded through personal income, corporate, and excise taxes. Federal and state support is shared based on the state's per capita income.

Rate setting formulas, procedures, and policies vary widely among states. All state Medicaid operations must be approved by the Centers for Medicare and Medicaid Services. The Medicaid program reimburses providers directly.

The Medicaid program covers inpatient and outpatient hospital services, physician services, diagnostic services, nursing care for older adults, home health care, preventative health screening services, and family planning services.

Workers' Compensation

First designed in 1911 to provide protection for employees that were injured on the job. This legislation provides continued income as well as paid medical expenses for employees injured while working. Workers' compensation is a joint federal and state program that is regulated at the state level. Recently case managers have assisted this process by monitoring the rehabilitation process and controlling potential abuse.

Employers with 10 or more employees or high risk employers must pay a percentage of each employee salary to the worker's compensation board of the state. The exact payment is based on the risk rating of the job or institution.

Reimbursement Coding

Current Procedural Terminology Codes

Current Procedural Terminology (CPT) codes are procedure codes used by physical therapists and other health care professionals to describe the interventions that were provided to a given patient. The majority of codes used by physical therapists are in the CPT 97000 series. Examples of commonly used CPT codes by physical therapists include: 97530 – Therapeutic Activities; 97035 – Ultrasound; 97012 – Traction, mechanical. CPT is a registered trademark of the American Medical Association.

International Classification of Diseases Codes

The International Classification of Diseases (ICD) codes are designed to describe a patient's infirmity through 17 categories based on etiology and affected anatomical systems. The codes consist of five distinct digits (e.g., 755.12). The first three digits indicate the basic diagnosis. The fourth digit and in some cases the fifth digit serve to differentiate the basic diagnosis or anatomical area affected. Physicians are required to make the medical diagnosis, however, in some cases a physical therapist may need to utilize the ICD manual to determine an appropriate ICD code. This action is within a physical therapist's scope of practice and would not be considered equivalent to making a medical diagnosis.

Chapter Eleven
Special Topics

Oncology

Oncology Terminology

Benign neoplasm: an abnormal cell growth that is usually slow growing and harmless; it closely resembles the adjacent tissue composition.

Cancer (malignancy, tumor, carcinoma): Cancer can be defined as groups of diseases characterized by uncontrolled cell proliferation with mutation and spreading of the abnormal cells. The etiology is based on the type and location of the cancer. The most common causes include cigarette smoking, diet and nutrition, chemical agents, physical agents, environmental causes, viral causes, and genetics.

Dysplasia: the process of normal change in shape, size, and type of normal cells.

Hyperplasia: an increase in cell number that may be normal or abnormal.

Malignant neoplasm: an abnormal cell growth that grows uncontrollably, invades and destroys adjacent tissues, and may metastasize to other sites and systems of the body.

Metaplasia: a change in a cell from one type to another that may be normal or abnormal.

Tumor (neoplasm): A tumor is an abnormal new growth of tissue that increases the overall tissue mass. Tumors are benign (non-cancerous) or malignant (cancerous) as well as primary or secondary. Primary tumors form from cells that belong to the area of the tumor. Secondary tumors grow from cells that have metastasized (spread) from another affected area within the body.

Tumor classification is defined by cell type, tissue of origin, amount of differentiation, benign versus malignant, and anatomic site.

Tissue and Tumor Classification

Tissue Classification	Examples	Tumor Classification
Epithelium Protect, absorb, and excrete	-Skin -Lines internal cavities -Mucous membrane -Lining of bladder	Carcinoma Glandular tissue- adenocarcinoma
Pigmented Cells	-Moles	Malignant Melanoma
Connective Tissues Elastic, collagen, fibrous	-Striated muscle -Blood vessels -Bone -Cartilage -Fat -Smooth muscle	Sarcoma Fibrosarcoma Liposarcoma Chondrosarcoma Osteosarcoma Hemangiosarcoma Leiomyosarcoma Rhabdomyosarcoma
Nerve Tissues Neurons, nerve fibers, dendrites, glial cells	-Brain -Nerves -Spinal cord -Retina	Astrocytoma Glioma Neurilemic sarcoma Neuroblastoma Retinoblastoma
Lymphoid Tissues	-Where ever lymph tissue is present throughout the body -Lymph nodes -Spleen -Can appear in stomach, intestines, skin, CNS, bone and tonsils	Lymphoma
Hematopietic Tissues	-Bone marrow -Plasma cells	Leukemia Myelodysplasia Myeloproliferative syndromes Multiple myeloma

General Signs and Symptoms of Cancer

C – Change in bowel/bladder routine

A – A sore that will not heal

U – Unusual bleeding/discharge

T – Thickening/lump develops

I – Indigestion or difficulty swallowing

O – Obvious change in wart/mole

N – Nagging cough/hoarseness

**Unexplained weight loss, fatigue, anorexia, anemia, pain, and/or weakness are other general symptoms that may indicate cancer

Staging

Staging of a malignancy is diagnosed through determining the extent of the disease, the lymph node involvement, and determining if metastases exist in other areas. Staging allows for appropriate treatment and course of intervention and can assist with predicting outcome and prognosis.

Leading Cause of Deaths

Male		Female	
Lung	31%	Lung	25%
Prostate	11%	Breast	15%
Colon	10%	Colon	11%
Pancreas	5%	Pancreas	6%
Leukemia	4%	Ovary	5%
Esophagus	3%	Non-Hodgkin's Lymphoma	4%
Liver	3%	Leukemia	4%
Bladder	3%	Uterine	2%
Kidney	3%	Brain	2%
Other	22%	Multiple Myeloma	2%
		Other	23%

* Cancer is the leading cause of death in the United States

* Data taken from the American Cancer Society, www.cancer.org

Diagnostic Tools

• Family history	• Pap smear
• Physical examination	• Blood tests
• Radiography	• Biopsy
• CT scan	• Mammography
• Bone scan	• Endoscopy
• Stool guaiac	• Isotope scan

Risk Factors

• Increasing age	• Poor diet
• Tobacco use	• Stress
• Alcohol use	• Occupational hazards
• Gender	• Ethnic background
• Virus exposure	• Genetic influence
• Environmental influence	• Sexual/reproductive behavior

Common Sites of Metastasis

• Lymph nodes	• Brain
• Liver	• Bone
• Lung	

Cancer Prevention

Primary Prevention	• Screening for high risk population • Elimination of modifiable risk factors • Chemoprevention-use of natural agents (i.e., teas, vitamins) to prevent cancer • Cancer vaccine
Secondary Prevention	• Early detection • Selective preventative pharmacological agents (e.g., Tamoxifen) • Multifactorial risk reduction
Tertiary Prevention	• Prevent disability that can occur secondary to cancer and its treatment • Manage symptoms • Limit complications

Types of Cancer

Skin Cancer

Basal Cell Carcinoma
- Slow growing
- Originates from epidermis
- Rarely metastasizes
- Sun exposure is a common cause
- Prognosis is good; can be cured

Squamous Cell Carcinoma
- Usually develops in sun-damaged skin
- Usually found in fair-skinned people
- Peak incidence at 60 years
- Can be difficult to diagnose
- Can metastasize
- Prognosis with treatment is excellent

Malignant Melanoma
- Originates from melanocytes
- Cutaneous melanoma can be classified as: superficial spreading, nodular, lentigo, maligna or acral lentiginous melanomas
- Peak incidence is between 40-60 years
- Risk factors include blonde/red hair, fair skin, blue eyes, sunburn easily
- Associated with intensity of sun exposure (as opposed to duration of exposure)
- Treatment requires surgical excision and radiation/chemotherapy
- Early diagnosis is vital to prognosis
- Can spread and metastasize quickly
- Metastases to the brain, lungs, liver, bone, skin, and CNS are fatal within 12 months
- 100% curable with early diagnosis

Breast Cancer
- Most common female malignancy, but can also occur in men
- Second leading cause of female death from cancer
- 70% of breast cancer occurs to patients over 50 years of age
- Risk factors include genetics, gender, age, menstrual history, and geography
- Presents as a lump; usually found by the woman
- Mass is typically firm, irregular, and non-painful
- Common metastases to the lymph nodes, lungs, bones, skin, and brain
- Treatment may include surgery, radiation, chemotherapy or hormonal manipulation
- Curable if diagnosed prior to metastases
- Survival rate decreases as the stage of the cancer increases

- If the cancer recurs, it is usually within two years of the initial diagnosis

Lung Cancer
- Cancer of the epithelium within the respiratory tract
- Most frequent cause of death from all cancers
- Incidence of death increases from age 45 and levels off at approximately 74 years of age
- Risk factors include cigarette smoking, environmental exposure, geographic location, occupational hazards, age, and family history
- Early symptoms include cough, sputum, and dyspnea
- Rapid metastasis can occur through the pulmonary vascular system, adrenal gland, brain, bone, and liver
- Poor prognosis in most cases secondary to expedited metastasis (less than 14% for a five year survival rate)

Pancreatic Cancer
- Fourth leading cause of death by cancer
- Cancer of the exocrine cells within the ducts (ductal adenocarcinoma) is the most common form of pancreatic cancer
- Peak incidence occurs during a person's 7th and 8th decades
- Most common in African American men
- Risk factors include tobacco use, gender, increasing age, and cholecystectomy
- Early symptoms are nondescript and include decreased appetite, abdominal pain, and weight loss
- Later symptoms include jaundice, obstruction, and back pain
- Metastasizes to the liver, lungs, pleura, colon, stomach, and spleen; poor prognosis

Brain Cancer
- Most primary cancers metastasize to the brain
- Primary CNS cancers rarely metastasize outside the CNS
- Signs and symptoms are based on location of the tumor within the brain
- Signs and symptoms include headache, seizures, increased intracranial pressure, cognitive and emotional impairment, and decreased motor and sensory function
- Symptoms progress rapidly
- Usually a poor prognosis with both primary brain cancer and brain metastases

Leukemia
- Malignant neoplasm of the white blood cells
- Replaces normal cells with lymphocytic or myelogenous cells
- Two acute forms, two chronic forms

- Main symptoms include anemia, infection, bruising/bleeding tendencies
- The five year survival rate has increased for acute leukemias to 75% for children and 44% for adults
- Chronic myelogenous leukemia has a less favorable prognosis due to limitations in treatment
- Chronic lymphocytic leukemia is fatal with no curative treatment
- Treatment can include chemotherapy, radiation, bone marrow transplant, stem cell transplant, and hormone therapy

Lymphoma

- Cancers that develop in the lymphatic system and occupy lymph tissues
- A painless lump is usually the first sign
- Lymphomas are categorized as Hodgkin's disease or non-Hodgkin's lymphoma
- Hodgkin's disease is distinguished by the presence of the Reed-Sternberg cells that are part of the tissue macrophage system
- Hodgkin's disease can metastasize to extralymphatic sites including the liver, bone marrow, spleen, and lungs
- Risk factors for Hodgkin's disease include association with Epstein Barre virus, immunosuppressant use, drug abuse, obesity, chronic or autoimmune diseases
- Hodgkin's disease is one of the most curable cancers depending on age, disease stage, overall health, and responsiveness to treatment at diagnosis
- Non-Hodgkin's lymphomas are solid tumors found within the lymphatic system
- Lymphomas are classified according to size, B-cell and T-cell markers, grading, and pattern of growth
- Risk factors for non-Hodgkin's lymphoma include exposure to benzene (i.e., cigarette smoke), auto emissions, pollution, and food containing high levels of polychlonnated biphenyls (i.e., meats, dairy, fish)
- Treatment options are based on the patient's age and staging classification and include chemotherapy, chemotherapy with radiation, stem cell transplant, and highly active antiretroviral therapy
- Prognosis of non-Hodgkin lymphoma varies based on classification, co-morbidities, and response to treatment

Multiple Myeloma

- A primary malignant neoplasm of plasma cells
- Most often found in bone marrow
- Initially found in bone marrow of flat bones will infiltrate other bone marrow and then other organs
- Slow progression with initial signs of bone pain, altered red blood cell, leukocyte, and platelet production
- Peak age of incidence is between 50 and 70 years

- Anemia, bleeding tendencies, and increased susceptibility to infection result
- The pre-symptomatic period of the disease can last from 5 to 20 years
- Treatment can include chemotherapy with high potency biphosphonates, stem cell therapy, bone marrow transplant
- Median duration of remission is three years
- Median length of survival is six years
- Currently, there is no curative treatment

Sarcoma (Bone Tumor)

- Most common bone tumors are osteosarcoma, chondrosarcoma, Ewing's sarcoma, and angiosarcoma
- Bone tumors are classified as osteoblastic or osteolytic
- Pain is the predominant sign; other signs include weight loss, failure to relieve pain, night pain, age, history of cancer, swelling, and fever
- Sarcomas usually metastasize to the lungs, liver, and other bones
- Diagnosis is made through biopsy; testing that assists diagnosis includes X-ray, MRI, and bone scan
- Treatment is based on staging of the cancer and ranges from radiation or chemotherapy to surgical excision or amputation
- Prognosis varies based on grade of malignancy and stage of tumor

Colon Cancer

- Adenocarcinoma is the primary cancer that affects the bowel
- Third leading cause of death from cancer for men and women
- Risk factors include genetic syndromes, increasing age, male gender, Crohn's disease, polyps, colitis, sedentary life style, cigarette smoking, and high fat diet
- Signs are not often seen in early stages; primary symptoms include a change in bowel habits, bright red blood noted during a bowel movement, and stomach pain
- Will metastasize to the liver, lungs, bone, and brain
- Treatment requires surgical removal of the tumor with adjunct chemotherapy or radiation
- Colostomy may be required
- Prognosis is good with early diagnosis when the cancer is contained
- Prognosis is poor if it has metastasized

Liver Cancer

- Hepatocellular carcinoma is the most common liver cancer
- Risk increases with age, especially after 60 years

- There is a link between HBV, hepatitis C, and hepatocellular cancer
- Risk factors include male gender, alcohol abuse, anabolic steroids, and oral contraceptives
- Symptoms are usually nondescript initially but can include gastrointestinal pain, abdominal distention, anorexia and/or weight loss, change in bowel habits, and jaundice
- Definitive diagnosis requires a liver biopsy
- Prognosis is currently at a five year survival rate of 35% with treatment; if treatment is unsuccessful, 4 to 6 months

Prostate Cancer

- Adenocarcinoma is the most common prostate cancer
- Second highest cause of death from cancer in men
- The majority of prostate cancer affects men over 50 years of age
- Risk factors include increased age, high fat diet, genetic predisposition, African American descent, and exposure to cadmium
- Can metastasize to the bladder, musculoskeletal system, lungs, and lymph nodes
- Most times this is asymptomatic until the cancer reaches the advanced stages
- Symptoms include urinary obstruction, pain, urgency, and decreased stream/flow of urine
- Diagnosis is found through prostate biopsy
- Treatment varies and can include surgical incision of the prostate gland, radiation, and hormonal therapy
- Prognosis is good with appropriate treatment, approximately 10% fatality rate from this diagnosis

Cervical Cancer

- Cervical cancer is slow growing
- The human papilloma virus is the primary cause of cervical cancer
- Other risk factors include smoking, maternal use of diethylstilbestrol (DES), African American ethnicity, oral contraceptive use, and certain sexually transmitted diseases
- Symptoms are not common during the early stages
- Symptoms can include abnormal bleeding, pelvic and low back pain, impairment with bladder and bowel function
- Annual cervical screening is recommended
- Diagnosis is made through a Pap test (smear)
- Treatment varies with the stage of the disease process and can include laser therapy, excision, cryotherapy, or hysterectomy with adjunct chemotherapy or radiation
- Prognosis is good with appropriate intervention

Oncology Treatment Options

Surgery

Surgery is used to resect and excise a neoplasm. Surgery is indicated only after consideration of the size, type, and location of the malignancy as well as the patient's age and overall health status. Surgery may be curative or palliative and usually requires a combination of other treatment modalities secondary to potential metastases. These adjunct therapies assist to alleviate all residual cancer cells. Common side effects include fatigue, pain, deformity, scar tissue formation, and infection.

Radiation

Radiation is administered as either ionizing radiation or particle radiation and can be delivered by teletherapy (external beam), brachytherapy (a sealed source) or system therapy (unsealed source). Radiation destroys the hydrogen bonds between the DNA strands within the cancer cells. Radiation may be used prior to surgical intervention to shrink a tumor and/or post-surgical intervention to ensure destruction of residual cancer cells. Radiation is most useful with localized cancer. Common side effects include headache, bone marrow suppression, skin reactions, neuropathy, visual disturbances, nausea, vomiting, urinary frequency, diarrhea, delayed wound healing, and infection.

Chemotherapy

Chemotherapy consists of a group of drugs that are administered to destroy cancer cells. Chemotherapeutic agents include alkylating agents, antimetabolite agents, steroid hormones, plant alkaloid agents, interferons, and anti-tumor antibiotics. Each class of chemotherapeutic agents has a different mechanism of action to destroy cancer cells. Chemotherapy is most useful with widespread cancer and metastatic cancer, but is also used to induce remission, cure and/or eradicate residual cancer cells. The drugs can be administered orally, subcutaneously, intramuscularly, intravenously or intracavitarily. Common side effects include nausea, vomiting, electrolyte imbalance, sexual dysfunction, hair loss, pain, and a decrease in platelet, red, and white blood cell counts.

Biotherapy (Immunotherapy)

Biotherapy utilizes various agents and/or techniques to change the relationship between the cancer and its host. Biologic response modifiers strengthen the person's biological response to the cancer cells. Common agents/procedures used with this treatment include interferons, interleukin-2, bone marrow transplant, stem cell transplant, monoclonal antibodies, hormonal therapy, and colony-stimulating factors. These forms of biotherapy are used in conjunction with other forms of curative cancer treatment (i.e., chemotherapy) in order to decrease unnecessary damage to the patient and support the overall therapeutic goals. Common side effects include fever, chills, nausea, vomiting, anorexia, central nervous system impairment, inflammatory reactions, leukopenia, and fatigue.

Antiangiogenic Therapy

Antiangiogenic therapy focuses on the use of thalidomide and its suppression of blood supply formation. It has had initial success in the treatment of multiple myeloma. There is research to support inhibition in the growth of primary tumors through blocking the process of tumor growth as opposed to destruction of an already formed mass.

Palliative Treatment (provide relief)

Palliative treatment for the management of cancer can include radiation, chemotherapy, physical therapy, chiropractics, acupuncture, alternative and homeopathic medicines, relaxation, biofeedback, pharmacological intervention, and hospice.

Oncology Profile

Examination

- Past medical history
- Risk factor profile
- History of current condition
- Medical management
- Precautions/contraindications
- Social history
- Medications
- Living environment
- Systems review
- Safety assessment
- Skin assessment
- Range of motion
- Motor assessment
- Endurance assessment
- Mobility skills
- Cancer pain assessment

Intervention

- Mobility training
- Positioning
- Therapeutic exercise (to tolerance)
- Energy conservation techniques
- Relaxation training
- Therapeutic modalities
- Assistive device/adaptive equipment training
- Wheelchair and orthotic prescription
- Pain management

Goals

- Maximize functional mobility
- Maximize strength
- Maximize endurance
- Maximize pain management techniques
- Maximize independence with adaptive equipment
- Maximize static and dynamic balance
- Maximize patient/caregiver competence with:
  - --Pain management/relaxation
  - --Use of adaptive equipment and orthotic devices
  - --Home exercise programs

Modality Contraindications in the Treatment of Cancer

Modality	Contraindications
Superficial heat Hot pack Paraffin Infrared Fluidotherapy	• Over irradiated areas • Over bleeding areas • Over inflammation • Over a tumor
Deep Heat Diathermy Ultrasound	• Over acute hemorrhage • Over growing epiphyses • Over inflammation • Over irradiated or insensitive skin • Over a tumor • Over implants
Cryotherapy Cold pack Ice massage Cold hydrotherapy Vapocoolant spray Cold compression	• Over dysvascular tissue/irradiated tissue • Impaired sensation to the treatment area • Delayed wound healing • Radiation or chemotherapy-induced nerve injury • When chemotherapy exacerbates-Raynaud's disease or peripheral vascular disease
Mechanical Agents Traction	• Presence of tumor • Presence of infection • Previous radiation therapy
Electrotherapy Neuromuscular electrical nerve stimulation TENS Acupuncture electrical stimulation	• Potential pathological fracture • Cardiopulmonary insufficiency • Deep bone pain

Treatment Guidelines

- ✓ A patient post-surgical skin grafting may require bed rest and bedside therapy per physician protocol
- ✓ Physical therapy is contraindicated while a patient is receiving radiation with implanted radioactive seeds
- ✓ Massage and heat are contraindicated over a radiated area for a minimum of 12 months
- ✓ Special care is required for a person undergoing radiation therapy in the areas marked as sites for treatment (where the beam radiation is delivered)
- ✓ It is important to notify the nurse/physician if a patient vomits during therapy, especially when the patient is taking antiemetic medication to control nausea and vomiting
- ✓ Always check the status of a patient undergoing chemotherapy regarding their level of toxicity and risk levels for contact with the other patients and staff
- ✓ Always modify treatment as necessary secondary to the side effects of medical treatment
- ✓ Always check physician orders prior to treatment of a patient with bone metastases for proper weight bearing status and clearance to perform mobility
- ✓ A physical therapist should minimize excessive shear force during mobility, especially over treatment areas
- ✓ Always check a patient's blood values daily, especially the platelet and hematocrit counts to determine if it is safe for the patient to be mobile and exercise
- ✓ Understanding the staging and grading of a patient's cancer and how the measure impacts the goals and anticipated outcomes
- ✓ Always encourage patient and family education in all aspects of care and mobility
- ✓ Exercise should be conducted at a range of 40-65% of the peak heart rate, heart rate reserve, VO_2 max or below the anaerobic threshold
- ✓ Perceived exertion should never exceed a 12 during exercise using the Borg's Rate of Perceived Exertion Scale
- ✓ Schedule therapeutic exercise during the day at the time of the patient's peak level of energy

Psychological Disorders

Affective Disorders

Affective disorders are classified by disturbances in mood or emotion. States of extreme happiness or sadness occur and mood can alternate without cause. These extreme emotions can become intense and unrealistic.

Depression
- Slower mental and physical activity
- Poor self-esteem
- Immobilized from everyday activities
- Sadness, hopelessness, and helplessness
- Desire to withdraw
- Delusions in severe cases

Mania
- Constantly active
- Impulses immediately expressed
- Unrealistic activity
- Elation and self-confidence
- Disagreement with a patient may produce patient aggression
- Disorganized thoughts and speech
- Very few patients are diagnosed with only a manic disorder

Bipolar
- Alternating periods of depression and mania
- Females are at greater risk
- Usually begins in a patient's twenties

Neuroses Disorders

Neuroses refer to a group of disorders that are characterized by individuals exhibiting fear and maladaptive strategies in dealing with stressful or everyday stimuli. Patients with neuroses are not dealing with psychosis, do not have delusions, and usually realize that they have a problem.

Obsessive-compulsive Disorder
- Obsessions – persistent thoughts that will not leave
- Compulsions – repetitive ritual behaviors the patient cannot stop performing
- Thoughts or ritual behaviors that interfere with daily living
- Unable to control irrational behavior
- Most commonly begins in young adulthood

Anxiety Disorder
- Constant high tension
- Overreacts in certain instances
- Presents with apprehension
- Chronic worry
- Acute anxiety attacks
  - --Lasts a few minutes in duration
  - --Excitation of the sympathetic autonomic nervous system
  - --Fear of impending doom or death
  - --Shortness of breath, heart palpitations, dizziness, nausea
  - --Initiated by unconscious and internal mechanisms

Phobia Disorder
- Excessive fear of objects, occurrences or situations
- Fear is considerably out of proportion and irrational
- Fear creates difficulty in everyday life
- Subclassifications include agorophobia, social phobia, and simple phobia
- May develop from traumatic experiences, observation, classical conditioning
- Simple phobias are the easiest to treat
  - --**Acrophobia:** fear of heights
  - --**Agorophobia:** fear of open spaces
  - --**Astraphobia:** fear of thunderstorms
  - --**Belonephobia:** fear of needles
  - --**Claustrophobia:** fear of being in closed-in places
  - --**Pathophobia:** fear of disease
  - --**Pyrophobia:** fear of fire
  - --**Zoophobia:** fear of animal(s)

Dissociative Disorders

Dissociative disorders develop when a person unconsciously dissociates (separates) one part of the mind from the rest.

Psychogenic Amnesia
- Produced by the mind
- No physical cause
- Forgets all aspects of the past

Multiple Personality
- A rare dissociative disorder
- Two or more independent personalities
- Each personality may or may not know about the other
- Causative factors are not understood
- Believed to allow a person to engage in behaviors that are against the patient's morality and normally produce guilt

Somatoform Disorders

Somatoform disorders are classified based on the physical symptoms present in each disorder.

Somatization Disorder
- Primarily in women
- Often chronic and long lasting
- Complaints of symptoms with no physiological basis
- Symptoms usually lead to medications and medical visits
- Symptoms alter the patient's life
- Resembles hypochondriasis disorder
- Has familial association

Conversion Disorder
- Physical complaints of neurological basis with no underlying cause
- Paralysis is the most common finding
- Other findings include deafness, blindness, paresthesia
- Freud believes this is mental anxiety transformed into physical symptoms
- Diagnosis can be made once testing is negative for physical ailments
- Both men and women can experience a conversion disorder

Hypochondriasis Disorder
- Excessive fear of illness
- Believes that minor illnesses or medical problems indicate a serious or life threatening disease

Schizophrenia Disorders

Schizophrenia disorders are psychotic in nature and present with disorganization of thought, hallucinations, emotional dysfunction, anxiety, and perceptual impairments. Causative factors include traumatic events, genetic inheritance, biochemical imbalances, and environmental influence.

Catatonic Schizophrenia
- Motor disturbances with rigid posturing
- Patients remain aware during episodes
- Episodes consist of uncontrolled movements
- Medications are required to regulate episodes

Paranoid Schizophrenia
- Delusions of grandeur
- Delusions of persecution
- May believe they possess special powers

Disorganized Schizophrenia
- Usually progressive and irreversible
- Inappropriate emotional responses
- Mumbled talking

Undifferentiated Schizophrenia
- May possess a mix of symptoms
- Does not classify into one category

Personality Disorders

A personality disorder is classified by observing a patient's pattern of behavior, dysfunctional view of society, and level of sadness. Personality disorders are usually ongoing patterns of dysfunctional behavior.

Psychopathic Personality
- Low morality
- Poor sense of responsibility
- No respect for others
- Impulsive behavior for immediate gratification
- High frustration
- Little guilt or remorse for all actions
- Inability to alter behavior even with punishment
- Expert liar

Antisocial Behavior
- Results from particular causes (e.g., need for attention or involvement in a gang)
- Usually have some concern for others
- Blames other institutions (e.g., family, school) for their actions
- Usually begins before 16 years of age
- Violates the rights of others
- Lacks responsibility and emotional stability

Narcissistic Behavior
- Incapable of loving others
- Self-absorbed
- Obsessed with success and power
- Unrealistic perception of self-importance

Borderline Behavior
- Instability in all aspects of life
- Can identify self from others as well as reality
- Uses projection, denial, defensiveness
- Intense and uncontrolled anger
- Chronic feelings of emptiness
- Unpredictable mood or behavior

Pharmacological Intervention for Psychiatric Management

Neuroleptic Agents	Traditional Agents
Used for short and long-term treatment of psychosis Used as tranquilizers or for sedation May produce hypotension, abnormal movements, over-sedation, blurred vision, and tics	Chlorpromazine (Thorazine) Prochlorperazine (Compazine) Fluphenazine (Prolixin) Haloperidol (Haldol) Droperidol (Inapsine) Thioridazine (Mellaril) **Atypical Agents** Risperidone (Risperdal) Quetiapine/Fumarate (Seroquel) Clozapine (Clozaril)
Antidepressant Agents	**Tricyclic (Tertiary Amine)**
Alleviate depression and/or anxiety; used in obsessive-compulsive disorder, bulimia and anorexia, social phobias, and post-traumatic stress disorders May produce weight gain, sedation, constipation, insomnia, cardiovascular issues, and orthostatic hypotension	Amitriptyline (Elavil) Doxepin (Sinequan) Trimipramine (Surmontil) **Tricyclic (Secondary Amine)** Desipramine (Norpramine) Nortriptyline (Pamelor) **(SSRI)-Selective Serotonin Reuptake Inhibitors** Fluoxetine (Prozac) Paroxetine (Paxil) Sertraline (Zoloft) Escitalopram (Lexapro) Fluvoxamine (Luvox) **Monoamine Oxidase Inhibitors (MAOI)** Phenelzine (Nardil) Tranylcypromine (Parnate) **Other Antidepressants** Maprotiline (Ludiomil) Bupropion (Wellbutrin) Trazodone (Desyrel) Venlafaxine (Effexor)

Pharmacological Intervention for Psychiatric Management(continued)

Sedative-Hypnotic Agents	Benzodiazepine Agents
Alleviate insomnia, frequent awakenings during sleep	Temazepam (Restoril)
	Triazolam (Halcion)
	Estazolam (Prosom)
	Fluorazepam (Dalmane)
May become addictive	**Nonbenzodiazepine Agents**
	Zolpidem (Ambien)
	Trazodone (Desyrel)
	Diphenhydramine (Benadryl)
Bipolar Disorder Agents	Lithium carbonate (Lithobid)
Act as mood stabilizer, controls manic episodes	Sodium dualproex (Depakote)
	Carbamazepine (Tegretol)
	Gabepentin (Neurontin)
	Vigabatrin (Sabril)
Anxiolytic Agents	**Benzodiazepine Agents**
Alleviate anxiety without significant sedation	Lorazepam (Ativan)
	Diazepam (Valium)
	Alprazolam (Xanax)
	Chlordiazepoxide (Librium)
May produce physical dependence or rebounding anxiety once medication is stopped	**Nonbenzodiazepine Agents**
	Buspirone (BuSpar)
	Doxepin (Sinequan)
	Hydroxyzine (Atarax)
	Propanolol (Inderal)

Obstetrics

Exercise and Pregnancy

Recommended exercise activities
- Swimming
- Walking
- Stretching
- Low impact aerobics
- Golfing
- Stationary cycling

Exercise activities to avoid
- High-level balance activities
- Skiing
- Water skiing
- Scuba diving
- Horseback riding
- Contact sports
- Skating
- Strenuous lifting

Pregnant women are encouraged to continue with exercise activity at a moderate rate during a low risk pregnancy. Guidelines permit women to remain at 50% to 60% of their maximal heart rate for approximately thirty minutes per session. Women must monitor their heart rate intermittently to ensure that they are maintaining their target heart rate. Non-weight bearing activities are preferred due to the continuous change in the center of gravity and balance. Loose clothing is advised to allow for adequate heat loss, and adequate fluids are required during exercise. Women should avoid becoming overtired and should not exercise in the supine position after the first trimester.

American College of Obstetricians and Gynecologists (ACOG) Recommendations for Exercise in Pregnancy and Postpartum

1. During pregnancy, women can continue to exercise and derive health benefits even from mild to moderate exercise routines. Regular exercise (at least three times per week) is preferable to intermittent activity.
2. Women should avoid exercise in the supine position after the first trimester. Such a position is associated with decreased cardiac output in most pregnant women. Since the remaining cardiac output will be preferentially distributed away from splanchnic beds (including the uterus) during vigorous exercise, such regimens are best avoided during pregnancy. Prolonged periods of motionless standing should also be avoided.
3. Women should be aware of the decreased oxygen available for aerobic exercise during pregnancy. They should be encouraged to modify the intensity of their exercise according to maternal symptoms. Pregnant women should stop exercising when fatigued and not exercise to exhaustion. Weight bearing exercises may under some circumstances be continued at intensities similar to those prior to pregnancy throughout pregnancy. Non-weight bearing exercises, such as cycling or swimming, will minimize the risk of injury and facilitate the continuation of exercise during pregnancy.
4. Morphologic changes in pregnancy should serve as a relative contraindication to types of exercise in which loss of balance could be detrimental to maternal or fetal well-being, especially in the third trimester. Further, any type of exercise involving the potential for even mild abdominal trauma should be avoided.
5. Pregnancy requires an additional 300 kcal/day in order to maintain metabolic homeostasis. Thus, women who exercise during pregnancy should be particularly careful to ensure an adequate diet.
6. Pregnant women who exercise in the first trimester should augment heat dissipation by ensuring adequate

hydration, appropriate clothing, and optimal environmental surroundings during exercise.

7. Many of the physiological and morphological changes of pregnancy persist four to six weeks postpartum. Thus, pre-pregnancy exercise routines should be resumed gradually based upon a woman's physical capability.

From American College of Obstetricians and Gynecologists. Exercise During Pregnancy and the Postpartum Period. (Technical Bulletin No. 189). Washington, DC, copyrights ACOG, February 1994, with permission.

Physiological Changes During Pregnancy

- Weight gain between 25 and 35 pounds
- Increased depth of respiration
- Increased tidal volume
- Increased minute ventilation
- Increased oxygen consumption per minute (15-20%)
- Abdominals become overstretched
- Ligaments become lax secondary to hormonal changes
- Joints may become hypermobile
- Increased blood volume (40-50%)
- Anemia may occur
- Hypotension in supine position during late pregnancy from pressure on the inferior vena cava
- Increased cardiac output (30-60%)

Postural Changes

- Change in the center of gravity
- Forward head posture
- Increased cervical lordosis
- Increased base of support in standing

Diastasis Recti

Diastasis recti is a separation of the rectus abdominis muscle along the linea alba that can occur during pregnancy. The exact cause is unknown, however, theories indicate biomechanical and hormonal changes in women may cause the separation. Testing should be performed on all pregnant women for diastasis recti prior to prescribing exercises that require the use of the abdominals. A therapist should place a hand horizontally over the umbilicus as the pregnant woman lies in a hooklying position. A patient is considered to have diastasis recti if the therapist detects a separation greater than the width of two fingers when the woman lifts her head and shoulders off the plinth. The therapist must note how many fingers fit into the separation and modify treatment accordingly. Diastasis recti requires stabilization and support with abdominal strengthening exercises. A newborn can also have diastasis recti secondary to incomplete development, however, in infants this condition usually resolves itself without intervention.

Pelvic Floor Weakness

The pelvic floor is comprised of a group of muscles that stretch between the pubis and coccyx and create the inferior stability of the pelvic cavity. The pubococcygeal muscles can become lax and over stretch during delivery or can become disrupted by an episiotomy. Weakness of the vaginal canal and stress incontinence are two problems that can result from childbirth and may require physical therapy intervention. Pubococcygeal or Kegel exercises should begin during pregnancy for prevention of pubococcygeal muscle weakness. The exercises require a patient to contract or squeeze as if she was stopping the flow of urine. The isometric contraction should be held five to ten seconds with complete relaxation after each contraction. Five to ten contractions should be performed in a series and three to four series should be performed each day.

Contraindications for Exercise During Pregnancy

- Pregnancy induced hypertension
- Preterm rupture of membrane
- Preterm labor during the prior or current pregnancy
- Incompetent cervix
- Persistent second to third trimester bleeding
- Intrauterine growth retardation

From American College of Obstetricians and Gynecologists. Exercise During Pregnancy and the Postpartum Period. (Technical Bulletin No. 189). Washington, DC, copyrights ACOG, February 1994, with permission.

Pediatrics

Developmental Gross and Fine Motor Skills	
Gross Motor Skills	**Fine Motor Skills**
Newborn to 1 Month:	

Prone
   Physiological flexion
   Lifts head briefly
   Head to side
 Supine
   Physiological flexion
   Rolls partly to side
 Sitting
   Head lag in pull to sit
 Standing
   Reflex standing and
   walking
	Regards objects in direct line of sight
	 Follows moving object to midline
	 Hands fisted
	 Arm movements jerky
	 Movements may be purposeful or random

Developmental Gross and Fine Motor Skills (continued)	
Gross Motor Skills	**Fine Motor Skills**
2 to 3 Months:	
Prone Lifts head 90 degrees briefly Chest up in prone position with some weight through forearms Rolls prone to supine *Supine* Asymmetrical tonic neck reflex (ATNR) influence strong Legs kick reciprocally Prefers head to side *Sitting* Head upright but bobbing Variable head lag in pull to sitting position Needs full support to sit *Standing* Poor weight bearing Hips in flexion, behind shoulders	Can see further distances Hands open more Visually follows through 180 degrees Grasp is reflexive Uses palmar grasp
4 to 5 Months:	
Prone Bears weight on extended arms Pivots in prone to reach toys *Supine* Rolls from supine to side position Plays with feet to mouth *Sitting* Head steady in supported sitting position Turns head in sitting position Sits alone for brief periods *Standing* Bears all weight through legs in supported stand	Grasps and releases toys Uses ulnar-palmar group

Gross Motor Skills	**Fine Motor Skills**
6 to 7 Months:	
Prone Rolls from supine to prone position Holds weight on one hand to reach for toy *Supine* Lifts head *Sitting* Lifts head and helps when pulled to sitting position Gets to sitting position without assistance Sits independently *Mobility* May crawl backward	Approaches objects with one hand Arm in neutral when approaching toy Radial-palmar grasp "Rakes" with fingers to pick up small objects Voluntary release to transfer objects between hands
8 to 9 Months:	
Prone Gets into hands-knees position *Supine* Does not tolerate supine position *Sitting* Moves from sitting to prone position Sits without hand support for longer periods Pivots in sitting position *Standing* Stands at furniture Pulls to stand at furniture Lowers to sitting position from supported stand *Mobility* Crawls forward Walks along furniture (cruising)	Develops active supination Radial-digital grasp develops Uses inferior pincer grasp Extends wrist actively Points with index finger Pokes with index finger Release of objects is more refined Takes objects out of container

Developmental Gross and Fine Motor Skills (continued)

Gross Motor Skills	Fine Motor Skills
10 to 11 Months:	
Standing Stands without support briefly Pulls to stand using half-kneel intermediate position Picks up object from floor from standing with support *Mobility* Walks with both hands held Walks with one hand held Creeps on hands and feet (bear walk)	Fine pincer grasp developed Puts objects into container Grasps crayon adaptively
12 to 15 Months:	
Mobility Walks without support Fast walking Walks backward Walks sideways Bends over to look between legs Creeps or hitches upstairs Throws ball in sitting position	Marks paper with crayon Builds tower using two cubes Turns over small container to obtain contents
16 to 24 Months:	
Squats in play Walks upstairs and downstairs with one hand held-both feet on step Propels ride-on toys Kicks ball Throws ball Throws ball forward Picks up toy from floor without falling	Folds paper Strings beads Stacks six cubes Imitates vertical and horizontal strokes with crayon on paper Holds crayon with thumb and fingers
2 Years:	
Rides tricycle Walks backward Walks on tiptoe Runs on toes Walks downstairs alternating feet Catches large ball Hops on one foot	Turns knob Opens and closes jar Able to button large buttons Uses child-size scissors with help Does 12 to 15 piece puzzles Folds paper or clothes

Preschool Age (3 to 4 Years):	
Throws ball 10 feet Walks on a line 10 feet Hops 2-10 times on one foot Jumps distances of up to two feet Jumps over obstacles up to 12 inches Throws and catches small ball Runs fast and avoids obstacles	Controls crayons more effectively Copies a circle or cross Matches colors Cuts with scissors Draws recognizable human figure with head and two extremities Draws squares May demonstrate hand preference
Early School Age (5 to 8 Years):	
Skips on alternate feet Gallops Can play hopscotch, balance on one foot, controlled hopping, and squatting on one leg Jumps with rhythm, control (jump rope) Bounces large ball Kicks ball with greater control Limbs growing faster than trunk allowing greater speed, leverage	Hand preference is evident Prints well, starting to learn cursive writing Able to button small buttons
Later School Age (9 to 12 Years):	
Mature patterns of movement in throwing, jumping, running Competition increases, enjoys competitive games Improved balance, coordination, endurance, attention span Boys may develop preadolescent fat spurt Girls may develop prepubescent and pubescent changes in body shape (hips, breasts)	Develops greater control in hand usage Learns to draw Handwriting is developed

Developmental Gross and Fine Motor Skills (continued)	
Gross Motor Skills	**Fine Motor Skills**
Adolescence (13 Years+):	
Rapid growth in size and strength, boys more than girls Puberty leads to changes in body proportions: center of gravity rises toward shoulders for boys, lower to hips for girls Balance and coordination skills, eye-hand coordination, endurance may plateau during growth spurt	Develops greater dexterity in fingers for fine tasks (knitting, sewing, art, crafts)

From Ratliffe KT: Clinical Pediatric Physical Therapy: A Guide for the Physical therapy Team. Mosby Company Inc., Philadelphia 1998, p.45-47, with permission.

Concepts of Development

Cephalic to Caudal: A person develops head and upper extremity control prior to trunk and lower extremity control. There is a general skill acquisition from the direction of head to toe.

Gross to Fine: A general trend for large muscle movement acquisition with progression to small muscle skill acquisition.

Mass to Specific: A general trend for a person to acquire simple movements and progress towards complex movements.

Proximal to Distal: A concept that uses the midline of the body as the reference point. Trunk control (midline stability) is acquired first with subsequent gain in distal control (extremities).

Pediatric Therapeutic Positioning

Proper positioning is essential to obtain maximum function for the pediatric population. Positioning is used for many purposes including facilitation of desired patterns of movement, inhibition of abnormal reflexes, normalization of tone, midline orientation, enhancement of respiratory capacity, pulmonary hygiene, maintaining skin integrity, and prevention of contractures.

Federal Legislation Affecting Health and Education for Children with Disabilities

Perkins Vocational and Applied Technology Act (enacted 1990)
Reauthorization and modification of the Education for all Handicapped Children (EHA). Provides free appropriate education in the least restrictive environment for individuals with disabilities from age 3 – 21.

IDEA Amendments (enacted 1991)
Reauthorized early intervention; established Federal Interagency Coordination Council.

Rehabilitation Act Amendments (enacted 1992)
Transition planning at high school graduation includes coordination of assistive technology services and rehabilitation system.

IDEA Amendments (enacted 1997)
Restructuring of IDEA into four distinct and individual parts.

Ideal Positioning

	Supine	**Prone**	**Sidelying**	**Sitting**
Pelvis and hips	Pelvis in line with trunk. Hips in 30 to 90 degrees of flexion. Neutral rotation of pelvis. Hips symmetrically abducted 10 to 20 degrees.	Pelvis in line with trunk. Hips in extension. Neutral rotation of pelvis. Hips symmetrically abducted 10-20 degrees.	Pelvis in line with trunk. Hips in flexion. Neutral rotation. Hips in 10 to 20 degrees abduction.	Pelvis in line with trunk. Hips at 90 degrees flexion. Neutral rotation of pelvis. Hips symmetrically abducted 10 to 20 degrees.

Ideal Positioning (continued)

	Supine	Prone	Sidelying	Sitting
Trunk	Straight. Shoulders in line with hips. Neutral rotation of trunk.	Straight. Shoulders in line with hips. Neutral rotation.	Straight. Shoulders in line with hips. Slight sidebending okay.	Straight. Shoulders over hips. Not rotated.
Head and neck	Head in neutral position. Facing forward. Slight cervical flexion.	Head in neutral position. Facing to one side. Slight cervical flexion.	Head in neutral position. Facing forward. Slight cervical flexion.	Head in neutral position. Facing forward. Head evenly on shoulders.
Shoulders and arms	Arms fully supported. Arms forward of trunk. Forearms rest on trunk or pillow.	Arms fully supported. Arms forward of trunk. Flexion at shoulders. Flexion at elbows.	Both arms supported. Lower arm forward, not lying on point of shoulders. Lower arm neutral rotation. Upper arm may have 0 to 40 degrees medial rotation.	Arms fully supported. Elbows in flexion. 0 to 45 degrees internally rotated shoulders.
Legs and feet	Knees supported in flexion. Feet held at 90 degrees.	Knees extended. Feet supported at 90 degrees.	Knees in flexion. Feet positioned at 90 degrees. Pillow between knees.	Knees at 90 degrees. Ankles at 90 degrees. Feet fully supported. Thighs fully supported.

From Ratliffe KT: Clinical Pediatric Physical Therapy: A Guide for the Physical Therapy Team. Mosby Inc., Philadelphia 1998, p.266, with permission.

Infant Reflexes and Possible Effects if Reflex Persists Abnormally

Primitive Reflex	Possible Negative Effect on Movement with Abnormal Persistence of Reflex
Asymmetrical Tonic Neck Reflex (ATNR)	
Stimulus: Head position, turned to one side **Response:** Arm and leg on face side are extended, arm and leg on scalp side are flexed, spine curved with convexity toward face side **Normal age of response:** Birth to 6 months	**Interferes with:** • Feeding • Visual Tracking • Midline use of hands • Bilateral hand use • Rolling • Development of crawling • Can lead to skeletal deformities (e.g., scoliosis, hip subluxation, hip dislocation)
Symmetrical Tonic Neck Reflex (STNR)	
Stimulus: Head position, flexion or extension **Response:** When head is in flexion, arms are flexed, legs extended. When head is in extension, arms are extended, legs are flexed **Normal age of response:** 6 to 8 months	**Interferes with:** • Ability to prop on arms in prone position • Attaining and maintaining hands-and-knees position • Crawling reciprocally • Sitting balance when looking around • Use of hands when looking at object in hands in sitting position

Infant Reflexes and Possible Effects if Reflex Persists Abnormally (cont.)

Primitive Reflex	Possible Negative Effect on Movement with Abnormal Persistence of Reflex
Tonic Labyrinthine Reflex (TLR)	
Stimulus: Position of labyrinth in inner ear—reflected in head position **Response:** In the supine position, body and extremities are held in extension; in the prone position, body and extremities are held in flexion **Normal age of response:** Birth to 6 months	Interferes with: • Ability to initiate rolling • Ability to prop on elbows with extended hips when prone • Ability to flex trunk and hips to come to sitting position from supine position • Often causes full body extension, which interferes with balance in sitting or standing
Galant Reflex	
Stimulus: Touch to skin along spine from shoulder to hip **Response:** Lateral flexion of trunk to side of stimulus **Normal age of response:** 30 weeks of gestation to 2 months	Interferes with: • Development of sitting balance • Can lead to scoliosis
Palmar Grasp Reflex	
Stimulus: Pressure in palm on ulnar side of hand **Response:** Flexion of fingers causing strong grip **Normal age of response:** Birth to 4 months	Interferes with: • Ability to grasp and release objects voluntarily • Weight bearing on open hand for propping, crawling, protective responses
Plantar Grasp Reflex	
Stimulus: Pressure to base of toes **Response:** Toe flexion **Normal age of response:** 28 weeks of gestation to 9 months	Interferes with: • Ability to stand with feet flat on surface • Balance reactions and weight shifting in standing
Rooting Reflex	
Stimulus: Touch on cheek **Response:** Turning head to same side with mouth open **Normal age of response:** 28 weeks of gestation to 3 months	Interferes with: • Oral-motor development • Development of midline control of head • Optical righting, visual tracking, and social interaction
Moro Reflex	
Stimulus: Head dropping into extension suddenly for a few inches **Response:** Arms abduct with fingers open, then cross trunk into adduction; cry **Normal age of response:** 28 weeks of gestation to 5 months	Interferes with: • Balance reactions in sitting • Protective responses in sitting • Eye-hand coordination, visual tracking
Startle Reflex	
Stimulus: Loud, sudden noise **Response:** Similar to Moro response but elbows remain flexed and hands closed **Normal age of response:** 28 weeks of gestation to 5 months	Interferes with: • Sitting balance • Protective responses in sitting • Eye-hand coordination, visual tracking • Social interaction, attention
Positive Support Reflex	
Stimulus: Weight placed on balls of feet when upright **Response:** Stiffening of legs and trunk into extension **Normal age of response:** 35 weeks of gestation to 2 months	Interferes with: • Standing and walking • Balance reactions and weight shift in standing • Can lead to contractures of ankles into plantar flexion

Infant Reflexes and Possible Effects if Reflex Persists Abnormally (cont.)

Primitive Reflex	Possible Negative Effect on Movement with Abnormal Persistence of Reflex
Walking (Stepping) Reflex	
Stimulus: Supported upright position with soles of feet on firm surface **Response:** Reciprocal flexion/extension of legs **Normal age of response:** 38 weeks of gestation to 2 months	**Interferes with:** ▪ Standing and walking ▪ Balance reactions and weight shifting in standing ▪ Development of smooth, coordinated reciprocal movements of lower extremities

From Ratliffe KT: Clinical Pediatric Physical Therapy: A Guide for the Physical Therapy Team. Mosby Inc., Philadelphia 1998, p.266, with permission.

Pediatric Assessment Tools

Instrument	Purpose	Other
Alberta Infant Motor Scale	--Identify components of motor development --Measure gross motor acquisition and skill maturation over time	--Use from birth to walking --Piper
Bayley Scale of Infant Development II	--Assessment of current developmental status using a mental scale, motor scale, and behavioral scale --Includes special populations	--Use from one month to 42 months --Bayley
Denver II	--Screen of four domains: personal-social, fine motor adaptive, language, and gross motor --Screens for developmental delay and need for further evaluation	--Use from two weeks to six years -Frankenburg
Functional Independence Measure for Children (WeeFim)	--Assesses and notes progression of functional independence --A measure of disability --Requires consistent performance of a skill	--Use from six months to seven years --Utilized by Uniform Data System (UDS)
Milani-Comparetti Motor Development Screening Test	--Measures functional motor skills and related reflexes --Demonstrates age appropriate responses through profile --Neuromotor delays	--Use from birth to two years --Milani-Comparetti, Gidoni
Movement Assessment of Infants	--Focus on infants that were treated in neonatal intensive care --Categories include muscle tone, reflexes, automatic reactions, and volitional movements --Identifies motor dysfunction and establishes baseline	--Use from birth to 12 months --Chandler, Swanson
Neonatal Behavioral Assessment	--Focus on interactive behavior, competence, and neurological status --Predictor of further neurological problems	--Use from three days to four weeks --Brazelton

Pediatric Assessment Tools (continued)

Instrument	Purpose	Other
Peabody Developmental Motor Scales	--Provides detailed assessment with instruction programming --Gross and fine motor scales --Identifies emergency skills --Does not require verbal language	--Use from birth to 83 months --Folio, Fewell
Pediatric Evaluation of Disability Inventory (PEDI)	--Assessment of functional skills --Designed for rehabilitation use --Includes areas of self care, mobility, social skills, level of assistance, and use of adaptive equipment	--Use from six months to 7.5 years --Haley

Pediatric Profile

Examination

- Past medical history
- History of current condition
- Social history (caregiver support)
- Medications
- Living environment
- Systems review
- Pediatric assessment tools
- Gross and fine motor skill acquisition
- Pathological reflexes
- Neurological assessment
- Strength
- Range of motion
- Respiratory assessment
- Postural tone assessment
- Reassessment of existing adaptive equipment, orthotics and splinting

Intervention

- Progression through pediatric milestones
- Therapeutic exercise
- Sensory integration
- Postural control
- Therapeutic positioning
- Therapeutic play
- Wheelchair and orthotic prescription
- Chest physical therapy
- Family/caregiver teaching
- Mobility training

Goals

- Maximize functional mobility
- Maximize range of motion
- Maximize strength and postural control
- Maximize patient/caregiver competence with:
  - --Home program
  - --Disease process and its progression
  - --Therapeutic positioning and handling
- Maximize independence with use of equipment

Pediatric Pathology

Cardiopulmonary

Asthma

Asthma is a reversible condition of airway hypersensitivity and bronchoconstriction within the lungs.

- **Causative factors** are extrinsic or intrinsic by nature. Extrinsic factors include allergens such as foods, animals, dust, smoke, and pollen. Intrinsic factors include exercise, stress, viral infections, and overall fatigue.
- **Characteristics** can range from mild to severe depending on the level of airway restriction. A mild asthma attack presents with wheezing, chest tightness, and slight shortness of breath. A severe asthma attack presents with dyspnea, flaring nostrils, diminished wheezing, anxiety, cyanosis, and the inability to speak. A severe attack left untreated will result in respiratory failure.
- **Treatment** includes pharmacological intervention using bronchodilators. Physical therapy management includes caregiver education, bronchial drainage and hygiene, breathing exercises, relaxation, endurance, and strength training.

Cystic Fibrosis

Cystic fibrosis is a disease of the exocrine glands that primarily affects the respiratory and gastrointestinal systems.

- The **causative factor** is a mutation of chromosome seven to include the cystic fibrosistransmembrane conductance regulator (CFTR). Cystic fibrosis is an autosomal recessive genetic disorder and a terminal disease.
- **Characteristics** change with the progression of the disease and include increased secretion of thick mucus, gastrointestinal distress, abnormal bowels, recurrent pulmonary infection, salty tasting skin, wheezing, productive cough, barrel chest, dyspnea, and progressive use of accessory muscles with respiration.
- **Treatment** has improved survival rates from seven years in the late 1960's to a mean age of 32 years today. Pharmacological interventions include antibiotics used to control pulmonary infections, nutritional supplements, pancreatic enzyme replacements, mucus thinning medications, and bronchodilators. Physical therapy treatment is essential and includes bronchial drainage, percussion, vibration, suctioning, breathing techniques, assisted cough, and ventilatory muscle training for optimal pulmonary function. General exercise is indicated to improve overall strength and endurance except with severe lung disease. Family involvement with a home program is vital for the child's ongoing pulmonary needs.

Patent Ductus Arteriosus

Patent ductus arteriosus is a disorder where the ductus arteriosus, which normally shunts blood in utero from the pulmonary artery directly to the descending aorta, fails to close shortly after birth.

- **Causative factors** for this condition include premature birth, respiratory distress syndrome, fetal alcohol syndrome, Trisomy 13 (Patau's syndrome), and Trisomy 18 (Edwards' syndrome).
- **Characteristics** of this condition depend on the size of the ductus. A small ductus may be asymptomatic where as a large ductus may present with tachycardia, respiratory distress, poor nutrition, weight loss, and congestive heart failure.
- Initial **treatment** attempts to non-surgically reduce the size of the ductus with use of diuretics and indomethacin when indicated. Surgical repair may be necessary for a large ductus or when initial management fails.

Respiratory Distress Syndrome (RDS)

Respiratory distress syndrome is a pulmonary condition seen in neonates born before 37 weeks of gestation. RDS is also known as hyaline membrane disease and is the leading cause of death in the neonate.

- **Causative factors** are due to the immaturity of the lungs and the inability to produce necessary levels of surfactant. This deficit results in increased alveolar tension, alveolar collapse, atelectasis, and difficulty breathing. Associated factors with RDS include being the second born twin, cesarean delivery, hypoxia, and acidosis.
- **Characteristics** are observed immediately as the infant works hard to breathe and re-inflate the collapsed lung. Tachypnea, flaring of the nostrils, use of accessory muscles, and respiratory distress are observed within one to two hours. Untreated, the infant lacks oxygen and presents with metabolic acidosis and acute respiratory failure.
- **Treatment** will vary and can include mechanical ventilation, supplemental oxygen, administration of artificial surfactant, nutritional support, bronchial drainage, and chest physical therapy. As a child recovers from RDS there is an increase in secretions from oxygen therapy and mechanical ventilation that requires short-term chest physical therapy.

Tetralogy of Fallot

Tetralogy of Fallot is the most common cyanotic heart defect where the following four abnormalities exist:
    Ventricular septal defect
    Right ventricular hypertrophy
    Aortic override of the interventricular septum
    Pulmonary stenosis

- The **causative factors** are congenital defect, association with Down syndrome and fetal alcohol syndrome.
- **Characteristics** vary depending on the extent of the defects and include dyspnea, hypoxia, failure to gain weight, cyanosis, and poor development.
- **Treatment** usually includes pharmacological intervention, reopening of the ductus arteriosus, or surgical reconstruction of the defects.

Musculoskeletal

Congenital Hip Dysplasia

Congenital hip dysplasia is a condition also known as developmental dysplasia. Presentation includes a malalignment of the femoral head with the acetabulum. The condition develops during the last trimester in utero.

- **Causative factors** may include cultural predisposition, malposition, and environmental and genetic influences.
- **Characteristics** include asymmetrical hip abduction with tightness and apparent femoral shortening of the involved side. Testing for this condition includes the Ortolani test, Barlow maneuver, and ultrasound.
- **Treatment** is dependent on age, severity, and initial attempts to reposition the femoral head within the acetabulum through the constant use of a harness,

bracing, splinting or traction. Open reduction with subsequent application of a hip spica cast may be required if conservative treatment fails. Physical therapy may be indicated after cast removal for stretching, strengthening, and caregiver education.

Congenital Limb Deficiencies

A congenital limb deficiency is a malformation that occurs in utero secondary to an impaired developmental course. Congenital limb deficiencies are classified as longitudinal or transverse.

- The **causative factor** of a longitudinal limb deficiency is an abnormality present at conception where a bone lacks potential to form. The causative factors of a transverse limb deficiency can include environmental factors, teratogen (thalidomide), trauma or infection.
- The primary **characteristic** of a longitudinal limb deficiency is a missing long bone such as the radius. A transverse limb deficiency is a limb that does not develop beyond a particular point.
- **Treatment** may focus on symmetrical movements, strengthening, range of motion, weight bearing activities, and prosthetic training.

Congenital Torticollis

Congenital torticollis is characterized by a unilateral contracture of the sternocleidomastoid musculature.

- Etiology is unknown, however, **causative factors** include malposition in utero, breech position in utero, and birth trauma. An infant is usually diagnosed within the first three weeks after birth.
- **Characteristics** include lateral flexion to the same side as the contracture, rotation toward the opposite side, and facial asymmetries.
- **Treatment** is usually conservative for the first year with emphasis on stretching, active range of motion, positioning, and caregiver education. Surgical management is indicated when conservative options have failed and the child is over one year of age. A surgical release followed by physical therapy may be indicated to for range of motion and proper alignment.

Legg-Calve-Perthes Disease

Legg-Calve-Perthes disease is characterized by degeneration of the femoral head due to a disturbance in the blood supply (avascular necrosis). The disease is self-limiting and has four distinct stages: condensation, fragmentation, re-ossification, and remodeling.

- **Causative factors** include trauma, genetic predisposition, synovitis, vascular abnormalities, and infection.
- **Characteristics** include pain, decreased range of motion, antalgic gait, and a positive Trendelenburg sign.

- **Treatment** methods may vary but the primary focus is to relieve pain, maintain the femoral head in the proper position, and improve range of motion. Physical therapy may be required intermittently for stretching, splinting, crutch training, aquatic therapy, traction, and exercise. Orthotic devices and surgical intervention may be indicated depending on classification and severity of the condition.

Osgood-Schlatter Disease

Osgood-Schlatter disease is a condition also known as traction apophysis that results from repetitive traction on the tibial tuberosity apophysis.

- The **causative factor** is the repeated tension to the patella tendon over the tibial tuberosity in young athletes, which results in a small avulsion of the tuberosity and swelling.
- **Characteristics** of this self-limiting condition include point tenderness over the patella tendon at the insertion on the tibial tubercle, antalgic gait, and pain with increasing activity.
- **Treatment** is usually conservative with focus on education, icing, flexibility exercises, and eliminating activities that place strain on the patella tendon such as squatting, running or jumping.

Osteogenesis Imperfecta

Osteogenesis imperfecta is a connective tissue disorder that affects the formation of collagen during bone development. There are four classifications of osteogenesis imperfecta that vary in levels of severity.

- The **causative factor** is genetic inheritance with type I and IV considered autosomal dominant traits, and types II and III considered autosomal recessive traits.
- **Characteristics** of this condition include pathological fractures, osteoporosis ("brittle bones"), hypermobile joints, bowing of the long bones, weakness, scoliosis, and impaired respiratory function.
- **Treatment** begins at birth with caregiver education on proper handling and facilitation of movement. Use of orthotics, active and symmetrical movements, positioning, functional mobility, and fracture management are essential areas of treatment. In severe cases where ambulation is not realistic, wheelchair prescription and training is indicated.

Scoliosis

Scoliosis is a lateral curvature of the spine that can be classified as infantile, juvenile, adolescent or adult.

- **Causative factors** include unknown etiology, altered development of the spine in utero, association with cerebral palsy, muscular dystrophy, other neuromuscular conditions and leg length discrepancy.
- **Characteristics** indicate whether a scoliosis is a structural or non-structural curve. A structural curve

cannot be corrected with active or passive movement and there is rotation of the vertebrae towards the convexity of the curve. This results in a rib hump over the thoracic region on the convex side of the curve. Asymmetries will be visually noted at the shoulders, scapulae, pelvis, and skinfolds. A non-structural curve will correct with lateral bending towards the apex of the curve. This type of curve is typically non-progressive with minimal rotation. The primary causative factor for a non-structural curve is a leg length discrepancy.

- **Treatment** is based on the type and severity of the curve, age, and previous management. Generally, curves that are less than 25 degrees require monitoring; curves between 25 and 40 degrees are treated with orthotic management and physical therapy intervention for posture, flexibility, respiratory function, and body mechanics. Curves that progress beyond 40 degrees require surgical intervention to improve spinal stability.

Talipes Equinovarus

Talipes equinovarus is a deformity of the ankle and foot also known as "clubfoot."

- **Causative factors** are unclear, however, theories postulate familial tendency, positioning in utero or defect in the ovum. This condition accompanies other neuromuscular abnormalities including spina bifida and arthrogryposis, and may result from the lack of movement that assists with repositioning in utero.
- **Characteristics** of this deformity involve adduction of the forefoot, various positioning of the hindfoot, and equinus at the ankle. Severe cases can include deformity of the lower leg.
- **Treatment** begins soon after birth and includes splinting and serial casting. The goal of intervention is to restore proper positioning of the foot and ankle. Failed management or severe involvement will require surgical intervention and subsequent casting.

Neurological

Arthrogryposis Multiplex Congenita

Arthrogryposis multiplex congenita is a non-progressive neuromuscular disorder that is estimated to occur during the first trimester in utero. The restriction in utero allows for fibrosis of muscles and structures within the joints.

- An exact etiology is unknown, but **causative factors** include poor movement during early development due to myopathic, neuropathic or joint abnormalities. The causative factor for a small percentage of children with this condition is genetic inheritance as an autosomal dominant trait.
- **Characteristics** include cylinder-like extremities with minimal definition, significant and multiple contractures, dislocation of joints, and muscle atrophy.

- The goal of **treatment** is to attain the maximum level of developmental skills through positioning, stretching, strengthening, splinting, and use of adaptive equipment. Significant family involvement is required for the home program. Surgical intervention may be indicated.

Cerebral Palsy

Cerebral palsy is an umbrella term used to describe movement disorders due to brain damage that are non-progressive and are acquired in utero, during birth or infancy. The brain damage decreases the brain's ability to monitor and control nerve and voluntary muscle activity.

- **Causative factors** before or during birth include a lack of oxygen, maternal infections, drug and alcohol abuse, placental abnormalities, toxemia, prolonged labor, prematurity, and Rh incompatibility. Causative factors that are seen in acquired cerebral palsy include meningitis, CVA, seizures, and head injury.
- **Characteristics** vary from mild and undetectable to severe loss of control accompanied by profound mental retardation. All types of cerebral palsy demonstrate abnormal muscle tone, impaired modulation of movement, presence of abnormal reflexes, and impaired mobility.

--Cerebral Palsy Primary Motor Patterns (mixed motor patterns exist):

Spastic - indicating a lesion in the motor cortex of the cerebrum; upper motor neuron damage

Athetoid - indicating a lesion involving the basal ganglia; cerebellum and cerebellar pathways

--Distribution of Involvement

Monoplegia - one extremity

Diplegia - primarily bilateral lower extremity involvement, however, upper extremities may be affected

Hemiplegia - unilateral involvement of the upper and lower extremities

Quadriplegia - involvement of the entire body

- **Treatment** of cerebral palsy is a lifelong process. Intervention includes ongoing family and caregiver education, normalization of tone, stretching, strengthening, motor learning and developmental milestones, positioning, weight bearing activities, and mobility skills. Splinting, assistive devices, and specialized seating may be indicated. Surgical intervention may be required for orthopedic management or reduction of spasticity.

Down Syndrome

Down syndrome is a genetic abnormality consisting of an extra twenty-first chromosome, termed trisomy 21.

- **Causative factors** include incomplete cell division of the 21st pair of chromosomes due to nondisjunction, translocation or mosaic classification. Advanced maternal age increases the risk of genetic imbalance.

- **Characteristics** of this syndrome include mental retardation, hypotonia, joint hypermobility, flattened nasal bridge, narrow eyelids with epicanthal folds, small mouth, feeding impairments, flat feet, scoliosis, congenital heart disease, and visual and hearing loss.
- **Treatment** should emphasize exercise and fitness, stability, maximizing respiratory function, and education for caregivers. Surgical intervention may be indicated for cardiac abnormalities.

Duchenne Muscular Dystrophy

Duchenne muscular dystrophy is a progressive disorder caused by the absence of the gene required to produce the muscle proteins dystrophin and nebulin. Without dystrophin and nebulin, cell membranes weaken, myofibrils are destroyed, and muscle contractility is lost. Fat and connective tissue eventually replace muscle, and death usually occurs from cardiopulmonary failure prior to age 25, usually in the teenage years.

- The **causative factor** for this disorder is inheritance as an X-linked recessive trait. The child's mother is a silent carrier and only male offspring will manifest the disease.
- **Characteristics** usually manifest between two and five years of age. Progressive weakness, disinterest in running, falling, toe walking, excessive lordosis, and pseudohypertrophy of muscle groups are common symptoms. Progressive impairment with ADLs and mobility begins around age five and the inability to ambulate follows.
- **Treatment** focuses on family and caregiver education, respiratory function, submaximal exercise, mobility skills, splinting, orthotics, and adaptive equipment. Medical management includes the use of immunosuppressants, steroids, and surgical intervention for orthopedic impairments.

Prader-Willi Syndrome

Prader-Willi syndrome is a genetic condition that is diagnosed by physical attributes and patterns of behavior rather than genetic testing.

- The **causative factor** is a partial deletion of chromosome 15.
- **Characteristics** include physical and behavioral attributes such as small hands, feet, and sex organs, hypotonia, almond shaped eyes, obesity, and a constant desire for food. This child will present with coordination impairments and mental retardation.
- **Treatment** includes postural control, exercise and fitness, and gross and fine motor skills training.

Spina Bifida

Spina bifida is a developmental abnormality due to insufficient closure of the neural tube by the 28th day of gestation. This defect usually occurs in the low thoracic, lumbar or sacral regions and affects the central nervous, musculoskeletal, and urinary systems.

- A single etiology has not been identified, however, **causative factors** include genetic predisposition, environmental influence, low levels of maternal folic acid, maternal hyperthermia, and certain classifications of drugs.

--Types of Spina Bifida

Spina Bifida Occulta - An impairment and non-fusion of the spinous processes of a vertebrae, however, the spinal cord and meninges remain intact. There is usually no associated disability.

Spina Bifida Cystica - Presents with a cyst-like protrusion through the non-fused vertebrae, which results in impairment.

--Forms of Spina Bifida Cystica

Meningocele - Herniation of meninges and cerebrospinal fluid into a sac that protrudes through the vertebral defect. The spinal cord remains within the canal.

Myelomeningocele - A severe form characterized by herniation of meninges, cerebrospinal fluid, and the spinal cord extending through the defect in the vertebrae. The cyst may or may not be covered by skin.

- **Characteristics** and associated impairments of myelomeningocele include motor loss below the level of defect in the spinal cord, sensory deficits, hydrocephalus, Arnold-Chiari Type II malformation, osteoporosis, clubfoot, scoliosis, tethered cord syndrome, latex allergy, bowel and bladder dysfunction, and learning disabilities.
- Initial **treatment** for this population prioritizes significant family teaching regarding positioning, handling, range of motion, and therapeutic exercise. Ongoing treatment in physical therapy includes range of motion, facilitation of developmental milestones, skin care, strengthening, balance and mobility training, adaptive equipment, splinting, orthotic prescription, and wheelchair prescription. Physical therapy is ongoing through adolescence and is based on the severity of impairments and needs of the child.

Spinal Muscular Atrophy (SMA)

Spinal muscular atrophy is a condition of progressive degeneration of the anterior horn cell.

--Categories of Spinal Muscular Atrophy

Acute Infantile SMA (Werdnig-Hoffmann disease) - Occurs between birth and two months of age.

Motor degeneration progresses quickly and life expectancy is less that one year.

Chronic Childhood SMA (type II muscular atrophy, chronic Werdnig-Hoffmann disease) - Presents after six months to one year and has slower progression than infantile SMA. Impairment is steady, however, a child can survive into adulthood.

Juvenile SMA (Kugelberg-Welander SMA) - Occurs later in childhood from 4-17 years of age. This population can also survive into adulthood.

- The **causative factor** of spinal muscular atrophy is an autosomal recessive genetic inheritance. Certain types of this disease involve a mutation on chromosome 5. Characteristics for all categories of the disease are the same, and vary in onset and speed of progression.
- **Characteristics** include progressive muscle weakness and atrophy, diminished or absent deep tendon reflexes, normal intelligence, intact sensation, and end stage respiratory compromise.
- **Treatment** includes positioning, vestibular and visual stimulation, and access to play. Treatment for the slower progressing categories is primarily supportive including educating caregivers, mobility training, and use of assistive devices and adaptive equipment.

Oncology

Astrocytoma

An astrocytoma is a classification that accounts for approximately fifty percent of pediatric brain tumors. The etiology of pediatric cancers is usually unknown.

- **Causative factors** include genetic predisposition, environmental influence, radiation and toxin exposure, and association with certain childhood disorders.
- There are two types of astrocytoma with **characteristics** as follows:
  Cerebellar - clumsiness, ataxic gait, headache, change in personality, and vomiting
  Supratentorial - headache, seizures, change in personality, visual impairments, and vomiting
- **Treatment** for *cerebellar* tumors consists of surgical resection with an 80-90% cure rate. Treatment for *supratentorial* tumors requires surgery to resect the tumor with radiation and/or chemotherapy.

Leukemia

Leukemia is a cancer of the blood that occurs when leukocytes change into malignant cells. These immature cells proliferate, accumulate in bone marrow, and ultimately cease the production of normal cells. This process will spread to lymph nodes, liver, spleen, and other areas of the body.

- The exact etiology is unknown, however, **causative factors** include environmental, chemical or toxin exposure, genetic predisposition, and viral association. There are many types of leukemia with acute lymphoblastic leukemia (ALL), and acute myelogenous leukemia (AML) occurring most frequently in children.
- **Characteristics** of these types include an abrupt onset with high fever, bleeding, enlarged lymph nodes and spleen, progressive weakness, fatigue, and painful joints. Blood work will indicate anemia, leukocyte count greater than 500,000 mm^3 and thrombocytopenia.
- **Treatment** will vary based on the type and degree of leukemia. Options include immunotherapy, cytotoxic agents, chemotherapy or radiation, and bone marrow transplant. Over 90% of patients with ALL achieve complete remission with treatment, while patients with AML achieve complete remission at a rate of 70-80%.

Neuroblastoma

A neuroblastoma is a tumor that initiates from primitive ectodermal cells of the neural plate and is found within the sympathetic nervous system, primarily seen in the adrenal glands or paraspinal ganglions. This is the most common malignant tumor seen in children.

- The etiology remains unknown, but **causative factors** include genetic predisposition, familial incidence, environmental influence, radiation and toxin exposure or viral association.
- **Characteristics** vary with the site and include an abdominal mass, change in personality, anemia, sweating, pain, and diarrhea.
- **Treatment** includes surgical resection, chemotherapy, and radiation. Prognosis is best for children diagnosed in the first year of life. In rare instances a neuroblastoma will spontaneously regress.

Non-Hodgkin's Lymphoma

Non-Hodgkin's lymphoma is a cancer of the lymphatic system with peak incidence between 7 - 10 years of age.

- The etiology is unknown, however, a likely **causative factor** is viral infection.
- **Characteristics** can differ from adults and include abdominal pain, swallowing issues, anemia, and swelling. Nodular histologies are rare in children.
- **Treatment** is dependent on the site and extent of the cancer and includes surgical resection, chemotherapy, and radiation.

Osteogenic Sarcoma

An osteogenic sarcoma is a cancer that occurs at the epiphyses of long bones. Osteogenic sarcoma is the most common form of bone cancer in children with a peak incidence between the ages of 10 to 20.

- **Causative factors** are unknown, however, there is a correlation between immunoincompetence and rate of tumor progression. Osteogenic sarcoma can metastasize quickly.

- **Characteristics** include presence of a mass, rapid metastases, and associated pain. Diagnosis can be made with a biopsy.
- **Treatment** includes amputation with proximal resection to ensure proper removal of affected tissue or surgical procedures that attempt to resect the tumor and salvage the limb. Chemotherapy is beneficial, however, radiation is not effective with this type of tumor.

Wilms' Tumor

Wilms' tumor is an embryonal adenomyosarcoma found in the kidney. Most cases are diagnosed between one and four years of age.

- **Causative factors** include genetic inheritance as an autosomal dominant disease or a non-inherited form with an unknown etiology.
- **Characteristics** include an abdominal mass, pain, hematuria, fever, nausea, and vomiting.
- **Treatment** includes resection of the kidney and the associated lymphatic tissue followed by chemotherapy and/or radiation. Dactinomycin is also administered due to the drug's antitumor properties. The five-year cure rate is approximately 75%.

Rheumatory

Juvenile Rheumatoid Arthritis

Juvenile rheumatoid arthritis (JRA) is the most common chronic rheumatic disease in children and presents with inflammation of the joints and connective tissues.

- The exact etiology is unknown, however, it is theorized that **causative factors** include an external source such as a virus, infection or trauma that may trigger an autoimmune response producing JRA in a child with a genetic predisposition.
- **Characteristics** depend on the classification of JRA. *Systemic juvenile rheumatoid arthritis* occurs in 10% to 20% of children with JRA and presents with acute onset, high fevers, rash, enlargement of the spleen and liver, and inflammation of the lungs and heart. *Polyarticular juvenile rheumatoid arthritis* accounts for 30-40% of children with JRA and presents with high female incidence, RF+ majority, and arthritis in more than five joints with symmetrical joint involvement. *Oligoarticular (Pauciarticular) juvenile rheumatoid arthritis* accounts for 40-60% of children with JRA and affects less than five joints with asymmetrical joint involvement. General characteristics include inflammation, malaise, pain with palpation and movement, stiffness, iritis, fever, and rash.
- **Treatment** includes pharmacological management to relieve inflammation and pain through NSAIDs, corticosteroids, and antirheumatic and immunosuppressive agents. Physical therapy

management includes passive and active range of motion, positioning, splinting and orthotic prescription, strengthening, endurance, weight bearing activities, postural training, and functional mobility. Pain management includes use of modalities such as paraffin, ultrasound, warm water, and cryotherapy. A realistic home program must be a constant priority. Surgical intervention may be indicated secondary to pain, contractures or irreversible joint destruction.

Models of Disability

The Nagi Model

Originally designed in 1965 by a social worker named Saad Nagi as an alternative to the medical model of disease. It describes health status as a product of the relationship between health and function and is defined by four primary concepts:

Pathology - An interruption or interference in the body's normal processes and the simultaneous efforts of the systems to regain homeostasis. Pathology occurs at the cellular level.

Impairment - The loss or abnormality at the tissue, organ or body system level. This can be of an anatomic, physiologic, mental or emotional nature. Each pathology will present with an impairment, however, impairments can exist without pathology (e.g., congenital defects). Impairments occur at the organ level.

Functional limitation - The inability to perform an action or skill in a normal manner due to an impairment. Functional limitations are at the level of the whole person.

Disability - Any restriction or inability to perform a socially defined role within a social or physical environment due to an impairment. Environmental barriers impose disability.

Example:

A patient with progressive weakness presents with paralysis of the trunk and lower extremities. The patient is diagnosed with a T12 spinal cord tumor. The patient utilizes a wheelchair for mobility and requires assistance with self-care. Prior to hospitalization the patient worked as a deliveryman.

Pathology - Spinal cord tumor at T12
Impairment - Loss of motor function below T12
Functional limitation - Unable to ambulate
Disability - Cannot continue to work as a deliveryman

The International Classification of Impairment, Disabilities, and Handicaps (ICIDH) Model

The World Health Organization (WHO) developed this model in 1980 with the focus on the long-term impact of non-fatal or chronic diseases. The model is defined by four primary concepts:

Disease - A biomechanical, physiological or anatomical abnormality within the body.

Impairment - The loss or abnormality of psychological, physiological or anatomical structure or function. Impairments occur at the organ level.

Disability - The inability to perform an activity in a normal manner due to an impairment. Disability occurs at the level of the whole person.

Handicap - The inability to perform in a social role due to social or environmental restrictions. Handicap occurs in a person-to-person or person-to-environment level. Handicap clearly separates environmental barriers and the person's ability to interact with the environment.

Example:

A 36-year-old female is diagnosed with multiple sclerosis. The patient resides alone and has recently utilized a wheelchair for mobility secondary to weakness and hypertonicity in her upper and lower extremities. She is no longer able to visit her brother who lives in a second floor apartment two blocks away.

Disease - Demyelination secondary to multiple sclerosis
Impairment - Weakness and tonal abnormalities in lower extremities
Disability - Unable to ambulate
Handicap - Unable to visit her brother who resides in the second floor apartment

Disablement Model

This model was designed by physical therapists appointed by the House of Delegates as the framework for the Guide to Physical Therapist Practice. This model rejects the medical model of disease and focuses on disablement using guidelines from the Nagi model. This model defines three primary concepts as they relate to physical therapy intervention.

Impairment - The loss or abnormality of physiological, psychological or anatomical structure or function.

Functional limitation - A restriction of the ability to perform in a competent manner. This occurs at the level of the whole person.

Disability - The inability to engage in roles in a particular social context and physical environment.

Example:

A 45-year-old right hand dominant female fell down a flight of stairs and sustained a compound fracture of the right humerus. She is currently casted and has difficulty with many self-care skills. She is employed in the data entry department of a local hospital.

Impairment - Fracture of the humerus
Functional limitation - Unable to get dressed
Disability - Cannot use the computer at work

Outcome Measurement Tools

Balance

Berg Functional Balance Scale

A tool designed to assess a patient's risk for falling. There are fourteen tasks, each scored on an ordinal scale from 0-4. These tasks include static, transitional, and dynamic activities in sitting and standing positions. The maximum score is a 56 with a score less than 45 indicating an increased risk for falling. This tool is used as a one-time examination or as an ongoing tool to monitor a patient who may be at risk for falls.

Functional Reach

A single task screening tool used to assess standing balance and risk of falling. A person is required to stand upright with a static base of support. A yardstick is positioned to measure the forward distance that a patient can reach without moving the feet. Three trials are performed and averaged together. The following are age related standard measurements for functional reach:

20 - 40 years – 14.5 - 17 inches
41 - 69 years – 13.5 - 15 inches
70 - 87 years – 10.5 - 13.5 inches

A patient that falls below the age appropriate range for functional reach has an increased risk for falling. The outcome measure demonstrates high test-retest correlation and intrarater reliability.

"Get Up and Go" Test

A functional performance screening tool used to assess a person's level of mobility and balance. The person initially sits in a supported chair with a firm surface, transfers to a standing position, and walks a few feet. The patient must then turn around without external support, walk back towards the chair, and return to a sitting position. The patient is scored based on amount of postural sway, excessive movements, reaching for support, side stepping, or other signs of loss of balance. The 5-point ordinal rating scale designates a score of one as normal and a score of five as severely abnormal. In an attempt to increase overall reliability the use of time was implemented. Patients who require over 20 seconds to complete the process may be at an increased risk for falling.

Romberg Test

An assessment of balance that positions the patient in unsupported standing, feet together, upper extremities folded, and eyes closed. A patient receives a grade of "normal" if they are able to maintain the position for 30 seconds.

Tinetti Performance Oriented Mobility Assessment

A tool used to screen patients and identify if there is an increased risk for falling. The first section assesses balance through sit to stand and stand to sit from an armless chair, immediate standing balance with eyes open and closed, tolerating a slight push in the standing position, and turning 360 degrees. A patient is scored from 0-2 in most categories with a maximum score of 16. The second section assesses gait at normal speed and at a rapid, but safe speed. Items scored in this section include initiation of gait, step length and height, step asymmetry and continuity, path, stance during gait, and trunk motion. A patient is scored either 0 to 1 or 0 to 2 with a maximum score of 12. The tool has a combined maximum total of 28 with the risk of falling increasing as the total score decreases. A total score less than 19 indicates a high risk for a fall.

Cognitive Assessment

Mini Mental State Examination

A tool designed to screen patients for cognitive impairment, psychoses or affective disorders. Each of the five sections: orientation, registration, attention and calculation, recall and language, and motor skills have multiple questions that receive one point for the correct answer or zero for the incorrect answer. There is a maximum score of 30 with a progressive level of cognitive impairment noted when a score of 24 or less is obtained.

Short Portable Mental Status Questionnaire

A ten item screening tool used to assess cognitive impairment primarily in the geriatric population. Orientation, short and long-term memory, practical skills,

and mathematical tasks are tested. The maximum score is ten with a score below eight indicating cognitive impairment. The lower the score below eight the more significant the cognitive impairment.

Coordination and Manual Dexterity

Frenchay Arm Test

A tool used to assess coordination and dexterity by performing five activities based on functional movement patterns. The activities include stabilizing and drawing lines with a ruler, manipulating a cylinder without dropping it, drinking from a glass, placing and removing a clothespin, and combing hair. A patient receives three attempts to complete each task. A score of one is noted for successful completion; a score of zero is noted for failure to complete the task.

Jebsen Hand Function Test

A tool designed to assess hand function using seven timed activities. These activities include writing a 24-letter sentence, turning cards, placing six small objects into a container, using a teaspoon to pick up five small items, stacking items, moving large lightweight items, and large heavy objects. Each activity is timed and the results are compared to normative data.

Peg Test

There are multiple tools that utilize a pegboard to assess dexterity including the Purdue Pegboard test, the nine-hole peg test, and the ten-hole peg test. These tools use the element of time for completion of the task and compare results to normative data.

Endurance

Borg Rating of Perceived Exertion Scale

A tool designed to measure perceived exertion, dyspnea, and exercise intensity. The original scale measures 6 to 20 points and the revised scale measures 0 to 10 points. The patient is instructed that a 6 (original) or 0 (new) corresponds to walking at a normal pace without fatigue. A score of 20 (original) or 10 (new) indicates high intensity exercise that cannot be completed due to exhaustion. After an activity a patient's score can indicate cardiopulmonary fatigue versus muscle fatigue. The score correlates with exercise intensity, heart rate, oxygen consumption, and blood lactate levels. Cardiopulmonary training effects can be seen with exercise intensity beginning at a 14 (original) or 4 to 5 (new) respectively. The scale is commonly used for patients with cardiovascular impairments.

Dyspnea Levels

A tool designed by Rancho Los Amigos Medical Center that attempts to rate the intensity and level of dyspnea that a patient experiences with activity. This ordinal scale consists of ratings from 0 to 4. A patient at level 0 is able to perform an activity and count to 15 without any additional breaths required. Levels 1, 2, and 3 require progressive extra breaths to count to 15. Level 4 indicates that the patient is unable to count while performing an activity. The test has not been shown to be valid, however, can be used to measure progress or decline during a course of rehabilitation.

Six-Minute Walk Test

A tool used to determine a patient's functional exercise capacity. The patient walks as far as he or she can for a timed six minutes with rest periods permitted as necessary. The tool is commonly used upon admission, discharge, and to monitor progress or decline throughout physical therapy. It allows for observation of heart rate and oxygen consumption during activity. This tool is administered to various populations including those with cardiac impairments, pulmonary disease, geriatrics with chronic conditions, and patients recovering from orthopedic surgical procedures.

Motor Recovery

Fugl-Meyer Assessment

An ordinal scale used to measure recovery post CVA. The framework is based on Brunnstrom's sequence of recovery. The five areas of assessment are joint movement and pain, balance, upper extremity motor function, sensation, and lower extremity motor function. Each item tested within an area is assigned a score from 0-3. The maximum combined score for upper extremity and lower extremity motor function is 100 and can be interpreted as a percentage of motor recovery. A score of 63 indicates approximately 63% return of motor function. This tool utilizes cumulative scoring for the entire assessment.

Montreal Evaluation

A tool that determines a patient's level of mobility by examining six specific areas in the following order: mental clarity, muscle tone, reflex activity, voluntary movement, automatic reactions, and pain. The construction of this tool utilized Bobath's NDT approach to neurological recovery. An ordinal scale of 0 to 3 is used for each item in each category. Muscle tone and active movements are examined separately, but scoring is cumulative for all areas. Each scored item includes multiple factors for a single score. This makes comparison of the individual scored items difficult.

Rivermead Motor Assessment

A tool based on the NDT approach to neurological recovery. The Rivermead Motor Assessment is divided into three major sections: gross function, leg and trunk, and arm. Each section is comprised of a subscale of tasks. These tasks increase in difficulty and are graded with a score of one for completion or zero for inability to perform the activity. The assessment possesses a high level of sensitivity when examining higher level patients and is reliable within one point.

Pain

McGill Pain Questionnaire

A pain assessment tool that is divided into four parts with a total of 70 questions.

Part 1 Patient marks on a drawing of the body to indicate area and type of pain (internal or external)

Part 2 Patient chooses one word that best describes the pain from each of the twenty categories

Part 3 Patient describes pattern of pain, factors that increase and relieve pain

Part 4 Patient rates the intensity of pain on a scale of zero to five

This tool can be used to establish a baseline, evaluate particular treatment regimens, and monitor progress. It is valid, reliable, and the most widely used pain assessment scale.

Numerical Rating Scale

A tool used to assess pain intensity by rating pain on a scale of 0-10 or 0-100. The 0 represents no discernable pain and the 10 or 100 represent the worst pain ever. The information is used as a baseline and should be reassessed at regular intervals in order to monitor progress. This scale is easy to administer, assess, and monitor.

Visual Analogue Scale

A tool used to assess pain intensity using a 10-15 cm line with the left anchor indicating "no pain" and the right anchor indicating "the worst pain you can have." The level of perceived pain is indicated on the line and is reassessed frequently over the course of physical therapy to record changes and progress, and to predict patient outcome. This scale can be highly sensitive if small increments such as millimeters are used to measure the patient's point of pain on the scale. The visual analogue scale is a valid tool if measurements are taken accurately.

Self-Care and ADL

Barthel Index

A tool designed to measure the amount of assistance needed to perform ten different activities with a total maximum score of 100. These activities include bowel management, bladder management, grooming, toilet use, feeding, transfers, mobility, dressing, stairs, and bathing. A score of 75-95 denotes mild impairment, 50-70 moderate impairment, 20-45 severe impairment, and below 20 indicates a very severe impairment. The index does not account for cognitive or safety issues and is not sensitive to higher level patients regarding their level of disability. It remains one of the oldest and most widely used tools that is reliable and possesses predictive validity.

Functional Independence Measure (FIM)

A tool that is primarily used in rehabilitation hospitals in order to determine a patient's level of disability and burden of care. This tool is part of the Uniform Data System for Medical Rehabilitation (UDS). A seven-point scale is utilized to examine 18 areas, which include self-care, sphincter control, transfers, locomotion, communication, and social cognitive activities. These items were designed based on the World Health Organization's Model of Disability. Scoring between a 1 and 5 denotes a level of dependence and between 6 and 7 a level of independence for a specific item. This tool is both valid and reliable and is used as a predictor of disability for the CVA population. The FIM is utilized on a larger scale to assess change within rehabilitation programs over time.

Katz Index of Activities of Daily Living

A nominal scale index used to identify self-care problems and the level of assistance required with the six areas of bathing, dressing, toileting, transfers, continence, and feeding. The score for each area is combined and the total score correlates with a letter grade scale (A through G). Each letter represents a level of ability with "A" representing independence in all six areas, the following letters representing increasing dependence, and "G" representing dependence in all six areas. This tool was originally intended only for inpatient and nursing home settings, however, it is now utilized with patients that require outpatient and community based services. It is a simple and quick assessment tool used to efficiently gather self-care information and predict outcome and need for ongoing assistance.

Pharmacology/Nutrition

Review of Systems: Side Effects/Subjective Complaints (In Order of Most Common Occurrence)

Gastrointestinal Distress: dyspepsia, heartburn, nausea, vomiting, abdominal pain, constipation, diarrhea, bleeding

• Salicylates	• Opioids	• β-Blockers
• Skeletal muscle relaxants	• ACE inhibitors	• Nitrates
• Antiarrhythmic agents	• Neuroleptics	• OCAs
• Theophylline	• NSAIDs	• Corticosteroids
• Calcium-channel blockers	• Diuretics	• Digoxin
• Cholesterol-lowering agents	• Estrogens and progestins	• Antiepileptic agents
• Antidepressants (TCAs and MAOIs, lithium)		

Pulmonary: bronchospasm, shortness of breath, respiratory depression

• Salicylates	• Opioids	• ACE inhibitors
• NSAIDs	• β-Blockers	

Central Nervous System: dizziness, drowsiness, insomnia, headaches, hallucinations, confusion, anxiety, depression, muscle weakness

• NSAIDs	• Opioids	• β-Blockers
• Nitrates	• Digoxin	• Antidepressants (TCAs and MAOIs)
• Antiepileptic agents	• Estrogens and progestins	• Skeletal muscle relaxants
• Corticosteroids	• Calcium-channel blockers	• ACE inhibitors
• Antianxiety agents	• Neuroleptics	• OCAs

Review of Systems: Side Effects/Subjective Complaints (continued) (In Order of Most Common Occurrence)

Dermatologic: skin rash, itching, flushing of face

- NSAIDs
- Nitrates
- Antiepileptics
- ACE inhibitors
- Estrogens and progestins

- β-Blockers
- Antiarrhythmic agents
- Corticosteroids
- Cholesterol-lowering agents

- Calcium-channel blockers
- OCAs
- Opioids
- MAOIs and lithium

Musculoskeletal: weakness, fatigue, cramps, arthritis, decreased exercise tolerance, osteoporosis

- Corticosteroids
- Antianxiety agents
- ACE inhibitors
- Neuroleptic agents

- Calcium-channel blockers
- Antidepressants
- Digoxin

- Diuretics
- β-Blockers
- Antiepileptic agents

Cardiac: bradycardia, ventricular irritability, AV block, CHF, PVCs, ventricular tachycardia

- Opioids
- TCAs
- Calcium-channel blockers

- β-Blockers
- Oral antiasthmatic agents
- Antiarrhythmic agents

- Digoxin
- Diuretics
- Neuroleptics

Vascular: claudication, hypotension, peripheral edema, cold extremities

- NSAIDs
- Nitrates
- Corticosteroids
- Antidepressants (TCAs and MAOIs)

- Diuretics
- Neuroleptics
- β-Blockers
- OCAs

- Calcium-channel blockers
- Estrogens and progestins
- ACE inhibitors

Genitourinary: sexual dysfunction, urinary retention, urinary incontinence

- Opioids
- OCAs
- Neuroleptics

- β-Blockers
- Diuretics
- Antidepressants (TCAs and MAOIs)

- Estrogens and progestins
- Antiarrhythmic agents

HEENT: tinnitus, loss of taste, headache, light-headedness, dizziness

- Salicylates
- Calcium-channel blockers
- Antiepileptic agents
- Nitrates
- Antidepressants (TCAs and MAOIs)

- Opioids
- Digoxin
- NSAIDs
- ACE inhibitors

- β-Blockers
- Antianxiety agents
- Skeletal muscle relaxants
- Antiarrhythmic agents

**Abbreviations: ACE, angiotensin-converting enzyme; MAOIs, monoamine oxidase inhibitors; NSAIDs, nonsteroidal anti-inflammatory drugs; OCAs, oral contraceptive agents; TCAs, tricyclic antidepressants.

From Boissonnault, WG: Examination in Physical Therapy Practice: Screening for Medical Disease. W.B. Saunders Company, Philadelphia 1995, p.350-351, with permission.

Vitamins

Vitamins are essential non-caloric nutrients that are required in small amounts for certain metabolic functions and cannot be manufactured by the body. Vitamins are most often classified as fat-soluble or water-soluble.

Fat-Soluble Vitamins

Fat-soluble vitamins include vitamins A, D, E, and K. After being absorbed by the intestinal tract, the vitamins are stored in the liver and fatty tissues. Fat-soluble vitamins require protein carriers to move through body fluids and excesses are stored in the body. Since they are not water-soluble, it is possible that the vitamins may reach toxic levels.

Vitamin A

Vitamin A is essential to the eyes, epithelial tissue, normal growth and development, and reproduction.

- **Common food sources** containing Vitamin A include green, orange, and yellow vegetables, liver, butter, egg yolks, and fortified margarine.
- **Symptoms of deficiency** include night blindness, rough and dry skin, and growth failure.
- **Symptoms of toxicity** include appetite loss, hair loss, and enlarged liver and spleen.

Vitamin D

Vitamin D increases the blood flow levels of minerals, notably calcium and phosphorus.

- **Common food sources** containing Vitamin D include fortified milk, fish oils, and fortified margarine.
- **Symptoms of deficiency** include faulty bone growth, rickets, and osteomalacia.
- **Symptoms of toxicity** include calcification of soft tissues and hypercalcemia.

Vitamin E

Vitamin E functions as an antioxidant in cell membranes and is especially important for the integrity of cells that are constantly exposed to high levels of oxygen such as the lungs and red blood cells.

- **Common food sources** containing Vitamin E include vegetable oils, wheat germ, nuts, and fish.
- **Symptoms of deficiency** include the breakdown of red blood cells, however, this is relatively rare in adults.
- **Symptoms of toxicity** include decreased thyroid hormone levels and increased triglycerides.

Vitamin K

Vitamin K is necessary for the synthesis of at least two of the proteins involved in blood clotting.

- **Common food sources** containing Vitamin K include dark green leafy vegetables, cheese, egg yolks, and liver.
- **Symptoms of deficiency** include hemorrhage and defective blood clotting.
- **Toxicity** has not been reported.

Water-Soluble Vitamins

Water-soluble vitamins are not stored in the body in any significant amount and therefore need to be included in the diet on a daily basis. Toxicity is less common than with fat-soluble vitamins.

Vitamin B_2 (Riboflavin)

Vitamin B_2 facilitates selected enzymes involved in carbohydrate, protein, and fat metabolism.

- **Common food sources** containing Vitamin B_2 include milk, green leafy vegetables, eggs, and peanuts.
- **Symptoms of deficiency** include inflammation of the tongue, sensitive eyes, and scaling of the skin.
- **Toxicity** has not been reported.

Vitamin B_3 (Niacin)

Vitamin B_3 facilitates several enzymes that regulate energy metabolism.

- **Common food sources** containing Vitamin B_3 include meats, whole grains, and white flour.
- **Symptoms of deficiency** include pellagra and gastrointestinal disturbances.
- **Symptoms of toxicity** include abnormal glucose metabolism, nausea, vomiting, and gastric ulceration.

Vitamin B_6 (Pyridoxine)

Vitamin B_6 is essential in the metabolism of proteins, amino acids, carbohydrates, and fat.

- **Common food sources** containing Vitamin B_6 include liver, red meats, whole grains, and potatoes.
- **Symptoms of deficiency** include peripheral neuropathy, convulsions, and depression.
- **Symptoms of toxicity** include sensory damage, numbness of the extremities, and ataxia.

Vitamin B_{12} (Cobalamin)

Vitamin B_{12} is essential for the functioning of all cells and aids in hemoglobin synthesis.

- **Common food sources** containing Vitamin B_{12} include meats, whole eggs, and egg yolks.
- **Symptoms of deficiency** include pernicious anemia and various psychological disorders.
- **Toxicity** has not been reported.

Vitamin C

Vitamin C assists the body to combat infections and facilitates wound healing. The vitamin is necessary for the development and maintenance of bones, cartilage, connective tissue, and blood vessels.

- **Common food sources** containing Vitamin C include citrus fruits, tomatoes, and cantaloupe.

- **Symptoms of deficiency** include anemia, swollen gums, loose teeth, and scurvy.
- **Symptoms of toxicity** include urinary stones, diarrhea, and hypoglycemia.

Biotin

Biotin is necessary for the action of many enzyme systems.

- **Common food sources** containing biotin include liver, meats, and milk.
- **Symptoms of deficiency** include anemia, depression, and muscle pain.
- **Toxicity** has not been reported.

Choline

Choline is a component of compounds necessary for nerve function and lipid metabolism.

- Choline is synthesized from methionine which is an amino acid.
- **Symptoms of deficiency** only occur when intake of methylamine is low.
- **Toxicity** has not been reported.

Folacin (Folic acid)

Folacin is involved in the formation of red blood cells and in the functioning of the gastrointestinal tract.

- **Common food sources** containing folacin include yeast, dark green leafy vegetables, and whole grains.
- **Symptoms of deficiency** include impaired cell division and alteration of protein synthesis.
- **Toxicity** has not been reported.

Pantothenic acid

Pantothenic acid is an integral component of complex enzymes involved in the metabolism of fatty acids.

- **Common food sources** containing pantothenic acid include liver, eggs, and whole grains.
- **Symptoms of deficiency** include headache, fatigue, and poor muscle coordination.
- **Symptoms of toxicity** include diarrhea.

Minerals

Minerals are organic elements that fulfill essential roles in metabolism.

Major Minerals

Calcium (Ca)

Calcium facilitates muscle contraction and relaxation, builds strong bones and teeth, and aids in coagulation.

- **Common food sources** containing calcium include milk, green leafy vegetables, and soy products.
- **Calcium deficiency** may lead to poor bone growth, rickets, osteomalacia, and osteoporosis.
- **Symptoms of toxicity** include kidney stones.

Chloride (Cl)

Chloride facilitates the maintenance of fluid and acid-base balance.

- **Common food sources** containing chloride include table salt, fish, and vegetables.
- **Chloride deficiency** may lead to a disturbance of acid-base balance.
- **Toxicity** has not been reported.

Magnesium (Mg)

Magnesium builds strong bones and teeth, activates enzymes, and helps regulate heartbeat.

- **Common food sources** containing magnesium include raw dark vegetables, nuts, soybeans, milk, and cheese.
- **Symptoms of deficiency** include confusion, apathy, muscle weakness, and tremors.
- **Symptoms of toxicity** include increased calcium excretion.

Phosphorus (P)

Phosphorus strengthens bones, assists in the oxidation of fats and carbohydrates, and aids in maintaining acid-base balance.

- **Common food sources** containing phosphorus include milk and milk products, meats, whole grains, and soft drinks.
- **Symptoms of deficiency** include weakness, stiff joints, and fragile bones.
- **Symptoms of toxicity** include muscle spasms.

Potassium (K)

Potassium maintains fluid and acid-base balance.

- **Common food sources** containing potassium include apricots, bananas, oranges, grapefruit, and milk.
- **Symptoms of deficiency** include impaired growth, hypertension, and diminished heart rate.
- **Symptoms of toxicity** include hyperkalemia and cardiac disturbances.

Sodium (Na)

Sodium facilitates the maintenance of acid-base balance, transmits nerve impulses, and helps control muscle contractions.

- **Common food sources** containing sodium include salt and milk.
- **Deficiency and toxicity** have not been reported.

Sulfur (S)

Sulfur facilitates enzyme activity and energy metabolism.

- **Common food sources** containing sulfur include meat, eggs, milk, and cheese.
- **Deficiency** is extremely rare.
- **Toxicity** has not been reported.

Trace Minerals

Chromium (Cr)

Chromium controls glucose metabolism.

- **Common food sources** containing chromium include whole grains, meats, and cheese.
- **Symptoms of deficiency** include weight loss and central nervous system abnormalities.
- **Symptoms of toxicity** include liver damage.

Cobalt (Co)

Cobalt is an essential component of vitamin B_{12} and functions to activate enzymes.

- **Common food sources** containing cobalt include figs, cabbage, and spinach.
- **Symptoms of deficiency** include pernicious anemia.
- **Symptoms of toxicity** include polycythemia and increased blood volume.

Copper (Cu)

Copper facilitates hemoglobin synthesis and lipid metabolism.

- **Common food sources** containing copper include shellfish, liver, meat, and whole grains.

- **Symptoms of deficiency** include anemia, central nervous system abnormalities, and abnormal electrocardiograms.
- **Symptoms of toxicity** include Wilson's disease.

Fluorine (F)

Fluorine aids in the formation of bones and teeth and prevents osteoporosis.

- **Common food sources** containing fluorine include fish and water.
- **Symptoms of deficiency** include increased susceptibility of dental cavities.
- **Symptoms of toxicity** include fluorosis.

Iodine (I)

Iodine assists with the regulation of cell metabolism and basal metabolic rate.

- **Common food sources** containing iodine include iodized salt and seafood.
- **Symptoms of deficiency** may include goiters.
- **Toxicity** has not been reported.

Iron (Fe)

Iron assists in the oxygen transport and cell oxidation.

- **Common food sources** containing iron include red meats and liver.
- **Symptoms of deficiency** include anemia.
- **Symptoms of toxicity** include hemochromatosis.

Manganese (Mn)

Manganese facilitates proper bone structure and functions as an enzyme component in general metabolism.

- **Common food sources** containing manganese include cereals and whole grains.
- There are no known **symptoms of deficiency.**
- **Toxicity** has not been reported.

Selenium (Se)

Selenium is a synergistic antioxidant with Vitamin E.
- **Common food sources** containing selenium include meat, eggs, milk, seafood, and garlic.
- **Symptoms of deficiency** include Keshan's disease.
- **Symptoms of toxicity** include physical defects of fingernails and toenails, nausea, and abdominal pain.

Molybdenum (Mo)

Molybdenum is a component of three enzymes necessary for normal cell functioning.

- **Common food sources** containing molybdenum include meats, whole grains, and dark green vegetables.
- **Symptoms of deficiency** include vomiting and tachypnea.
- **Toxicity** has not been reported.

Zinc (Zn)

Zinc aids in immune function and cell division.

- **Common food sources** containing zinc include seafood, liver, milk, cheese, and whole grains.
- **Symptoms of deficiency** include depressed immune functions and impaired skeletal growth.
- **Symptoms of toxicity** include anemia, nausea, and vomiting.

Unit Three

Clinical Application Templates

The clinical application template allows candidates to explore many of the elements of patient/client management for a wide variety of medical conditions. Although candidates have been exposed to a variety of medical conditions during their clinical education experiences it is unlikely they have been exposed to the vast number of medical conditions commonly encountered on the examination. By utilizing the clinical application templates students can broaden their experience base and as a result be better prepared to answer examination questions.

This section presents 50 different clinical application templates. Candidates are encouraged to review the templates and carefully reflect on the presented information. Candidates should attempt to make this activity an active learning exercise and resist the urge to simply read each of the templates. For example, let's assume that a candidate was reviewing a clinical application template on an anterior cruciate ligament sprain. In each category of the clinical application template candidates should assess their knowledge by asking specific questions. Two specific examples for the tests and measures section are listed below:

When reviewing range of motion, candidates should ask themselves the following:

- What is normal range of motion at the knee?
- Which type of end-feel would be considered normal for knee flexion and extension?
- Where should the axis, moving arm, and stationary arm of the goniometer be aligned when measuring range of motion?
- Where should the therapist stabilize when conducting the measurement?

When reviewing joint integrity and mobility, candidates should ask themselves the following:

- Which special test or tests would be the most appropriate to assess the ligamentous integrity of the anterior cruciate ligament?
- Describe the process for administering the special test?
- What finding would be indicative of a positive test?

By engaging in this type of active learning exercise, candidates are able to further assess their level of preparedness for the examination. Although some candidates may be quite comfortable reviewing selected clinical application templates, many candidates learn that they lack necessary content in many others. For example, do you feel adequately prepared to discuss the patient/client management of each of the following diagnoses: amyotrophic lateral sclerosis, cystic fibrosis, cerebrovascular accident, and rotator cuff tendonitis. Prior to taking the actual examination candidates should have some reasonable level of comfort discussing each of the 50 clinical application templates included in this unit.

Candidates should not rely solely on the presented clinical application templates and instead should utilize the template format to review a variety of other medical conditions. This type of active learning is best performed by a small group of candidates with a given candidate acting as the facilitator. In this manner students can share their individual clinical experience with the group and at the same time benefit from the knowledge of their classmates.

*The clinical application template was adapted from a document by the Academy of Specialty Boards entitled "Preparing Items that Measure More than Recall." The document was originally designed to help item writers develop sample questions for the Physical Therapy Specialty Examinations.

Clinical Application Templates

Achilles Tendon Rupture

Diagnosis:

What condition produces a patient's symptoms?
Rupture of the Achilles tendon normally occurs within one to two inches above its tendinous insertion on the calcaneus. A patient will present with symptoms secondary to the rupture and discontinuity of the Achilles tendon.

An injury was most likely sustained to which structure?
The Achilles tendon is the largest and strongest tendon in the human body and is formed from the tendinous portions of the gastrocnemius and soleus muscles coalescing above the insertion on the calcaneal tuberosity. Theories suggest that an Achilles tendon rupture usually occurs in an Achilles tendon that has undergone degenerative changes. The degenerative changes will begin with hypovascularity in the Achilles tendon area. The impaired blood flow in combination with repetitive microtrauma creates degenerative changes within the tendon and as a result makes the tendon more susceptible to injury.

Inference:

What is the most likely contributing factor in the development of this condition?
An Achilles tendon rupture occurs most frequently when pushing off of a weight bearing extremity with an extended knee, through unexpected dorsiflexion while weight bearing or with a forceful eccentric contraction of the plantar flexors. Participation in sports that require quick-changing footwork such as softball, tennis, basketball, and football are high-risk activities. Other contributing factors include poor stretching routine, tight calf muscles, improper shoe wear during high risk activities, and altered biomechanics at the foot during activities (such as a flattened arch). A person over 30 years of age is at a higher risk for rupture secondary to the decrease in blood flow to the area of the tendon associated with aging. A person with a history of corticosteroid injections to the tendon may also have a predisposition for rupture. The highest incidence for rupture is in individuals between 30 and 50 years of age that usually have no history of calf or heel pain and commonly participate in recreational activities.

Confirmation:

What is the most likely clinical presentation?
A patient with an Achilles tendon rupture will present with swelling over the distal tendon, a palpable defect in the tendon above the calcaneal tuberosity, and pain and weakness with plantar flexion. The patient may limp and will often complain that during the injury there was a snap or a pop that was associated with the severe pain. A patient will not be able to stand on their toes and in a prone position will not demonstrate any passive plantar flexion with squeezing of the affected calf muscle (the Thompson test). A complete rupture will result in a palpable gap in the tendon prior to the insertion.

What laboratory or imaging studies would confirm the diagnosis?
Confirmation of an Achilles tendon rupture should utilize x-ray to rule out an avulsion fracture or bony injury. MRI can be used to locate the presence and severity of the tear or rupture.

What additional information should be obtained to confirm the diagnosis?
Diagnosis of an Achilles tendon rupture relies on patient history of the event and a positive Thompson's test. Patient history usually reveals a popping sound and a release from the back of the ankle. Physical examination and palpation reveal a discontinuity within the tendon. The O'Brien needle test may be used by the physician to confirm the rupture.

Examination:

What history should be documented?
Important areas to explore include mechanism of present injury, past medical history, medications, current health status, social history and habits, occupation, living environment, and social support system.

What test/measures are most appropriate?
Anthropometric characteristics: circumferential measurements for edema, palpation to determine ankle effusion
Arousal attention, and cognition: examine mental status, learning ability, memory, motivation
Assistive and adaptive devices: potential utilization of crutches
Gait, locomotion, and balance: safety with/without an assistive device during gait; biomechanics of gait
Integumentary integrity: assessment of sensation
Joint integrity and mobility: special tests such as Thompson's test
Muscle performance: strength assessment, characteristics of muscle contraction
Pain: pain perception assessment scale
Range of motion: active and passive range of motion
Sensory integration: assessment of proprioception and kinesthesia

Self-care and home management: assessment of functional capacity

What additional findings are likely with this patient?

An Achilles tendon rupture is more common in men and in individuals that do not consistently exercise, but are the "weekend warriors." There are risks and benefits to both philosophies of treatment (non-operative and operative) and the physician usually determines the course of treatment on a patient-by-patient basis accounting for the patient's age, activity level, and comorbidities.

Management:

What is the most effective management of this patient?

Medical management of a ruptured Achilles tendon incorporates immobilization through casting or a surgical approach for repair or reconstruction. Pharmacological intervention is not necessary for this condition except to relieve pain through NSAIDs, acetaminophen or narcotics depending on physician preference and patient profile. Non-surgical treatment includes serial casting for approximately ten weeks followed by the use of a heel lift to ensure maximal healing without stress on the tendon for three to six months. Physical therapy begins when the cast is removed. If a patient requires surgical intervention then a cast or a brace is required for six to eight weeks. Physical therapy intervention is primarily the same for surgical and non-surgical patients and includes range of motion, stretching, icing, assistive device training, endurance programming, gait training, strengthening, plyometrics, and skill specific training. Modalities, pool therapy, and other cardiovascular equipment may assist in the recovery of functional motion and endurance.

What home care regimen should be recommended?

A home care regimen is vital to the success of a patient's recovery. A program must be based on a patient's post-operative impairments and follow the physician's post-surgical protocol. A home program generally incorporates icing and elevation early in the rehabilitation process. A patient is required to continue a home program throughout the six to seven months of rehabilitation. Other areas of focus include range of motion, strengthening, gait, endurance activities, and high-level skill and sport specific tasks.

Outcome:

What is the likely outcome of a course in physical therapy?

Physical therapy should begin after surgical intervention or when the cast is removed from a non-surgical patient. Assuming an unremarkable recovery, a patient should return to their previous functional level within six to seven months.

What are the long-term effects of the patient's condition?

A patient that manages the Achilles tendon rupture without surgery and allows the tendon to heal on its own has a higher rate of rerupture (40% rerupture the tendon) compared to a patient that has surgical repair of the tendon (0-5% rerupture the tendon). An advantage to non-surgical management is a reduced risk of infection from surgery. However, it may result in an incomplete return of functional performance. A patient that has surgical intervention has a decreased risk for reinjury and a higher rate of return to athletic activities.

Comparison:

What are the distinguishing characteristics of a similar condition?

Achilles tendonitis can be an acute or chronic condition due to repetitive microtrauma that builds scar tissue in the area over time. A patient initially feels an aching sensation after activity and progresses to pain with walking. There may be localized tenderness and swelling in the area. In the acute stage a patient should utilize anti-inflammatory medications, rest for 2-3 weeks and use a heel lift. In the chronic stage the symptoms and pain may last beyond six weeks. Examination often reveals a thickened and nodular Achilles tendon. Surgical intervention may be warranted at this stage.

Clinical Scenarios:

Scenario One

A 32-year-old female is playing soccer in a recreational league. A physical therapist that assists the team observes her kick the ball and then fall to the ground. The therapist examines the patient in the training room and finds that the patient has some plantar flexion in a non-weight bearing position, but is unable to plantar flex the foot while weight bearing. The patient states that something popped while running and palpation indicates a separation in the Achilles tendon.

Scenario Two

A 46-year-old male is referred to physical therapy status post surgical reconstruction of a left Achilles tendon rupture. The patient has been casted for one week and has been using axillary crutches for household mobility. The patient has no significant past medical history. He is employed as a truck driver and resides in a one-story home. The patient sustained the injury while playing tennis.

Adhesive Capsulitis

Diagnosis:

What condition produces a patient's symptoms?

Adhesive capsulitis (also known as "frozen shoulder") is an enigmatic shoulder disorder characterized by inflammation and fibrotic thickening of the anterior joint capsule of the shoulder. The inflamed capsule becomes adherent to the humeral head and undergoes contracture. This condition is characterized by the symptoms of limitation in glenohumeral motion and pain.

An injury was most likely sustained to which structure?

Adhesive capsulitis is classified as primary or secondary. Primary adhesive capsulitis occurs spontaneously and secondary adhesive capsulitis results from an underlying condition. Inflammation within the joint capsule causes fibrous adhesions to form and the capsule to thicken. A decrease in space within the capsule leads to a decrease of synovial fluid and further irritation to the glenohumeral joint.

Inference:

What is the most likely contributing factor in the development of this condition?

Primary adhesive capsulitis has no known etiology; however, it is associated with conditions such as diabetes mellitus, hypothyroidism or cardiopulmonary conditions. Secondary adhesive capsulitis can result from trauma, immobilization, reflex sympathetic dystrophy, rheumatoid arthritis, abdominal disorders, and psychogenic disorders. Orthopedic intrinsic disorders that may initiate this process include supraspinatus tendonitis, partial tear of the musculotendinous cuff and bicipital tendonitis. Adhesive capsulitis occurs more in the middle-aged population with females having a greater incidence than males.

Confirmation:

What is the most likely clinical presentation?

Data regarding the prevalence and incidence of adhesive capsulitis is lacking. According to a published study adhesive capsulitis occurs in 2% of the population within the United States and in 11% of individuals that are diagnosed with diabetes mellitus. A small percentage of patients (10-15%) develop bilateral adhesive capsulitis. Adhesive capsulitis is characterized by restricted active and passive range of motion at the glenohumeral joint. Characteristics of the acute phase include pain that radiates below the elbow and awakens the patient at night. Passive range of the shoulder is limited during this phase due to pain and guarding. During the chronic phase pain is usually localized around the lateral brachial region, the patient is not awakened by pain, and passive range is limited due to capsular stiffness. Pain is present with a loss of glenohumeral motion, restricted elevation, and lateral rotation.

What laboratory or imaging studies would confirm the diagnosis?

An arthrogram can assist with the diagnosis of adhesive capsulitis by detecting a decreased volume of fluid within the joint capsule. The glenohumeral joint normally holds approximately 16-20 ml of fluid; however, adhesive capsulitis decreases the size of the capsule so it holds only 5-10 ml of fluid. Other tests should only be performed for differential diagnosis.

What additional information should be obtained to confirm the diagnosis?

The diagnosis of adhesive capsulitis is confirmed from clinical evaluation and past medical history. The patient may present with the greatest restriction of glenohumeral motion in abduction and lateral rotation but all planes of motion are usually affected. There is tightness within the anteroinferior joint capsule, pain with stretching, and restriction with passive and active range of motion.

Examination:

What history should be documented?

Important areas to explore include past medical and surgical history, medications, family history, current symptoms, current health status, social history and habits, occupation, leisure activities, and social support system.

What test/measures are most appropriate?

Anthropometric characteristics: circumferential measurements of bilateral upper extremities
Arousal, attention, and cognition: examine mental status, learning ability, memory, motivation
Community and work integration: analysis of community, work, and leisure activities
Cranial nerve integrity: assessment of muscle innervation by the cranial nerves, dermatome assessment
Environmental, home, and work barriers: analysis of current and potential barriers or hazards
Integumentary integrity: skin assessment, assessment of sensation

Joint integrity and mobility: assessment of hyper- and hypomobility of a joint, soft tissue swelling and inflammation
Muscle performance: strength assessment, muscle tone assessment
Pain: pain perception assessment scale, visual analog scale, assessment of muscle soreness
Posture: analysis of resting and dynamic posture
Range of motion: active and passive range of motion
Self-care and home management: assessment of functional capacity

What additional findings are likely with this patient?

A patient with adhesive capsulitis may encounter muscle spasms around the shoulder secondary to muscle guarding. A loss of reciprocal arm swing may be seen and disuse muscle atrophy may occur over time. A thorough examination must be completed to rule out concomitant systemic, rheumatologic, inflammatory, metastatic or infectious disorders.

Management:

What is the most effective management of this patient?

Medical management varies with adhesive capsulitis. Adhesive capsulitis is a self-limiting process that can take over 12 months in its course. Pharmacological intervention should emphasize the control of pain through acetaminophen, longer acting analgesics, NSAIDs or narcotics. A physician may inject the shoulder with corticosteroids to assist with recovery of motion. Surgical intervention to break up adhesions or release muscles adhered to the capsule is a last resort if conservative management fails. Physical therapy intervention during the acute phase includes icing or superficial heat, gentle joint mobilization, progressive strengthening, pendulum exercises, and isometric strengthening. During the chronic phase physical therapy intervention and goals may also include ultrasound, grade III and IV mobilization, increasing the extensibility of the joint capsule, and techniques such as PNF to restore painless functional range of motion.

What home care regimen should be recommended?

A home care regimen during the acute phase should include some self-stretching but avoid abduction secondary to the risk of damage to subacromial tissue. Once the patient enters the chronic phase the program should emphasize self-stretching, progressive exercises, posture management, PNF and other exercises such as pendulum exercises and "wall climbing" to assist with improving range of motion.

Outcome:

What is the likely outcome of a course in physical therapy?

Physical therapy is usually prescribed on an outpatient basis for three to five months after diagnosis. Adhesive capsulitis usually follows a nonlinear pattern of recovery. Spontaneous recovery is said to take 12-24 months in duration.

What are the long-term effects of the patient's condition?

Most patients are able to fully recover over time, but an estimated 7-14% of patients experience some permanent loss of range of motion at the shoulder joint. This loss is frequently asymptomatic and may not impair a patient's functional ability.

Comparison:

What are the distinguishing characteristics of a similar condition?

Acute bursitis is characterized by pain that is intense and sometimes throbbing over the lateral brachial region. This condition may arise secondary to calcific tendonitis. Active and passive motion in all directions is limited by pain. Abduction greater than 60 degrees and flexion greater than 90 degrees usually produces severe pain. Acute bursitis lasts for only a few days and unlike adhesive capsulitis this condition will usually resolve itself within a few weeks.

Clinical Scenarios:

Scenario One

A 29-year-old was diagnosed with primary adhesive capsulitis and referred to outpatient physical therapy. The patient is self-employed as an artist and enjoys outdoor activities. Past medical history includes diabetes mellitus since age six and a femur fracture 11 months ago. The patient noticed reduced range of motion and an increase in pain over the last few weeks.

Scenario Two

A 53-year-old female fell off her bike six months ago while cycling in a road race and sustained an injury to her shoulder complex. The patient attempted to immobilize her arm in a sling for two weeks. The patient states that she was unable to regain functional motion in her shoulder once she stopped using the sling. She saw a physician who diagnosed her with "frozen shoulder." The patient is limited to 10 degrees lateral rotation and 95 degrees of shoulder flexion.

Alzheimer's Disease

Diagnosis:

What condition produces a patient's symptoms?
Alzheimer's disease is a progressive neurological disorder that results in deterioration and irreversible damage within the cerebral cortex and subcortical areas of the brain. The loss of neurons results from the breakdown of several processes that would normally sustain the brain cells.

An injury was most likely sustained to which structure?
Neurons that are normally involved with acetylcholine transmission deteriorate within the cerebral cortex of the brain. Postmortem biopsy reveals neurofibrillary tangles within cytoplasm, amyloid plaques, and cerebral atrophy. Amyloid plaques contain fragmented axons, altered glial cells, and cellular waste that result in an inflammatory response that provides further damage to the nervous system. Amyloid can also cause atrophy of the smooth muscle of the arteries of the brain, predisposing them to rupture.

Inference:

What is the most likely contributing factor in the development of this condition?
The exact etiology of Alzheimer's disease is unknown; however, hypothesized causes include lower levels of neurotransmitters, higher levels of aluminum within brain tissue, genetic inheritance, autoimmune disease, abnormal processing of the substance amyloid, and virus. Approximately 4.5 million individuals are living with Alzheimer's disease in the United States. The risk of developing Alzheimer's disease increases with age and there is a higher incidence in women. The prevalence of Alzheimer's disease is 6% of individuals over 65 and 20% of individuals over 80 years of age.

Confirmation:

What is the most likely clinical presentation?
Alzheimer's disease is initially noted by a change in higher cortical functions characterized by subtle changes in memory, impaired concentration, and difficulty with new learning. These symptoms progress in the early stages and there is a loss of orientation, word finding difficulties, emotional lability, depression, poor judgment, and impaired ability to perform self-care skills. During the middle stages of Alzheimer's disease the patient will develop behavioral and motor problems characterized by neurological symptoms such as aphasia, apraxia, perseveration, agitation, and violent or socially unacceptable behavior that can include wandering. Eventually all ability to learn is lost and long-term memory also disappears. End-stage

Alzheimer's disease is characterized by severe intellectual and physical destruction. Patients in this stage will present with vegetative symptoms including incontinence, functional dependence, the inability to speak, and seizure activity.

What laboratory or imaging studies would confirm the diagnosis?
Alzheimer's disease presently cannot be confirmed until a postmortem biopsy reveals the neurofibrillary tangles and amyloid plaques. MRI can be used to assess any abnormalities or signs of atrophy within the brain that is associated with Alzheimer's disease or to rule out other medical conditions. Single photon emission computed tomography (SPECT) may be used to determine brain activity and predict potential for Alzheimer's disease. Blood work, urine, and spinal fluid may be required to rule out other diseases that may cause signs of dementia.

What additional information should be obtained to confirm the diagnosis?
A physical examination, neurological examination, and neuropsychological testing are required for diagnosis of probable Alzheimer's disease. The patient must demonstrate at least two deficits of cognition, memory, and related cognitive functioning with the absence of all other brain disease or disturbances in consciousness that may contribute to the identified deficits. Family history and symptoms may provide insight into the expected speed of progression of the disease.

Examination:

What history should be documented?
Important areas to explore include past medical history, family history, history of current symptoms, current health status, living environment, social history and habits, occupation, and social support system.

What test/measures are most appropriate?
Aerobic capacity and endurance: assessment of vital signs at rest and with activity
Arousal, attention, and cognition: examine mental status, learning ability, memory, motivation, Mini-Mental State Examination, level of consciousness
Assistive and adaptive devices: analysis of components and safety of a device
Environmental, home, and work barriers: analysis of current and potential barriers or hazards
Gait, locomotion, and balance: static and dynamic balance in sitting and standing, safety during gait with/without an assistive device, Functional Ambulation Profile, Berg Balance Scale

Motor function: equilibrium and righting reactions, coordination, physical performance scales
Muscle performance: strength assessment
Posture: analysis of resting and dynamic posture
Range of motion: active and passive range of motion
Reflex integrity: assessment of deep tendon and pathological reflexes (e.g., Babinski, ATNR)
Self-care and home management: assessment of functional capacity, Functional Independence Measure (FIM), Barthel Index

What additional findings are likely with this patient?

A patient with end-stage Alzheimer's disease is at high risk for infection and pneumonia. These patients may experience complications from a persistent vegetative state such as contractures, decubiti, fracture, and pulmonary compromise.

Management:

What is the most effective management of this patient?

Medical management of Alzheimer's disease may include pharmacological intervention during the early stages of the disease process. Medications are administered to inhibit acetylcholinesterase, alleviate cognitive symptoms, and control behavioral changes. Drug therapies are usually short-term in effect lasting six to nine months. Tacrine (Cognex), donepezil (Aricept), and rivastigmine (Exelon) are common pharmacological agents used to treat Alzheimer's disease; however, the side effects can be substantial. Physical therapy management should focus on maximizing the patient's remaining function and providing family and caregiver education. The therapist should attempt to create an emotional and physical environment that provides the patient with the opportunity to experience success. Modifying the layout of the patient's living space in order for the patient to easily find items is one example of creating an environment that encourages success. Safety with functional mobility and gait training may be indicated in the early stages of the disease. Later stages may require ongoing caregiver education regarding assistance with mobility, range of motion, and positioning. Many patients require a long-term care facility that specializes in Alzheimer's disease secondary to personality changes, aggressive behavior, and end-stage complications.

What home care regimen should be recommended?

During the early stages of Alzheimer's disease a patient should continue with activity as tolerated and utilize a memory book or other compensatory strategies at home. As the disease progresses, a patient will rely on caregiver support to assist with a daily exercise program. The patient should be encouraged to exercise, ambulate, and participate in everyday activities such as folding laundry, making beds, and assisting with dinner in order to avoid restlessness and wandering.

Outcome:

What is the likely outcome of a course in physical therapy?

Physical therapy may be indicated intermittently throughout the course of the disease; however, the therapy will not alter or cease the progression of the disease process.

What are the long-term effects of the patient's condition?

Alzheimer's disease is a chronic and progressive disorder and is the fourth leading cause of death in adults. The typical course of the disease averages between seven and eleven years. The leading cause of death of a patient with Alzheimer's disease is infection or dehydration.

Comparison:

What are the distinguishing characteristics of a similar condition?

Multi-infarct dementia produces symptoms in a step-like manner secondary to ongoing cerebral infarcts. This form of dementia is usually found in patients that are over 70 years of age and is more common in males. Hypertension is a primary risk factor and depression is common. A patient may also experience neurological deficits such as hemiplegia and emotional lability.

Clinical Scenarios:

Scenario One

A 65-year-old female is referred to physical therapy for gait disturbances. The patient resides alone and drives on a regular basis. During the initial examination the patient reveals that she is sometimes confused when driving. The patient complains that she has difficulty managing her time around the house and requires an extended amount of time to get ready in the morning.

Scenario Two

A 79-year-old male is seen by a physical therapist in an Alzheimer's residential facility. The physician recommends gait training with a walker. The patient enjoys walking around the unit; however, he has fallen several times within the last month.

Amyotrophic Lateral Sclerosis

Diagnosis:

What condition produces a patient's symptoms?
Amyotrophic lateral sclerosis (ALS) is a chronic degenerative disease that produces both upper and lower motor neuron impairments. Demyelination, axonal swelling, and atrophy within the cerebral cortex, premotor areas, sensory cortex, and temporal cortex cause the symptoms of ALS.

An injury was most likely sustained to which structure?
Rapid degeneration and demyelination occur in the giant pyramidal cells of the cerebral cortex and affect areas of the corticospinal tracts, cell bodies of the lower motor neurons in the gray matter, anterior horn cells, and areas within the precentral gyrus of the cortex. The rapid degeneration causes denervation of muscle fibers, muscle atrophy, and weakness.

Inference:

What is the most likely contributing factor in the development of this condition?
The exact etiology of ALS is unknown (90% of all cases); however, there are multiple theories of causative factors that include genetic inheritance as an autosomal dominant trait, a slow acting virus, metabolic disturbances, and theories of toxicity of lead and aluminum. Familial ALS occurs in 5-10% of all cases. Risk for ALS is higher in men and usually occurs between 40 to 70 years of age.

Confirmation:

What is the most likely clinical presentation?
Early clinical presentation of ALS may include both upper and lower motor neuron involvement. Early lower motor neuron signs include asymmetric muscle weakness, cramping, and atrophy that are usually found within the hands. Muscle weakness due to denervation eventually causes significant fasciculations, atrophy and wasting of the muscles. The weakness spreads throughout the body over the course of the disease and generally follows a distal to proximal path. Upper motor neuron symptoms occur due to the loss of inhibition of the muscle. Incoordination of movement, spasticity, clonus, and a positive Babinski reflex are some of the indicators of upper motor neuron involvement. Bulbar involvement is characterized by dysarthria, dysphagia, and emotional lability. Initially a person may have either upper or lower motor neuron involvement, but eventually both categories are affected. A patient with ALS will exhibit fatigue, oral motor impairment, fasciculations, spasticity, motor paralysis, and eventual respiratory paralysis.

What laboratory or imaging studies would confirm the diagnosis?
There are multiple tests used to assist with diagnosing ALS. Electromyography assesses fibrillation and muscle fasciculations. Muscle biopsy verifies lower motor neuron involvement rather than muscle disease and a spinal tap may reveal a higher protein content in some patients with ALS. CT scan will appear normal until late in the disease process.

What additional information should be obtained to confirm the diagnosis?
Diagnosis relies heavily on symptoms that determine both upper and lower motor neuron involvement. A patient that presents with motor impairment without sensory impairment is a primary indicator of ALS. Definitive diagnosis also first requires a physician to rule out other neurological conditions such as multiple sclerosis, spinal cord tumors, progressive muscular dystrophy, Lyme disease, and syringomyelia. In 1990 the World Federation of Neurology established four categories for diagnosis of ALS: Suspected ALS, Possible ALS, Probable ALS, and Definite ALS. Each category has specific criteria for diagnosis.

Examination:

What history should be documented?
Important areas include past medical history, family history, history of current symptoms, current health status, living environment, social history and habits, occupation, and social support system.

What test/measures are most appropriate?
Aerobic capacity and endurance: assessment of vital signs at rest and with activity, perceived exertion scale
Anthropometric characteristics: weight and height
Arousal, attention, and cognition: examines mental status, learning ability, memory, motivation
Assistive and adaptive devices: analysis of components and safety of a device
Environmental, home, and work barriers: analysis of current and potential barriers or hazards
Gait, locomotion, and balance: static and dynamic balance in sitting and standing, safety during gait with/without an assistive device
Motor function: motor assessment scales, coordination, equilibrium and righting reactions
Muscle Performance: strength assessment, muscle endurance, muscle tone assessment, muscle atrophy
Neuromotor development and sensory integration: analysis of reflex movement patterns, assessment of involuntary movements, sensory integration tests, gross and fine motor skills

> Posture: analysis of resting and dynamic posture
> Range of motion: active and passive range of motion
> Reflex integrity: assessment of deep tendon and pathological reflexes (e.g., Babinski, ATNR)
> Self-care and home management: Barthel Index
> Ventilation, respiration, and circulation: respiratory muscle strength, accessory muscle utilization, assessment of cough

What additional findings are likely with this patient?

During the initial stages of ALS there are various effects on the body. Progression of the disease allows for significant deterioration within the brain and spinal cord and a patient may exhibit paralysis of vocal cords, swallowing impairment, contractures, decubiti, and breathing difficulty that requires ventilatory support. Throughout the course of ALS, however, sensation, eye movement, and bowel and bladder function remain preserved.

Management:

What is the most effective management of this patient?

Effective management of ALS is based on supportive care and symptomatic therapy. Pharmacological intervention may include riluzole (Rilutek). This drug appears to have an effect on the progression of the disease process, however, its long-term effects are unknown. Symptomatic therapy may include anticholinergic, antispasticity, and antidepressant medications. Physical, occupational, speech, respiratory, and nutritional therapies may be warranted. Physical therapy intervention should focus on the quality of life and should include a low-level exercise program, range of motion, mobility training, assistive/adaptive devices, wheelchair prescription, bronchial hygiene, and energy conservation techniques. Patient, family, and caregiver training are very important as the disease continues to progress.

What home-care regimen should be recommended?

A home care regimen for a patient with ALS must consider the rate of disease progression and level of respiratory involvement. Goals should focus on maximizing the patient's functional capacity. A low-level exercise program may be indicated as long as the patient does not exercise to fatigue and promote further weakness. Family involvement is encouraged to support the patient through the course of the disease and assist with mobility, pacing skills, energy conservation techniques, and overall safety. During the later part of the disease the family and caregivers must

be competent with positioning, bronchial hygiene, range of motion, and assistance with mobility.

Outcome:

What is the likely outcome of a course in physical therapy?

Physical therapy intervention may assist with current issues, however, therapy does not hinder progression of ALS. Therapeutic goals will consider disease progression and focus on teaching for the patient and caregivers.

What are the long-term effects of the patient's condition?

ALS is usually a rapidly progressing neurological disease with an average course of two to five years with 20-30% of patients surviving longer than five years. Research indicates that although there is no structured course of this disease process, if a patient is diagnosed before 50 years of age the disease is usually longer in course. Death usually occurs from respiratory failure.

Comparison:

What are the distinguishing characteristics of a similar condition?

Muscular dystrophy (MD) is the term for a group of inherited disorders that are progressive and exhibit degeneration of muscles without sensory or neural impairment. Progressive weakness occurs to the muscle fibers secondary to the absence of dystrophin within the skeletal muscles. This group of disorders presents early in life and usually shortens life expectancy. Disuse atrophy, muscle deterioration, contractures, and cardiac and respiratory weakness are common characteristics of this disease process. A patient with MD usually dies from respiratory/cardiac complications secondary to the primary disease process.

Clinical Scenarios:

Scenario One

A 56-year-old male is diagnosed with ALS and presents with mild atrophy of the hand. The patient owns his own business as a painter and wants to continue working for as long as he can. The patient is referred to physical therapy for a home exercise program.

Scenario Two

A 60-year-old female is referred to physical therapy secondary to a left CVA. The patient was also diagnosed with ALS two years ago, requires the use of a wheelchair for mobility, and occasionally chokes while eating. The patient has assistance at home from her husband who is in good health.

Ankylosing Spondylitis

Diagnosis:

What condition produces a patient's symptoms?
Ankylosing spondylitis (AS), also known as Marie-Strumpell disease, is a systemic condition that is characterized by inflammation of the spine and larger peripheral joints. The chronic inflammation causes destruction of the ligamentous-osseous junction with subsequent fibrosis and ossification of the area.

An injury was most likely sustained to which structure?
AS primarily affects the sacroiliac joint, intervertebral disks, spine, costovertebral and apophyseal joints, connective tissue, and larger peripheral joints (hips, knees, and shoulders). Ossification can occur within all affected joints resulting in pain and deformity.

Inference:

What is the most likely contributing factor in the development of this condition?
AS is a progressive systemic disorder with uncertain etiology. Research supports the possibility of genetic inheritance combined with environmental influence. Gender, race, age, and genealogy are all factors to consider regarding risk for developing AS. A person born with a histocompatibility antigen HLA-B27 has a high risk for the disease. Approximately 80-90% of patients with AS are HLA-B27 positive, but only 2% of individuals that are HLA-B27 positive develop AS. HLA-B27 is found in 8.5% of Caucasians and only 2.5% of African Americans. Men are at a two to three time greater risk than women and onset is typically seen between twenty and forty years of age.

Confirmation:

What is the most likely clinical presentation?
A patient with early AS will present with recurrent and insidious episodes of low back pain, morning stiffness, impaired spinal extension, and limited range of motion in the affected joints for over a three-month period of time. As the disease progresses pain will become severe, consistent, and extending to the midback, and sometimes towards the neck. The natural lumbar curve will eventually flatten due to muscle spasms. Other manifestations include fixed flexion at the hips, spinal kyphosis, fatigue, weight loss, and peripheral joint involvement. If the costovertebral joints are affected a patient will present with impaired chest mobility, compromised breathing, and decreased vital capacity.

What laboratory or imaging studies would confirm the diagnosis?
X-ray of the spine may be negative in the initial stage of AS but with progression will reveal areas of erosion, demineralization, calcification, and syndesmophyte formation (ossification of the outside of the intervertebral disks). In the later stages of the disease x-ray will reveal fusion of the sacroiliac joint, calcification of apophyseal joints and spinal ligaments, and a bamboo appearance of the spine. Blood work can be used to rule out other diseases and assists with the diagnosis since the majority of patients with AS possess the HLA- B27 antigen and approximately 40% have an elevated erythrocyte sedimentation rate.

What additional information should be obtained to confirm the diagnosis?
Physical examination may reveal joint tenderness, pain, and/or limitation of the sacroiliac joint and the spine. Family inheritance and a thorough history of a patient's symptoms assist with the diagnosis of AS.

Examination:

What history should be documented?
Important areas to explore include past medical history, medications, current health status, family inheritance, living environment, occupation, leisure activities, social history and habits, and social support system.

What test/measures are most appropriate?
Anthropometric characteristics: baseline height measurement, circumferential chest measurements during inspiration
Arousal, attention, and cognition: examine mental status, learning ability, memory, motivation
Assistive and adaptive devices: analysis of components and safety of a device
Community and work integration: analysis of community, work, and leisure activities
Environmental, home, and work barriers: analysis of current and potential barriers or hazards
Ergonomics and body mechanics: analysis of dexterity and coordination
Gait, locomotion, and balance: assessment of static and dynamic balance in sitting and standing, safety during gait, Functional Ambulation Profile, analysis of wheelchair management
Joint integrity and mobility: assess hypomobility and limitation of a joint, Wright-Schober test for spinal mobility
Muscle performance: strength assessment
Pain: pain perception assessment scale
Posture: analysis of resting and dynamic posture

Range of motion: active and passive range of motion
Reflex integrity: assessment of deep tendon and pathological reflexes (e.g., Babinski, ATNR)
Self-care and home management: assessment of functional capacity
Sensory integrity: assessment of sensation
Ventilation, respiration, and circulation: analysis of thoracolumbar movement and chest expansion during breathing, measurement of vital capacity

What additional findings are likely with this patient?

Long-term AS will present with progressive symptoms and multiple complications. Iritis, uveitis, osteoporosis, fracture, atlantoaxial subluxation, and complete spinal fusion can occur in severe longstanding cases of AS. Pericarditis, cardiac pathology, pulmonary fibrosis, cardiac arrhythmias, amyloidosis, and aortic insufficiency have also been noted as potential complications.

Management:

What is the most effective management of this patient?

The goals of medical management are to reduce inflammation, maintain functional mobility, and relieve pain. Pharmacological intervention may include NSAIDs, disease-modifying drugs such as methotrexate, analgesics, and specifically Indomethacin to relieve pain. Physical therapy intervention should include postural exercises emphasizing extension, general range of motion, pain management, and energy conservation techniques. Low-impact and aerobic exercise with emphasis on extension and rotation are appropriate for a patient with AS. High-impact and flexion exercises are contraindicated. Patient education should include posture retraining, positioning for sleeping, and lifting techniques. Excessive exercise should be avoided as it can increase the inflammatory response and injury. Swimming is a highly recommended activity. Surgical intervention is rarely indicated to correct or stabilize a musculoskeletal deformity.

What home care regimen should be recommended?

A home care regimen for a patient with AS should include a daily low-impact therapeutic exercise program. Range of motion should focus on spinal movement in all directions. The patient requires a firm sleeping surface and competence with proper positioning and use of pillows to maintain optimal alignment. Ongoing breathing exercises and posture retraining will assist with overall level of function.

Outcome:

What is the likely outcome of a course in physical therapy?

Physical therapy cannot modify the progression of AS; however, it may assist to alleviate pain and improve a patient's functional capacity. A patient may require physical therapy on an intermittent basis for secondary complications throughout the disease process.

What are the long-term effects of the patient's condition?

AS progresses slowly over a fifteen to twenty-five year period and may remain isolated to the spine and sacroiliac joint or spread to larger peripheral joints. Stiffness and joint limitation are common long-term effects of AS that can negatively impact a patient's functional mobility. The extent of disability varies greatly with only 1% of patients experiencing complete remission. Normal course includes periods of exacerbations and remissions. Hip disease with AS is a marker for a severe form of AS and is more likely to occur in a patient that is diagnosed at a young age.

Comparison:

What are the distinguishing characteristics of a similar condition?

Sjogren's syndrome, like AS, is classified as a spondylarthropathy. Sjogren's is a chronic arthritis and autoimmune disease that also can affect several organs. Lymphocytes attack healthy tissues and organs and are usually found in combination with RA or lupus. Postmenopausal women are affected most often with over two to four million individuals in the United States living with the disease. It does not have a cure, but can be managed through medications, exercise, and proper nutrition. Exercise should follow general guidelines for the treatment of RA.

Clinical Scenarios:

Scenario One

A 28-year-old male is seen in physical therapy shortly after being diagnosed with AS. The patient complains of sacroiliac pain and tenderness. The patient has a negative family history and is currently employed as a high school maintenance technician.

Scenario Two

A 60-year-old female is seen in physical therapy with advanced AS. The patient has bilateral hip flexion contractures and kyphosis. The patient resides alone and receives daily assistance from her two sisters who live locally. The patient has previously refused recommendations to utilize an assistive device for ambulation.

Anterior Cruciate Ligament Sprain – Grade III

Diagnosis:

What condition produces a patient's symptoms?
The anterior cruciate ligament (ACL) extends from the anterior intracondylar region of the tibia to the medial aspect of the lateral femoral condyle in the intracondylar notch. The ligament prevents anterior translation of the tibia on the fixed femur and posterior translation of the femur on the fixed tibia. The ACL is a broad cord that has long collagen strands that permits up to 500 pounds of pressure prior to rupture. The ligament has a poor blood supply and does not have the ability to heal a complete tear. Injuries to the ACL most commonly occur during hyperflexion, rapid deceleration, hyperextension or landing in an unbalanced position.

An injury was most likely sustained to which structure?
A grade III ACL sprain refers to a complete tear of the ligament with excessive laxity. Tears of the anterior cruciate ligament most often occur in the midsubstance of the ligament and not at the ligament's attachment on the femur or tibia. Laxity rarely occurs solely in a straight plane and instead is often classified as anterolateral or anteromedial.

Inference:

What is the most likely contributing factor in the development of this condition?
Participation in athletic activities requiring high levels of agility (soccer, basketball, volleyball) and contact sports increases the incidence of an ACL injury. Recent studies indicate that women involved in selected athletic activities experienced significantly higher ACL injury rates (estimated two to eight times higher) than their male counterparts. There are many hypothesized reasons for this finding but to date a definitive answer has not been identified. Causative factors for ACL disruption include body movement and positioning, muscle strength, joint laxity, Q angle, and a narrow intercondylar notch.

Confirmation:

What is the most likely clinical presentation?
Epidemiological studies estimate that approximately 1:3000 individuals sustain an ACL injury annually in the United States with the peak incidence occurring between 14 and 29 years of age. This age group corresponds to an overall higher activity level, which increases the risk of injury. A grade III ACL sprain is characterized by significant pain, effusion, and edema that significantly limits range of motion. The patient may be unable to bear weight on the involved extremity resulting in dependence on an assistive device. Ligamentous testing reveals visible laxity in the knee and may exacerbate the patient's pain level.

What laboratory or imaging studies would confirm the diagnosis?
MRI is the preferred imaging tool to identify the presence of an ACL tear and possible disruption of other soft tissue structures such as ligaments and menisci. X-rays may be used to rule out a fracture.

What additional information should be obtained to confirm the diagnosis?
Subjective reports such as hearing a loud pop or feeling as though the knee buckled is often associated with a complete tear of the anterior cruciate ligament. Special tests such as the Lachman, anterior drawer, and pivot shift test can be used to confirm the diagnosis. It is important to perform all special tests bilaterally.

Examination:

What history should be documented?
Important areas to explore include mechanism of present injury, current symptoms, past medical history, medications, living environment, social history and habits, and social support system.

What test/measures are most appropriate?
Anthropometric characteristics: knee effusion and lower extremity circumferential measurements
Arousal, attention, and cognition: examine mental status, learning ability, memory, motivation
Assistive and adaptive devices: analysis of components and safety of a device, potential utilization of crutches
Gait, locomotion, and balance: safety during gait with an assistive device
Integumentary integrity: assessment of sensation (pain, temperature, tactile), skin assessment
Joint integrity and mobility: special tests for ligaments and menisci, Lachman and reverse Lachman test, anterior drawer test, palpation of structures, joint play, soft tissue restrictions, joint pain
Muscle performance: strength and active movement assessment, resisted isometrics, muscle contraction characteristics, muscle endurance
Orthotic, protective, and supportive devices: utilization of bracing, taping or wrapping, foot orthotic assessment
Pain: pain perception assessment scale
Range of motion: active and passive range of motion
Self-care and home management: assessment of functional capacity
Sensory integrity: proprioception and kinesthesia

What additional findings are likely with this patient?

Approximately two-thirds of the time the ACL is torn there is an accompanying meniscal tear. The collateral ligaments can also be involved although not as commonly as the menisci. When all three structures (ACL, MCL, and medial meniscus) are damaged it is referred to as the "unhappy triad."

Management:

What is the most effective management of this patient?

Management of a patient following a grade III ACL sprain includes controlling edema, increasing range of motion, strengthening, and improving the fluidity of gait. For patients electing to have surgery the patellar tendon is the most commonly utilized graft for intraarticular reconstruction. Patients often initially present with a knee immobilizer and crutches to protect the reconstructed ligament. Specific parameters are difficult to identify since many orthopedic surgeons utilize very specific protocols. Physical therapy management in the initial post-operative phase includes protecting the integrity of the graft, controlling edema, and improving range of motion. Specific intervention activities include pain modulation, patellar mobility, active range of motion exercises, gait activities, and quadriceps exercises. As patients progress in their rehabilitation program treatment begins to focus on strengthening activities emphasizing closed-chain exercises and selected functional activities. Closed-chain exercises are considered more desirable than open-chain exercises since they minimize anterior translation of the tibia. Patients should be required to complete a functional progression prior to returning to unrestricted athletics. For patients opting for a conservative (non-operative) approach, it is necessary to begin an aggressive strengthening program once the acute phase of the injury has subsided.

What home care regimen should be recommended?

The home care regimen should consist of range of motion, strengthening, palliative care, and functional activities as warranted based on the results of the patient examination and course (operative versus non-operative) of treatment.

Outcome:

What is the likely outcome of a course in physical therapy?

It is possible that with an aggressive strengthening program and/or activity modification patients may be able to participate in light to moderate athletic activities without formal surgical reconstruction. Patients electing to have surgery can expect to return to their previous functional level in four to six months.

What are the long-term effects of the patient's condition?

Patients that sustain a complete tear of the ACL and elect not to have reconstructive surgery will likely be at increased risk for instability and subsequent deterioration of joint surfaces.

Comparison:

What are the distinguishing characteristics of a similar condition?

A grade III posterior cruciate ligament (PCL) sprain is less common than an ACL sprain. The most common mechanism of injury for a PCL sprain is a "dashboard" injury or forced knee hyperflexion as the foot is plantar flexed. A grade III PCL injury will typically produce effusion, posterior tenderness, and a positive posterior drawer test. Knee extension is often limited due to the effusion and stretching of the posterior capsule and gastrocnemius. The rehabilitation program typically emphasizes strengthening of the quadriceps muscles. Individuals with an isolated PCL sprain may not exhibit any functional performance limitations and as a result, surgical intervention is far less common than with an ACL sprain. A PCL sprain alters the arthrokinematics of the knee joint and as a result a patient will be susceptible to degenerative changes such as arthritis.

Clinical Scenarios:

Scenario One

A 16-year-old gymnast sustains a grade I ACL injury after landing awkwardly on her left leg during a vault. The patient is two days status post injury and has mild effusion in the involved knee. The patient is a competitive gymnast and needs to compete in a regional meet in slightly less than four weeks.

Scenario Two

A 35-year-old male is referred to physical therapy after injuring his knee in a softball game. The patient reports tearing the ACL ten years ago in a skiing accident. The patient is active, however, reports more recent episodes of instability. The physician notes significant arthritic changes in the involved knee including diminished joint space.

Breast Cancer

Diagnosis:

What condition produces a patient's symptoms?
Breast cancer's primary symptom is a painless mass within the breast tissue. This mass is composed of malignant altered cells that proliferate and spread without control. A malignancy can occur anywhere within the breast tissue; however, the lump is usually found directly behind the areola in men and is usually located behind the areola or in the outer upper quadrant of the breast in women. There may or may not be generalized discomfort in the area of the mass.

An injury was most likely sustained to which structure?
Injury occurs initially at the cellular level within the breast tissue. Breast cancer either begins in the lobules which are the milk producing glands or in the ducts that bring the milk to the nipples. Breast cancer can spread into the lymphatic system and will commonly metastasize to the brain, lungs, bones, adrenals, and liver.

Inference:

What is the most likely contributing factor in the development of this condition?
The etiology of breast cancer is unknown; however, estrogen is believed to have some relationship to the disease process. Risk factors include gender, age, young menarche, late menopause, family history of breast cancer, high alcohol intake, high fat diet, radiation exposure, and past history of cancer. Breast cancer can occur in both males and females; however, males account for less then 1% of all breast cancer cases.

Confirmation:

What is the most likely clinical presentation?
Breast cancer has a median and mean age between 60 and 61 years of age. Breast cancer makes up approximately 30% of all female cancers and is the second leading cause of death in female cancers within the United States. Approximately 70% of all breast cancer occurs in women over the age of 50. A patient with breast cancer will present with a lump in the breast that is noticed by a physician (10%) or by the patient through self-examination (90%). Breast cancer is initially otherwise asymptomatic. As the disease progresses the breast may become painful, change shape, bleed from the nipple, and dimple over the area of the mass. Symptoms associated with metastases may include bone pain, upper extremity edema, and weight loss.

What laboratory or imaging studies would confirm the diagnosis?
Mammography is used to detect the location and growth of a mass; however, definitive diagnosis of breast cancer is made only after microscopic examination of a suspected mass by needle or excision biopsy. Ultrasound can also be used to detect if a lump is filled with fluid or a solid mass. Sentinel lymph node mapping is used upon diagnosis to identify exact lymph node involvement.

What additional information should be obtained to confirm the diagnosis?
Additional information such as family history of cancer, past medical history, and history of self-examination is helpful in support of a definitive diagnosis. This information is usually obtained prior to mammography and biopsy.

Examination:

What history should be documented?
Important areas to explore include past medical history, family history of cancer, medications, current health status, social history and habits, hand dominance, occupation, living environment, and social support system.

What test/measures are most appropriate?
Aerobic capacity and endurance: assessment of vital signs at rest and with activity
Anthropometric characteristics: upper extremity circumferential measurements
Arousal, attention, and cognition: examine mental status, learning ability, memory, motivation
Community and work integration: analysis of community, work, and leisure activities
Gait, locomotion, and balance: assess static/dynamic balance in sitting and standing, safety during gait
Integumentary integrity: assessment for potential infection of surgical incision
Muscle performance: strength assessment
Pain: pain perception assessment scale, visual analog scale
Range of motion: active and passive range of motion
Self-care and home management: assessment of self-care and home management skills, assessment of functional capacity, Barthel Index
Sensory integrity: assessment of superficial and combined sensations, proprioception, and kinesthesia

What additional findings are likely with this patient?

Additional findings are dependent on the stage of the cancer (I, II, III, IV) and course of treatment. If a patient has undergone surgical resection or mastectomy the patient may experience pain, edema, fatigue, and psychological issues. Patients that are diagnosed with advanced breast cancer may experience pleural effusion, pathological fractures, and spinal compression.

Management:

What is the most effective management of this patient?

The medical management of breast cancer is based on the size and the stage of the mass and corresponding involvement of the lymph nodes. Surgical management may range from excision of the mass (lumpectomy) to total radical mastectomy with axillary dissection. Chemotherapy, radiation therapy, and hormone therapies may be used in isolation or after a surgical procedure. Physical therapy may be indicated to assist with lymphedema management, post-surgical breathing exercises, positioning, pain management, strengthening and endurance activities, range of motion exercises, massage, intermittent compression, and patient education.

What home care regimen should be recommended?

A home care regimen should include education, positioning, and techniques to manage lymphedema. Range of motion exercises, energy conservation techniques, as well as general exercise and endurance activities should continue on a regular basis at home.

Outcome:

What is the likely outcome of a course in physical therapy?

Physical therapy may be indicated for post-surgical management to assist with impairments and promote independence with self-care and functional skills.

What are the long-term effects of the patient's condition?

The long-term effects of breast cancer are varied. The risk of recurrence is always present and should be monitored closely. Post-surgical lymphedema may persist and require ongoing home management. Overall prognosis and ten-year survival rates for women is over 85% for stage I disease; 66% for stage II; 36% for stage III; and 7% for stage IV disease. The survival rate decreases as the tumor progresses and lymph nodes become involved. Overall mortality has decreased 1-2% annually within the United States secondary to changes in lifestyle, improved self-examination, earlier diagnosis, and better treatment.

Comparison:

What are the distinguishing characteristics of a similar condition?

Fibrocystic breast disease (mammary dysplasia) usually occurs in both breasts and is characterized by nodular lumps within the breast tissue. The cysts are benign and become tender immediately prior to menstruation. Fibrocystic breast disease is the most common breast disorder occurring in 89 per 100,000 women. Other symptoms include aching and burning within the breast. Symptoms normally disappear after menstruation is over. Although benign, fibrocystic breast disease increases a patient's risk for breast cancer later in life.

Clinical Scenarios:

Scenario One

A 65-year-old female is seen by a physical therapist 24 hours after total mastectomy. The patient was active prior to the surgery and walked for exercise two miles everyday. The patient's past medical history is positive for fibrocystic breast disease, diabetes mellitus, and skin cancer. The patient reports pain with coughing. The patient resides alone in a retirement village and lost her husband to cancer last year. She has three supportive children that reside in the local area.

Scenario Two

A 45-year-old female is referred to outpatient physical therapy with lymphedema secondary to stage III breast cancer and radical mastectomy three months ago. The patient is fatigued and anxious about the increased size of her arm and limitation in range of motion. The patient runs a daycare center out of her home and is active in her church. Past medical history includes endometriosis and pharmacological treatment for depression.

Carpal Tunnel Syndrome

Diagnosis:

What condition produces a patient's symptoms?

The carpal tunnel is created by the transverse carpal ligament, the scaphoid tuberosity and trapezium, the hook of the hamate and pisiform, and the volar radiocarpal ligament and volar ligamentous extensions between the carpal bones. The median nerve, four flexor digitorum profundus tendons, four flexor digitorum superficialis tendons, and the flexor pollicis longus tendon pass through the carpal tunnel. Carpal tunnel syndrome (CTS) occurs as a result of compression of the median nerve where it passes through the carpal tunnel.

An injury was most likely sustained to which structure?

The median nerve is injured by compression within the carpal tunnel at the wrist. Normal tissue pressure within the tunnel is seven to eight mm Hg but CTS can result in pressure above 30 mm Hg, which further increases with flexion and extension of the wrist. The increase in pressure produces ischemia in the nerve. This results in sensory and motor disturbances in the median nerve distribution of the hand.

Inference:

What is the most likely contributing factor in the development of this condition?

Any condition such as edema, inflammation, tumor or fibrosis may cause compression of the median nerve within the carpal tunnel and result in ischemia. The exact etiology of CTS is unclear; however, conditions that produce inflammation of the carpal tunnel that can contribute to CTS include repetitive use, rheumatoid arthritis, pregnancy, diabetes, trauma, tumor, hypothyroidism, and wrist sprain or fracture. Other etiologies include a congenital narrowing of the tunnel and vitamin B6 deficiency.

Confirmation:

What is the most likely clinical presentation?

Approximately five million individuals in the United States are diagnosed with CTS. Most patients are diagnosed between 35 and 55 years of age with prevalence in women. A patient with CTS will initially present with sensory changes and paresthesia along the median nerve distribution in the hand. It may also radiate into the upper extremity, shoulder, and neck. Symptoms include night pain, weakness of the hand, muscle atrophy, decreased grip strength, clumsiness, and decreased wrist mobility. Initially, muscle atrophy is often noted in the abductor pollicis brevis muscle and progresses to the thenar muscles.

What laboratory or imaging studies would confirm the diagnosis?

Electromyography and electroneurographic studies can be used to diagnose a motor conduction delay along the median nerve within the carpal tunnel. MRI is sometimes used to identify inflammation of the median nerve, altered tendon or nerve positioning within the tunnel or thickening of the tendon sheath.

What additional information should be obtained to confirm the diagnosis?

Physical examination, history, and review of symptoms are extremely important when diagnosing CTS. Provocation testing such as a positive Tinel's sign, a positive Phalen's test, and a positive tethered median nerve stress test along with the other symptoms will assist to confirm the diagnosis.

Examination:

What history should be documented?

Important areas to explore include past medical history, medications, history of symptoms, current health status, occupation, living environment, social history and habits, leisure activities, and social support system.

What test/measures are most appropriate?

Anthropometric characteristics: wrist and hand circumferential measurements

Arousal, attention, and cognition: examine mental status, learning ability, memory, motivation

Community and work integration: analysis of community, work, and leisure activities

Environmental, home, and work barriers: analysis of current and potential barriers or hazards

Ergonomics and body mechanics: analysis of dexterity and coordination

Integumentary integrity: skin and nailbed assessment, assessment of sensation

Joint integrity and mobility: assessment of hypomobility of a joint, assessment of soft tissue swelling/inflammation, Tinel's sign, Phalen's test, tethered median nerve stress test

Muscle performance: strength assessment including hand musculature

Orthotic, protective, and supportive devices: potential utilization of bracing or splinting

Pain: pain perception assessment scale

Range of motion: active and passive range of motion

Self-care and home management: assessment of functional capacity

What additional findings are likely with this patient?

Advanced CTS can present with muscle atrophy of the hand, radiating pain in the forearm and shoulder, and nerve damage with motor and sensory loss. Unrelieved compression creates initial neurapraxia with some demyelination of the axons. This results in eventual axonotmesis and wallerian degeneration within the nerve distribution. The patient may present with ape hand deformity caused by atrophy of the thenar musculature and first two lumbricals. Research indicates that approximately 50% of cases include bilateral involvement.

Management:

What is the most effective management of this patient?

A patient with CTS will initially receive conservative management including local corticosteroid injections, splinting, and physical therapy management. Recent pharmacological intervention has included Methylprednisolone injected proximally to the tunnel. Research indicates a 77% relief of symptoms from this method after 30 days. Physical therapy is one aspect of conservative management and includes splinting, carpal mobilization, and gentle stretching. Biomechanical analysis and adaptation of a patient's occupation, work place, leisure activities, and living environment may be necessary. If conservative treatment fails the patient may require surgery to release the carpal ligament and decompress the median nerve. Newer surgical techniques allow for smaller incisions, less manipulation of the nerve, and are highly successful for long-term relief of symptoms. Post-surgical physical therapy intervention should include the use of moist heat with electrical stimulation, iontophoresis, cryotherapy, gentle massage, desensitization of the scar, tendon gliding exercises, and active range of motion. A patient should initially avoid wrist flexion and a forceful grasp. After four weeks a patient can progress with active wrist flexion, gentle stretching, putty exercises, light progressive resistive exercise, and continued modification of body mechanics. Radial deviation against resistance should be avoided due to the tendency for irritation and inflammation. Post-surgical rehabilitation usually lasts six to eight weeks.

What home care regimen should be recommended?

A home care regimen should consist of continued stretching and strengthening exercises. The patient must be competent and compliant regarding the use of a splint and follow all work and leisure modifications.

Outcome:

What is the likely outcome of a course in physical therapy?

Physical therapy intervention should improve a patient's condition and decrease symptoms of CTS within four to six weeks. If conservative treatment fails and the patient requires surgical intervention, rehabilitation may last six to eight weeks.

What are the long-term effects of the patient's condition?

CTS can have minor effects on some patients while having debilitating effects on others. The overall long-term effects are dependent on the degree of involvement, the amount of permanent damage, and the level of success with conservative or surgical management. It is possible to have no long-term effects from this condition if the patient responds positively to physical therapy and the rehabilitation process. Other patients may be left with permanent motor and sensory impairments along the median nerve distribution.

Comparison:

What are the distinguishing characteristics of a similar condition?

Compression in the tunnel of Guyon occurs with inflammation to the ulnar nerve between the hook of the hamate and the pisiform. This condition occurs from tasks such as leaning during extended handwriting, leaning on bike handles while riding, repetitive gripping activities or trauma. The patient will present with paresthesias along the ulnar distribution, weakness and atrophy of the hypothenar musculature, decreased mobility of the pisiform, and impaired grip strength. This condition can be treated with conservative management or surgical intervention.

Clinical Scenarios:

Scenario One

A 26-year-old female is seen in physical therapy with a diagnosis of bilateral CTS. The patient has not been treated previously for this syndrome and is employed as a telephone sales specialist. The patient complains of pain in her hands, numbness when sleeping and while performing at work, and muscle soreness in both hands.

Scenario Two

A 45-year-old male with CTS is referred to physical therapy ten days after surgical decompression. The patient's post-operative routine includes resting the hand, using a splint, icing, and elevation. Minimal edema is noted at the wrist. The patient is anxious to return to work.

Central Cord Syndrome

Diagnosis:

What condition produces a patient's symptoms?
Central cord syndrome (CCS) is an incomplete spinal cord lesion that most often results from a cervical hyperextension injury. Symptoms are secondary to damage to the central aspect of the spinal cord. CCS usually occurs from a fall but can occur from other forms of trauma such as a motor vehicle accident.

An injury was most likely sustained to which structure?
The spinal cord sustains bleeding into the central gray matter that causes damage to the centrally located cervical tracts. Injury is caused by a ligamentum flavum (hyperextension) injury or otherwise from anterior compression of the cord due to osteophyte formation. Studies often reveal axonal disruption in the lateral columns at the level of injury with preservation of the gray matter.

Inference:

What is the most likely contributing factor in the development of this condition?
The most common mechanism of injury for CCS is a hyperextension injury of the cervical spine. Other potential contributing factors in the development of CCS include cervical spondylosis, narrowing or congenital defect of the spinal canal, tumor, rheumatoid arthritis or syringomeylia. CCS predominantly affects the population over 50 years of age with a greater incidence in men.

Confirmation:

What is the most likely clinical presentation?
CCS presents with motor loss that is greater in the upper extremities than the lower extremities and is most severe distally in the upper extremities. This presentation is due to the damage that occurs within the central location of the spinal cord. Sensory loss found below the level of the lesion is usually limited but can be variable. Lumbar, thoracic, and cervical components proceed medially in order towards the center of the spinal cord. Sacral segments are usually unaffected since they are located laterally within the spinal cord. Bowel and bladder functions resolve in 55-85% of patients with CCS after six months.

What laboratory or imaging studies would confirm the diagnosis?
MRI is used to assess spinal cord impingement from bone or disk. CT scan of the spine will assess spinal canal compromise and the degree of impingement.

X-rays can be utilized to assess potential fractures, dislocations, and degree of spondylolitic deterioration.

What additional information should be obtained to confirm the diagnosis?
Diagnosis is made using results of MRI, CT scan, and X-ray findings. Information may be obtained from past medical history and mechanism of injury that usually supports the diagnosis of CCS.

Examination:

What history should be documented?
Important areas to explore include past medical history, medications, family history, current symptoms, mechanism of injury, social history and habits, occupation, leisure activities, and social support system.

What test/measures are most appropriate?
Aerobic capacity and endurance: autonomic responses to positional changes, assessment of vital signs at rest/activity

Arousal, attention, and cognition: examine mental status, learning ability, memory, motivation

Assistive and adaptive devices: analysis of components and safety of a device, wheelchair prescription

Community and work integration: analysis of community, work, and leisure activities

Environmental, home, and work barriers: analysis of current and potential barriers or hazards

Gait, locomotion, and balance: static and dynamic balance in sitting and standing, safety during gait with/without an assistive device, Berg Balance Scale, Tinetti Performance Oriented Mobility Assessment, wheelchair management

Integumentary integrity: skin assessment, American Spinal Injury Association (ASIA)-Standard Neurological Classification of Spinal Cord Injury Sensory Examination

Motor function: equilibrium and righting reactions, posture and balance in sitting

Muscle performance: ASIA-Standard Neurological Classification of Spinal Cord Injury Motor Examination, muscle tone examination

Neuromotor development and sensory integration: analysis of reflex movement patterns

Pain: assessment of neuropathic pain

Posture: analysis of resting and dynamic posture

Range of motion: active and passive range of motion

Reflex integrity: assessment of deep tendon and pathological reflexes (e.g., Babinski, ATNR)

Self-care and home management: assessment of functional capacity, Functional Independence Measure (FIM), Barthel Index
Ventilation, respiration, and circulation: breathing patterns, auscultation of the lungs and heart

What additional findings are likely with this patient?

Each patient with CCS will present differently based on location and extent of injury to the spinal cord. Potential side effects and complications include autonomic dysreflexia, spasticity, neurogenic bladder and bowel, allodynia, and pressure ulcers.

Management:

What is the most effective management of this patient?

Rehabilitation services are initiated once the patient is medically stable. Medical management should include physiatry, physical therapy, occupational therapy, vocational counseling, and social services. Methylprednisolone should be administered within eight hours of injury to assist with neurologic recovery. Other pharmacological intervention may include blood pressure medication to combat autonomic dysreflexia, antispasticity medication for treatment of spasticity, anticonvulsants for treatment of neurogenic pain, prophylactic anticoagulants, and antidepressants if warranted. Physical therapy intervention should include patient and caregiver education, range of motion, strengthening, endurance activities, balance retraining, proximal stabilization exercises, and functional mobility based on the patient's current functional status. Adaptive devices may be required to assist with overall mobility. If a patient ambulates, a platform attachment walker may initially be indicated since hand function is usually poor for grasp. Surgical intervention is rare but may be indicated if compression within the spinal cord persists or progress ceases without cause.

What home care regimen should be recommended?

A home care regimen should include a continuation of exercise, endurance, and functional mobility training based on the patient's current functional abilities. Outpatient physical therapy may be warranted and should modify the home program as necessary.

Outcome:

What is the likely outcome of a course in physical therapy?

Physical therapy can assist a patient with CCS to attain maximum functional outcome based on level and extent of injury. Overall outcome, however, is based on age, motivation, compliance, and extent of injury.

What are the long-term effects of the patient's condition?

CCS is the most common incomplete spinal cord lesion and accounts for approximately 30% of overall incomplete tetraplegia. Statistics indicate 77% of patients with CCS will ambulate, 53% will gain bowel and bladder control, and 42% regain some hand function. Older patients do not tend to recover as well as younger ones. Favorable long-term prognostic factors for a good outcome include early hand function, improvement of strength in all extremities during the inpatient stay, and little to no lower extremity involvement.

Comparison:

What are the distinguishing characteristics of a similar condition?

Anterior cord syndrome (ACS) normally affects two-thirds of the spinal cord and can occur from a cervical flexion injury or anterior spinal artery embolisation. There is a complete loss of motor function as well as pain and temperature below the level of the lesion due to damage of the spinothalamic and corticospinal tracts. Preservation of the posterior columns allow for intact vibration and proprioception. ACS has the worst prognosis for all the spinal cord syndromes with only 10-15% of patients achieving functional recovery.

Clinical Scenarios:

Scenario One

A 22-year-old female is admitted to the rehabilitation floor with CCS secondary to a MVA. She has some motion in her lower extremities, shoulders, and trace motion at the elbows. She only wants to practice walking and refuses therapy for any other treatment. She also is currently refusing any form of adaptive equipment for use during ambulation and with dressing. The patient is currently living with her friend and planned to move out of state in six weeks. She is employed as a teacher assistant at a local middle school.

Scenario Two

A 79-year-old male is diagnosed with CCS after being admitted through the emergency room secondary to a fall down his basement steps. He complains of severe neck pain and currently is not able to initiate movement in all four extremities. He is anxious and wants to return home to his second floor apartment as soon as he can. He misses his wife of 60 years who he has cared for since her stroke three years ago.

Cerebral Palsy

Diagnosis:

What condition produces a patient's symptoms?
Cerebral palsy (CP) is an umbrella term used to describe a group of non-progressive movement disorders that result from brain damage. CP has an incidence of 2-4:1,000 births and is the most common cause of permanent disability in children.

An injury was most likely sustained to which structure?
There is a wide variety of neurological damage that can occur with injury. Autopsy reports have indicated lesions that include hemorrhage below the lining of the ventricles, damage to the central nervous system that caused neuropathy and anoxia, and hypoxia that caused encephalopathy. Hypoxic and ischemic injuries disrupt normal metabolism that results in global damage to the developing fetus. CP is classified by neurological dysfunction and extremity involvement. Spastic CP involves upper motor neuron damage; athetoid CP involves damage to the cerebellum, cerebellar pathways or both.

Inference:

What is the most likely contributing factor in the development of this condition?
The etiology may be multifactorial and is sometimes unknown. Risk factors are categorized as prenatal (80%) or perinatal and postnatal (20%) cases. Prenatal risk factors include Rh incompatibility, hypothyroidism, maternal malnutrition, infection, diabetes, and chromosome abnormalities. Perinatal factors include multiple or premature births, breech delivery, low birth weight, prolapsed cord, placenta abruption, and asphyxia. Postnatal factors include CVA, head trauma, neonatal infection, and brain tumor. The most common causative factor of CP is prenatal cerebral hypoxia.

Confirmation:

What is the most likely clinical presentation?
CP is the second most common neurological impairment seen in children (following mental retardation). CP is a neuromuscular disorder of posture and controlled movement; however, clinical presentation is highly variable based on the area and extent of CNS damage. A child may present with high tone, low tone or athetoid movement. CP is classified as monoplegia (one involved extremity), hemiplegia (unilateral involvement of the upper and lower extremities), and quadriplegia (involvement of all extremities). CP is also classified as mild, moderate, and severe. General characteristics include motor delays, abnormal muscle tone and motor control, reflex abnormalities, poor postural control, high risk for hip dislocations, and balance impairments. Intellect, vision, hearing, and perceptual skills are usually altered in conjunction with CP. All other characteristics of CP are classification dependent.

What laboratory or imaging studies would confirm the diagnosis?
If CP is suspected through clinical findings, including seizures, an electroencephalography (EEG) may be performed. X-ray of the hip may rule out hip dislocation; blood and urine tests can be used to investigate a metabolic cause of CP. Observation usually will diagnose CP secondary to the observed outward characteristics.

What additional information should be obtained to confirm the diagnosis?
Diagnosis of CP is regularly confirmed through an extensive neurological evaluation, patient observation, and patient history including developmental progress, and the presence of pathological reflexes. Differential diagnosis is performed to rule out other potential disorders.

Examination:

What history should be documented?
Important areas to explore include past medical history, risk factors, maternal course of pregnancy, medications, family history, current characteristics, social history, and social support system.

What test/measures are most appropriate?
Aerobic capacity and endurance: assessment of vital signs at rest and with activity, auscultation of the lungs
Arousal, attention, and cognition: examine mental status, learning ability, memory, motivation
Assistive and adaptive devices: analysis of components and safety of a device
Environmental, home, and work barriers: analysis of current and potential barriers or hazards
Gait, locomotion, and balance: static/dynamic balance
Integumentary integrity: skin assessment, assessment of sensation
Joint integrity and mobility: assessment of hyper- and hypomobility of a joint
Motor function: equilibrium and righting reactions, coordination, posture and balance, sensorimotor integration, Barthel Index, Bayley Scale of Infant Development, Bruininks-Oseretsky Test of Motor Proficiency, Alberta Infant Motor Scale, Pediatric Evaluation of Disability Inventory

Muscle performance: muscle tone assessment, strength assessment if appropriate
Neuromotor development and sensory integration: analysis of reflex movement patterns, assessment of involuntary movements, sensory integration tests, gross and fine motor skills, developmental milestones
Orthotic, protective, and supportive devices: analysis of components of a device
Pain: adapted pain scale
Posture: analysis of resting and dynamic posture
Range of motion: active and passive range of motion, assessment of contractures
Reflex integrity: assessment of deep tendon and pathological reflexes (e.g., Babinski, ATNR, Moro)
Sensory integrity: proprioception and kinesthesia
Ventilation, respiration, and circulation: breathing patterns, respiratory strength, accessory muscle utilization

What additional findings are likely with this patient?

Specific additional findings are dependent on the classification and extent of CP. Generally, complications can include aspiration, pneumonia, contractures, scoliosis, and constipation. Mental retardation and epilepsy are present in 50-60% of children diagnosed with CP. Common comorbidities include learning disabilities, seizure disorders, vision and hearing impairments, bowel and bladder dysfunction, microcephalus, and hydrocephalus. Secondary impairments may include psychosocial issues for the patient and family members.

Management:

What is the most effective management of this patient?

Effective medical management of CP requires a life-long team approach. Pharmacological intervention may require antianxiety, antispasticity, and anticonvulsant medications. Physical therapy for CP often uses neurodevelopmental treatment and sensory integration techniques. Treatment should include normalization of tone, patient and caregiver education, motor learning, developmental milestones, positioning, stretching, strengthening, balance, and mobility skills. Adaptive equipment, specialized wheelchair seating, and orthotic prescription may be indicated. Surgical management may be required and include hip correction, contracture release, motor point block, dorsal rhizotomy or correction of scoliosis.

What home care regimen should be recommended?

A home care regimen for a patient with CP is also a life-long process that will require ongoing modification to meet the progression of goals. Family and caregiver involvement is vital for patients with moderate to severe CP. A home program may include patient and caregiver education, exercise, positioning, stretching, mobility training, and strengthening.

Outcome:

What is the likely outcome of a course in physical therapy?

Physical therapy will attempt to maximize a patient's level of current function and prevent secondary loss. If a patient is going to ambulate, this will usually occur by the age of eight. The ability or inability to ambulate will have a large impact on the direction and goals of therapeutic intervention.

What are the long-term effects of the patient's condition?

CP is a non-progressive, but permanent condition. The long-term effects and overall functional outcome depend on the extent of injury, associated impairments, and caregiver support. Prognosis for mild to moderate CP is a near normal life span. Fifty percent of children with severe CP die by the age of ten.

Comparison:

What are the distinguishing characteristics of a similar condition?

Arthrogryposis multiplex congenita (AMC) occurs in utero and is also considered to be non-progressive. AMC is considered a neuromuscular syndrome and is classified into three forms. The infant is born with multiple contractures and may have fibrous bands that developed in place of muscle. A patient with AMC should have a normal life expectancy and is usually of normal intelligence. It is usually difficult for these individuals to live independently due to their level of physical disability.

Clinical Scenarios:

Scenario One

A two-year-old female diagnosed with moderate spastic quadriplegia is seen in physical therapy. She is delayed in developmental milestones and beginning to acquire contractures. The parents are very supportive and the child appears happy and cooperative. The child's chart indicates normal intelligence.

Scenario Two

A nine-year-old male is seen in physical therapy at the request of his parents. The patient is diagnosed with moderate low tone quadriplegia, has minimal impairments with intelligence, and has acquired a 30-degree left thoracic scoliosis. The parents requested the evaluation since the child remains nonambulatory.

Cerebrovascular Accident

Diagnosis:

What condition produces a patient's symptoms?
Cerebrovascular accident (CVA) occurs when there is an interruption of cerebral circulation that results in cerebral insufficiency, destruction of surrounding brain tissue, and subsequent neurological deficit. The ischemia occurs from either a stroke in evolution (the infarct slowly progresses over one to two days) or as a completed stroke (an abrupt infarct with immediate neurological deficits).

An injury was most likely sustained to which structure?
CVA results from prolonged ischemia to an artery within the brain. This condition can cause subsequent neurological damage relative to the size and location of the infarct. Disruption of blood flow to a certain artery will lead to damage of a specific area of the brain and its functions. There are different types of CVA that include ischemic stroke (thrombus, embolus, lacunar) and hemorrhagic stroke (intracerebral, subdural, subarachnoid).

Inference:

What is the most likely contributing factor in the development of this condition?
The primary risk factors for CVA are classified as modifiable and non-modifiable. Modifiable factors include hypertension, atherosclerosis, heart disease, diabetes, elevated cholesterol, smoking, and obesity. Hypertension is the most prevalent modifiable cause of CVA. Non-modifiable risk factors include age, race, family history, and sex. Age constitutes the greatest risk for CVA, in fact 73% of patients sustaining a stroke are greater than 65 years of age.

Confirmation:

What is the most likely clinical presentation?
The incidence for an initial CVA is 114:100,000 persons or 750,000 individuals that have a first CVA in the United States per year. It is estimated there are four million stroke survivors living today. The clinical presentation of a CVA is determined by the location and extent of the infarct. Typical characteristics can include hemiplegia or hemiparesis, sensory, visual, and perceptual, impairments, balance abnormalities, dysphagia, aphasia, cognitive deficits, incontinence, and emotional lability.

What laboratory or imaging studies would confirm the diagnosis?
Computed tomography can confirm an area of infarct in the brain and its vascular origin; however, it can present as negative for up to a few days after the event. MRI allows for the diagnosis of ischemia within the brain almost immediately after onset. Positron emission tomography (PET) can provide information regarding cerebral perfusion and cell function. Ultrasonography identifies areas of diminished blood flow in vessels and angiography may identify a clot and determine if surgical intervention is necessary.

What additional information should be obtained to confirm the diagnosis?
A chest x-ray may be warranted to rule out lung disease, while an electrocardiogram is used to examine potential cardiac abnormalities. Diagnosis is usually based upon patient history, physical and neurological examinations, symptoms, and diagnostic testing.

Examination:

What history should be documented?
Important areas to explore include past medical history, medications, risk factor profile, current health status, social history and habits, occupation, living environment, and social support system.

What test/measures are most appropriate?
Arousal, attention, and cognition: examine mental status, learning ability, memory, motivation, Mini-Mental State Exam, Boston Diagnostic Aphasia Examination
Assistive and adaptive devices: analysis of components and safety of a device
Gait, locomotion, and balance: static and dynamic balance in sitting and standing, safety during gait with an assistive device, Berg Balance Scale, Tinetti Performance Oriented Mobility Assessment, Functional Ambulation Profile
Integumentary integrity: skin and sensation assessment
Motor function: equilibrium and righting reactions, coordination, motor assessment scales
Muscle performance: muscle tone assessment, assessment of active movement, Stroke Rehabilitation Assessment of Movement (STREAM)
Neuromotor development and sensory integration: assess involuntary movements, sensory integration, gross and fine motor skills, reflex movement patterns
Orthotic, protective, and supportive devices: analysis of components of a device, analysis of movement while wearing a device
Posture: analysis of resting and dynamic posture
Pain: pain perception assessment scale
Range of motion: active and passive range of motion
Reflexes: assessment of pathological reflexes (e.g., Babinski, ATNR)

Self-care and home management: assessment of functional capacity, Rankin Scale, NIH Stroke Scale, Functional Independence Measure (FIM)
Sensory integrity: proprioception and kinesthesia

What additional findings are likely with this patient?

A patient with a left CVA may present with weakness or paralysis to the right side, impaired processing, heightened frustration, aphasia, dysphagia, motor apraxia, and right hemianopsia. A patient with a right CVA may present with weakness or paralysis to the left side, poor attention span, impaired awareness and judgment, memory deficits, left inattention, emotional lability, impulsive behavior, and left hemianopsia. Coma and death are the most severe consequences of a CVA. It is common for patients post CVA to have residual complications and deficits that persist.

Management:

What is the most effective management of this patient?

Medical management will initially include medically stabilizing the patient through medication and surgical intervention. Pharmacological intervention can include thrombolytic agents, anticoagulants (contraindicated for hemorrhagic CVA), diuretics, antihypertensives, and potential long-term use of aspirin. Respiratory care must also be a priority during acute rehabilitation. Physical therapy during the acute phase focuses on: positioning, pressure relief, sensory awareness and integration, ROM, weight bearing, facilitation, muscle re-education, balance, and postural control. The physical therapist is responsible for implementing the most appropriate therapeutic strategies based on the degree of impairment. There are many approaches to neurological rehabilitation that include, but are not limited to: Bobath's Neuromuscular Developmental Treatment (NDT), motor control, Brunnstrom's Movement Therapy in Hemiplegia, Rood, and Kabat, Knott, and Voss' Proprioceptive Neuromuscular Facilitation (PNF). Many therapists integrate facets from multiple approaches based on the patient's response to selected interventions.

What home care regimen should be recommended?

Approximately 75% of patients that have experienced a CVA return home at various levels of functional mobility. The majority of patients require ongoing therapy services part of their home care regimen. A therapeutic program should be designed for a patient to continue at home independently or with the required level of assistance. Fall prevention, control of spasticity, endurance training, and optimizing functional mobility are important components of a successful home program.

Outcome:

What is the likely outcome of a course in physical therapy?

A patient that experiences neurological deficits due to a CVA may require physical therapy to assist with motor re-education, sensory stimulation, and functional mobility. The outcome is dependent on the patient's overall health, level of cognition and motivation, motor recovery, residual deficits, and family support.

What are the long-term effects of the patient's condition?

The effects of a CVA can be quite diverse ranging from spontaneous recovery to permanent disability requiring compensatory strategies and techniques in order to function. The first three months of recovery typically reveals the most measurable neurologic recovery and is usually a good indicator of the long-term outcome. Long-term outcome is based on several factors including: the site and extent of CVA, premorbid status, age, potential for plasticity of the nervous system, and motivation. Research indicates that a patient can continue to improve the control of movement and show progress for an average of two to three years post CVA.

Comparison:

What are the distinguishing characteristics of a similar condition?

A transient ischemic attack (TIA) is also characterized by diminished blood supply to the brain; however, it is transient. Although the patient may present with similar symptoms of a CVA, the symptoms last for only a brief period of time. Unlike a CVA, the TIA does not cause permanent residual neurological deficits. A TIA is an indication, however, of future risk for a CVA.

Clinical Scenarios:

Scenario One

A 43-year-old male is diagnosed with a left hemorrhagic CVA due to an aneurysm of the middle cerebral artery. The patient resides with his wife and two teenage sons.

Scenario Two

A 79-year-old female is diagnosed with a right CVA involving the anterior cerebral artery. The patient was unconscious for two days and is functioning at a very low-level. The patient was residing in an independent living facility where she had meals provided for her in the dining area.

Cystic Fibrosis

Diagnosis:

What condition produces a patient's symptoms?
Cystic fibrosis (CF) is an inherited disease that affects the ion transport of the exocrine glands resulting in impairment of the hepatic, digestive, respiratory, and reproductive systems. The disease causes the exocrine glands to overproduce thick mucus (that causes subsequent obstruction), overproduce normal secretions or overproduce sodium and chloride.

An injury was most likely sustained to which structure?
CF affects multi-systems within the body; however, the respiratory and gastrointestinal systems are usually the most involved in the disease process. There is an underlying impermeability of epithelial cells to chloride that results in viscosity of mucous gland secretions within the lungs, sweat glands, pancreas, and intestines. CF creates an elevation of sodium chloride and pancreatic enzyme insufficiency.

Inference:

What is the most likely contributing factor in the development of this condition?
CF is an autosomal recessive genetic disorder (both parents are carriers of the defective gene) and is located on the long arm of chromosome seven. This disorder creates an abnormality in the CF transmembrane conductance regulator (CFTR) protein. CFTR normally is involved with the process that allows for chloride to pass through the plasma membrane of epithelial cells. It is estimated that 5% of the population carry a recessive gene for CF.

Confirmation:

What is the most likely clinical presentation?
CF is the most common lethal genetic disorder affecting Caucasian children in the United States. Incidence is estimated at 1:2,500 births for Caucasians compared to 1:17,000 births for African Americans. CF can be diagnosed shortly after birth, however, it is sometimes not diagnosed for years. The most consistent symptom is the finding of high concentrations of sodium and chloride in the sweat. Parents will notice a salty taste when kissing their child. Other symptoms vary depending on the systems that are affected by the disease and the course of progression. These systems include pulmonary, gastrointestinal, digestive (liver, intestinal, pancreatic), genitourinary, and musculoskeletal impairments. Early symptoms may include a persistent cough, salty skin, sputum production, wheezing, poor weight gain, and recurrent infections.

What laboratory or imaging studies would confirm the diagnosis?
Neonates' meconium can be tested as a screening tool for increased albumin. The quantitative pilocarpine iontophoresis sweat test is the sole diagnostic tool in determining the presence of CF. Sodium and chloride amounts greater than 60 mEq/l (standard value is 40 mEq/l) is a positive diagnosis for CF. The sweat test should be performed twice to ensure accuracy.

What additional information should be obtained to confirm the diagnosis?
Additional information in the diagnosis of CF is found through a positive family history, genetic screening of the parents, a previous diagnosis of failure to thrive, and in the manifestation of symptoms.

Examination:

What history should be documented?
Important areas to explore include past medical history (if diagnosed after birth), medications, current health status, developmental milestones, living environment, and social support system.

What test/measures are most appropriate?
Aerobic capacity and endurance: assessment of vital signs at rest and with activity, perceived exertion scale
Arousal, attention, and cognition: examine mental status, learning ability, memory, motivation
Assistive and adaptive devices: analysis of components and safety of a device
Integumentary integrity: skin assessment, sweat test findings, clubbing of the digits
Muscle performance: active motion strength assessment
Posture: analysis of resting and dynamic posture, especially thorax and shoulder girdle
Range of motion: active and passive range of motion, chest wall mobility
Self-care and home management: functional capacity
Ventilation, respiration, and circulation: assess cough and clearance of secretions, pulmonary function testing (FEV_1 and FVC), pulse oximetry, auscultation of the lungs, accessory muscle utilization and vital capacity

What additional findings are likely with this patient?
The most common complication of CF is an exacerbation of obstructive pulmonary disease. Pulmonary function testing results in a decreased forced expiratory volume (FEV_1) and forced vital capacity (FVC). The functional residual capacity (FRC) and residual volume (RV) become increased. Hypoxemia and hypercapnia develop due to the alteration in

perfusion. Chronic pulmonary infections and poor absorption often lead to barrel chest, pectus carinatum, and kyphosis deformities. Approximately 90% of patients have pancreatic enzyme deficiency, degeneration, and eventual progressive fibrosis of the pancreas. This process interferes with digestion and absorption of nutrients. Airway obstruction can cause pulmonary hypertension, atelectasis, pneumonia, and lung abscess. Severe complications can include cirrhosis, diabetes mellitus, pneumothorax, cardiac pathology, pancreatitis, cor pulmonale, and intestinal obstruction.

Management:

What is the most effective management of this patient?

Medical management of CF is a multidisciplinary approach that should focus on the quality of life, providing emotional and psychosocial support, and controlling symptoms. Nutritional support is necessary throughout the patient's life to ensure adequate nutrition. Pharmacological intervention is required to treat infections, thin mucus secretions, replace pancreatic enzymes, reduce inflammation, and assist with breathing. Psychological counseling is indicated as needed. Gene therapy is experimental and attempts to correct the defect in CF cells. Physical therapy intervention is essential for management of the disease. Chest physical therapy should be performed several times per day and includes bronchial drainage, percussion, vibration, breathing and assistive cough techniques, and ventilatory muscle training. Posture training, mobilization of the thorax, and breathing exercises must be incorporated into the overall program. A patient may also be trained to use autogenic drainage, a positive expiratory pressure (PEP) device or Flutter valve therapy to assist with independent bronchial drainage. General exercise and stretching are indicated to optimize overall function. Family and patient education are vital to the survival of the patient.

What home care regimen should be recommended?

A home care regimen for a patient with CF requires an ongoing routine performing postural drainage and chest physical therapy several times each day. Family members are trained to provide this ongoing support at home. Mechanical percussors may be used to ease the time and energy spent on manual percussion by the care provider. Mechanical percussors also offer the patient control and independence with treatment. Physical conditioning including exercise and endurance training are indicated except with severe lung disease. Exercise programs may improve pulmonary function, increase maximal work capacity, improve mucus expectoration, and increase self-esteem.

Outcome:

What is the likely outcome of a course in physical therapy?

A patient with CF will require intermittent physical therapy throughout his or her life. The goals of physical therapy are to maximize secretion clearance from the lungs, optimize pulmonary function, and maximize the patient's quality of life.

What are the long-term effects of the patient's condition?

CF is a terminal disease; however, the median age of death has increased to 32 years of age due to early detection and comprehensive management. The most common cause of death for patients with CF remains respiratory failure. A child that initially presents with gastrointestinal symptoms generally has a good clinical course whereas a child that initially presents with pulmonary symptoms is more likely to clinically deteriorate at a faster pace. Males generally have a better prognosis than females.

Comparison:

What are the distinguishing characteristics of a similar condition?

There is no other respiratory disease that is similar to the etiology of CF. However, chronic obstructive pulmonary disease (COPD) has similar lung characteristics. COPD is characterized by altered pulmonary function tests, difficulty with expiration, cough, sputum production, and physical damage to specific portions of the lungs. Chest physical therapy and pharmacological intervention are indicated for moderate to advanced COPD.

Clinical Scenarios:

Scenario One

A four-week-old infant is referred to physical therapy after being diagnosed with CF. The infant has a pleasant disposition and does not have any observable discomfort; however, the parents are very anxious. The patient has three siblings that do not have CF disease.

Scenario Two

A 26-year-old female with CF is referred to physical therapy with a severe respiratory infection. The patient recently moved into an apartment with her boyfriend and works 30 hours per week in a hair salon. Prior to the infection the patient was living at home and was able to manage the disease with occasional assistance from family members. The physical therapy referral is for chest physical therapy.

Degenerative Spondylolisthesis

Diagnosis:

What condition produces a patient's symptoms?
Spondylolisthesis is the forward slippage of one vertebra on the vertebra below. There are several types of spondylolisthesis classified by the actual cause for the slippage. Classifications include congenital, isthmic, degenerative, post-traumatic, and pathologic spondylolisthesis. Degenerative spondylolisthesis (DS) is caused by the weakening of joints that allows for forward slippage of one vertebral segment on the one below due to degenerative changes. These changes include segmental ligamentous instability and hypertrophic subluxating facet joints which can result in stenosis of the spinal canal.

An injury was most likely sustained to which structure?
The most common site of DS is the L4-L5 level. The slippage causes cauda equina symptoms secondary to stenosis of the canal. It is theorized that ischemia and poor nourishment secondary to the stenosis deprives the associated spinal nerves and results in pain. The L5 nerve root is compressed in an L4-L5 olisthesis. Other structures that can be irritated include the intervertebral disk, posterior and anterior longitudinal ligaments, and vertebral periosteum and bone.

Inference:

What is the most likely contributing factor in the development of this condition?
DS is caused by arthritis and degenerative changes in the spine. The intervertebral disk looses some of its ability to resist motion and as a result the vertebral facets increase in size and develop bone spurs to compensate. This condition can actually produce spinal stenosis and weaken the spine itself resulting in the slippage of a vertebrae. Since all structures of the spine remain intact the slippage is usually limited due to the secondary bony restraints of the spine.

Confirmation:

What is the most likely clinical presentation?
DS usually affects individuals over 50 years of age. It is more common with African Americans and women also have a higher incidence of occurrence than men. Back pain is a primary symptom that is said to increase with exercise, lifting overhead, prolonged standing, getting out of bed or a car, walking up stairs or an incline, and positioning in extension. The pain may be severe and radiate depending on the area of stenosis secondary to the vertebral slippage. Sensory and motor loss may be significant and follow a myotomal and/or dermatomal distribution. Most patients do not have significant neurologic deficits, however, a few do experience severe changes.

What laboratory or imaging studies would confirm the diagnosis?
Plain radiographs of the vertebral column are adequate to confirm the diagnosis of DS. CT scan or MRI may be indicated to rule out any other contributing conditions or to further assess nerve impingement.

What additional information should be obtained to confirm the diagnosis?
Physical and neurological examinations in combination with a full medical history usually provide adequate information for probable diagnosis; however, X-rays are required for definitive diagnosis of DS.

Examination:

What history should be documented?
Important areas to explore include past medical history and previous testing, medications, family history, current symptoms, current health status, social history and habits, occupation, leisure activities, and social support system.

What test/measures are most appropriate?
Arousal, attention, and cognition: examine mental status, learning ability, memory, motivation
Assistive and adaptive devices: analysis of components and safety of a device
Community and work integration: analysis of community, work, and leisure activities
Environmental, home, and work barriers: analysis of current and potential barriers or hazards
Ergonomics and body mechanics: analysis of dexterity and coordination, evaluation of proper lifting techniques
Gait, locomotion, and balance: static and dynamic balance in sitting and standing, safety during gait with/without an assistive device, Functional Ambulation Profile
Joint integrity and mobility: assessment of hyper- and hypomobility of a joint, soft tissue swelling and inflammation
Muscle performance: strength assessment
Pain: pain perception assessment scale, visual analog scale, assessment of muscle soreness
Posture: analysis of resting and dynamic posture
Range of motion: active and passive range of motion
Reflex integrity: assessment of deep tendon and pathological reflexes (e.g., Babinski, ATNR)
Self-care and home management: assessment of functional capacity
Sensory integrity: assessment of sensation

What additional findings are likely with this patient?

A patient with DS may or may not have additional slippage of the vertebra over time. If the slippage of the vertebra worsens it does not necessarily correspond to an increase in symptoms. Symptoms may increase with or without marked degenerative changes and vice versa. A patient that does experience ongoing neurological deficits will require surgical intervention regardless of the amount of slippage.

Management:

What is the most effective management of this patient?

Medical management of a patient diagnosed with DS should initially include education, medication, activity modification, and physical therapy intervention. Pharmacological intervention should include NSAIDs to decrease acute inflammation. Corticosteroids may be indicated for severe symptoms. Epidural steroid injections and selective nerve root injections are sometimes indicated if oral medications fail. Activity modification and rest should be instituted to further allow inflammation to subside and improve overall symptoms. Long-term bed rest, however, should be avoided. Once the acute phase has subsided physical therapy should begin. William's flexion exercises should be performed to strengthen the abdominals and reduce lumbar lordosis. Back school, modalities, postural education, and other exercises that provide core stabilization and increase flexibility should be included in the patient's program. External support such as bracing or wearing of a corset may relieve intradiscal pressure. Surgical intervention is only indicated if conservative treatment fails, the pain becomes disabling or significant neurological impairment exists. Surgical intervention usually involves decompression with or without spinal fusion.

What home care regimen should be recommended?

A patient with DS should initially take NSAIDs and decrease overall activities to allow for a reduction in the acute symptoms. Once a patient is able to tolerate physical therapy the home care regimen should include prescribed exercises to improve abdominal strength and core stabilization, flexibility exercises, and proper positioning. Goals for the home program are to alleviate pain and improve function. A patient should only modify the home program per physical therapist instruction.

Outcome:

What is the likely outcome of a course in physical therapy?

The majority of patients with DS are successful with conservative treatment that may include physical therapy, home program, bracing, and use of NSAIDs as needed.

What are the long-term effects of the patient's condition?

The long-term effects of DS vary based on progression and advancement of the slipped vertebrae and/or progression of symptoms. Some patients may be able to manage pain and maintain function without any further associated pathology. If symptoms continue to progress, then surgical intervention may be required.

Comparison:

What are the distinguishing characteristics of a similar condition?

Congenital spondylolisthesis is the slippage of one vertebra on the vertebra below due to an anomaly or defect in the fusion of the neural arch. This usually occurs in the upper sacral vertebral arches or at the L5 level. The condition is usually diagnosed during the growth spurts between 12 and 16 years of age. Patients are normally pain free prior to this point and begin to express complaints of back pain, "sciatica" pain, and other symptoms. There is a strong genetic association found in this type of spondylolisthesis.

Clinical Scenarios:

Scenario One

A 65-year-old female is seen in physical therapy with a diagnosis of L5 degenerative spondylolisthesis. She complains of pain in her back that can occasionally radiate down her left leg. She resides with her husband in their two-story home and works part-time at a grocery store as a clerk. She also enjoys gardening but has been having a difficult time with all activities in the last eight weeks secondary to pain.

Scenario Two

A 74-year-old male two weeks status post spinal fusion is examined in a nursing home. The patient was diagnosed six months ago with DS, shortly after he began to exhibit neurological symptoms. The physician prescribes physical therapy daily to improve strength and functional independence.

Down Syndrome

Diagnosis:

What condition produces a patient's symptoms?
Down syndrome (trisomy 21) occurs when there is an error in cell division either through nondisjunction (95%), translocation (4%) or mosaicism (1%) and the cell nucleus results in 47 chromosomes. Nondisjunction occurs when faulty cell division results in three specific chromosomes instead of two and extra chromosomes are then replicated for every cell. Translocation occurs when part of a chromosome breaks off during cell division and attaches to another chromosome. The total number of chromosomes remains 46 but Down syndrome exists. Mosaicism occurs right after fertilization when nondisjunction occurs in the initial cell divisions. This results in a mixture of cells with 46 and 47 chromosomes.

An injury was most likely sustained to which structure?
The pair of 21st chromosomes is responsible for Down syndrome when nondisjunction, translocation or mosaicism occurs during cell division.

Inference:

What is the most likely contributing factor in the development of this condition?
The exact etiology of Down syndrome is currently unknown. Some theories suggest that an increase in maternal age (and age of the oocyte) may cause predisposition to errors in meiosis. Environmental factors such as virus, paternal age, medical exposure, reproductive medications, and intrinsic predispositions have been associated with Down syndrome.

Confirmation:

What is the most likely clinical presentation?
Down syndrome occurs once in every 800-1,000 live births. In the United States there are approximately 350,000 individuals living with Down syndrome. Down syndrome is the most common cause of mental retardation. Other clinical manifestations include hypotonia, flattened nasal bridge, almond-shaped eyes, abnormally shaped ears, Simian line (palmar crease), epicanthal folds, enlargement of the tongue, congenital heart disease, developmental delay, and a variety of musculoskeletal disorders.

What laboratory or imaging studies would confirm the diagnosis?
During pregnancy a female can be tested for Alpha-fetoprotein, human chorionic gonadotropin, and unconjugated estrogen levels (the triple screen). Three diagnostic studies include chorionic villus sampling, amniocentesis or percutaneous umbilical blood sampling. Detection of Down syndrome occurs in approximately 60-70% of the women tested that are carrying a baby with Down syndrome. After birth a chromosome analysis called a karyotype can be performed to confirm the suspected diagnosis.

What additional information should be obtained to confirm the diagnosis?
In most cases diagnosis of Down syndrome is made through the physical attributes that are present at birth. Chromosomal testing is also used to determine the exact chromosomal pathogenesis.

Examination:

What history should be documented?
Important areas to explore include past medical history including cardiac status, family history, history of seizures, current health status, physical attributes, developmental delay, and social support system.

What test/measures are most appropriate?
Arousal, attention, and cognition: mental status, learning ability, memory, intelligence testing
Environmental, home, and work barriers: analysis of current and potential barriers or hazards
Ergonomics and body mechanics: analysis of dexterity and coordination
Gait, locomotion, and balance: static and dynamic balance in sitting and standing, safety during gait with/without an assistive device
Integumentary integrity: skin and sensation assessment
Joint integrity and mobility: assessment of hyper- and hypomobility of a joint, ligamentous laxity
Motor function: equilibrium and righting reactions, motor assessment scales, coordination, posture and balance in sitting, assessment of sensorimotor integration, Peabody Developmental Motor Scales
Muscle performance: strength and tone assessment
Neuromotor development and sensory integration: analysis of reflex movement patterns, assessment of involuntary movements, sensory integration tests, gross and fine motor skills, Bayley Scales of Infant Development
Posture: analysis of resting and dynamic posture
Range of motion: active and passive range of motion
Reflex integrity: assessment of deep tendon and pathological reflexes (e.g., Babinski, ATNR)
Self-care and home management: assessment of functional capacity, WEE-FIM

Ventilation, respiration, and circulation: assessment of cough and clearance of secretions, breathing patterns, respiratory muscle strength, accessory muscle utilization and vital capacity, perceived exertion scale, pulse oximetry, palpation of pulses, pulmonary function testing, auscultation of the lungs and heart

What additional findings are likely with this patient?

There are many associated impairments that a child with Down syndrome may inherit. Potential manifestations and secondary complications that are associated with Down syndrome include atlantoaxial instability, sensory, hearing, and visual impairments, umbilical hernia, respiratory compromise, and Alzheimer's disease. Persons with Down syndrome also have an increased incidence of celiac disease, epilepsy, constipation, as well as blood, dermatologic, and musculoskeletal disorders.

Management:

What is the most effective management of this patient?

Medical management of Down syndrome is a team approach that requires life long intervention and should be directed toward the specific medical and developmental goals. The overall goal of treatment is to achieve maximum potential and level of function. Pharmacological intervention is based on a particular characteristic or complication such as leukemia or a seizure disorder. Physical therapy intervention plays an important role in the treatment of Down syndrome. Developmental delay, hypotonia, laxity of the ligaments, and poor strength are key areas for the focus of physical therapy treatment. A child with Down syndrome will also require learning strategies based on his or her level of mental retardation. Children with Down syndrome regularly have significant verbal-motor impairments when they verbally respond to a stimulus. Physical therapy will not accelerate developmental milestones, but help the patient avoid compensatory patterns with static positioning and mobility.

What home care regimen should be recommended?

A home care regimen should be multifaceted with caregivers being proficient with all aspects of care. A routine of exercise is highly important for a child with Down syndrome in order to avoid inactivity and obesity. Positioning and handling are key components in order to maximize proper alignment and to minimize pathological reflexes, malalignment, and instability.

Outcome:

What is the likely outcome of a course in physical therapy?

Physical therapy will assist a child by teaching optimal movement patterns during developmental activities and by improving strength. Physical therapy will be indicated on an intermittent basis based on level of function and secondary complications. Strengthening and endurance activities should be encouraged within a home program.

What are the long-term effects of the patient's condition?

Individuals with Down syndrome today have a longer life expectancy secondary to advances in medical care; however, it is still less than standard life expectancy. Higher mortality results from issues such as congenital heart defects and gastrointestinal anomalies. Immune system dysfunction, repeated respiratory infections, onset of leukemia, pulmonary hypertension, and complications from Alzheimer's disease all contribute to a higher overall mortality rate compared to the general population. Approximately 80% of patients with Down syndrome reach the age of 55.

Comparison:

What are the distinguishing characteristics of a similar condition?

Prader-Willi syndrome is a genetic disorder that occurs when there is a partial deletion of chromosome 15. Characteristics include hypotonia, difficulties with feeding during infancy, short stature, excessive appetite, and obesity through childhood. Learning disabilities also exist.

Clinical Scenarios:

Scenario One

A six-month-old boy with Down syndrome is evaluated for outpatient physical therapy. Moderate hypotonia exists and the child does not roll or sit with support. The child's chart indicates atlantoaxial instability with minimal subluxation between C1 and C2. The boy's parents are supportive but both work full-time and are concerned about the competence of the daycare provider.

Scenario Two

A 12-year-old-girl with Down syndrome is seen in physical therapy two times per week at her school. The child is status post right femur fracture and the cast was taken off two weeks ago. The physician orders strengthening and cardiovascular endurance activities. The child has mild scoliosis and minimal learning deficits. The child is moderately obese and complains of pain consistently during treatment.

Duchenne Muscular Dystrophy

Diagnosis:

What condition produces a patient's symptoms?
Duchenne muscular dystrophy (DMD) is a progressive neuromuscular degenerative disorder that manifests symptoms once fat and connective tissue begin to replace muscle that has been destroyed by the disease process. The mutation of the dystrophin gene causes the symptoms of DMD.

An injury was most likely sustained to which structure?
A patient with DMD is born with a mutation in the dystrophin gene Xp21 that normally codes for the muscle membrane protein dystrophin. This gene is found on the X-chromosome and since it is a recessive trait, only males are affected while females are carriers. The lack of dystrophin allows for damage within the sarcolema with contraction of the muscle. The mutated gene causes weakening of cell membranes, destruction of myofibrils, and loss of muscle contractility. The destroyed muscle cells are replaced with fatty deposits.

Inference:

What is the most likely contributing factor in the development of this condition?
The etiology of DMD is inheritance as an X-linked recessive trait. The mother is the silent carrier of this disorder. Since it is a recessive trait, only male offspring will manifest the disorder while female offspring become carriers.

Confirmation:

What is the most likely clinical presentation?
The incidence of DMD in the United States is 20-35:100,000 live male births. Diagnosis of DMD usually occurs between two and five years of age. The first symptoms include a waddling gait, proximal muscle weakness, clumsiness, toe walking, excessive lordosis, pseudohypertrophy of the calf and other muscle groups, and difficulty climbing stairs. DMD primarily affects the shoulder girdle musculature, pectorals, deltoids, rectus abdominis, gluteals, hamstrings, and calf muscles, and is initially identified when a child begins to have difficulty getting off the floor; needing to use the Gowers' maneuver. During this technique a patient uses his hands to stabilize and walk up his legs in order to attain an upright posture. Approximately one-third of patients have some form of learning disability secondary to the dystrophin abnormalities. The disabilities usually present as subtle cognitive and/or behavioral deficits. There is usually rapid progression of this disease with the inability to ambulate by ten to twelve years of age.

What laboratory or imaging studies would confirm the diagnosis?
Electromyography is used to examine the electrical activity within the muscles. A muscle biopsy can be performed to determine the absence of dystrophin and evaluate the muscle fiber size. DNA analysis and high serum creatinine kinase levels in the blood also assist with confirming the diagnosis.

What additional information should be obtained to confirm the diagnosis?
Clinical examination, current symptoms, and family history are used to assist in the diagnosis, the type, and progression of the disease. Definitive diagnosis is made from clinical findings along with EMG and muscle biopsy results.

Examination:

What history should be documented?
Important areas to explore include past medical history, family history, medications, current symptoms, current health status, living and school environment, and social support system.

What test/measures are most appropriate?
Anthropometric characteristics: circumferential measurements to monitor muscle atrophy
Aerobic capacity and endurance: assessment of vital signs at rest and with activity
Arousal, attention, and cognition: examine mental status, learning ability, memory, motivation
Assistive and adaptive devices: analysis of components and safety of a device
Environmental, home, and work barriers: analysis of current and potential barriers or hazards
Gait, locomotion, and balance: static and dynamic balance in sitting and standing, safety during gait with/without an assistive device
Joint integrity: assessment of hypermobility and hypomobility of a joint, assessment of deformity
Muscle performance: assessment of active movement
Orthotic, protective, and supportive devices: analysis of components of a device, analysis of movement while wearing a device
Pain: pain perception assessment scale
Posture: analysis of resting and dynamic posture
Range of motion: active and passive range of motion, contracture assessment
Ventilation, respiration, and circulation: breathing patterns, respiratory muscle strength, accessory muscle utilization, pulmonary function testing

What additional findings are likely with this patient?

Additional findings occur with progression of the disease. Disuse atrophy, contractures, scoliosis, inability to ambulate, weight gain/obesity, cardiac and respiratory impairments, musculoskeletal deformity, and gastrointestinal dysfunction are the most common findings. Respiratory problems and scoliosis progress once the child is utilizing a wheelchair.

Management:

What is the most effective management of this patient?

Medical management of DMD focuses on maintaining function of the unaffected musculature for as long as possible. Pharmacological intervention may include glucocorticoids and immunosuppressant medications. Physical therapy intervention is initially indicated to assist a young child with progression through the developmental milestones. Once a child presents with impairments, physical therapy should focus on maintaining available strength, encouraging mobility, adapting to the loss of function, and promoting family involvement in a home program. Manual muscle testing and range of motion should be evaluated on a consistent basis to determine the pattern and rate of disability. Orthotic prescription, adaptive devices, and wheelchair prescription are areas that will require attention during the course of the disease. Respiratory care will also become a vital part of the plan of care as the patient weakens and strength diminishes. As DMD progresses, treatment will include range of motion, prevention of contracture/deformity, positioning, pain management, breathing exercises and postural drainage, and the use of a wheelchair or adaptive equipment. Ongoing emotional support for the child/family is necessary.

What home care regimen should be recommended?

A home care regimen relies on family involvement for a successful home program. Proper positioning, range of motion, submaximal exercise, and breathing exercises are all important aspects that assist a child to maintain function for as long as possible.

Outcome:

What is the likely outcome of a course in physical therapy?

Physical therapy is an important aspect in the care of a child with DMD; however, it will not alter the degenerative process of the disease. The goals of physical therapy throughout the course of the disease are to maintain present function, adapt to the progressive loss of mobility skills, and educate the patient and family. It is the role of the physical therapist to ensure that full and proper training has been completed on all aspects of a patient's care to ensure the highest level of function.

What are the long-term effects of the patient's condition?

DMD is a progressive disorder that occurs early in childhood and progresses rapidly. DMD usually affects the cardiac muscle in the later stages of the disease. Death occurs primarily from cardiopulmonary complications due to cardiac muscle involvement or respiratory muscle dysfunction. Death usually takes place by the time a patient is a teenager, or less frequently into their 20's.

Comparison:

What are the distinguishing characteristics of a similar condition?

Facioscapulohumeral dystrophy (FSHD), also known as Landouzy-Dejerine dystrophy, is a form of muscular dystrophy that is also inherited but the exact genetic origin is unclear. This disease presents later in a child's life, usually between seven and twenty years of age. Characteristics include facial and shoulder girdle weakness, weakness lifting the arms over the head, and difficulty closing the eyes. This disease is more common in males than females. The females tend to be carriers of the disorder. Life span remains normal.

Clinical Scenarios:

Scenario One

A three-year-old male was recently diagnosed with DMD. The mother reports that the child can ambulate, but prefers to be carried. The child crawls up the stairs and has been falling more frequently. The patient has two sisters at home and resides in a two-story home. At present, both parents work full-time and the child is enrolled in a home daycare.

Scenario Two

A 12-year-old male diagnosed with DMD is referred to physical therapy secondary to increased weakness and frequent falls. The patient is currently ambulating with bilateral Lofstrand crutches. There is evidence of pseudohypertrophy and a mild plantar flexion contracture. The patient's mother is concerned that he is at risk for serious injury while ambulating at school.

Emphysema

Diagnosis:

What condition produces a patient's symptoms?
Emphysema is the condition of pathologic accumulation of air in the lungs found with chronic obstructive pulmonary disease (COPD). There are three classifications of emphysema that include centrilobular emphysema, panlobular emphysema, and paraseptal emphysema. Emphysema results from a long history of chronic bronchitis, recurrent alveolar inflammation or from genetic predisposition of a congenital alpha 1-antitrypsin deficiency.

An injury was most likely sustained to which structure?
Emphysema results from a non-reversible injury and destruction of elastin protein within the alveolar walls. This process causes permanent enlargement of the air spaces distal to the terminal bronchioles within the lungs. Anatomical changes include loss of elastic recoil, excessive airway collapse during exhalation, and chronic obstruction of airflow. Progression of the disease includes further destruction of the alveolar walls, collapse of the peripheral bronchioles, and impaired gas exchange. Emphysema causes pockets of air to form between the alveolar spaces, (known as blebs), and within the lung parenchyma (known as bullae). This results in an increase in dead space within the lungs that diminishes gas exchange.

Inference:

What is the most likely contributing factor in the development of this condition?
The primary risk factors for the development of emphysema include chronic bronchitis, lower respiratory infections, cigarette smoking, and genetic predisposition. Environmental influence includes air pollution and other airborne toxins. The risk of acquiring emphysema increases with age.

Confirmation:

What is the most likely clinical presentation?
COPD is the second leading cause of disability in individuals under 65 years of age worldwide. There are two million individuals in the United States diagnosed with emphysema (and another 14 million with some form of COPD). Emphysema can be asymptomatic until middle age and is most often diagnosed between 55 and 60 years of age. Centrilobular emphysema usually destroys the bronchioles in the upper lungs while the alveolar sacs usually remain intact. Panlobular emphysema destroys the air spaces of the acinus and is usually found in the lower lungs. Paraseptal emphysema destroys the alveoli in the lower lobes resulting in blebs along the lung periphery. Symptoms of emphysema worsen with the progression of the disease and include a persistent cough, wheezing, difficulty breathing especially with expiration, and an increased respiration rate. Advanced disease symptoms include increased use of accessory muscles, severe dyspnea, cor pulmonale, and cyanosis.

What laboratory or imaging studies would confirm the diagnosis?
X-ray is utilized to visually evaluate the shape and spacing of the lungs. Other imaging studies include a planogram to detect bullae and a bronchogram to evaluate mucus ducts and detect possible enlargement of the bronchi. Arterial blood gases may indicate a decreased PaO_2.

What additional information should be obtained to confirm the diagnosis?
A physical examination, thorough patient history (including cigarette smoking), and pulmonary function tests are required for diagnosis. Pulmonary function testing will result in impaired forced expiratory volume (FEV_1), vital capacity (VC), and forced vital capacity (FVC). Total lung capacity (TLC), residual volume (RV), and functional residual capacity (FRC) will be increased.

Examination:

What history should be documented?
Important areas to explore include past medical history, history of smoking, medications, current health status, social history and habits, occupation, living environment, and social support system.

What test/measures are most appropriate?
Aerobic capacity and endurance: assessment of vital signs at rest and with activity, perceived exertion scale, Six-Minute Walk Test, Three Minute Step Test
Arousal, attention, and cognition: examine mental status, learning ability, memory, motivation
Assistive and adaptive devices: analysis of components and safety of a device
Environmental, home, and work: analysis of current and potential barriers or hazards
Gait, locomotion, and balance: static and dynamic balance in sitting and standing, safety during gait with/without an assistive device
Muscle performance: strength assessment, assessment of active movement and muscle endurance
Posture: analysis of resting and dynamic posture
Self-care and home management: functional capacity

<u>Ventilation, respiration, and circulation</u>: assessment of thoracoabdominal movement, auscultation of vesicular sounds/potential rhonchi, pulse oximetry, pulmonary function testing, accessory muscle utilization

What additional findings are likely with this patient?

A patient with emphysema may present with a barrel chest appearance, an increased subcostal angle, rounded shoulders secondary to tight pectorals, rosy skin coloring, and may utilize pursed-lip breathing to assist with ventilation. Patients will also have high rates of anxiety associated with difficulty breathing and may present with claustrophobia, insomnia, and depression. Complications such as the formation and rupture of bullae and blebs can lead to pneumothorax. Cor pulmonale is a serious complication that can occur with advanced emphysema.

Management:

What is the most effective management of this patient?

Medical management of a patient with emphysema includes pharmacological intervention, oxygen therapy, and physical therapy. Pharmacological intervention promotes bronchodilation, improved oxygenation, and ventilation. Drugs such as oral/inhaled bronchodilators, anti-inflammatory agents, mucolytic expectorants, mast cell membrane stabilizers, and antihistamines may be used in the treatment of emphysema. Preventative immunizations against influenza and pneumonia are also recommended. Physical therapy intervention is based on the severity of the disease process and can include general exercise and endurance training, breathing exercises including pursed-lip breathing, ventilatory muscle strengthening, chest wall exercises, and patient education on posture, airway secretion clearance, and energy conservation techniques. Pulse oximetry should be used to monitor a patient's oxygen saturation during activities and exercise. This will assist with patient education and deter the effects of hypoxemia. Chest physical therapy is required during advanced stages of emphysema.

What home care regimen should be recommended?

The home care regimen should include breathing strategies and exercises, energy conservation, pacing techniques, and general strength and endurance training.

Outcome:

What is the likely outcome of a course in physical therapy?

A patient with emphysema may require physical therapy intermittently as the disease progresses. The goals of physical therapy are to maximize the patient's functional abilities and optimize pulmonary function.

What are the long-term effects of the patient's condition?

Emphysema is a chronic progressive disease process. Patients require ongoing medical care and intermittent physical therapy intervention. Life expectancy decreases to less than five years with severe expiratory slowing measured at a rate of <1L of air during forced expiratory volume (FEV_1).

Comparison:

What are the distinguishing characteristics of a similar condition?

Bronchiectasis is inherited or acquired and is characterized by chronic inflammation and dilation of bronchi and destruction of the bronchial walls. This disease is associated with chronic bacterial infections and is an extreme form of bronchitis. Incidence within the United States is low. Bronchiectasis has a higher risk for development in patients with cystic fibrosis, sinusitis, Kartagener's syndrome, and endobronchial tumors. Characteristics include a chronic cough with sputum, hemoptysis, wheezing, dyspnea, and recurrent respiratory infections. Primary treatment includes physical therapy, bronchodilators, and antibiotics.

Clinical Scenarios:

Scenario One

A 65-year-old male is referred to physical therapy after recently being diagnosed with emphysema. The patient works in an oil refinery part-time and manages a small dairy farm. The patient's past medical history is negative for smoking and consists of recurrent respiratory infections and chronic cough. The patient complains of shortness of breath with exertion, however, pulmonary function testing indicates only minimal impairment in lung volumes.

Scenario Two

A 75-year-old female requires physical therapy for management of emphysema. The patient has a history of smoking cigarettes for over 40 years and continues to smoke approximately one pack per day. The patient has an oxygen saturation rate of 94% at rest and requires two liters of oxygen with exertion. The patient has moderate impairment in pulmonary function testing and a persistent cough. The patient presently resides in a two-story home and assists with the care of her disabled husband.

Fibromyalgia Syndrome

Diagnosis:

What condition produces a patient's symptoms?

Fibromyalgia syndrome (FMS) is classified as a rheumatology syndrome or a nonarticular rheumatic condition. Pain is the primary symptom caused by tender points within muscles, tendons, and ligaments.

An injury was most likely sustained to which structure?

The exact etiology of FMS is unknown. Theories suggest potential biochemical, metabolic or immunologic pathology. Researchers believe it to be multifactorial in origin and suggest a link to a dysfunction within the stress system, autonomic nervous system, immune system and/or reproductive and hormone systems.

Inference:

What is the most likely contributing factor in the development of this condition?

Since the exact etiology of FMS is unknown there is speculation linking many factors to the development of this condition. Factors include diet, sleep disorders, viral infections, psychological distress, occupational and environmental factors, hypothyroidism, trauma, and potential hereditary links. Many individuals diagnosed with FMS note multiple causative factors, however, there are individuals diagnosed with FMS that possess none of the theorized causative factors.

Confirmation:

What is the most likely clinical presentation?

The American College of Rheumatology's data indicates that there are approximately six million individuals living with FMS making it the most common musculoskeletal disorder in the United States. FMS has a greater incidence in females (almost 75% of the cases) and can affect any age but most frequently is diagnosed between 14 and 68 years of age. FMS is diagnosed when a patient exhibits the criteria authored by the American College of Rheumatology. There is a widespread history of pain that exists in all four quadrants of the body (above and below the waist), axial pain is present, and there is pain in at least 11 of 18 standardized "tender point" sites. These sites include the occiput, low cervical area, trapezius, supraspinatus, second rib, lateral epicondyle, gluteal area, greater trochanter, and the knee. The patient may also complain of fatigue, memory and visual impairment, sleep disturbances, irritable bowel syndrome, headaches, and anxiety/depression.

What laboratory or imaging studies would confirm the diagnosis?

FMS has been commonly misdiagnosed as myofascial pain, systemic lupus erythematosus, fibrocytis, and chronic fatigue syndrome. There are no specific tests used to diagnose FMS. Radiographs are negative and blood work often appears normal except for a possible alteration in the levels of substance P. This substance is a chemical involved with pain transmission. Image studies and other lab testing are performed only for differential diagnosis.

What additional information should be obtained to confirm the diagnosis?

FMS is diagnosed according to the criteria from the American College of Rheumatology. A dolorimeter is used for reliability when testing the tender points by providing a consistent pressure (4 kg/cm^2). If the patient meets the criteria and has experienced symptoms for greater than three months then a patient may be diagnosed with FMS. Diagnostic written tools that can assist with diagnosis include the Beck Depression Inventory and the Fibromyalgia Impact Questionnaire.

Examination:

What history should be documented?

Important areas to explore include past medical history, medications, family history, current symptoms, current health status, social history and habits, occupation, leisure activities, and social support system.

What test/measures are most appropriate?

Aerobic capacity and endurance: assessment of vital signs at rest and with activity, perceived exertion scale, pulse oximetry, auscultation of the lungs

Arousal, attention, and cognition: examine mental status, learning ability, memory, motivation

Community and work integration: analysis of community, work, and leisure activities

Environmental, home, and work barriers: analysis of current and potential barriers or hazards

Ergonomics and body mechanics: analysis of dexterity and coordination

Gait, locomotion, and balance: static and dynamic balance in sitting and standing, safety during gait

Integumentary integrity: skin assessment, assessment of sensation

Joint integrity and mobility: assessment of hyper- and hypomobility of a joint, effusion, edema

Muscle performance: strength assessment, muscle tone assessment

Neuromotor development and sensory integration: analysis of reflex movement patterns, assessment of involuntary movements, sensory integration tests, gross and fine motor skills
Pain: pain perception assessment scale, visual analog scale, assessment of muscle soreness and tender points
Posture: analysis of resting and dynamic posture
Range of motion: active and passive range of motion
Self-care and home management: assessment of functional capacity

What additional findings are likely with this patient?

The aforementioned symptoms can progress over time. Certain symptoms intensify and cause the patient to lose functional independence secondary to increased pain, decreased range of motion, and severe fatigue.

Management:

What is the most effective management of this patient?

FMS is best treated with a multidisciplinary approach including education, medical management, and exercise. Medical management will attempt to normalize various dysfunctions of the autonomic nervous system, hormonal imbalances, and metabolic abnormalities. Physicians must address sleep disorders (which can be common) and pharmacological intervention based on symptoms. Psychotherapy may be warranted for anxiety or depression and must incorporate stress management and coping strategies into the plan of care. Physical therapy intervention may include relaxation techniques, energy conservation, gentle stretching, moist heat, ultrasound, posture and body mechanics, biofeedback, and exercise to tolerance. Aquatic therapy is recommended to improve a patient's fitness level and an ergonomic evaluation should be performed at the patient's work place. This population should not work through pain. They require short exercise sessions initially (three to five minutes) due to a low tolerance for exertion.

What home care regimen should be recommended?

A home care regimen should include short duration exercise, aquatic therapy (if indicated), energy conservation strategies, the use of proper positioning, proper body mechanics, and gentle stretching. Patient education is the key to success. Exercises that strain muscles such as weight lifting should be avoided. A comprehensive plan should also include lifestyle management, nutritional support, and stress management.

Outcome:

What is the likely outcome of a course in physical therapy?

A patient with FMS may benefit from multidisciplinary intervention. Patient compliance with a home program increases the overall success rate. In many cases symptoms can remain unchanged even with intervention and patient compliance. A percentage of patients will report improvement in areas of fatigue, sleep, and self-reported pain.

What are the long-term effects of the patient's condition?

FMS is presently not "curable." Many patients that have mild symptoms do not require multidisciplinary intervention and have a good long-term outcome. The majority of patients diagnosed with FMS exhibits moderate levels of symptoms and usually continue to experience these symptoms for years or even their entire lifetime.

Comparison:

What are the distinguishing characteristics of a similar condition?

Myofascial pain syndrome (MPS) is often misdiagnosed for FMS. MPS is characterized by trigger points rather than tender points and lacks associated symptoms. MPS is a localized musculoskeletal condition that is specific to a muscle. FMS on the other hand is a systemic condition. MPS is usually caused by overuse, reduced muscle activity or repetitive motions.

Clinical Scenarios:

Scenario One

A 32-year-old female recently diagnosed with FMS is seen in physical therapy. Her chief complaints are fatigue, pain throughout her body, and difficulty with sleeping which has effected her employment as a mail carrier. She has been on disability for the last six months and under a physician's care for depression.

Scenario Two

A 45-year-old construction worker is referred to physical therapy with diagnosis of FMS. His history reveals mild symptoms for the last year. He has seen specialists and was diagnosed last week by a rheumatologist. He is positive for 12 tender points and denies any sleep disturbances or other medical history. He is currently working and appears motivated for therapy.

Full-Thickness Burn

Diagnosis:

What condition produces a patient's symptoms?
Full-thickness burns can be caused by thermal (fire, hot fluids, steam), chemical (acid, alkalis, vesicants) or electrical (lightning, high voltage, faulty wiring) agents. This severe burn causes immediate cellular and tissue death and subsequent vascular destruction. The patient will experience primary and secondary symptoms secondary to the extent and area of injury.

An injury was most likely sustained to which structure?
A full-thickness burn indicates complete destruction of the epidermis, dermis, hair follicle, and nerve endings within the dermis; and also affects the subcutaneous fat layer and underlying muscles, resulting in red blood cell destruction. There is irreversible damage sustained to all epithelial elements.

Inference:

What is the most likely contributing factor in the development of this condition?
The National Burn Information Exchange indicates that 75% of burns are a direct result of the patient's actions. There are approximately two million individuals burned annually with 70,000 hospitalized and 6,000-7,000 deaths. There is higher risk for burns in one to five-year-olds as well as individuals over 70 years of age. Burns are currently the third leading cause of accidental death in all age categories with males having a higher overall frequency of injury.

Confirmation:

What is the most likely clinical presentation?
A full-thickness burn is characterized by a variable appearance of deep red, black or white coloring. Eschar forms from necrotic cells and creates a dry and hard layer that requires debridement. Edema is present at the site of injury and in surrounding tissues. Hairs within the region of the burn are easily pulled from the follicle due to the destruction. An area of full-thickness burn does not have sensation or pain due to destruction of free nerve endings; however, there may be pain from adjacent areas that experience partial-thickness burns. During the initial stages the patient will experience thermoregulation impairment, shortness of breath, electrolyte disturbances, poor urine output, and variation in level of consciousness.

What laboratory or imaging studies would confirm the diagnosis?
Blood work should include a complete blood count, electrolytes, blood urea nitrogen, creatinine, bilirubin, and arterial blood gases. This will indicate baseline data, systemic changes, level of shock, and metabolic complications. Bronchoscopy and pulmonary function tests may be indicated to assess airway damage and pulmonary insufficiency.

What additional information should be obtained to confirm the diagnosis?
Diagnosis is primarily based on observation and assessment regarding the extent and depth of the burn. The rule of nines and the Lund-Browder charts grossly approximate the percentage of the body affected by a burn.

Examination:

What history should be documented?
Important areas to explore include past medical history, mechanism of injury, medications, family history, type and percentage of burn, current symptoms and health status, social history and habits, occupation, leisure activities, and social support system.

What test/measures are most appropriate?
Aerobic capacity and endurance: assessment of vital signs, perceived exertion scale, pulse oximetry
Anthropometric characteristics: circumferential measurements of affected areas
Arousal, attention, and cognition: examine mental status, learning ability, memory, motivation
Cranial nerve integrity: dermatome assessment
Gait, locomotion, and balance: static and dynamic balance in sitting and standing
Integumentary integrity: sensation assessment, assessment of burn, size, color, eschar, hair follicle integrity, wound mapping
Joint integrity and mobility: assessment of contracture, hypomobility of joints, soft tissue swelling
Muscle performance: strength and tone assessment
Pain: pain perception assessment scale, visual analog scale to the area of the burn and surrounding tissues
Posture: analysis of resting and dynamic posture
Range of motion: active and passive range of motion
Reflex integrity: assessment of deep tendon and pathological reflexes (e.g., Babinski, ATNR)
Self-care and home management: functional capacity, Functional Independence Measure (FIM)
Ventilation, respiration, and circulation: cough and clearance of secretions, auscultation of the lungs, breathing patterns, respiratory muscle strength, accessory muscle utilization, vital capacity, pulse oximetry and palpation, pulmonary function testing

What additional findings are likely with this patient?

A patient with a full-thickness burn will present with multiple secondary effects based on the mechanism of the burn, size of the burn, and location of the burn. Infection, hypertrophic scarring, and contractures are the most common complications. Other secondary damage may include impairments of the cardiovascular system, renal system, gastrointestinal system, respiratory system and/or immune system. Damage to these vital areas can result in metabolic disorders, acidosis, sepsis, and dehydration.

Management:

What is the most effective management of this patient?

The initial management includes medically stabilizing the patient followed by a full assessment of primary and secondary damage. This emergent phase lasts 48-72 hours and concludes with regaining capillary permeability and hemodynamic stability. An autograft procedure is usually required for full-thickness burns. The rehabilitation phase is a long-term commitment that includes all aspects of functional recovery. Physical therapy intervention begins immediately following skin grafting and includes wound care, pulmonary exercises, positioning, splinting, and immobilization for the first three to five days. A therapist will also provide education regarding skin care, positioning, and contracture prevention. Early ambulation and mobility activities should be incorporated as soon as possible in order to decrease complications such as atelectasis, pneumonia, and contracture. Continued physical therapy management will involve edema control, monitoring of any elastic garments, massage, stretching, hydrotherapy, ROM, debridement, relaxation techniques, progressive exercise, ambulation, and functional mobility training.

What home care regimen should be recommended?

A patient must continue with the established splinting and positioning schedule at home. Physical therapy may initially be warranted for continued pulmonary management, stretching, and functional mobility. A home program is vital to the patient's continued success and should include strengthening exercises, massage, scar management, positioning, and stretching. As the patient progresses, participation in wound management, activities of daily living, and functional activities should be incorporated into the daily routine.

Outcome:

What is the likely outcome of a course in physical therapy?

Patient outcome is dependent on location, extent, and secondary complications of the burn. Physical therapy will provide the patient with education for an ongoing therapeutic program. Therapeutic exercise, stretching, compression garments, and other modalities will enhance the probability of a positive outcome.

What are the long-term effects of the patient's condition?

The mortality rate has decreased over the last two decades due to improvement in burn care, prevention of infection, and advances in grafting procedures. Mortality rates are highest for children under four and adults over 65 years of age. Overall prognosis is dependent on factors such as cardiac pathology, alcoholism, peripheral vascular disease, and obesity. Other factors that also require consideration are: depression, social and emotional shock, and level of difficulty reintegrating into a daily routine (with employment, spouse, children, community). Long-term outcome is also based on the extent of secondary effects such as scarring and contractures. Garments may be worn up to two years after injury. Without significant complications a patient should achieve independence within a few months post injury.

Comparison:

What are the distinguishing characteristics of a similar condition?

A partial-thickness burn damages the epidermis and the papillary layer of the dermis (the dermis remains largely intact). This burn presents with blister formation, bright red coloring, intact blanching, moderate edema, and pain. The burn will heal without surgical intervention within seven to ten days with minimal to no scarring noted.

Clinical Scenarios:

Scenario One

A 32-year-old female six weeks status post full-thickness burns to 50% of her right arm and 70% of her right leg is referred to physical therapy. She wears compression garments and has decreased range of motion. She resides alone in a two-story home and is employed as a cook.

Scenario Two

A three-year-old boy is referred to physical therapy 48 hours after an autograft for a full-thickness burn on the left side of his thorax. The chart review notes the mechanism of injury as pulling a cup of coffee off a table. Other medical history includes developmental delay, seizures, and hydrocephaly.

Guillain-Barre Syndrome

Diagnosis:

What condition produces a patient's symptoms?
Guillain-Barre syndrome (GBS) or acute polyneuropathy is a temporary inflammation and demyelination of the peripheral nerves' myelin sheaths, potentially resulting in axonal degeneration. GBS results in motor weakness in a distal to proximal progression, sensory impairment, and possible respiratory paralysis.

An injury was most likely sustained to which structure?
The autoantibodies of GBS attack segments of the myelin sheath of the peripheral nerves. The infecting organism is of similar structure to molecules found on the surface of myelin sheaths. The antibodies produced attack both the organism of infection as well as the Schwann cells due to the similar structure. This decreases nerve conduction velocity and results in weakness or paralysis of the involved muscles. The demyelination that is initiated at Ranvier's nodes occurs secondary to macrophage response and inflammation; and as a result, destruction of the myelin. The body responds to this process and attempts to repair the damage through Schwann cell division and myelinization of the damaged nerves. Motor fibers are predominantly affected.

Inference:

What is the most likely contributing factor in the development of this condition?
The exact etiology of GBS is unknown; however, it is hypothesized to be an autoimmune response to a previous respiratory infection, influenza, immunization or surgery. Viral infections, Epstein-Barr syndrome, cytomegalovirus, bacterial infections, surgery, and vaccinations have been associated with the development of GBS.

Confirmation:

What is the most likely clinical presentation?
GBS can occur at any age, however, there is a peak in frequency in the young adult population and again in adults that are between their fifth and eighth decades. Incidence is slightly greater in males than females and in Caucasians than African Americans with an overall incidence of 1.7:100,000 within the United States. A patient with GBS will initially present with distal symmetrical motor weakness and will likely experience mild distal sensory impairments and transient paresthesias. The weakness will progress towards the upper extremities and head. The level of disability

usually peaks within two to four weeks after onset. Muscle and respiratory paralysis, absence of deep tendon reflexes, and the inability to speak or swallow may also occur. GBS can be life threatening if there is respiratory involvement. There are multiple subtypes of GBS, but the classic type involves acute onset of symptoms with peak impairment within four weeks, followed by a two to four week static period and gradual recovery that can take months to years.

What laboratory or imaging studies would confirm the diagnosis?
GBS can be diagnosed through a cerebrospinal fluid sample that contains high protein levels and little to no lymphocytes. Electromyography will result in abnormal and slowed nerve conduction.

What additional information should be obtained to confirm the diagnosis?
A physical and neurological examination, strength testing, and a review of relevant medical history are all important in the diagnosis of GBS. The National Institute of Neurologic and Communicative Disorders and Stroke has established criteria to assist with the diagnosis of GBS.

Examination:

What history should be documented?
Important areas to explore include past medical, family, and surgical history, recent illness, medications, immunizations, current symptoms and health status, social history and habits, occupation, living environment, and social support system.

What test/measures are most appropriate?
Aerobic capacity and endurance: vital signs at rest/activity, responses to positional changes
Arousal, attention, and cognition: examine mental status, learning ability, memory, motivation
Assistive and adaptive devices: analysis of components and safety of a device
Cranial nerve integrity: assessment of muscles innervation by the cranial nerves, dermatome assessment
Community and work integration: analysis of community, work, and leisure activities
Gait, locomotion, and balance: static and dynamic balance in sitting and standing, safety during gait with/without an assistive device, Berg Balance Scale, Tinetti Performance Oriented Mobility Assessment, analysis of wheelchair management
Integumentary integrity: skin and sensation assessment

Motor function: equilibrium and righting reactions, coordination, motor assessment scales

Muscle performance: strength and tone assessment

Orthotic, protective, and supportive devices: potential utilization of bracing

Pain: pain perception assessment scale

Range of motion: active and passive range of motion

Reflex integrity: assessment of deep tendon and pathological reflexes

Self-care and home management: assessment of functional capacity

Ventilation, respiration and circulation: pulmonary function tests, assessment of cough and secretions

What additional findings are likely with this patient?

The extent of impairment for each patient depends on the clinical course of the GBS. The patient may also experience bladder weakness, deep muscle pain, and autonomic nervous system involvement including arrhythmia, tachycardia, postural hypotension, heart block, and absent reflexes. Up to 30% of patients require mechanical ventilation during the acute stage. Respiratory assistance can last as long as 50-60 days.

Management:

What is the most effective management of this patient?

Medical management of a patient with GBS may require hospitalization for treatment of symptoms. Pharmacological intervention often includes immunosuppressive and analgesic/narcotic medications. Corticosteroids are controversial and usually contraindicated. Cardiac monitoring, plasma exchange (through plasmaphoresis), and mechanical ventilation may be required. A tracheostomy may be performed for ventilation. Physical, occupational, and speech therapies are indicated to facilitate neurological rehabilitation. Physical therapy should be initiated upon admission to the hospital with focus on passive range of motion, positioning, and light exercise. During the acute stage a physical therapist must limit overexertion and fatigue to avoid exacerbation of symptoms. As the patient progresses, intervention may include orthotic, wheelchair or assistive device prescription, exercise and endurance activities, family teaching, functional mobility and gait training, and progressive respiratory therapy. The therapeutic pool may be indicated to initiate movement without the effects of gravity.

What home-care regimen should be recommended?

A home care regimen should include breathing exercises and incentive spirometry for respiratory involvement. A patient, along with the caregiver, must continue with therapeutic exercise, ongoing functional mobility training, and endurance activities as tolerated.

Outcome:

What is the likely outcome of a course in physical therapy?

Physical therapy may assist with recovery, but it cannot alter the course of the disease. Physical therapy intervention may be required on an ongoing basis to assist with recovery that can last from 3-12 months.

What are the long-term effects of the patient's condition?

GBS is an autoimmune response that varies in severity from person to person. Recovery is slow and can last up to two years after onset. Although most patients experience full recovery, statistics indicate that 20% have remaining neurologic deficits, and 3-5% of patients die from respiratory complications.

Comparison:

What are the distinguishing characteristics of a similar condition?

Polyneuropathy is a progressive condition that affects the nerves. The most common etiology is metabolic conditions such as diabetes mellitus. Polyneuropathy develops slowly, bilaterally, and symmetrically. The first symptom is often sensory impairment of the distal lower extremities. Pain, diminished deep tendon reflexes, and motor loss are other symptoms of this condition that is marked by exacerbations and remissions. Medical management will focus on stabilizing the underlying metabolic condition.

Clinical Scenarios:

Scenario One

A 25-year-old female has been hospitalized for one week with a diagnosis of GBS. The patient's strength assessment reports 3-/5 bilateral hip strength, 2+/5 bilateral knee strength, and 2-/5 bilateral ankle strength. The patient is anxious to improve and is eager to begin physical therapy. The patient resides alone in a second floor apartment and works as a bank teller.

Scenario Two

A 43-year-old male was admitted to the hospital one month ago with GBS. The patient had significant paralysis and was ventilator dependent. The patient began to improve two weeks ago and was taken off the ventilator. The patient was in good health prior to admission and worked as an independent international sales representative. The patient is diabetic and has a history of alcoholism. He is divorced with no children.

Human Immunodeficiency Virus

Diagnosis:

What condition produces a patient's symptoms?
The human immunodeficiency virus (HIV) is a retrovirus that initially invades and destroys cells within the immune system; specifically CD4+ T-lymphocytes (T-cells). This virus also affects monocytes, macrophages, and B-cells. Once the T-cells decrease beyond a specific level a patient will begin to demonstrate symptoms of the HIV infection.

An injury was most likely sustained to which structure?
HIV infects T-cells within the immune system. Other cells that eventually house HIV include monocytes, macrophages, microglia, cervical cells, and epithelial cells of the GI tract. HIV uses and destroys these cells that possess the antigen CD4 on their surface in order to replicate HIV, and as a result the immune system becomes weaker and unable to function.

Inference:

What is the most likely contributing factor in the development of this condition?
HIV is transmitted through contact with blood, semen, vaginal secretions, and breast milk. Contact can be sexual, perinatal or through contact with blood or body fluids that carry infected cells. Risk factors for contracting HIV include unprotected sexual relations, intravenous drug use or mother to fetus transmission. The top three largest risk factors for contracting HIV are homosexual male sex (46% of HIV cases), intravenous drug use (25% of HIV cases), and heterosexual sex (11%).

Confirmation:

What is the most likely clinical presentation?
The incidence of newly diagnosed cases of HIV is approximately 40,000 per year within the United States (decreased from 150,000 new cases yearly during the mid-1980s). A patient will not immediately present with any symptoms after the initial transmission of the infection. A patient may actually be "symptom free" for one to two years post infection or may exhibit flu-like symptoms including rash and fever. HIV immediately begins a latent phase where replication of the virus is minimal. The three phases of this disease process include asymptomatic HIV, symptomatic HIV, and acquired immunodeficiency syndrome (AIDS). The T-cell count will begin to decrease during the "asymptomatic" phase; however, symptoms will not appear until the count decreases to a certain level. Manifestations of HIV may lead to other infections, malignancies, neurological dysfunction, dementia, and cardiac pathologies.

What laboratory or imaging studies would confirm the diagnosis?
HIV is diagnosed through various blood tests such as the enzyme-linked immunosorbent test or Western blot test. Once diagnosed the lab results can also assist with classifying the stage of HIV infection.

What additional information should be obtained to confirm the diagnosis?
Definitive diagnosis is made through blood tests; however, the physician should ascertain accurate medical and social history. Accurate drug use and sexual partner history will allow for appropriate patient education in order to cease the spread of the virus. A positive diagnosis will allow the patient to notify others at risk.

Examination:

What history should be documented?
Important areas to explore include past medical history, medications, family history, current symptoms, current health status, social history and habits, occupation, leisure activities, and social support system.

What test/measures are most appropriate?
Aerobic capacity and endurance: assessment of vital signs, perceived exertion scale, auscultation of the lungs
Arousal, attention, and cognition: examine mental status, learning ability, memory, and level of motivation
Community and work integration: analysis of community, work, and leisure activities
Environmental, home, and work barriers: analysis of current and potential barriers or hazards
Gait, locomotion, and balance: static and dynamic balance in sitting and standing, safety during gait with/without an assistive device, Tinetti Performance Oriented Mobility Assessment, analysis of wheelchair management
Integumentary integrity: skin assessment and sensation assessment
Motor function: equilibrium and righting reactions, motor assessment scales, coordination, posture and balance in sitting, assessment of sensorimotor integration, physical performance scales
Muscle performance: strength assessment, muscle tone assessment
Pain: pain perception assessment scale
Range of motion: active and passive range of motion

Reflex integrity: assessment of deep tendon and pathological reflexes (e.g., Babinski, ATNR)
Self-care and home management: assessment of functional capacity
Ventilation, respiration, and circulation: pulmonary function testing, breathing patterns, perceived exertion scale, assessment of cough

What additional findings are likely with this patient?

The Centers for Disease Control classifies HIV into three categories based on the T-cell count. Symptoms and secondary illnesses occur as the T-cell count decreases. The onset of AIDS occurs when the T-cell count falls below 200 cells per mm^3 (normal ranges 650-1,200 cells) or when one of 26 specific AIDS defining disorders is present or both. A patient may experience musculoskeletal, neuromuscular, cardiopulmonary, integumentary, and other impairments secondary to HIV.

Management:

What is the most effective management of this patient?

Early detection is important so that pharmacological intervention can be initiated and slow progression of the virus. There is no cure for HIV; however, proper medical intervention can allow this virus to remain a manageable chronic condition. Medical management will institute antiretroviral therapy (HAART) when T-cells drop below 500 mm^3. The goal of drug therapy is to significantly decrease the virus' ability to replicate, and therefore, decrease the progression of the disease. Drugs may include nucleoside analogs, protease inhibitors, and non-nucleoside reverse transcriptase inhibitors. Physical therapy intervention may be indicated during the course of HIV/AIDS due to secondary impairments. Physical therapy goals and intervention would include the promotion of optimal fitness, flexibility, energy conservation, stress management, ADL equipment, relaxation, aquatic therapy, modalities, positioning, pain management, breathing exercises, and neurological rehabilitation.

What home care regimen should be recommended?

A patient with HIV must follow a home regimen including medication, proper nutrition and sleep, and fitness in order to remain as healthy as possible. A physical therapy home program can also minimize the negative effects on functional ability and improve the overall independence and quality of life.

Outcome:

What is the likely outcome of a course in physical therapy?

Physical therapy may be warranted for periods of time throughout the progression of HIV/AIDS. Physical therapy cannot alter the progression of the virus, but can foster improvement in functional mobility, conditioning, and overall independence.

What are the long-term effects of the patient's condition?

There are currently 42 million individuals around the world living with HIV/AIDS. There is presently no cure for HIV/AIDS; however, with early combination therapies patients are surviving longer and living more productive lives. Studies indicate that psychosocial factors influence progression of the virus as well as survival. Presently, the leading cause of death is kidney failure secondary to the extended drug therapies.

Comparison:

What are the distinguishing characteristics of a similar condition?

Hepatitis B (HBV) is a form of viral hepatitis that produces inflammation and damage to the liver. Like HIV, hepatitis B is transmitted parenterally through intravenous drug use, sexual relations, blood transfusions, perinatal transmission or dialysis. A vaccine is available for prevention and blood tests are used for diagnosis. Approximately 95% of those infected with HBV fully recover; however, 10% of these become carriers. Some of the carriers develop chronic liver disease and may die prematurely.

Clinical Scenarios:

Scenario One

A 19-year-old female is seen in outpatient physical therapy secondary to weakness and balance impairments. She was diagnosed with HIV two years ago but the physician believes that she was infected at least one to two years prior to diagnosis by IV drug use. Her T-cell count is 404 mm^3 using HIV drug therapies.

Scenario Two

A 58-year-old male was diagnosed with AIDS one year ago and has lost significant weight. He presents with general muscle atrophy and is having difficulty with ambulation and ADLs. The patient is referred to physical therapy for adaptive and assistive devices. He lives with his partner in a ranch style home and is on medical disability.

Huntington's Disease

Diagnosis:

What condition produces a patient's symptoms?
Huntington's disease (HD), also known as Huntington's chorea, is a neurological disorder of the CNS and is characterized by degeneration and atrophy of the basal ganglia (specifically the striatum) and cerebral cortex within the brain.

An injury was most likely sustained to which structure?
HD affects the basal ganglia and cerebral cortex of the brain. The ventricles of the brain become enlarged secondary to atrophy of the basal ganglia and there is extensive loss of small and medium sized neurons. There appears to be an overall decrease in the quantity and activity of gamma-aminobutyric acid (GABA) and acetylcholine neurons that are produced in these areas. The identified neurotransmitters become deficient and are unable to modulate movement. Loss of neurons creates dysfunction in inhibition that results in the symptoms of chorea, bradykinesia, and rigidity. The thalamus is also believed to contribute to the movement disorders associated with the disease process.

Inference:

What is the most likely contributing factor in the development of this condition?
HD is genetically transmitted as an autosomal dominant trait with the defect linked to chromosome four and to the gene identified as IT-15. The disease is usually perpetuated by a person that has children prior to the normal onset of symptoms and without knowledge that he/she possesses the defective gene. Genetic testing is able to identify the defective gene for HD prior to the onset of symptoms.

Confirmation:

What is the most likely clinical presentation?
The prevalence of HD is approximately 4-8:100,000 in North America with 25,000 individuals diagnosed with HD in the United States. The average age for developing symptoms ranges between 35 and 55 years; however, symptoms can develop at any age. HD is a disease that produces a movement disorder, affective dysfunction, and cognitive impairment. The patient will initially present with involuntary choreic movements and a mild alteration in personality. Unintentional facial expressions such as a grimace, protrusion of the tongue, and elevation of the eyebrows are common. As the disease progresses gait will become ataxic and a patient will experience choreoathetoid movement of the extremities and the trunk. Speech disturbances and mental deterioration are

common. Late stage HD is characterized by a decrease in IQ, dementia, depression, dysphagia, incontinence, inability to ambulate or transfer, and progression from choreiform movements to rigidity.

What laboratory or imaging studies would confirm the diagnosis?
Magnetic resonance imaging (MRI) or computed tomography (CT scan) may indicate atrophy or abnormalities within the cerebral cortex as well as the basal ganglia. Positron-emission tomography (PET) may be used to augment other testing and obtain information regarding blood flow, oxygen uptake, and metabolism of the brain. A DNA marker study may be administered to determine if the autosomal dominant trait is present for HD.

What additional information should be obtained to confirm the diagnosis?
A physical examination, review of symptoms, and family history are important components in the diagnosis of HD.

Examination:

What history should be documented?
Important areas to explore include past medical history, medications, family history, current symptoms, health status, social history/habits, occupation, living environment, and support system.

What test/measures are most appropriate?
Aerobic capacity and endurance: assessment of vital signs at rest and with activity
Arousal, attention, and cognition: examine mental status, learning ability, memory, motivation
Gait, locomotion, and balance: static/dynamic balance in sitting/standing, safety during gait, Functional Reach Test, Tinetti Performance Oriented Mobility Assessment, Functional Ambulation Profile
Motor function: equilibrium/righting reactions, coordination
Muscle performance: strength and tone assessment, tremor assessment, testing for dysdiadochokinesia
Neuromotor development and sensory integration: analysis of reflex movement patterns, assessment of involuntary movements
Posture: analysis of resting and dynamic posture
Range of motion: active and passive range of motion
Self-care and home management: assessment of functional capacity, Functional Independence Measure (FIM), Barthel Index

What additional findings are likely with this patient?

Dementia and other psychological changes usually occur after neurological symptoms appear. The emotional disorder worsens with progression and may require admission to a psychiatric facility for severe depression and/or suicidal attempts. Secondary complications that can occur from symptoms of HD include loss of range of motion, deformity, pain, communication breakdown, aspiration and choking, and fatigue and weakness from weight loss.

Management:

What is the most effective management of this patient?

Medical management of HD requires a team approach including genetic, psychological, and social counseling for the patient and family. Education regarding disease process, coping strategies, and genetic consequences should initiate immediately following diagnosis. Medical treatment will focus on symptoms and pharmacological management for HD is usually initiated once choreiform movement impairs a patient's functional capacity. Drug classes such as anticonvulsants and antipsychotics may assist as these block dopamine transmission; however, have very serious side effects. Commonly utilized drugs include Perphenazine, Haloperidol (Haldol), and Reserpine. Physical, occupational, and speech therapy interventions may be warranted intermittently throughout the course of the disease and should focus on current problems with mobility and self-care skills. Physical therapy should maximize endurance, strength, balance, postural control, and functional mobility. Intervention should focus on motor control and utilize techniques including coactivation of muscles, trunk stabilization, the use of biofeedback, and relaxation in attempt to maintain a patient's functional status. Patient education should include prone lying, stretching, prevention of deformity and contracture, and safety with mobility. As the disease progresses, the degree of dementia will influence treatment and goals. The physical therapist must continue to emphasize family involvement and caregiver teaching. As the patient continues to lose function the caregiver will require education regarding posture, seating, assistance with transfers, mobility, and the use of adaptive equipment.

What home care regimen should be recommended?

A home care regimen should include an exercise routine, functional mobility skills, relaxation techniques, range of motion, stretching exercises, and endurance activities. Participation in a home care regimen can assist to maintain the optimal quality of life during the progression of the disease process.

Outcome:

What is the likely outcome of a course in physical therapy?

Physical therapy is recommended on an intermittent basis throughout the course of the disease. Physical therapy will not prevent further degeneration; however, it will maximize the patient's functional potential and safety. The goal of physical therapy is to attain an optimal functional outcome within the limitations of the disease process.

What are the long-term effects of the patient's condition?

HD is a chronic progressive genetic disorder that is fatal within 15 to 20 years after clinical manifestation. Late stages of the disease result in total physical and mental incapacitation. The patient usually requires an extended care facility due to the burden of care and physical, cognitive, and emotional dysfunction.

Comparison:

What are the distinguishing characteristics of a similar condition?

Athetoid (dyskinetic) cerebral palsy is a non-progressive motor disorder caused by central nervous system damage specifically to the basal ganglia. Clinical manifestations include slow and involuntary movements, choreiform movements, severe dysarthria, and an increased risk of aspiration pneumonia. The involuntary movements will increase with stress and fatigue and subside with sleep. Physical therapy intervention should focus on motor control and mobility deficits in order to attain the highest level of functioning.

Clinical Scenarios:

Scenario One

A 48-year-old attorney is referred for physical therapy home services. The patient was diagnosed with HD two years ago and resides in a two-story home. The patient has a significant other and they reside together. The patient's primary complaint is a loss of balance while ambulating. The patient refuses to utilize an assistive device.

Scenario Two

A 45-year-old female is referred to physical therapy. She was diagnosed with HD seven years ago and has recently fallen multiple times. According to family members the patient is short-tempered, irritable, and occasionally demonstrates poor judgment. The physician requests physical therapy for an evaluation and home program.

Juvenile Rheumatoid Arthritis

Diagnosis:

What condition produces a patient's symptoms?
Juvenile rheumatoid arthritis (JRA) is a form of arthritis found in children less than 16 years of age. JRA causes inflammation and stiffness to multiple joints for a period of greater than six weeks. The inflammatory process affects the tissues surrounding the affected synovial joints causing symptoms of JRA.

An injury was most likely sustained to which structure?
JRA, like adult rheumatoid arthritis, is an autoimmune disorder that occurs when the immune cells mistakenly begin to attack the joints and organs causing local and systemic effects throughout the body. The severity of ongoing injury is based on the specific classification and subtype of the disease.

Inference:

What is the most likely contributing factor in the development of this condition?
The etiology for JRA is currently unknown. Research postulates that JRA develops in children with a genetic predisposition for the disease. The predisposition may be triggered by environmental factors or a viral or bacterial infection. Girls have a higher incidence of JRA; and it is found to begin most commonly in the toddler or adolescent.

Confirmation:

What is the most likely clinical presentation?
JRA is an umbrella term for three specific classifications and subtypes of childhood arthritis. Classification is based on the number of joints involved, symptoms, presence of the rheumatoid factor (RF) or antinuclear antibody (ANA), and systemic involvement. General symptoms include persistent joint swelling, pain, and stiffness. Pauciarticular JRA involves four or less joints, is asymmetric, and is usually a mild form of JRA. This is the most common form of JRA and accounts for 50% of the cases; with girls under eight most likely to develop this subtype. ANA can also be found in 20-30% of patients and correlates with eye disease. Polyarticular JRA involves more than four joints, is usually symmetrical, involves the joints of the hands and feet as well as larger joints, and has potential for severe destruction. This subtype accounts for 30-40% of the cases and children may have the IgM rheumatoid factor (RF) similar to adult RA. Systemic JRA accounts for 10-20% of the cases and is otherwise known as Still's disease. Onset includes a high fever, chills, and a rash that may last for weeks, followed by severe myalgia and polyarthritis.

This form presents with severe extraarticular manifestations including anemia, hepatosplenomegaly, lymphadenopathy, pericarditis, and myocarditis. Most children in this subtype are negative for RF or ANA antibodies. About 25% experience severe and unremitting arthritis.

What laboratory or imaging studies would confirm the diagnosis?
There is not a single test to identify the presence of JRA. Blood tests may include serum evaluation to measure inflammation and detect RF, ANA or HLAB27 (human leukocyte antigen). Only a small percentage of patients with JRA possess RF or ANA. An erythrocyte sedimentation rate (ESR or "sed rate") may also indicate rheumatic disease. Other tests or procedures may be used to rule out other conditions such as Lyme disease, lupus, infection, and cancers.

What additional information should be obtained to confirm the diagnosis?
Diagnosis is made largely through physical examination, a patient's past and present medical status, and meeting the criteria set forth by the American Rheumatoid Association regarding the diagnosis and classification of JRA.

Examination:

What history should be documented?
Important areas to explore include past medical history, medications, family history, current symptoms, current health status, social history and habits, leisure activities, and social support system.

What test/measures are most appropriate?
Aerobic capacity and endurance: vital signs at rest and with activity, timed walk, aerobic endurance, VO_2 max
Anthropometric characteristics: circumferential measurements of all affected joints
Arousal, attention, and cognition: examine mental status, learning ability, memory, motivation
Assistive and adaptive devices: analysis of components and safety of a device
Environmental and home barriers: analysis of current and potential barriers or hazards
Ergonomics and body mechanics: analysis of dexterity and coordination
Gait, locomotion, and balance: static/dynamic balance in sitting and standing, visual inspection of gait with and without shoes, timed walk, gait over level and unlevel surfaces, footprint analysis and videography
Integumentary integrity: skin and sensation assessment

Joint integrity and mobility: active joint count, joint effusion, articular tenderness

Motor function: equilibrium and coordination

Muscle performance: break testing of isometric contractions, manometer method of strength testing, dynamic muscle strength using repetition maximum (only if pain free)

Neuromotor development and sensory integration: analysis of reflex movement patterns, assessment of involuntary movements, sensory integration tests, gross and fine motor skills

Orthotic, protective, and supportive devices: analysis of components and movement using a device

Pain: Pediatric Pain Questionnaire (PPQ), visual analog scale

Posture: analysis of resting and dynamic posture, scoliosis screening

Range of motion: active/passive range of motion for extremities, active motion only for cervical spine, angular deformities and joint play assessments

Self-care and home management: Pediatric Evaluation of Disability Inventory (PEDI), Child Health Assessment Questionnaire (CHAQ), Juvenile Arthritis Functional Status Index (JASI)

What additional findings are likely with this patient?

Potential complications are dependent on the subtype of JRA and the presence (or absence) of RF or ANA. Joint swelling, stiffness, and pain are the most common symptoms. Eye inflammation and development of iritis/uveitis can be a significant complication. Some patients have periods of exacerbations and remissions while other patient's symptoms will persist.

Management:

What is the most effective management of this patient?

A pediatric rheumatologist is ideal to direct a multidisciplinary team in the complex care of JRA. Primary goals of treatment are to maintain a high level of physical functioning and quality of life. Pharmacological intervention may include NSAIDS, immunosuppressive medications, disease-modifying antirheumatic drugs, and corticosteroids. Physical therapy intervention is a key component and should include range of motion, exercise, and pain control. Functional mobility, strengthening, endurance, and aerobic training will assist a patient in overall function. Range of motion exercises, modalities, splints and orthotics, patient/family education, and the integration of recreational activities should optimize the quality of life. Surgical intervention is sometimes warranted for severe contractures or irreversible joint destruction. Soft tissue release, supracondylar osteotomy, and arthroplasty are the most common surgical procedures.

What home care regimen should be recommended?

A home care regimen should provide an individualized exercise program. The program should be simple and take no more than 20 minutes to complete in order to optimize compliance. Swimming is also a beneficial activity for a child with JRA.

Outcome:

What is the likely outcome of a course in physical therapy?

Physical therapy may be indicated periodically throughout a patient's childhood based on symptoms and complications. Ongoing education and revision of a home program is vital to promote patient compliance. Physical therapy outcome is variable depending on the severity of the patient's symptoms.

What are the long-term effects of the patient's condition?

Long-term effects of JRA are dependent on subtype, symptoms, and any complications encountered. Some patients "outgrow" JRA and are not affected as adults while others experience pain and other manifestations of the disease on a consistent and long-term basis.

Comparison:

What are the distinguishing characteristics of a similar condition?

Infectious bacterial arthritis most often develops within a joint secondary to systemic corticosteroid use, trauma, HIV or alcohol/drug abuse. If treated immediately, long-term prognosis is good. If left uncontrolled, toxemia and septicemia can be fatal. Inflammation and pannus within the synovium erodes articular cartilage. There is an acute onset of swelling, tenderness, and loss of range of motion. A child will usually not bear weight through the involved joint.

Clinical Scenarios:

Scenario One

A 12-year-old boy diagnosed with systemic JRA is seen in physical therapy two days status post soft tissue release of the bilateral heel cords. The patient primarily uses a wheelchair for mobility.

Scenario Two

A six-year-old girl is seen in physical therapy shortly after diagnosis of pauciarticular JRA two months ago. The patient's primary complaint is pain in the right ankle with any weight bearing activity. The patient enjoys playing outside and participates in soccer in the fall.

Lateral Epicondylitis

Diagnosis:

What condition produces a patient's symptoms?
Lateral epicondylitis (tennis elbow) is characterized by inflammation or degenerative changes at the common extensor tendon that attaches to the lateral epicondyle of the elbow. The primary symptom of this condition is pain.

An injury was most likely sustained to which structure?
Repeated overuse of the wrist extensors, particularly the extensor carpi radialis brevis can produce tensile stress and result in microscopic tearing and damage to the extensor tendon. Other muscles that can be affected include the extensor digitorum, extensor carpi radialis longus, and extensor carpi ulnaris.

Inference:

What is the most likely contributing factor in the development of this condition?
The exact etiology is uncertain, however, repetitive wrist action against resistance during extension and supination appear to produce this condition. Over time inflammation of the periosteum may develop with formation of adhesions. The continued microtrauma does not allow for proper healing and will continue to injure the tissues. This pattern is best seen while hitting a backhand in tennis; however, overuse with painting, hand tools, gardening, and any repeated activity that involves forceful wrist extension can result in lateral epicondylitis. Men are more likely to develop lateral epicondylitis and it is also more common for individuals in their late 30's and 40's secondary to the normal loss of the extensibility of connective tissue with age.

Confirmation:

What is the most likely clinical presentation?
A typical patient with lateral epicondylitis is usually between the third and fifth decades of life and has unilateral involvement of the elbow. Lateral epicondylitis presents with pain along the lateral aspect of the elbow especially over the lateral epicondyle that sometimes radiates into the dorsum of the hand. The pain will increase with wrist flexion with elbow extension, resisted wrist extension, and resisted radial deviation. The patient may also have difficulty holding or gripping objects and insufficient forearm functional strength. Range of motion of the elbow usually remains normal; however, may be limited in severe cases. The patient will have localized tenderness over the lateral epicondyle and may present with localized swelling.

The pain usually increases with activity and is noted at night.

What laboratory or imaging studies would confirm the diagnosis?
No lab or imaging studies are required to diagnose lateral epicondylitis. X-ray or MRI may be used to rule out other conditions. Electrodiagnostic tests are only beneficial if there is radial nerve involvement.

What additional information should be obtained to confirm the diagnosis?
Lateral epicondylitis is usually diagnosed based on history, physical examination of the extremity, and several manual maneuvers that specifically identify the presence of lateral epicondylitis. An increase in pain at the lateral epicondyle with resisted wrist extension confirms the pathology of the extensor carpi radialis brevis.

Examination:

What history should be documented?
Important areas to explore include past medical history, medications, family history, current symptoms, current health status, social history and habits, occupation, leisure and sport activities, and social support system.

What test/measures are most appropriate?
Anthropometric characteristics: circumferential measurements of the forearm
Arousal, attention, and cognition: examine mental status, learning ability, memory, motivation
Community and work integration: analysis of community, work, and leisure activities
Environmental, home, and work barriers: analysis of current and potential barriers or hazards
Integumentary integrity: skin assessment, assessment of sensation
Joint integrity and mobility: assessment of hyper- and hypomobility of a joint, soft tissue swelling and inflammation, quality of movement of the elbow complex, provocative tests for lateral epicondylitis including Cozen's/test 1, Mills/test 2, Tennis Elbow test
Muscle performance: strength assessment, muscle tone assessment, grip test dynamometer
Orthotic, protective, and supportive devices: potential utilization of bracing, splinting
Pain: pain perception assessment scale, visual analog scale, assessment of muscle soreness
Posture: analysis of resting and dynamic posture
Range of motion: active and passive range of motion of bilateral upper extremities
Reflex integrity: assessment of deep tendon reflexes

<u>Self-care and home management</u>: assessment of functional capacity

What additional findings are likely with this patient?

If the patient is involved in tennis or some other potential overuse activity there should be remediation and modification in training, technique, and equipment to minimize the chance of recurrence.

Management:

What is the most effective management of this patient?

Medical management initially treats the pain and inflammation through protection, rest, ice, compression, and elevation. During the initial phase the patient should avoid all activities that aggravate the injury. Pharmacological intervention should include NSAIDs to alleviate pain and inflammation. Modalities may also be used such as phonophoresis with hydrocortisone or iontophoresis with dexamethasone. On occasion, resting splints may be used during the acute stage to relieve tension of the involved muscles. Physical therapy intervention should initiate stretching and strengthening to improve flexibility and increase functional activities. All exercise must remain pain free. Other modalities including electrical stimulation and cryotherapy may be beneficial. Strengthening should include elbow, wrist, and hand exercises. As a patient progresses resistive, isokinetic, and sport-specific exercises should be introduced. Counter-force bracing in the form of a forearm band may be indicated to reduce the degree of tension in the region of the muscular attachment. A patient should wean from the brace, prior to the completion of rehabilitation so the patient does not depend on it or use it as a replacement for rehabilitation.

What home care regimen should be recommended?

A home care regimen should include the same therapeutic program the patient performs during physical therapy. Patient education should include modification of all activities that exacerbate the symptoms. It is imperative that the patient not rush or advance beyond the parameters of the home program as it will exacerbate the condition. A patient must avoid all activities that produce pain and use ice, elevation, and rest as needed.

Outcome:

What is the likely outcome of a course in physical therapy?

Physical therapy may be indicated for one to three months with goals of regaining appropriate strength, flexibility, and endurance while reducing inflammation and pain of the involved muscles. Overall outcome is favorable and a patient should be able to return to all previous functional activities without restrictions.

What are the long-term effects of the patient's condition?

Lateral epicondylitis will commonly recur; however, continued stretching and exercise will decrease the risk of future recurrence. If conservative treatment does not improve symptoms after two to three months surgical intervention may be indicated.

Comparison:

What are the distinguishing characteristics of a similar condition?

Medial epicondylitis (golfer's or swimmer's elbow) results from repeated microtrauma to the flexor carpi radialis and/or the humeral head of the pronator teres during pronation and wrist flexion. There is pain with resisted wrist flexion and resisted pronation and point tenderness over the medial epicondyle. Treatment is similar in protocol to lateral epicondylitis; however, is directed at the appropriate location. Complete immobilization is never recommended, however, counter-force bracing or splinting may be indicated.

Clinical Scenarios:

Scenario One

A 27-year-old tennis player is seen in physical therapy diagnosed with right lateral epicondylitis. The patient plays in a competitive league and recently changed his instructor and increased the number of games played per week. He complains of pain and point tenderness over the lateral epicondyle. He is very frustrated, as this pain has had a large impact on his ability to win games.

Scenario Two

A 42-year-old female diagnosed with right lateral epicondylitis has been seen in physical therapy for four weeks. She has a past medical history that includes reflex sympathetic dystrophy two years ago in the right upper extremity and status post hysterectomy three months ago. She has not had any relief of pain and states that she cannot hold anything in her right hand. She enjoys gardening and works at a vegetable farm, but does not want to decrease any of her current activities.

Lymphedema Post-Mastectomy

Diagnosis:

What condition produces a patient's symptoms?
Lymphedema following a mastectomy is termed secondary lymphedema and is the result of damage to the lymphatic nodes and vessels during surgery. Excessive accumulation of lymph fluid within the soft tissues is caused by an excess load of lymph fluid or inadequate transport capacity within the lymphatic system secondary to the loss of homeostasis.

An injury was most likely sustained to which structure?
The lymphatic system is damaged as a result of the mastectomy, the surgical removal of the breast, whereby the lymphatic nodes and vessels are removed or damaged. The lymph system is unable to compensate, the lymph vessels dilate, and the valve flaps are not able to fully stop lymph flow. This allows for backflow of lymph into the tissues. This chain reaction causes further injury, chronic inflammation and progression including fibrosis, hypoxia within the tissues, and an increase risk of infection.

Inference:

What is the most likely contributing factor in the development of this condition?
The most likely contributing factor in the development of lymphedema following a mastectomy is the damage and/or removal of the axillary lymph nodes and vessels in an attempt to prevent the spread of breast cancer. If the lymphatic nodes have not been removed but have received radiation they may stop functioning due to chronic inflammation, fibrosis, and scarring. Globally, the parasitic infection called filariasis is the most common cause of secondary lymphedema. The virus is carried by mosquitoes in regions such as Africa, India, and Malaysia. Other causes include severe infection, crush injuries, burns or repeated pregnancies. There are an estimated three million new cases of secondary lymphedema each year with approximately 30% of breast cancer survivors affected by this condition. Primary lymphedema statistics indicate 15% of cases present at birth and 75% of the cases are acquired from adolescence through midlife years. Females are affected more than males with a 4:1 ratio.

Confirmation:

What is the most likely clinical presentation?
The clinical presentation of lymphedema includes edema in an affected area/extremity that increases with dependent positioning. The patient usually does not experience pain but rather a tight or heavy sensation. Lymphedema is classified into three stages that present differently based on the severity of the condition. Stage I is characterized by pitting edema that reduces with elevation overnight and does not exhibit any fibrotic changes. Stage II is identified by some fibrotic changes that begin to occur and increase in non-pitting edema that does not reduce with elevation. Stage III is characterized with skin changes, frequent infections, and severe edema that is non-pitting and fibrotic.

What laboratory or imaging studies would confirm the diagnosis?
Diagnosis is confirmed through history, observation, and several diagnostic tools to rule out other potential disorders. A Doppler study of the affected area is able to rule out a deep vein thrombosis. A CT scan or MRI may be performed before treatment of lymphedema is initiated to rule out malignancy. A lymphoscintigram is a nuclear medicine procedure that tests the function of the lymphatic system.

What additional information should be obtained to confirm the diagnosis?
A medical evaluation should include a thorough history including all illnesses, hospitalizations, and surgeries. History should be noted regarding the current edema and its course. Date of onset, progression, and symptoms associated with the edema are important to attain and note in the patient's record.

Examination:

What history should be documented?
Important areas to explore include past medical history and surgical history, medications, history of swelling, family history, current symptoms, current health status, living environment, social history and habits, occupation, and social support system.

What test/measures are most appropriate?
Aerobic capacity and endurance: assessment of vital signs at rest and with activity, perceived exertion scale, pulse oximetry, auscultation of the lungs
Anthropometric characteristics: circumferential and volumetric measurements of involved areas, skinfold measurements
Arousal, attention, and cognition: examine mental status, learning ability, memory, motivation
Community and work integration: analysis of community, work, and leisure activities
Environmental, home, and work barriers: analysis of current and potential barriers or hazards
Gait, locomotion, and balance: static and dynamic balance in sitting and standing, safety during gait with/without an assistive device

Integumentary integrity: skin assessment, assessment of sensation, nailbed assessment
Joint integrity and mobility: soft tissue swelling and inflammation
Muscle performance: strength and tone assessment
Pain: pain perception assessment scale
Range of motion: active and passive range of motion
Self-care and home management: assessment of functional capacity
Ventilation, respiration, and circulation: assessment of brachial and radial pulses, capillary refill assessment

What additional findings are likely with this patient?

Additional findings are based on the etiology, stage, and progression of the lymphedema. Complications can include ulcer formation, increased risk for fungal and bacterial infections, loss of range, fatigue, and fibrotic edema with atrophic skin changes. If left untreated a patient could progress to stage III "lymphostatic elephantiasis."

Management:

What is the most effective management of this patient?

Effective medical management of secondary lymphedema may involve pharmacological intervention or natural substances that increase proteolysis and macrophage activity; however, there is no particular class of drugs that can "cure" lymphedema. Surgery is used in the treatment of severe lymphedema but only achieves limited results since the cause remains unchanged. Physical therapy intervention usually follows a treatment approach termed combined decongestive physiotherapy (CDP). The philosophy of lymphatic management includes patient education in skin care, hygiene, bandaging, self-massage, and exercise. Therapeutic intervention should focus on manual lymph drainage, short stretch compression bandages, retrograde massage, exercise, compression therapy, and use of a mechanical pump. Care must be taken, however, not to exceed 45 mm Hg during compression therapy since a greater pressure can damage or collapse the lymphatic walls.

What home care regimen should be recommended?

A home care regimen is vital to the success of the CDP treatment of lymphedema. A patient must understand and comply with skin care, bandaging, self-massage, lymphatic drainage techniques, compression therapy, and an exercise program. Each patient must also understand the lifetime precautions that can increase lymphedema such as sunburn, air travel, excessive exercise, poor nutrition, and obesity.

Outcome:

What is the likely outcome of a course in physical therapy?

Comprehensive lymphedema intervention such as CDP has shown significant reduction in lymphedema during treatment and continued reduction with an ongoing home program over time.

What are the long-term effects of the patient's condition?

Lymphedema is progressive if left untreated but can be managed through intervention and education. Patients must comply with a home program and must remain aware of all activities that place the patient at an increased risk for lymphedema.

Comparison:

What are the distinguishing characteristics of a similar condition?

Lipedema is a condition where there appears to be swelling throughout the bilateral lower extremities from the hips to the ankle joints. This swelling is actually subcutaneous adipose tissue. This condition is sometimes confused with lymphedema but does not affect the lymphatic system. It most often occurs in women with hormonal disorders and is believed to have a family history in approximately 20% of the cases. Medical management treats the hormonal imbalance and assists with nutritional guidance to allow for effective weight management.

Clinical Scenarios:

Scenario One

A 39-year-old female post right mastectomy secondary to malignancy develops lymphedema in her right arm four months after surgery. She resides alone and is employed as a web design consultant. She complains of heaviness in the arm, but denies pain. She was referred by her oncologist for outpatient physical therapy.

Scenario Two

A 68-year-old male is seen in physical therapy with stage II lymphedema in his right lower extremity. He underwent a total hip replacement two months ago and states immediate swelling and discomfort. His history includes multiple abdominal surgeries with edema present after each surgery. He presents with non-pitting edema that does not reduce with elevation.

Medial Collateral Ligament Sprain – Grade II

Diagnosis:

What condition produces a patient's symptoms?

The medial collateral ligament (MCL) connects the medial epicondyle of the femur to the medial tibia and as a result resists medially directed force at the knee. The MCL is the primary stabilizer of the medial side of the knee against valgus force and lateral rotation of the tibia (especially during knee flexion). This extra-articular ligament is a thick and flat band which attaches proximally on the medial femoral condyle and extends to the medial surface of the tibia approximately six centimeters below the joint line. A common mechanism of injury is a direct blow against the lateral surface of the knee causing valgus stress and subsequent damage to the medial aspect of the knee.

An injury was most likely sustained to which structure?

The medial collateral ligament is comprised of two parts. A deep part of the ligament attaches to the cartilage meniscus and the superficial part attaches further down the joint. A grade II injury of the MCL is characterized by partial tearing of the ligament's fibers resulting in joint laxity when the ligament is stretched. Often the medial capsular ligament is involved in a grade II sprain of the MCL.

Inference:

What is the most likely contributing factor in the development of this condition?

Individuals participating in contact activities requiring a high level of agility are particularly susceptible to a MCL injury. Mechanism of injury is usually a blow to the outside of the knee joint causing excess force to the medial side of the joint. The MCL can also be injured by a twisting of the knee. Muscle weakness resulting in poor dynamic stabilization may also increase the incidence of this type of injury.

Confirmation:

What is the most likely clinical presentation?

A patient with a grade II MCL injury will likely present with an inability to fully extend and flex the knee, pain and significant tenderness along the medial aspect of the knee, possible decrease in strength, potential loss of proprioception, and an antalgic gait. There is typically discernable laxity with valgus testing, instability of the joint, and slight to moderate swelling around the knee. More severe swelling may be indicative of meniscus or cruciate ligament involvement.

What laboratory or imaging studies would confirm the diagnosis?

MRI is a non-invasive imaging technique that can be utilized to view soft tissue structures such as ligaments. The imaging technique is extremely expensive and therefore may not be commonly employed on an individual with a suspected MCL injury without other extenuating circumstances.

What additional information should be obtained to confirm the diagnosis?

A valgus stress test is a technique designed to detect medial instability in a single plane. The examiner applies a valgus stress at the knee while stabilizing the ankle in slight lateral rotation. The test is often performed initially in full extension and then in 30 degrees of flexion. A patient with a grade II MCL sprain may exhibit 5-15 degrees of laxity with valgus stress at 30 degrees of flexion.

Examination:

What history should be documented?

Important areas to explore include mechanism of present injury, current symptoms, past medical history, medications, living environment, occupation, social history and habits, and social support system.

What test/measures are most appropriate?

Anthropometric characteristics: palpation to determine knee effusion, lower extremity circumferential measurements

Arousal, attention, and cognition: examine mental status, learning ability, memory, motivation

Assistive and adaptive devices: analysis of components and safety of a device, potential utilization of crutches

Community and work integration: analysis of community, work, and leisure activities

Environmental, home, and work barriers: analysis of current and potential barriers or hazards

Gait, locomotion, and balance: safety during gait with an assistive device

Integumentary integrity: assessment of sensation (pain, temperature, tactile), skin assessment

Joint integrity and mobility: special tests for ligaments and menisci, valgus stress test, palpation of structures, joint play, soft tissue restrictions, joint pain

Muscle performance: strength assessment, assessment of active movement, resisted isometrics, muscle contraction characteristics, muscle endurance

Orthotic, protective, and supportive devices: potential utilization of bracing, taping or wrapping

Pain: pain perception assessment scale, visual analog scale

Range of motion: active and passive range of motion
Self-care and home management: assessment of functional capacity
Sensory integrity: assessment of proprioception and kinesthesia

What additional findings are likely with this patient?

Anterior cruciate ligament and/or meniscal damage often accompanies a grade II MCL injury. As a result it is often prudent to perform special tests directed at these particular structures. The MCL normally has a good secondary support system with weight bearing forces compressing the medial side of the joint and adding to the overall stability of the joint. This allows the structures to be protected after injury along with use of a brace.

Management:

What is the most effective management of this patient?

Medical management for a grade II MCL sprain usually involves conservative management including R.I.C.E. (rest, icing, compression, and elevation). Pharmacological intervention is directed towards pain management through acetaminophen or NSAIDs. The patient may utilize a full-length knee immobilizer or a hinge brace and crutches to limit weight bearing through the involved lower extremity for initial rehabilitation. Physical therapy intervention should be directed towards increasing range of motion in the involved extremity and beginning light resistive exercises. Range of motion exercises may include heel slides or stationary cycling without resistance. Resistive exercises should be directed towards the quadriceps and may include isometrics and closed kinetic chain exercises. Functional activities such as gait and stair climbing should be incorporated into the treatment program. Superficial modalities and electrical stimulation may be utilized to combat pain and inflammation. Transverse friction massage may be applied to the healing ligament so it does not adhere to surrounding and adjacent structures. Care must be taken not to massage the proximal attachment of the MCL due to potential bony periosteal disruption. A patient should be required to complete a functional progression prior to returning to unrestricted activity.

What home care regimen should be recommended?

The home care regimen should consist of range of motion, strengthening, palliative care, and functional activities as warranted based on the results of the patient examination. The use of crutches should continue until the patient can adequately extend the knee joint.

Outcome:

What is the likely outcome of a course in physical therapy?

A grade II MCL sprain should progress fairly quickly if no other structures (ACL or meniscus) are involved. A patient should be able to return to their previous functional level within four to eight weeks following the injury.

What are the long-term effects of the patient's condition?

Proper healing time and rehabilitation management should allow the patient to return to all forms of activity once the patient demonstrates full range of motion, ambulation without a limp, no visual swelling, and competence with all agility testing. If the patient has residual laxity from the injury the patient may be susceptible to reinjury.

Comparison:

What are the distinguishing characteristics of a similar condition?

A grade II lateral collateral ligament injury differs from a MCL injury in several ways. The lateral collateral ligament attaches proximally on the lateral femoral condyle and runs distally and posteriorly to insert on the head of the fibula. Lateral collateral ligament injuries are far less common than MCL injuries. Management should focus on the same general goals (range of motion, strengthening, palliative care, and functional activities) as those outlined for the MCL injury.

Clinical Scenarios:

Scenario One

A 17-year-old male is diagnosed with a left grade III MCL sprain and a small tear in the medial meniscus. The patient was playing football when he was tackled and hit at the knee. The patient has no significant past medical history and plans to participate in football at the collegiate level.

Scenario Two

A 20-year-old college field hockey player complains of knee pain after being diagnosed with a grade I MCL sprain. The patient is mildly tender to palpation over the medial joint line and exhibits trace effusion. The patient has no significant past medical history and would like to return to athletic competition as soon as possible.

Multiple Sclerosis

Diagnosis:

What condition produces a patient's symptoms?
Multiple sclerosis (MS) produces patches of demyelination that decreases the efficiency of nerve impulse transmission. Symptoms vary based on the location and the extent of demyelination.

An injury was most likely sustained to which structure?
Multiple sclerosis is characterized by demyelination of the myelin sheaths that surround nerves within the brain and spinal cord. Myelin breakdown results in plaque development, decreased nerve conduction velocity, and eventual failure of impulse transmission. Lesions are scattered throughout the central nervous system and do not follow a particular pattern.

Inference:

What is the most likely contributing factor in the development of this condition?
The exact etiology of MS is unknown. Genetics, viral infections, and environment all have a role in the development of MS. It is theorized that a slow acting virus initiates the autoimmune response in individuals that have environmental and genetic factors for the disease. The incidence of MS is higher in Caucasians between the ages of 20 and 35 years and is nearly twice as common in women as in men. There is also a higher incidence of MS in temperate climates.

Confirmation:

What is the most likely clinical presentation?
The prevalence of MS differs by geographic area, sex, and race. In the United States the prevalence is 30-80:100,000 with 250,000-350,000 current cases. The highest incidence is 20-35 years of age; however, MS can occur at any age. MS can be classified as relapsing-remitting MS (85%), secondary-progressive MS, primary-progressive MS or progressive-relapsing MS. The clinical presentation varies based on the type of disease, the location, extent of demyelination, and degree of sclerosis. Initial symptoms can include visual problems, paresthesias and sensory changes, clumsiness, weakness, ataxia, balance dysfunction, and fatigue. The clinical course usually consists of periods of exacerbations and remissions; however, the degree of neurologic dysfunction and subsequent recovery will follow typical patterns of the specific type of MS. The frequency and intensity of exacerbations may indicate the speed/course of the disease process.

What laboratory or imaging studies would confirm the diagnosis?
There is not a single testing procedure to diagnose MS early in the disease. MRI may assist with observation and establishing a baseline for lesions, evoked potentials may demonstrate slowed nerve conduction, and cerebrospinal fluid can be analyzed for an elevated concentration of gamma globulin and protein levels.

What additional information should be obtained to confirm the diagnosis?
Clinical presentation and reliable patient history of symptoms are vital in the diagnosis of MS. Guidelines indicate that a clinically definitive diagnosis of MS can be made if a person experiences two separate attacks and shows evidence of two separate lesions. Other diagnoses (having specific criteria) include: laboratory-supported definite MS, clinically probable MS, and laboratory-supported probable MS.

Examination:

What history should be documented?
Important areas to explore include past medical history, history of symptoms, medications, current health status, social history and habits, occupation, living environment, and social support system.

What test/measures are most appropriate?
Aerobic capacity and endurance: assessment of vital signs at rest and with activity
Arousal, attention and cognition: examine mental status, learning ability, memory, and motivation, Mini-Mental State Examination
Assistive and adaptive devices: analysis of components and safety of a device
Community and work integration: analysis of community, work, and leisure activities
Gait, locomotion, and balance: static/dynamic balance in sitting/standing, Tinetti Performance Oriented Mobility Assessment, Berg Balance Scale
Motor function: assessment of dexterity and coordination; assessment of postural, equilibrium, and righting reactions; gross and fine motor skills
Muscle performance: strength and tone assessment, tremor assessment, muscle endurance, Modified Fatigue Impact Scale
Neuromotor development and sensory integration: analysis of reflex movement patterns
Pain: pain perception assessment scale
Posture: resting/dynamic posture, potential contracture
Range of motion: active and passive range of motion

What additional findings are likely with this patient?

A low percentage of patients experience benign MS and have little to no long-term disability. The majority experience progressive degeneration through periods of exacerbations and remissions. As the disease advances exacerbations leave greater ongoing disability and the length of remissions decrease. Ongoing symptoms can include emotional lability, depression, dementia, psychological problems, spasticity, tremor, weakness, paralysis, sexual dysfunction, and loss of bowel and bladder control.

Management:

What is the most effective management of this patient?

Management of MS includes pharmacological, medical, and therapeutic intervention. The goal of medical treatment of MS is to lessen the length of exacerbations and maximize the health of the patient.

Pharmacological intervention is quite complex and can include ABC drugs (approved in the treatment of MS) that are classified as immunomodulatory medications. Physical, occupational, and speech therapies are indicated throughout the clinical course of the disease and well as nutritional and psychological counseling. Physical therapy intervention includes regulation of activity level, relaxation and energy conservation techniques, normalization of tone, balance activities, gait training, core stabilization and control, and adaptive/assistive device training. Patient and caregiver education regarding safety, energy conservation, patterns of fatigue, and the use of adaptive devices is vital to the quality of life.

What home care regimen should be recommended?

A home care regimen should include a submaximal exercise/endurance program. Exercise in the morning when the patient is rested is advisable to avoid fatigue. The patient may need frequent rest periods throughout the day and may benefit from breaking a task into smaller steps to avoid fatigue. Ongoing ambulation and mobility activities are important to maintain endurance and prevent disuse atrophy. Aquatic therapy may also be indicated as it is beneficial to this population.

Outcome:

What is the likely outcome of a course in physical therapy?

Physical therapy is indicated intermittently throughout the clinical course of MS with the goal of maximizing

functional capacity and the quality of life. Physical therapy will not alter the progression of the disease process but rather treat the current symptoms and assist the patient to attain the highest level of function. Factors that influence exacerbations include heat, stress, infection, trauma, and pregnancy.

What are the long-term effects of the patient's condition?

MS is generally a progressive degenerative disease process that creates permanent damage and disability. Factors that influence exacerbations include heat, stress, and trauma. Most patients live with MS for many years and die from secondary complications such as disuse atrophy, pressure sores, contractures, pathological fractures, renal infection, and pneumonia. If left untreated 50% of patients will require a wheelchair within 15 years post diagnosis. Overall mortality rate and long-term outcome correlates to age at diagnosis, number of attacks and exacerbations, frequency and duration of remissions, and type of MS. Suicide is also seven times greater when compared to the same age control group without MS.

Comparison:

What are the distinguishing characteristics of a similar condition?

Dystonia is a neurologic syndrome that presents with involuntary and sustained muscle contractions that cause repetitive movements. Idiopathic dystonia has a genetic basis and accounts for two-thirds of all cases. Secondary dystonia usually results from brain damage or CNS damage. There are no definitive tests to diagnose dystonia. Treatment is based on current symptoms and includes pharmacological intervention, physical therapy, and occasional surgical intervention. Prognosis is based on age of onset and spontaneous remission occurs in 25-30% of the cases.

Clinical Scenarios:

Scenario One

A 28-year-old female has had visual difficulty, urinary urgency, tingling, and upper extremity weakness on two separate occasions recently. The patient has an aunt with MS; however, has no other significant medical history. The patient was referred to physical therapy by her primary physician.

Scenario Two

A 42-year-old male with MS is referred to physical therapy. The patient has experienced several exacerbations and remissions with full recovery in the past. The patient presently appears to have an exacerbation of symptoms including excessive fatigue. He lives alone and works in a library.

Myocardial Infarction

Diagnosis:

What condition produces a patient's symptoms?
Myocardial infarction (MI) occurs when there is poor coronary artery perfusion, ischemia, and subsequent necrosis of the cardiac tissue usually due to thrombus, arterial blockage or atherosclerosis. The location and severity of the infarct will determine symptoms and the overall acute clinical picture.

An injury was most likely sustained to which structure?
A MI produces ischemia and subsequent necrosis to a portion of the myocardium. The extent of the damage to the myocardium is dependent on the duration of ischemia and on the thickness of the tissue involved. A transmural MI involves the full-thickness of the myocardium while a nontransmural MI involves the subendocardial area (inner third of the myocardium). The myocardium has three zones that form concentric circles around the point of infarct termed: zone of infarct, zone of hypoxic injury, and zone of ischemia. Thrombosis of the anterior descending branch of the left coronary artery is the most common location of infarct and affects the left ventricle. A right coronary artery thrombosis can result in an infarct of the posteroinferior portion of the left ventricle and potentially affect the right ventricular myocardium.

Inference:

What is the most likely contributing factor in the development of this condition?
The primary risk factors for MI include patient or family history of heart disease, smoking, physical inactivity, stress, hypertension, elevated cholesterol, diabetes mellitus, and obesity. The use of cocaine, aortic stenosis or coronary artery dissection may also cause a MI. It has been documented that a MI will occur more frequently in the morning hours and during the November to December holiday season.

Confirmation:

What is the most likely clinical presentation?
MI occurs in 1.5 million individuals each year within the United States with a mortality rate of 500,000 deaths annually. Approximately two-thirds of patients experience prodromal symptoms days to weeks before the event, including unstable angina, shortness of breath, and fatigue. A patient that is experiencing a MI will initially present with deep pain or pressure in the substernal area. The pain may or may not radiate to the jaw and down the left arm or to the back. The patient cannot alleviate the pain with rest or nitroglycerin and the pain may last for hours. The patient is usually anxious, pale, sweating, fatigued, and may present with nausea and vomiting. Symptoms of a MI frequently do not follow a typical pattern, especially in females. There are also instances of a silent MI where no symptoms are noted.

What laboratory or imaging studies would confirm the diagnosis?
The primarily tool to detect a MI is a 12-lead electrocardiogram. An inverted T wave indicates myocardial ischemia, elevated ST segment indicates acute infarction, and a depressed ST segment indicates a pending subendocardial or transmural infarction. A blood serum analysis can be utilized to determine the level of selected cardiac enzymes. The level of selected enzymes such as creatine phosphokinase (CPK), aspartate transferase (AST), and lactic dehydrogenase (LDH) can be dramatically altered during and after a MI. A complete blood count (CBC), chest radiograph, radionuclide imaging, and amylase level may be ordered to assist with the diagnosis.

What additional information should be obtained to confirm the diagnosis?
Additional information in the diagnosis of a MI is found through the manifestation of symptoms (see clinical presentation) and clinical examination including a thorough past medical history and history of current symptoms.

Examination:

What history should be documented?
Important areas to explore include past medical history, family history, medications, current health status, living environment, social history and habits, occupation, and social support system.

What test/measures are most appropriate?
Aerobic capacity and endurance: vital signs at rest and during activity, palpation of pulses, perceived exertion scale, electrocardiogram analysis, auscultation of the heart and lungs, pulse oximetry
Arousal, attention, and cognition: examine mental status, learning ability, memory, motivation
Assistive and adaptive devices: analysis of components and safety of a device
Environmental, home, and work: analysis of current and potential barriers or hazards
Gait, locomotion, and balance: assessment of static and dynamic balance in sitting and standing, safety during gait with/without an assistive device
Muscle performance: strength assessment through active movement only (no manual muscle testing)

Pain: pain perception scale, visual analog scale
Posture: analysis of resting and dynamic posture
Self-care and home management: assessment of functional capacity, Barthel Index
Ventilation, respiration, and circulation: ventilation, respiration, and circulation; assessment of pulses

What additional findings are likely with this patient?

A patient status post MI is at risk for complications that include arrhythmias, hypotension, pericarditis, impaired cardiac output, pulmonary edema, congestive heart failure, pericarditis, cardiogenic shock, recurrent infarction and sudden death. Arrhythmias occur in 90% of patients post MI and are caused by ischemia, ANS impairment, electrolyte imbalances, conduction defects, and other chemical imbalances.

Management:

What is the most effective management of this patient?

Initial medical management of a MI is to stabilize the patient and initiate pharmacological intervention to hinder the evolution of the MI. Anticoagulants, beta-blockers, thrombolytic agents, angiotensin-converting enzyme inhibitors, vasodilators, and estrogen (in women) may be used. Once stable, the patient is managed through a cardiac rehabilitation program. Surgical intervention including angioplasty, stenting, endarterectomy, and bypass grafting may be indicated based on the underlying cause of the MI. Exercise testing is performed within three days of the MI in order to establish baseline guidelines for patients that are cleared to exercise and do not exhibit any arrhythmias or angina. Physical therapy intervention usually follows a multi-phase cardiac rehabilitation program and continues in an outpatient setting once the patient is discharged from the hospital. Low-level therapeutic exercise, functional activities, relaxation, breathing techniques, endurance training, and continuous monitoring of vital signs are key components this program. Patient education regarding reduction of risk factors, return to activity, and commitment to fitness and health are also important to the success of physical therapy intervention.

What home care regimen should be recommended?

A home care regimen should follow the guidelines indicated for each phase of cardiac rehabilitation. A patient must continue with safe exercise, and integration of risk factor reduction. Symptom recognition and nutritional strategies are also important in a daily routine.

Outcome:

What is the likely outcome of a course in physical therapy?

Cardiac rehabilitation is recommended status post MI. The patient should start in the coronary care unit (CCU) and progress through each of the phases of cardiac rehabilitation. The goal is successful completion of a cardiac rehabilitation program allowing the patient to resume all activities of daily living and recreational pursuits. Upon completion the patient should possess self-management skills associated with symptoms/risk factors of heart disease.

What are the long-term effects of the patient's condition?

A patient that has experienced a MI may be able to return to all previous activities after successful completion of a cardiac rehabilitation program. A patient must continue to reduce the modifiable risk factors and maintain an appropriate level of exercise in order to limit a possible subsequent MI. Long-term outcome is dependent on prior functional ability, the extent and damage to the heart, and factors that negatively affect prognosis such as age, cardiovascular disease, hypotension, the presence of comorbidities, and an abnormal treadmill exercise test.

Comparison:

What are the distinguishing characteristics of a similar condition?

Angina pectoris is a myocardial ischemic disorder that occurs when there is an oxygen deficit to the coronary arteries. Coronary artery disease accounts for 90% of all cases of angina. Angina is classified as stable, post-infarction, Prinzmetal's, resting, unstable, nocturnal or variant. Symptoms often occur during exertion and include chest pain that may radiate. Rest or nitroglycerin normally provides relief of the symptoms. Treatment of the underlying cause is essential to prevent further damage to the heart.

Clinical Scenarios:

Scenario One

A 51-year-old male is referred to a phase I cardiac rehabilitation program after a transmural MI two days ago. The patient has hypertension, high cholesterol, smokes, and is obese. The patient currently supervises a local automobile dealership. The patient is divorced and lives in a two-story home.

Scenario Two

A 78-year-old female is status post nontransmural MI. The patient is very active and plays golf. The patient's past medical history includes treatment for a cardiac arrhythmia, obesity, and diabetes mellitus. The physician referred the patient for cardiac rehabilitation.

Osteogenesis Imperfecta

Diagnosis:

What condition produces a patient's symptoms?
Osteogenesis Imperfecta (OI) is a rare congenital disorder of collagen synthesis that affects all connective tissue in the body. The genetic defect affects collagen-producing genes and reduces production of collagen from 20-50%. There are many mutations identified and various underlying causes that combine to produce the phenotypic expression of OI in a patient.

An injury was most likely sustained to which structure?
The genes for type I collagen production (COL1A1 and COL1A2) have been identified as the genes that become mutated and result in OI. Since collagen production is vital throughout the body, bones and all forms of connective tissue are compromised. OI can also compromise growth, hearing, cardiopulmonary function, and joint integrity.

Inference:

What is the most likely contributing factor in the development of this condition?
Most children inherit OI from parents as either an autosomal dominant or autosomal recessive trait. Twenty-five percent of the time the genetic defect occurs by spontaneous mutation of the genes. Statistics estimate that 30 to 50 thousand individuals are living with OI in the United States.

Confirmation:

What is the most likely clinical presentation?
OI is classified into four types and has a wide range of clinical presentations ranging from normal appearance with mild symptoms to severe involvement that is fatal during infancy. Type I is the mildest form where a child has near normal growth and appearance with frequency of fractures usually ceasing after puberty. The patient experiences mild or moderate fragility, but most times without deformity. This patient will usually present with blue sclerae, easy bruising, triangular face, and possible hearing loss. Type II is the most severe form where a child dies in utero or by early childhood. This child has significant fragility of connective tissue, experiences multiple fractures with extreme deformities, and has a soft skull. Type III is severe but these children present with greater ossification of the skull. Type III characteristics include significant growth, retardation, progressive deformities, ongoing fractures, severe osteoporosis, triangular face, blue sclerae, and significant limitations with functional mobility. Type IV is usually a milder course that involves mild to moderate fragility and osteoporosis

(but greater than type I). The patient will experience fractures easily prior to puberty, but some children improve at that time. Type IV may or may not have a shorter stature, will have bowing of long bones, a barrel shape of their rib cage, possible hearing loss, brittle teeth, and will present with near normal sclerae. These children have a near normal life expectancy.

What laboratory or imaging studies would confirm the diagnosis?
A skin biopsy is used to examine the collagen and determine what type of OI is present. X-rays and bone scans may be used for evidence of deformities and old fractures. Bone densitometry may also be used to measure bone mass and estimate the risk of fracture for specific sites within the body. The diagnosis is made through these tests and in combination with the examination and history.

What additional information should be obtained to confirm the diagnosis?
Diagnosis should be determined based on physical examination, family and personal medical history, and testing described in the above paragraph.

Examination:

What history should be documented?
Important areas to explore include past medical history including falls, medications, family history, current symptoms and health status, and social support system.

What test/measures are most appropriate?
Arousal, attention, and cognition: examine mental status, learning ability, memory, motivation
Environmental, home, and work barriers: analysis of current and potential barriers or hazards
Ergonomics and body mechanics: analysis of dexterity and coordination
Gait, locomotion, and balance: static/dynamic balance in sitting/standing, safety during gait with/without an assistive device, analysis of wheelchair management
Integumentary integrity: skin and sensation assessment
Joint integrity and mobility: assessment of hyper- and hypomobility of a joint
Muscle performance: strength assessment of active motion, muscle tone assessment
Neuromotor development and sensory integration: reflex movement patterns and involuntary movements, sensory integration tests, gross/fine motor skills
Orthotic, protective, and supportive devices: analysis of components of a device, analysis of movement while wearing a device

<u>Pain</u>: pain perception assessment scale, visual analog scale, assessment of muscle soreness
<u>Posture</u>: analysis of resting and dynamic posture, scoliosis assessment
<u>Range of motion</u>: active range of motion only
<u>Self-care and home management</u>: assessment of functional capacity

What additional findings are likely with this patient?

Children with OI often have delayed developmental milestones secondary to ongoing fractures with immobilization, hypermobility and laxity of joints, and poorly developed muscles. Most Type I children are community ambulators, approximately 57% of Type IV are household ambulators and 26% are community ambulators, and only 26% of Type III become household ambulators.

Management:

What is the most effective management of this patient?

Medical management is directed at controlling the symptoms of OI. General goals include maximizing independence with mobility, improving optimal bone mass and muscle strength, and prevention of fractures and deformities. Pharmacological interventions have been studied, but have not shown any strong effect. Children should not be given steroids since it may deplete bone and increase fragility. Nutritional counseling and strong dental care are important in the management of OI. Lightweight orthotics may be indicated early to support the extremities, assist with ambulation, encourage weight bearing, and prevent fractures. Physical therapy intervention initially focuses on parent handling techniques, recognition of fractures, positioning, and activities that facilitate safe movement. Treatment of a child with OI should incorporate developmental activities, strengthening, positioning, weight bearing, and the use of mobility aids (scooters, riding toys or wheelchair). Swimming is also a good alternative for strengthening and exercise. All strengthening exercises should avoid rotational forces, placing weights/resistance near a joint, and using long lever arms. Surgical procedures known as "rodding" may also be indicated if a child has more than two fractures to the same bone within six months or if the angle of the long bone would not allow for stable ambulation.

What home care regimen should be recommended?

A home care regimen will be successful if parents are competent with many of the relevant aspects of care. Handling techniques, recognition of fractures, precautions and contraindications, standing program,

and exercise through activities are all key components of a home program for a child with OI. A child needs to continue to move and exercise in a safe fashion in order to optimize strength and bone mass.

Outcome:

What is the likely outcome of a course in physical therapy?

Physical therapy may be required intermittently over the course of the patient's childhood depending on the severity of OI and the secondary complications. Physical therapy must also update a home program for optimal therapeutic results. Physical therapy may be in an outpatient setting or through the school system. The physical therapist should work closely with the physician and caregivers for comprehensive care.

What are the long-term effects of the patient's condition?

A patient with OI has outcome potential based on the type of disorder, symptoms, and secondary complications encountered. A strong predictor of a child's ability to ambulate in the future also lies in the child's ability to sit by ten months of age. Some children live normal lives with minimal involvement while others use power wheelchairs for mobility and experience multiple secondary complications.

Comparison:

What are the distinguishing characteristics of a similar condition?

Arthrogryposis multiplex congenita (AMC) is a non-progressive neuromuscular disorder that results from multiple conditions that ultimately limit fetal movement in an intact skeleton and cause multiple congenital contractures at birth. Children are also born with muscle atrophy and weakness, and articular rigidity. Primary forms of AMC include contracture syndromes, amyoplasia, and distal arthrogryposis. Some children will ambulate and others will require wheelchairs for mobility.

Clinical Scenarios:

Scenario One

A nine-month-old boy is seen in physical therapy with Type IV OI. He currently has a cast on his left lower extremity due to a femur fracture. His mother wants to learn activities in sitting and handling techniques that would help her son.

Scenario Two

A 12-year-old female is seen by a school therapist. She underwent intramedullary rod placement in her right femur six weeks ago. She has type III OI and uses a wheelchair. She also presents with a 45 degree thoracic scoliosis and bowing in her upper extremities.

Osteoporosis

Diagnosis:

What condition produces a patient's symptoms?
Osteoporosis is a metabolic bone disorder where the rate of bone resorption accelerates while the rate of bone formation slows down; osteoclast activity exceeds osteoblast activity. This reduction of bone mass decreases the overall bone density and strength. Primary osteoporosis includes classifications such as idiopathic osteoporosis, involutional (senile) osteoporosis, and postmenopausal osteoporosis. Secondary osteoporosis occurs due to a primary disease process or as a result of taking certain medications.

An injury was most likely sustained to which structure?
Osteoporosis primarily affects trabecular bone in a postmenopausal patient; however, primarily seen in both trabecular and cortical bone in the geriatric population. Impaired bone formation due to declining osteoblast function in addition to the loss of calcium and phosphate salts within the bone structure cause brittle and porous bones that easily fracture. All bones can be affected with fractures of the vertebrae, distal radius/ulna, and femoral neck being the most common.

Inference:

What is the most likely contributing factor in the development of this condition?
The exact cause of primary osteoporosis is unknown; however, there are risk factors that include inadequate dietary calcium, smoking, excessive caffeine, high intake of alcohol or salt, small stature, Caucasian race, inactive lifestyle, family history or history of chronic disease. Secondary osteoporosis may be caused by prolonged drug therapies of heparin or corticosteroid use, endocrine disorders, malnutrition, and other disease processes. Postmenopausal osteoporosis targets women approximately 50-60 years of age. Involutional (senile) osteoporosis usually targets men and women >70 years of age. Idiopathic osteoporosis can occur in both genders at all ages.

Confirmation:

What is the most likely clinical presentation?
Osteoporosis is the most frequently seen metabolic bone disease that affects approximately 10 million individuals within the United States. The prevalence is expected to increase with the increase in the aging population. A patient diagnosed with osteoporosis may complain of low thoracic or lumbar pain, experience compression fractures of the vertebrae, and complain of back pain. Vertebral and other crush fractures may occur with little to no trauma. Pain is acute and increases with weight bearing and palpation. A patient may also present with deformities such as kyphosis, Dowager's hump, a decrease in height, and other postural changes.

What laboratory or imaging studies would confirm the diagnosis?
There is not an accurate measure of overall bone strength or standards for routine screening that have been established; however, X-rays are taken to investigate the amount of degeneration and the decrease in density of a particular area. A bone mineral density test accounts for 70% of bone strength and is the easiest way to determine osteoporosis. A photon absorptiometry is used to measure bone mass particularly of the vertebrae, hips, and extremities. Quantitative CT scans may be used to aid diagnosis by examining the bone density of the spine.

What additional information should be obtained to confirm the diagnosis?
Differential diagnosis including lab testing and urinalysis must exclude other disease processes through examination and testing. A patient's past medical history, current symptoms, and type and location of pain all play a role in diagnosing osteoporosis.

Examination:

What history should be documented?
Important areas to explore include past medical history, medications, family history, current symptoms, current health status, social history and habits, occupation, leisure activities, and social support system.

What test/measures are most appropriate?
Aerobic capacity and endurance: assessment of vital signs at rest and with activity, perceived exertion scale
Arousal, attention, and cognition: examine mental status, learning ability, memory, motivation
Assistive and adaptive devices: analysis of components and safety of a device
Environmental, home, and work barriers: analysis of current and potential barriers or hazards
Ergonomics and body mechanics: analysis of dexterity and coordination
Gait, locomotion, and balance: static and dynamic balance in sitting and standing, safety during gait with/without an assistive device, Berg Balance Scale, functional capacity evaluation
Integumentary integrity: skin and sensation assessment
Motor function: coordination, posture/balance in sitting
Muscle performance: strength of active range of motion only

Pain: pain perception scale, visual analog scale
Posture: analysis of resting and dynamic posture
Range of motion: active range of motion
Self-care and home management: assessment of functional capacity

What additional findings are likely with this patient?

Once osteoporosis progresses in severity it can affect areas other than weight bearing bones such as the skull, long bones, and ribs. Spontaneous fractures and skeletal deformities may increase due to the continuing bone loss. A single fracture significantly increases the risk for subsequent fractures and skeletal deformities such as kyphosis.

Management:

What is the most effective management of this patient?

Effective management of osteoporosis includes vitamin and pharmaceutical supplements, proper nutrition, education and physical therapy intervention. Hormone replacement therapy is recommended for postmenopausal patients. Calcium supplements, vitamin D, Raloxifene, and Fosamax (prevents bone resorption) may be recommended in the treatment of osteoporosis. Physical therapy intervention should include patient education regarding exercise, positioning, pain management, nutrition, and fall prevention. Physical therapy should include an exercise program that emphasizes weight bearing activities as tolerated. A patient may require a corset or lumbar support if at risk for vertebral fractures and many patients will require training with an assistive device. Aquatic therapy will assist with conditioning, however, should not replace weight bearing activities. Surgical intervention may be indicated for a patient requiring fracture stabilization.

What home care regimen should be recommended?

The home care regimen for osteoporosis includes a consistent home exercise program that combines exercise, walking, and other activities within a patient's tolerance. Exercise is crucial to slowing the bone resorption process and increasing bone development. Patients should be educated to avoid heavy resistive exercise, excessive flexion during exercise or household activities, and the use of ballistic movements. Light resistance such as small dumbbells or Theraband can be used with caution after consulting with the physician.

Outcome:

What is the likely outcome of a course in physical therapy?

Physical therapy should prescribe an exercise program that the patient can follow independently. Patient education should allow for independent decision making regarding proper nutrition and activities that incorporate precautions and fall prevention techniques. This level of patient competency should assist in decreasing the risk of fractures and other complications. Physical therapy cannot cease the process, but can empower the patient to effectively manage this bone disorder.

What are the long-term effects of the patient's condition?

Osteoporosis will create thin and porous bones that will fracture easily and result in direct and indirect complications. Deformity and pain can become long-term effects of osteoporosis. Early detection and management of osteoporosis is important to the long-term effects of the disease.

Comparison:

What are the distinguishing characteristics of a similar condition?

Paget's disease (osteitis deformans) is a chronic bone disease of unknown etiology where there is thickened, spongy, and abnormal bone formation. Large multinucleated osteoblasts, fibrous tissue, and thickened lamellae and trabeculae form and create weak and brittle bones. Bone pain, headache, hearing loss, fatigue, and stiffness are some early characteristics of Paget's disease. Progression of the disease includes bowing of long bones, an increase in skull size, bone deformities, and fractures (especially of the vertebrae).

Clinical Scenarios:

Scenario One

A 63-year-old female is seen in outpatient physical therapy for a home exercise program. She is postmenopausal and does not take hormone replacement therapy. She has been recently diagnosed with osteoporosis and X-rays revealed three old vertebral fractures. The patient's major complaints are pain and stiffness.

Scenario Two

A 92-year-old male was admitted to the hospital for internal fixation of a femoral neck fracture. The patient's history reveals osteoporosis, diabetes, and anxiety. He wants to be discharged home to care for his cat. The physician orders are for physical therapy two times per week with the goal of returning home alone.

Parkinson's Disease

Diagnosis:

What condition produces a patient's symptoms?

Parkinsonism syndrome is used to describe a group of disorders within subcortical gray matter of the basal ganglia that produces a similar disturbance of balance and voluntary movements. This syndrome occurs as a secondary effect or disorder from another disease process. Parkinson's disease is a primary degenerative disorder and is characterized by a decrease in production of dopamine (neurotransmitter) within the corpus striatum portion of the basal ganglia. The degeneration of the dopaminergic pathways creates an imbalance between dopamine and acetylcholine. This process produces the symptoms of Parkinson's disease.

An injury was most likely sustained to which structure?

Injury occurs to the subcortical gray matter within the basal ganglia, specifically the substantia nigra and the corpus striatum. The basal ganglia stores the majority of dopamine and is responsible for modulation and control of voluntary movement. A patient with Parkinson's disease exhibits degeneration of dopaminergic neurons that results in depletion of dopamine production within the basal ganglia. Change in the neurochemical production damages the complex loop between the basal ganglia and the cerebrum.

Inference:

What is the most likely contributing factor in the development of this condition?

Primary Parkinson's disease has an unknown etiology and accounts for the majority of patients with Parkinsonism. Contributing factors that can produce symptoms of Parkinson's disease include genetic defect, toxicity from carbon monoxide, excessive manganese or copper, carbon disulfide, vascular impairment of the striatum, encephalitis, and other neurodegenerative diseases such as Huntington's disease or Alzheimer's disease.

Confirmation:

What is the most likely clinical presentation?

There are approximately 500,000 individuals affected by Parkinsonism and about 42% of these are diagnosed specifically with Parkinson's disease. The risk for developing Parkinson's disease increases with age and 1:100 are affected over the age of 75. The majority of patients are between 50 and 79 years of age and approximately 10% are diagnosed before 40 years. The majority of patients with Parkinson's disease will initially notice a resting tremor in the hands (sometimes called a pill-rolling tremor) or feet that increases with stress and disappears with movement or sleep. Early in the disease process a patient may attribute symptoms to "old age" such as balance disturbances, difficulty rolling over and rising from bed, and impairment with fine manipulative movements seen in writing, bathing and dressing. A patient's symptoms slowly progress and often include hypokinesia, sluggish movement, difficulty with initiating (akinesia) and stopping movement, festinating and shuffling gait, bradykinesia, poor posture, dysphagia, and "cogwheel" or "lead pipe" rigidity of skeletal muscles. Patients may also experience "freezing" during ambulation, speech, blinking, and movements of the arms. A patient with Parkinson's disease will also have a mask-like appearance with no facial expression.

What laboratory or imaging studies would confirm the diagnosis?

There is no laboratory or imaging studies that initially diagnose Parkinson's disease. CT scan or MRI may be used to rule out other neurodegenerative diseases and obtain a baseline for future comparison.

What additional information should be obtained to confirm the diagnosis?

Definitive diagnosis is difficult during the early stages of the disease. Parkinson's disease is believed to progress slowly over 25 to 30 years prior to the onset of pharmacological intervention. Diagnosis is made from patient history, history of symptoms, and differential diagnosis to rule out other potential disorders. There are evaluation tools that are utilized to classify a patient by stage of the disease process.

Examination:

What history should be documented?

Important areas to explore include past medical history, medications, current symptoms, current health status, social history and habits, occupation, living environment, and social support system.

What test/measures are most appropriate?

Aerobic capacity and endurance: assessment of vital signs at rest and with activity

Arousal, attention, and cognition: examine mental status, learning ability, memory, motivation, and Mini-Mental State Examination

Environmental, home, and work barriers: analysis of current and potential barriers or hazards

Gait, locomotion, and balance: static and dynamic balance in sitting and standing, Functional Reach Test, Tinetti Performance Oriented Mobility Assessment,

Berg Balance Scale, outcome measurement tools, safety with/without an assistive device during gait

Joint integrity and mobility: analysis of quality of movement, examine joint hypermobility and hypomobility

Motor function: assessment of dexterity, coordination and agility, assessment of postural, equilibrium, and righting reactions

Muscle performance: strength assessment, muscle tone assessment, and tremor assessment

Posture: analysis of resting and dynamic posture

Range of motion: active and passive range of motion

Self-care and home management: functional capacity, Barthel Index, safety assessments, Parkinson's disease Questionnaire (PDQ-39)

Sensory integration: assessment of combined sensation, assessment of proprioception and kinesthesia

Ventilation, respiratory, and circulation: assessment of chest wall mobility, expansion, and excursion

What additional findings are likely with this patient?

Since Parkinson's disease is a progressive condition there are ongoing physical and cognitive impairments. A patient may develop a stooped posture and an increased risk for falling. Progression of the disease may result in dysphagia, difficulty with speech, and pulmonary impairment. Greater attention is required for skin care once nutrition and mobility are further compromised. Many patients with Parkinson's disease die from complications of bronchopneumonia.

Management:

What is the most effective management of this patient?

The medical management of Parkinson's disease relies heavily on pharmacological intervention. Dopamine replacement therapy, (Levodopa, Sinemet, Madopar) is the most effective treatment in reducing the symptoms of Parkinson's disease such as movement disorders, bradykinesia, rigidity, and tremor. Antihistamines, anticholinergics, and antidepressants are also utilized. Physical, occupational, and speech therapies may be warranted intermittently throughout the course of the disease. Physical therapy intervention should include maximizing endurance, strength, and functional mobility. Verbal cueing and oral/visual feedback are effective tools to use with this population. Family teaching, balance activities, gait training, stretching, trunk rotation activities, assistive device training, relaxation techniques, and respiratory therapy are all important components in the treatment of Parkinson's disease. Psychological and nutritional counseling are recommended.

What home care regimen should be recommended?

A home care regimen should include an exercise routine, functional mobility skills, the use of relaxation techniques, range of motion and stretching exercises, and endurance activities. A competent caretaker is vital to the success of the home program and must continuously motivate the patient to continue with mobility and endurance activities in order to avoid deleterious effects of the disease process.

Outcome:

What is the likely outcome of a course in physical therapy?

Physical therapy is recommended on an intermittent basis throughout the course of the disease and will focus on current symptoms that arise. Physical therapy will not prevent further degeneration or cure the movement disorder; however, it will assist the patient to maximize their level of function and quality of life.

What are the long-term effects of the patient's condition?

Parkinson's disease does not significantly alter a patient's lifespan if the patient is diagnosed with a generalized form between 50 and 60 years of age. As the disease progresses, however, there will be an exacerbation of all symptoms and significant loss of mobility. The inactivity and deconditioning allows for complications and eventual death.

Comparison:

What are the distinguishing characteristics of a similar condition?

Wilson's disease is inherited as an autosomal recessive trait and causes a defect in the metabolism of copper. The accumulation of copper within erythrocytes, the liver, the brain, and kidneys produces the associated degenerative changes. The patient presents with hepatic insufficiency, tremor, choreoathetoid movements, dysarthria, and progressive rigidity.

Clinical Scenarios:

Scenario One

A 35-year-old female is sent to physical therapy shortly after being diagnosed with Parkinson's disease. She is presently having difficulty maintaining a grasp on items from an assembly line at work and complains of frequently tripping.

Scenario Two

A 42-year-old male was diagnosed with Parkinson's disease four years ago. The patient requires physical therapy to reassess gait and prescribe an assistive device. The son states that the patient sits a great deal at home and lacks motivation to engage in exercise.

Patellofemoral Syndrome

Diagnosis:

What condition produces a patient's symptoms?
Patellofemoral syndrome is caused by an abnormal tracking of the patella between the femoral condyles. The tracking problem places increased and misdirected forces between the patella and femur. This most commonly occurs when the patella is pulled too far laterally during knee extension.

An injury was most likely sustained to which structure?
Patellofemoral syndrome causes damage to the articular cartilage of the patella. The damage can range from softening of the cartilage to complete cartilage destruction resulting in exposure of subchondral bone.

Inference:

What is the most likely contributing factor in the development of this condition?
The exact etiology of patellofemoral syndrome is unknown; however, it is extremely common during adolescence, is more prevalent in females than males, and has a direct association with the activity level of the patient. In an older population patellofemoral syndrome is often associated with osteoarthritis. Additional factors associated with patellofemoral syndrome include patella alta, insufficient lateral femoral condyle, weak vastus medialis obliquus, excessive pronation, excessive knee valgus, and tightness in lower extremity muscles (the iliotibial, hamstrings, gastrocnemius, and vastus lateralis).

Confirmation:

What is the most likely clinical presentation?
A patient with patellofemoral syndrome often describes a gradual onset of anterior knee pain following an increase in physical activity. The pain is characteristically located behind the patella (retropatellar pain) and may be exacerbated with activities that increase patellofemoral compressive forces (stair climbing, jumping) and also with prolonged static positioning (sitting with the knee flexed at 90 degrees as in a car, plane, theatre). Point tenderness is common over the lateral border of the patella and crepitus may be elicited when the patella is manually compressed into the trochlear groove. Visible quadriceps atrophy may be noted in the involved lower extremity particularly along the vastus medialis obliquus. The patient may also complain of burning pain when sitting for prolonged periods of time or when ascending stairs.

What laboratory or imaging studies would confirm the diagnosis?
Laboratory or imaging studies are not commonly used to diagnose patellofemoral syndrome. X-rays are often used to rule out a fracture, examine the configuration of the patellofemoral joint, and identify potential osteophytes, joint space narrowing, patella alta, and arthritic changes. Arthrogram and arthroscopy can be used to examine the articular cartilage.

What additional information should be obtained to confirm the diagnosis?
Special tests such as Clarke's sign can be useful when attempting to confirm the diagnosis. The test is performed by applying pressure immediately proximal to the upper pole of the patient's patella. The physician/therapist then asks the patient to isometrically contract the quadriceps. A positive test is indicated by a failure to fully contract the quadriceps or by the presence of retropatellar pain. The test should be performed at varying degrees of flexion and extension. It is helpful to determine the patient's Q angle and examine the alignment of the patient's feet, as these factors can contribute to the causative factors.

Examination:

What history should be documented?
Important areas to explore include past medical history, medications, current symptoms and health status, social history, occupation/recreational activities, living environment, and social support system.

What test/measures are most appropriate?
Anthropometric characteristics: knee effusion, lower extremity circumferential measurements
Arousal, attention, and cognition: examine mental status, learning ability, memory, motivation
Assistive and adaptive devices: components and safety of a device, potential utilization of crutches
Environmental, home, and work barriers: analysis of current and potential barriers or hazards
Gait, locomotion, and balance: safety during gait with an assistive device
Integumentary integrity: assessment of sensation (pain, temperature, tactile), skin assessment
Joint integrity and mobility: Clarke's sign, patella grind test (active and passive), dynamic patella tracking, patella glide test, palpation of structures, joint play, soft tissue restrictions, joint pain
Muscle performance: strength assessment, assessment of active movement, resisted isometrics, muscle contraction characteristics, muscle endurance

Orthotic, protective, and supportive devices: potential utilization of bracing, taping or wrapping
Pain: pain perception assessment scale
Range of motion: active and passive range of motion
Self-care and home management: functional capacity
Sensory integrity: proprioception and kinesthesia

What additional findings are likely with this patient?

Patients diagnosed with patellofemoral syndrome often have an increased Q angle. The normal Q angle is 13 degrees in males and 18 degrees in females. The Q angle is measured using the anterior superior iliac spine, the midpoint of the patella, and the tibial tubercle. Differential diagnosis should rule out other problems such as referred pain from the hip, Osgood-Schlatter syndrome, neuroma, patellar tendonitis, plica syndrome, and infection of the knee joint.

Management:

What is the most effective management of this patient?

Medical management of patellofemoral syndrome is usually successful with conservative measures; surgical intervention is rare. Pharmacological intervention may include acetaminophen, NSAIDs, and steroid injections into the joint. Physical therapy management includes controlling edema, stretching, strengthening, improving range of motion, and activity modification.
Mobilization activities to increase medial glide can be beneficial to increase the flexibility of the lateral fascia. Strengthening activities emphasizing the vastus medialis obliquus in non-weight bearing and weight bearing positions are recommended. Biofeedback can be a useful tool in order to selectively train the muscle. Stretching activities should emphasize the hamstrings, iliotibial band, tensor fasciae latae, and rectus femoris. Strengthening activities may include quadriceps setting exercises, straight leg raising and mini-squats incorporating the hip adductors. Exercises such as deep squats should be avoided since they will tend to aggravate the patient's condition. Patellar taping to improve the position and tracking of the patella during dynamic activities can be useful to limit irritation.

What home care regimen should be recommended?

The home care regimen should consist of range of motion, strengthening, stretching, palliative care, and functional activities. An active patient must decrease their level of activities to relieve the additional stress placed on the patellofemoral joint. A patient must also comply with recommendations for proper footwear and orthotics to improve alignment and lessen aggravation of symptoms, specifically knee pain.

Outcome:

What is the likely outcome of a course in physical therapy?

A patient with patellofemoral syndrome that undergoes conservative management may be able to return to their previous functioning within four to six weeks.

What are the long-term effects of the patient's condition?

Prognosis for a full recovery is good with successful conservative management; however, failure to adequately address the cause of the patellofemoral syndrome will likely result in a patient's condition further deteriorating. The patient may experience increased irritation of the patellofemoral joint that further impacts their ability to participate in activities of daily living. Periodic exacerbations of the condition most commonly due to an increased activity level may require further physical therapy intervention.

Comparison:

What are the distinguishing characteristics of a similar condition?

Patellar tendonitis is an overuse condition characterized by inflammatory changes of the patellar tendon. The condition is most prevalent in athletes who participate in activities requiring repetitive jumping skills. The primary complaint is often pain over the anterior portion of the superior tibia with activities such as jumping or ascending/descending stairs. Patients may also experience pain after prolonged sitting and often exhibit point tenderness at the superior pole of the patella tendon. Management of patellar tendonitis incorporates many of the same interventions as patellofemoral syndrome such as range of motion, stretching, and palliative care.

Clinical Scenarios:

Scenario One

A 14-year-old female is referred to physical therapy with patellofemoral syndrome. The patient has mild edema and is sensitive to light touch over the anterior surface of the knee. The patient reports gaining ten pounds and expresses that she is willing to do "anything" to improve her present condition.

Scenario Two

A 45-year-old male is referred to physical therapy after experiencing anterior knee pain for the last week. The patient is 19 weeks status post ACL reconstruction and has recently returned to a softball league. The patient reports an insidious onset of pain and insists that he has been faithful to his home program. A note from the referring physician confirms that the integrity of the graft is fine and he suspects patellofemoral syndrome.

Plantar Fasciitis

Diagnosis:

What condition produces a patient's symptoms?
The plantar fascia is a thin layer of tough connective tissue that supports the arch of the foot. Plantar fasciitis is an inflammatory process of the plantar fascia (or aponeurosis) at its origin on the calcaneus. Plantar fasciitis is a chronic overuse condition that develops secondary to repetitive stretching of the plantar fascia through excessive foot pronation during the loading phase of gait. This results in stress at the calcaneal origin of the plantar fascia.

An injury was most likely sustained to which structure?
Injury can occur to the plantar fascia itself and cause microtearing, inflammation, and pain. The abductor hallucis, flexor digitorum brevis, and quadratus plantae muscles share the same origin on the medial tubercle of the calcaneus and may also become inflamed and irritated.

Inference:

What is the most likely contributing factor in the development of this condition?
Factors that contribute to the development of plantar fasciitis include excessive pronation during gait, tightness of the foot and calf musculature, obesity, and possessing a high arch. A person participating in endurance sports such as running and dancing or a person with an occupation that requires prolonged walking or standing has an increased risk for plantar fasciitis. It is believed that development of plantar fasciitis results from a combination of predisposing factors. Although it is more common in the middle-age population, it also occurs in younger individuals, but usually in combination with calcaneal apophysitis.

Confirmation:

What is the most likely clinical presentation?
A patient with plantar fasciitis presents with severe pain in the heel when first standing up in the morning (when the fascia is contracted, stiff, and cold). This pain has also been reported to radiate proximally up the calf and/or distally to the toes. This is the most common symptom that relates directly to the diagnosis of plantar fasciitis and in one study was expressed in over 84% of cases. Pain typically subsides for a few hours during the day, but increases with prolonged activity or when the patient has been non-weight bearing and resumes a weight bearing posture. Pain has also been described by patients as "pain that moves around." A patient will typically experience point tenderness and pain with palpation over the calcaneal insertion of the plantar fascia. There may be bony growths in the plantar fascia near its insertion. Plantar fasciitis is usually unilateral and tightness in the Achilles tendon is found in the majority of the patients.

What laboratory or imaging studies would confirm the diagnosis?
Plantar fasciitis is initially treated based on symptoms and physical examination. If pain persists after six to eight weeks of physical therapy intervention, MRI may be used to confirm the diagnosis. Other diagnostic tools may include x-ray and bone scan to rule out a stress fracture, rheumatology work up to rule out systemic etiology, and EMG testing to rule out nerve entrapment.

What additional information should be obtained to confirm the diagnosis?
A thorough history and biomechanical assessment of the foot, observation of the fat pad, examination for Achilles tendon tightness, analysis of footwear, and gait disturbances all assist in diagnosing plantar fasciitis.

Examination:

What history should be documented?
Important areas to explore include mechanism of current injury, training routine, past medical history, medications, social history and habits, occupation, living environment, and social support system.

What test/measures are most appropriate?
Anthropometric characteristics: circumferential measurements of affected area or extremity
Arousal, attention, and cognition: examine mental status, learning ability, memory, motivation
Community and work integration: analysis of community, work, and leisure activities
Environmental, home, and work barriers: analysis of current and potential barriers or hazards
Gait, locomotion, and balance: biomechanical analysis of gait during walking and running (if appropriate), footprint analysis, dynamic plantar pressure distribution
Integumentary inspection: assessment of sensation, skin assessment
Joint integrity and mobility: assessment of swelling, inflammation, and joint restriction
Muscle performance: strength assessment, muscle endurance
Pain: pain perception scale, visual analog scale
Orthotic, protective, and supportive devices: potential utilization of taping or use of cushions

Posture: analysis of resting and dynamic posture
Range of motion: active and passive range of motion
Sensory integrity: assessment of proprioception and kinesthesia
Self-care and home management: assessment of functional capacity

What additional findings are likely with this patient?

Bony hypertrophy can occur at the origin of the plantar fascia resulting in a heel spur. Plantar fasciitis is a relative of heel spur syndrome, but is not the same condition. Heel spurs develop initially as calcium deposits that form due to the repetitive stress and inflammation in the plantar fascia.

Management:

What is the most effective management of this patient?

Medical and pharmacological management of a patient with plantar fasciitis usually requires local corticosteroid injections or anti-inflammatory medications to reduce inflammation within the plantar fascia. Physical therapy intervention consists of ice massage, deep friction massage, shoe modification, heel insert application, foot orthotic prescription, modification of activities to include non-weight bearing endurance activities, and a gentle stretching program of the Achilles tendon and plantar fascia. Muscle strengthening exercises for the intrinsic and extrinsic muscles should be implemented once the acute symptoms have subsided. During the acute phase the patient must also modify activities and rest the affected foot. Heel cup prescription and casting may also be indicated.

What home care regimen should be recommended?

A home care regimen for a patient with plantar fasciitis should include ongoing strengthening and stretching exercises (especially stretching of the gastrocnemius and medial fascial band in the morning and prior to and after exercise), maintenance of a fitness program, the use of proper footwear, and the use of foot orthotics and heel inserts if warranted. Night tension splints may be indicated if symptoms persist.

Outcome:

What is the likely outcome of a course in physical therapy?

Conservative physical therapy intervention on an outpatient basis in combination with a consistent home program should allow the patient to return to a more functional level within eight weeks. Total resolution of symptoms can take up to twelve months. Physical therapy, orthotic prescription, splinting, pharmacological injections, and physician follow-up are all components of the treatment program that may be required for a positive outcome.

What are the long-term effects of the patient's condition?

A patient previously diagnosed with plantar fasciitis is at an increased risk for recurrence; however, successful conservative management, compliance with a home program, and proper footwear will decrease the incidence of any negative long-term effects. If conservative management fails the patient may require surgical intervention; however, this option is relatively rare. Approximately 10% of patients can develop persistent, chronic, and disabling symptoms.

Comparison:

What are the distinguishing characteristics of a similar condition?

The tarsal tunnel is the region where the tibial nerve passes between the medial malleolus and the calcaneus. The tibial nerve splits into the medial and lateral plantar nerves while still traversing in the tunnel along with other nerves in this region. Tarsal tunnel syndrome is characterized by pain that is experienced with weight bearing, but not with direct palpation to the plantar fascia. Characteristics of tarsal tunnel syndrome include complaints of numbness, burning pain, tingling, and paresthesias at the heel. Etiology consists of entrapment and compression of the posterior tibial nerve or plantar nerves within the tarsal tunnel due to inflammation or thickening of the flexor retinaculum.

Clinical Scenarios:

Scenario One

A 19-year-old male athlete is referred to physical therapy with bilateral heel pain. The physician has ruled out systemic disorders and diagnosed bilateral mechanical plantar fasciitis. The athlete is a swimmer and began running cross-country last fall. The patient is otherwise healthy, but wants to return to athletic activities as soon as possible.

Scenario Two

A 56-year-old female is referred to physical therapy with left plantar fasciitis. The patient is mildly obese and works the night shift at a paper mill. She stands at her station throughout the shift and is required to walk between the two buildings every hour. The patient has a history of mild asthma and a cardiac murmur. She is anxious to obtain relief from her symptoms since she feels that her employment may be jeopardized .

Reflex Sympathetic Dystrophy

Diagnosis:

What condition produces a patient's symptoms?
Reflex sympathetic dystrophy (RSD), also known as complex regional pain syndrome type I (occurring subsequent to trauma) or complex regional pain syndrome type II (associated with peripheral nerve injury) is usually found in an extremity that has experienced some form of trauma. Symptoms result from a disturbance in the functioning of the sympathetic nervous system. The increase in sympathetic activity causes a release of norepinephrine in the periphery and subsequent vasoconstriction of blood vessels. This results in pain and an increase in sensitivity to peripheral stimulation.

An injury was most likely sustained to which structure?
RSD results from injured sensory nerve fibers at one somatic level that initiates sympathetic efferent activity that affects many segmental levels. The extremity of origin sustains injury as well as areas adjacent to the extremity.

Inference:

What is the most likely contributing factor in the development of this condition?
The exact etiology of RSD is unknown; however, predisposing factors include trauma, surgery, CVA, TBI, repetitive motion disorders, and lower motor neuron and peripheral nerve injuries. RSD is reported to occur following 5% of all injuries. While many cases of RSD resolve, others progress and become a disabling disorder. RSD can affect all age groups but is most likely found in the age group of 35-60 years with females three times more likely to be affected by RSD than males.

Confirmation:

What is the most likely clinical presentation?
A patient with RSD will experience intense, burning, and chronic pain in the affected extremity that will eventually spread proximally. Early in the syndrome the degree of pain is greater than expected based on the amount of trauma that the tissue sustained. Edema, thermal changes, discoloration, stiffness, and dryness are seen during stage I (acute stage) of RSD. Progression to stage II (dystrophic stage) is characterized by worsening and constant pain, continued edema, and trophic skin changes. X-rays may reveal bone loss, osteoporosis, and subchondral bone erosion in the affected extremity. Stage III (atrophic stage) is characterized by pain that continues

to spread, hardened edema, decreased limb temperature, and atrophic changes to fingertips or toes. X-rays at this stage may reveal demineralization and ankylosis. Motor disorders such as tremor, spasms, and atrophy may also be present throughout each stage of RSD.

What laboratory or imaging studies would confirm the diagnosis?
Imaging studies that can assist with the diagnosis of RSD include X-rays, thermographic studies, a three-phase bone scan, and laser Doppler flowmetry.

What additional information should be obtained to confirm the diagnosis?
RSD is diagnosed primarily through a complete physical examination and a patient's complete medical history including a history and course of illness.

Examination:

What history should be documented?
Important areas to explore include past medical history, medications, family history, current symptoms, current health status, social history and habits, occupation, leisure activities, and social support system.

What test/measures are most appropriate?
Anthropometric characteristics: circumferential measurements of affected area or extremity
Arousal, attention, and cognition: examine mental status, learning ability, memory, motivation
Environmental, home, and work barriers: analysis of current and potential barriers or hazards
Gait, locomotion, and balance: static and dynamic balance in sitting and standing, safety during gait
Integumentary integrity: skin assessment, assessment of sensation, skin temperature changes
Joint integrity and mobility: assessment of hyper- and hypomobility of a joint, soft tissue swelling
Motor function: motor assessment scales, assessment of sensorimotor integration, physical performance scales
Muscle performance: strength assessment, muscle tone assessment
Pain: pain perception scale, visual analog scale, assessment of muscle soreness, McGill Pain Questionnaire
Reflex integrity: assessment of deep tendon and pathological reflexes
Posture: analysis of resting and dynamic posture
Range of motion: active and passive range of motion
Sensory integrity: assessment of proprioception and kinesthesia
Self-care and home management: assessment of functional capacity

What additional findings are likely with this patient?

RSD will affect a patient's function throughout the progression of this neurovascular syndrome. RSD may progress to the point of bone demineralization and joint ankylosis (seen in stage III). Muscle atrophy, contractures, spasms, and incoordination will also contribute to functional decline. Depression and anxiety are also frequently seen and require medical attention. Malingering for secondary gain has been documented in some cases and should be monitored by the rehabilitation team.

Management:

What is the most effective management of this patient?

RSD requires prolonged medical management. Treatment is based on identifying the underlying cause and stage of RSD at the time of diagnosis. Pharmacological intervention may include NSAIDs and corticosteroids for pain relief in early stages. Amitriptyline may be used for sleep and calcium channel blockers used for increasing peripheral circulation. Baclofen has been used as a long-term intervention to assist motor function. Biphosphanate administration is warranted in later stages to combat bone loss. Surgical interventions such as sympathetic blocks or a sympathectomy are used to alleviate pain. Physical therapy intervention is a key component in the management of RSD. Pain control, patient education, skin care, joint mobilization, desensitization, and functional activity training are vital to the program. Modalities, pool therapy, relaxation training, and a home program all assist a patient with management of this syndrome.

What home care regimen should be recommended?

A home program is vital to the management of RSD. Stretching and ROM, light weight bearing activities, ice and/or heat, TENS, and light exercise for conditioning are all key components of a home program. The patient must be educated and encouraged to use the involved extremity as tolerated. Edema management using a pump or compression garments may be indicated. Functional activities must also be encouraged.

Outcome:

What is the likely outcome of a course in physical therapy?

Overall prognosis is better for a patient that begins treatment early in the cycle of the disease process. Physical therapy attempts to break the pain cycle and allows for a patient to continue with functional activities. Outcome is also dependent on a patient's motivation to maintain all aspects of a home program.

What are the long-term effects of the patient's condition?

RSD can spontaneously resolve or can continue with ongoing symptoms that can last for years or follow a pattern of remissions and recurring symptoms that develop from subsequent injuries. A patient's long-term outcome is dependent on how early the RSD was detected and treated. Research indicates a better prognosis if treatment is initiated within the first six months of the disease process.

Comparison:

What are the distinguishing characteristics of a similar condition?

Sympathetically maintained pain (SMP) is a pain syndrome that is maintained by sympathetic efferent activity and is caused by a partial peripheral nerve lesion. SMP occurs less than RSD and is characterized by pain that is produced by a non-painful stimulus, vasomotor disturbances, and trophic changes. These symptoms remain localized to the affected nerve and the pain can usually be temporarily alleviated by sympathetic nerve block. Physical therapy intervention is warranted to assist with pain control through the use of modalities.

Clinical Scenarios:

Scenario One
A 39-year-old female is seen in physical therapy with stage I (acute) RSD. The patient complains of burning pain in her left arm and presents with mild edema. The patient injured her shoulder two months ago. Past medical history includes being diagnosed with fibromyalgia two years ago. She is a team manager for a photography company and works approximately 50 hours per week.

Scenario Two
A 62-year-old female is evaluated in physical therapy. She was diagnosed with RSD 13 months ago. She complains of significant pain in her right lower extremity and cannot walk without a walker. She has both hip and knee flexion contractures and significant swelling of the affected lower extremity.

Restrictive Lung Disease

Diagnosis:

What condition produces a patient's symptoms?
Restrictive lung disease (RLD) is a classification of disorders caused by a pulmonary or extrapulmonary restriction that produces impairment in lung expansion and an abnormal reduction in pulmonary ventilation. There are multiple conditions that can cause restrictive lung disease. Many symptoms are common regardless of the underlying etiology and other symptoms are disease-specific.

An injury was most likely sustained to which structure?
Pulmonary restriction of the lungs can be caused by tumor, interstitial pulmonary fibrosis, scarring within the lungs, and pneumonia. Extrapulmonary restrictions of the lungs include pleural effusion, chest wall stiffness, structural abnormality, postural deformity, respiratory muscle weakness, and central nervous system injury.

Inference:

What is the most likely contributing factor in the development of this condition?
There are varying etiologies for the group of disorders that cause restrictive lung disease. Musculoskeletal etiology includes scoliosis, pectus excavatum or other chest wall deformity, rib fractures, ankylosing spondylitis, and kyphosis. Pulmonary etiology includes idiopathic pulmonary fibrosis, pneumonia, pleural effusion, sarcoidosis, hyaline membrane disease, and tumor within the lungs. Other etiologies include inhalation of toxic fumes, drug therapy, asbestos, rheumatoid arthritis, systemic lupus erythematosus, muscular dystrophy, spinal cord injury, obesity, neurologic, and neuromuscular diseases.

Confirmation:

What is the most likely clinical presentation?
The clinical presentation varies based on the underlying cause or disease process. The pathogenesis of RLD includes a decrease in lung and chest wall compliance, decrease in lung volumes and an increase in the work of breathing. Generally, restrictive lung disease is characterized by a reduction of lung volumes (total lung capacity, vital capacity, inspiratory reserve volume, tidal volume, expiratory reserve volume, and inspiratory capacity) due to impaired lung expansion. A patient with restrictive lung disease will present with decreased chest mobility, decreased breath sounds, shortness of breath, hypoxemia, a rapid and shallow respiratory pattern (tachypnea), respiratory muscle weakness, ineffective cough, and increased use of accessory muscles.

What laboratory or imaging studies would confirm the diagnosis?
A chest radiograph is utilized to evaluate lung structure and evidence of fibrosis, infiltrates, tumor, and deformity. Arterial blood gas analysis may indicate a decrease in PaO_2.

What additional information should be obtained to confirm the diagnosis?
Pulmonary function testing will result in impaired vital capacity (VC), forced vital capacity (FVC), and total lung capacity (TLC). The patient will usually present with normal residual volume (RV) and expiration flow rates. Expiratory reserve volume (ERV) and functional residual capacity (FRC) are often decreased. Arterial blood gas analysis examines the presence of hypoxemia and hypocapnia.

Examination:

What history should be documented?
Important areas to explore include past medical history, medications, current health status, social history and habits, occupation, living environment, and social support system.

What test/measures are most appropriate?
Aerobic capacity and endurance: assessment of vital signs at rest and with activity, perceived exertion scale, pulse oximetry, auscultation of the lungs
Arousal, attention, and cognition: examine mental status, learning ability, memory, motivation
Assistive and adaptive devices: analysis of components and safety of a device
Environmental, home, and work barriers: analysis of current and potential barriers or hazards
Gait, locomotion, and balance: static and dynamic balance in sitting and standing, safety during gait with/without an assistive device, Berg Balance Scale, Tinetti Performance Oriented Mobility Assessment, Functional Ambulation Profile
Motor function: assessment of dexterity, coordination and agility, assessment of postural, equilibrium, and righting reactions
Muscle performance: strength assessment, active movement
Posture: analysis of resting and dynamic posture
Range of motion: active and passive range of motion
Self-care and home management: assessment of functional capacity

Ventilation, respiration, and circulation: auscultation of breath sounds, thoracoabdominal movement, pulmonary function testing, perceived exertion scale, assessment of cough and clearance of secretions

What additional findings are likely with this patient?

A patient with restrictive lung disease may become incapable of deep inspiration due to poor lung expansion. As restrictive lung disease progresses respiratory muscle fatigue will lead to impaired alveolar ventilation and carbon dioxide retention. A patient will initially present with exertional dyspnea and progress to dyspnea at rest if the restriction progresses.

Hypoxemia, pulmonary hypertension, cor pulmonale, severe decrease in oxygenation, and ventilatory failure are complications and outcomes of advanced restrictive lung disease.

Management:

What is the most effective management of this patient?

Medical management of restrictive lung disease includes treatment of the underlying cause through pharmacological intervention, physical therapy, and potential surgical intervention. Physical therapy intervention is based on the severity of the condition, but is consistently oriented toward the goals of maximizing gas exchange and obtaining maximal functional capacity. Physical therapy intervention may include body mechanics, posture training, diaphragm and ventilatory muscle strengthening, relaxation and energy conservation techniques, and the use of these techniques during functional mobility. Breathing exercises, coughing techniques, and airway secretion clearance are often components of a comprehensive care plan.

What home care regimen should be recommended?

A home care regimen should include breathing strategies and exercises, proper positioning, energy conservation and pacing techniques, general strengthening and endurance activities, and postural awareness with mobility. Low-level general strengthening and endurance training are indicated as tolerated.

Outcome:

What is the likely outcome of a course in physical therapy?

Physical therapy intervention is specific to the underlying cause of the restrictive lung disease. Outcome is based on the etiology of the restrictive lung disease and patient response to physical therapy intervention. Treatment goals should include improving oxygenation and obtaining the maximal level of functioning.

What are the long-term effects of the patient's condition?

Long-term effects from restrictive lung disease are also specific to the underlying cause. Some disorders require surgical intervention that alleviates the condition while other conditions are progressive and irreversible. Some patients with end-stage disease may be candidates for lung transplantation, however, most eventually progress to ventilatory failure. Idiopathic pulmonary fibrosis is a restrictive lung disease that has a high mortality rate within four to six years of diagnosis whereas many conditions that cause restrictive lung disease are alleviated through appropriate management.

Comparison:

What are the distinguishing characteristics of a similar condition?

Tuberculosis is an infectious and inflammatory systemic disease that can result in restrictive lung disease. The disease is a chronic pulmonary and extrapulmonary disease that causes fibrosis within the lungs. It is caused by the mycobacterium tuberculosis (tubercle bacillus) and transmitted through infected airborne droplets that are inhaled. Pulmonary symptoms include fatigue, weakness, an initial non-productive cough, and dyspnea with exertion. The disease also can affect other systems within the body including the lymph nodes and organs.

Pharmacological intervention is the primary means of treating a patient with tuberculosis.

Clinical Scenarios:

Scenario One

A 32-year-old male shows signs of restrictive lung disease. The patient is slightly short of breath with activity, has difficulty with deep inspiration, and complains of a non-productive cough. The patient had prolonged exposure to asbestos at his last place of employment and is under a physician's care. The physician referred the patient to physical therapy to improve the patient's general pulmonary status.

Scenario Two

A 65-year-old female is seen in physical therapy for restrictive lung disease secondary to the removal of a benign tumor from the left lung. The patient reports having difficulty breathing, limited inhalation capability, and a productive cough. The patient has not been able to perform self-care and home activities secondary to breathing difficulties and relies solely on her 72-year-old husband.

Rheumatoid Arthritis

Diagnosis:

What condition produces a patient's symptoms?
Rheumatoid arthritis (RA) is a systemic autoimmune disorder of the connective tissue that is characterized by chronic inflammation within synovial membranes, tendon sheaths, and articular cartilage. The acute and chronic inflammatory changes produce the symptoms of this condition.

An injury was most likely sustained to which structure?
Smaller peripheral joints are usually the first to be affected by RA; however, all connective tissue may become involved. Inflammation is present within the synovial membrane and granulation tissue forms as a result of the synovitis. The granulation tissue and protein degrading enzymes erode articular cartilage resulting in destruction, adhesions, and fibrosis within the joint.

Inference:

What is the most likely contributing factor in the development of this condition?
The etiology of RA is unknown; however, there appears to be evidence of genetic predisposition with viral or bacterial triggers. Approximately 80% of individuals diagnosed with RA possess a positive rheumatoid factor (RF). RF represents the presence of autoantibodies that conflict with immunoglobulin antibodies found in the blood. The incidence of RA in women is three times greater than the incidence in men.

Confirmation:

What is the most likely clinical presentation?
RA affects approximately 1-2% of the population within the United States or two million individuals (1.5 million women, 600,000 men). This condition is characterized by periods of exacerbations and is diagnosed most frequently between 30 and 50 years of age. RA will vary in onset and progression from patient to patient. Onset of RA may be sudden or develop over a period of weeks. Early characteristics include fatigue, bilateral involvement, tenderness of smaller joints, and low-grade fever. Patients often experience pain with motion, stiffness including prolonged morning stiffness, and progression of symptoms to larger synovial joints. In late stages of the disease the heart can become affected and deformities, subluxations, and contractures can occur.

What laboratory or imaging studies would confirm the diagnosis?
Blood work assists with the diagnosis of RA through evaluation of the rheumatoid factor (RF), white blood cell count, erythrocyte sedimentation rate, hemoglobin, and hematocrit values. A synovial fluid analysis evaluates the content of synovial fluid within a joint. X-rays can be used to evaluate the joint space and the extent of decalcification.

What additional information should be obtained to confirm the diagnosis?
Physical examination and patient history of symptoms are required to confirm the diagnosis. The American Rheumatoid Association has designed diagnostic criteria for RA that can be used as a guide to determine a definite, possible, probable or classic diagnosis.

Examination:

What history should be documented?
Important areas to explore include past medical history, family history, medications, current symptoms and health status, living environment, social history and habits, occupation, and social support system.

What test/measures are most appropriate?
Aerobic capacity and endurance: assessment of vital signs at rest and with activity, timed walk, $VO_{2\,max}$
Anthropometric characteristics: circumferential measurements of all affected joints
Arousal, attention, and cognition: examine mental status, learning ability, memory, motivation
Community and work integration: analysis of community, work, and leisure activities
Ergonomics and body mechanics: analysis of dexterity and coordination
Environmental, home, and work barriers: analysis of current and potential barriers or hazards
Gait, locomotion, and balance: safety during gait with/without an assistive device, Functional Ambulation Profile, gait over level/unlevel surfaces, visual inspection of gait with and without shoes
Integumentary integrity: skin and sensation assessment
Joint integrity and mobility: assessment of joint hypomobility, soft tissue inflammation, presence of deformity, active joint count, articular tenderness
Motor function: equilibrium and righting reactions, motor assessment scales, coordination, posture and balance in sitting, physical performance scales
Muscle performance: break testing of isometric contractions, manometer method of strength testing

Orthotic, protective, and supportive devices: potential utilization of bracing, analysis of movement while wearing a device
Pain: pain perception assessment scale
Range of motion: active and passive range of motion
Self-care and home management: assessment of functional capacity
Sensory integrity: assessment of sensation, proprioception, and kinesthesia

What additional findings are likely with this patient?

Extraarticular manifestations with RA can include pericarditis, anemia, tearing of tendons and musculature, osteoporosis, swan neck and/or boutonniere deformities, compression neuropathies, peripheral neuropathies, depression, pleurisy, skin changes, and anorexia.

Management:

What is the most effective management of this patient?

Early medical management of a patient with RA is critical to improve the long-term outcomes of the disease. Medical treatment will focus on pain relief, reduction of edema, and preservation of joint integrity. Pharmacological intervention is required to decrease inflammation and retard the progression of the disease. NSAIDs, corticosteroids, and disease-modifying medications such as methotrexate are indicated. Physical therapy management during the acute stage or exacerbation includes patient education regarding regular rest, pain relief, relaxation, positioning, joint protection techniques, splinting, energy conservation, and body mechanics. Treatment may include gentle massage, hydrotherapy, hot pack, paraffin or cold modalities, gentle isometrics, and instruction in the use of assistive devices. Treatment during the acute stage should avoid resistive exercise, deep heating modalities, and any form of active stretching since these activities will further exacerbate the arthritis. Physical therapy management during the chronic stage or remission focuses on improving overall functional capacity, endurance, and strength. Treatment consists of low-impact conditioning through swimming or the stationary bicycle. Gentle stretching may be indicated to maintain available range of motion; however, aggressive stretching is contraindicated.

What home care regimen should be recommended?

A home care regimen for a patient with RA must maintain a delicate balance between activity and rest. The patient should perform low-level exercise, utilize relaxation and energy conservation techniques, and use splints as needed. The patient should recognize when total rest is indicated due to an acute exacerbation.

Outcome:

What is the likely outcome of a course in physical therapy?

Physical therapy cannot halt the progression of RA; however, it can improve a patient's ability to function. Physical therapy may be indicated intermittently throughout the disease process with goals that focus on pain relief, relaxation, improving motion, and preventing deformity.

What are the long-term effects of the patient's condition?

RA is a chronic disease process that currently does not have a known cure, progresses at a varied rate, creates irreversible damage and deformity, and results in disability. As the disease progresses there is bilateral and symmetrical involvement of joints. Systemic effects include insomnia, fatigue, and organ involvement including the heart and lungs.

Comparison:

What are the distinguishing characteristics of a similar condition?

Osteoarthritis is a chronic degenerative condition that usually develops secondary to repetitive trauma, disease or obesity. The hyaline cartilage in the joint softens and breaks apart allowing bone-to-bone contact that results in joint deformity, crepitus, impaired range of motion, and pain. Pain typically increases with prolonged activity. Joints become swollen and tender and joint deformity develops. Men and women are equally affected by osteoarthritis. Surgical procedures including osteotomy and joint replacement may be indicated if conservative treatment is unsuccessful.

Clinical Scenarios:

Scenario One

A 38-year-old female diagnosed with RA is seen in an outpatient clinic. The patient history reveals fatigue and malaise for two to three weeks and pain in the fingers and wrists. The patient has difficulty caring for herself at home and is on medical leave from her job. The patient does not have any other significant past medical history and resides alone.

Scenario Two

A 74-year-old male diagnosed with RA is treated by a physical therapist. The patient presents with multi-joint involvement, deformities of the hands and feet, poor endurance, stiffness, and pain. The patient is ambulatory, however, is currently in a wheelchair secondary to pain from an exacerbation. The patient is oriented and has a history of COPD.

Rotator Cuff Tendonitis

Diagnosis:

What condition produces a patient's symptoms?

Repetitive overhead activities can produce impingement of the supraspinatus tendon immediately proximal to the greater tubercle of the humerus. The impingement is caused by an inability of a weak supraspinatus muscle to adequately depress the head of the humerus in the glenoid fossa during elevation of the arm. As a result the humerus translates superiorly due to the disproportionate action of the deltoid muscle. Primary impingement occurs from intrinsic or extrinsic factors within the subacromial space. Secondary impingement describes symptoms that occur from poor mechanics or instability at the shoulder joint.

An injury was most likely sustained to which structure?

The supraspinatus muscle has the most commonly involved tendon in rotator cuff tendonitis. The muscle originates on the supraspinatus fossa of the scapula and inserts on the greater tubercle of the humerus. Bicipital and infraspinatus tendonitis as well as bursitis may also co-exist as other contributing factors.

Inference:

What is the most likely contributing factor in the development of this condition?

Individuals participating in activities that require excessive overhead activity such as swimming, tennis, baseball, painting, and other manual labor activities are at increased risk for rotator cuff tendonitis. Excessive use of the upper extremity following a prolonged period of inactivity also can produce this condition. Statistically individuals from 25-40 years of age are the most likely to develop this condition.

Confirmation:

What is the most likely clinical presentation?

A patient with rotator cuff tendonitis often reports difficulty with overhead activities and a dull ache following periods of activity. The patient may experience a feeling of weakness and identify the presence of a painful arc of motion most commonly occurring between 60 and 120 degrees of active abduction. The patient usually presents with pain with palpation of the musculotendinous junction of the involved muscle and/or with stretching or resisted contraction of the muscle. Pain often increases at night resulting in difficulty sleeping on the affected side. The patient will often have difficulty with dressing and repetitive shoulder motions such as lifting, reaching, throwing, swinging or pushing and pulling with the involved upper extremity.

What laboratory or imaging studies would confirm the diagnosis?

Magnetic resonance imaging can be used to identify the presence of rotator cuff tendonitis; however, due to the high cost it is not commonly employed prior to the initiation of formal treatment. X-rays with the shoulder laterally rotated can be used to identify the presence of calcific deposits or other bony abnormalities.

What additional information should be obtained to confirm the diagnosis?

A number of specific special tests including the empty can test, Jobe test, Neer impingement test, and Hawkins-Kennedy impingement test can be used to confirm the presence of rotator cuff tendonitis or impingement.

Examination:

What history should be documented?

Important areas to explore include past medical history, family history, medications, history of symptoms, current health status, living environment, social history and habits, occupation, and social support system.

What test/measures are most appropriate?

Anthropometric characteristics: upper extremity circumferential measurements
Arousal, attention, and cognition: examine mental status, learning ability, memory, motivation
Assistive and adaptive devices: analysis of components and safety of a device
Community and work integration: analysis of community, work, and leisure activities
Integumentary integrity: skin assessment, assessment of sensation
Joint integrity and mobility: soft tissue swelling and inflammation, assessment of joint play, palpation of the joint, empty can test, Neer impingement test, Hawkins-Kennedy impingement test
Motor function: posture and balance
Muscle performance: strength assessment
Pain: pain perception assessment scale
Posture: analysis of resting and dynamic posture
Range of motion: active and passive range of motion
Reflex integrity: assessment of deep tendon reflexes
Self-care and home management: assessment of functional capacity

What additional findings are likely with this patient?

Rotator cuff tendonitis often presents in association with impingement syndrome. Impingement syndrome typically involves the supraspinatus tendon, glenoid labrum, long head of the biceps, and subacromial bursa. It is extremely difficult to determine through examination the level of involvement of each of the identified structures.

Management:

What is the most effective management of this patient?

Medical management of acute rotator cuff tendonitis usually includes pharmacological intervention and physical therapy. Pharmacological intervention will focus on pain relief through analgesics and NSAIDs. Acute physical therapy intervention guidelines should include cryotherapy, activity modification, range of motion, and rest. As the acute phase subsides the patient is often instructed in strengthening exercises. Since the rotator cuff muscles are dependent on adequate blood supply and oxygen tension it is essential that all range of motion and strengthening exercises are pain free. Range of motion exercises using a pulley system or a cane can serve as an effective intervention. Strengthening exercises are initiated with the arm at the patient's side in order to prevent the possibility of impingement. Elastic tubing or handheld weights are often the preferred equipment of choice. It is important for the entire rotator cuff to be strong prior to initiating overhead activities. Shoulder shrugs and push-ups with the arms abducted to 90 degrees can effectively be used to strengthen the upper trapezius and serratus anterior. This type of activity promotes elevation of the acromion without direct contact with the rotator cuff.

What home care regimen should be recommended?

The home care regimen should consist of range of motion, strengthening, palliative care, and functional activities as warranted based on the results of the patient examination.

Outcome:

What is the likely outcome of a course in physical therapy?

A patient with rotator cuff tendonitis should be able to return to their previous level of functioning with conservative management within four to six weeks. Outcome can be dependent, however, on the patient's classification of stage I, II or III impingement syndrome. Stage I is usually found in the population less than 25 years of age and consists of localized inflammation, edema and minimal bleeding around the rotator cuff. Stage II represents progressive deterioration of the tissues surrounding the rotator cuff

and is common in 25 to 40-year-old patients. Stage III represents the end-stage and is usually found in patients over 40 years of age. There is usually disruption and/or rupture of numerous soft tissue structures.

What are the long-term effects of the patient's condition?

Failure to adequately treat rotator cuff tendonitis may necessitate significant activity modification or more aggressive surgical management such as subacromial decompression. Prolonged inflammation of the rotator cuff tendon may facilitate eventual tearing of the rotator cuff musculature.

Comparison:

What are the distinguishing characteristics of a similar condition?

A rotator cuff tear is usually the result of repetitive microtrauma but can also result suddenly from a single traumatic event. Partial tears often occur in a younger population while complete tears more commonly occur in older individuals. The mechanism of injury is often a fall on an outstretched arm or a sudden strain applied to the shoulder during pushing or pulling activities. Diagnosis is made through MRI to identify the tear. Surgical repair of the rotator cuff is often required and may be done with arthroscopy or through a traditional open technique. The shoulder is usually protected by a sling and small abduction pillow for the first six weeks post surgery. Rehabilitation and return to full function can take upwards of six months; heavy lifting may be restricted for six to twelve months following surgery.

Clinical Scenarios:

Scenario One

A 23-year-old female diagnosed with rotator cuff tendonitis is referred to physical therapy after experiencing pain while swimming the breaststroke in a competitive swim meet one week ago. The patient participates on a school swim team and a private club and practices four to six times a week. A few days after experiencing the shoulder pain the patient was back in the pool; however, was unable to return to her previous training regimen.

Scenario Two

A 45-year-old male employed as a pipe fitter is referred to physical therapy after subacromial decompression. The patient is one week status post surgery and is anxious to "test" his involved shoulder. Prior to surgery the patient was placed on "light duty." It has been six months since the patient was able to perform his job without restrictions. The patient presently denies any pain in the involved shoulder.

Sciatica Secondary to a Herniated Disk

Diagnosis:

What condition produces a patient's symptoms?
A herniated disk is an intervertebral disk that bulges and protrudes posterolaterally against a nerve root. Sciatica is the diagnosis of compression of the sciatic nerve (L4, L5, S1, S2, S3) secondary to a herniated disk causing a patient's symptoms. Other causes for sciatica include tumor, infection, spondylolisthesis, narrowing of the canal, and blood clots.

An injury was most likely sustained to which structure?
As a patient get older there are natural and significant alterations in the composition of the intervertebral disks and supporting structures. In a herniated disk the nucleus pulposus has bulged posterolaterally secondary to a weakening of the outer annulus fibrosis and posterior longitudinal ligament. The sciatic nerve experiences an inflammatory response and subsequent damage secondary to the compression from the herniated disk.

Inference:

What is the most likely contributing factor in the development of this condition?
The most common contributing factor for this condition is the natural aging process. Each decade the composition of the annulus fibrosus and nucleus pulposus is altered and decreases in overall stability. Once there is adequate structural breakdown within the disk a patient becomes a high risk for injury. A "normal mechanical load on a normal disk" is now an "excessive load on a compromised disk." As expected, sciatica secondary to a herniated disk is most often seen in patients between 40 and 60 years of age.

Confirmation:

What is the most likely clinical presentation?
Sciatica is characterized by low back and gleuteal pain that typically radiates down the back of the thigh along the sciatic nerve distribution. Sciatic pain occurs from nerve root compression and can be dull, aching or sharp. Pain may have a sudden onset or develop gradually over time. Early sciatica may involve discomfort or pain limited to the low back and gleuteal region. Leg pain can become greater than the back pain and can radiate the entire length of the nerve to the toes. The patient may also experience: intermittent numbness and tingling localized to the dermatomal distribution, limited thoracolumbar range of motion in all planes, tenderness to palpation at the segment of herniation, and muscle guarding.

What laboratory or imaging studies would confirm the diagnosis?
Radiologic testing of the spine and electrophysiologic studies are initially performed to assist with diagnosis. Other imaging may include myelogram, discography, CT scan or MRI. Blood work may assist with differential diagnosis.

What additional information should be obtained to confirm the diagnosis?
A full examination should be performed that includes history (trauma, osteoporosis, corticosteroid use), functional assessment, inspection, palpation, and special tests. The straight leg raise test will reproduce symptoms in the case of a herniated disk. The exam should also include testing for non-organic back pain to rule out psychological factors.

Examination:

What history should be documented?
Important areas to explore include past medical history and treatment, history of trauma and accidents, medications, family history, current symptoms, current health status, social history and habits, occupation, leisure activities, and social support system.

What test/measures are most appropriate?
Arousal, attention, and cognition: examine mental status, learning ability, memory, motivation
Assistive and adaptive devices: analysis of components and safety of a device
Community and work integration: analysis of community, work, and leisure activities
Environmental, home, and work barriers: analysis of current and potential barriers or hazards
Ergonomics and body mechanics: analysis of dexterity and coordination
Gait, locomotion, and balance: static and dynamic balance in sitting and standing, Functional Ambulation Profile
Integumentary integrity: skin assessment, assessment of sensation, dermatome testing of the lower extremities
Joint integrity and mobility: assessment of hyper- and hypomobility of a joint, soft tissue swelling and inflammation
Muscle performance: strength assessment, resisted isometrics, straight leg raise testing
Pain: Oswestry Function Test, McGill Pain Questionnaire, visual analog scale
Posture: analysis of resting and dynamic posture
Range of motion: active and passive movement of the spine, combined movements, segmental mobility testing

Reflex integrity: assessment of deep tendon and pathological reflexes (clonus)
Self-care and home management: assessment of functional capacity, Functional Independence Measure

What additional findings are likely with this patient?

Sciatica will produce pain that increases with certain positions due to an increase in intradiskal pressure. Pain will increase in a sitting position or when lifting, forward bending or twisting. Sneezing and coughing can also exacerbate the pain. Although a patient may want to stop all activity to relieve pain, prolonged bed rest is contraindicated and will not relieve pain on a long-term basis.

Management:

What is the most effective management of this patient?

Medical management of sciatica due to a herniated disk includes short-term bed rest, overall reduction of intradiskal pressure, patient education, physical therapy, medications, and in rare instances surgical intervention. Pharmacological intervention will incorporate NSAIDs initially to relieve pain followed by epidural injections of cortisone and local anesthetics that may be indicated for temporary relief; however, do not alter the root of the problem. Physical therapy intervention should include patient education on positioning and biomechanics, pain management, traction, heat, lumbar stabilization exercises, McKenzie exercises, stretching, and endurance activities. Swimming, stationary bicycling and walking are indicated within tolerance. Lifting, squatting, and climbing are contraindicated due to the significant increase in intradiskal pressure. Most herniations will spontaneously decrease in size with conservative treatment. Research indicates that the majority of patients improve with two to four months of conservative treatment; however, approximately 2% of patients undergo surgery. Common surgical intervention may include laminectomy, discectomy, chemonucleolysis, laser discectomy or laminotomy.

What home care regimen should be recommended?

A home care regimen should include ongoing caution regarding positioning and constant effort to decrease intradiskal pressure. A home exercise program including stabilization exercises is indicated as well as other aerobic/endurance activities to tolerance.

Outcome:

What is the likely outcome of a course in physical therapy?

Most patients improve with conservative treatment over a two to four month period. Physical therapy intervention combined with a consistent home program will provide the patient with the necessary tools to relieve pain and improve function.

What are the long-term effects of the patient's condition?

Sciatica secondary to a herniated disk can be corrected through rest and physical therapy intervention. Healing of the disk can also occur and scarring can reinforce the posterior aspect and annular fibers so that it is protected from further protrusion. Restoration of functional mobility is plausible; however, surgical intervention may be required if neurological symptoms increase or no progress is made with conservative measures.

Comparison:

What are the distinguishing characteristics of a similar condition?

Spinal stenosis is another condition that can be a causative factor of sciatica. Symptoms that would indicate spinal stenosis include lower extremity weakness with or without sciatica, back and leg pain after ambulating a short distance, increasing symptoms with continued ambulation, and relief of symptoms through flexion. Radiologic results reveal disk narrowing and degenerative spondylolisthesis. Surgery is only recommended as a last resort when conservative treatment fails.

Clinical Scenarios:

Scenario One

A 42-year-old female is referred to physical therapy with an L5 herniated disk and sciatica. The patient injured her back skiing three months ago. She presently works 50 hours per week at a daycare facility. Current symptoms include radiating pain down the left leg, a "feeling of weakness," and an inability to sleep at night due to pain.

Scenario Two

A 65-year-old male has been seen in physical therapy for three months with sciatica secondary to a L4 herniated disk. The patient states that he experiences constant pain. The physical therapist questions the patient's overall compliance with his established home exercise program. The physician orders are prescribed as physical therapy three times per week.

Scoliosis

Diagnosis:

What condition produces a patient's symptoms?
A patient with scoliosis presents with a lateral curvature of the spine. The curvature is usually found in the thoracic or lumbar vertebrae and can be associated with kyphosis or lordosis. The curvature of the spine may be towards the right or towards the left and rotation of the spine may or may not occur. Typically, the rotation will occur towards the convex side of the major curve.

An injury was most likely sustained to which structure?
The injury or deformity begins when the vertebrae of the spine deviate from the normal vertical position. The curvature disrupts normal alignment of the ribs and muscles and can create compensatory curves that attempt to keep the body in proper alignment. The vertebral column, rib cage, supporting ligaments, and muscles are all affected by a scoliosis of the spine.

Inference:

What is the most likely contributing factor in the development of this condition?
Idiopathic scoliosis, termed for its unknown etiology, accounts for approximately 80% of all cases. Upwards of 1:10 children are affected by some form of scoliosis with 1:4 requiring treatment for the curvature. The age of onset determines the subset of classification as infantile (0 to 3), juvenile (four to puberty), adolescent (12 for girls and 14 for boys) or adult (skeletal maturation) scoliosis. Non-structural scoliosis is a reversible curve that can change with repositioning. This type of curve is non-progressive and is usually caused by poor posture or leg length discrepancy. Structural scoliosis cannot be corrected with movement and can be caused by congenital, musculoskeletal, and neuromuscular reasons. Contributing factors of a structural curve include altered development of the spine in utero, association with neuromuscular diseases (cerebral palsy, muscular dystrophy, congenital defect of the vertebrae), and inheritance as an autosomal dominant trait. Research indicates a predisposition for scoliosis with a multifactorial etiology.

Confirmation:

What is the most likely clinical presentation?
A patient with a structural curve will present with asymmetries of the shoulders, scapulae, pelvis, and skinfolds. Juvenile idiopathic scoliosis is characterized by a thoracic curve with convexity towards the right. This curve may progress quickly and develop compensatory curves above and below. As the curve progresses there will be a rib hump posteriorly over the thoracic region on the convex side of the curve. The patient does not typically experience pain or other subjective symptoms until the curve has progressed. Adolescent scoliosis of greater than 30 degrees is seen more in females than males (10:1). Adult scoliosis affects approximately 500,000 adults in the United States. Curves that are less than 20 degrees rarely cause a person to experience significant problems or impairments.

What laboratory or imaging studies would confirm the diagnosis?
X-rays should be taken in an anterior and lateral view with the patient standing and with the patient bending over. A device called a scoliometer can be used to measure the angle of trunk rotation. The Cobb method can be used to determine the angle of curvature. A bone scan or MRI can be used to determine and rule out conditions such as infections, neoplasms, spondylolysis, disk herniations or compression fractures.

What additional information should be obtained to confirm the diagnosis?
Physical examination allows visual inspection of the curvature and physical asymmetries. A scoliometer can assist with measurement and the examiner can determine if the curve is non-structural or structural.

Examination:

What history should be documented?
Important areas to explore include past medical history, family history, medications, current health status, living environment, school activities, and social support system.

What test/measures are most appropriate?
Aerobic capacity and endurance: assessment of vital signs at rest and with activity, perceived exertion scale
Arousal, attention, and cognition: examine mental status, learning ability, memory, motivation
Ergonomics and body mechanics: analysis of dexterity and coordination
Integumentary integrity: skin and sensation assessment
Gait, locomotion, and balance: static and dynamic balance in sitting and standing, safety during gait with/without an assistive device, analysis of wheelchair management
Joint integrity and mobility: assessment of hyper- and hypomobility of a joint
Muscle performance: strength assessment

Orthotic, protective, and supportive devices: analysis of components of a device, analysis of movement while wearing a device
Pain: assessment of muscle soreness
Posture: analysis of resting and dynamic posture
Range of motion: active and passive range of motion
Self-care and home management: assessment of functional capacity

What additional findings are likely with this patient?

Common postural findings with scoliosis include increased spacing between the elbow and trunk during standing, leg length discrepancy, uneven shoulder and hip heights, and prominence on one side of the pelvis or breast (due to rotation of the curve). If a progressive scoliosis is untreated the deformity can increase to an angle in excess of 60 degrees and cause pulmonary insufficiency, significant pain, impairment in lung capacity, and degenerative changes including arthritis and disk pathology. Early screening, detection and treatment are necessary to control the curvature and avoid surgical intervention.

Management:

What is the most effective management of this patient?

Medical management of scoliosis is based on the type and severity of the curve, patient age, and previous management. Patients with scoliosis may utilize electrical stimulation to alleviate pain and biofeedback for education with proper posture and positioning. A patient with scoliosis that is less than 25 degrees should be monitored every three months. Breathing exercises and a strengthening program for the trunk and pelvic muscles are indicated. A patient with scoliosis that ranges between 25 and 40 degrees requires a spinal orthosis and physical therapy intervention for posture, flexibility, strengthening, respiratory function, and proper utilization of the spinal orthosis. A patient with scoliosis that is greater than 40 degrees usually requires surgical spinal stabilization. One method to surgically correct scoliosis is through posterior spinal fusion and stabilization with a Harrington rod. Physical therapy intervention after surgical fusion is indicated for breathing exercises, posture, flexibility, general strengthening, and respiratory muscle strengthening.

What home care regimen should be recommended?

A home care regimen is based on the type and severity of the curve. Exercise, stretching, posture, and flexibility are important components of an exercise program.

Outcome:

What is the likely outcome of a course in physical therapy?

Physical therapy intervention should improve a patient's condition through patient education and therapeutic exercise. Physical therapy may be indicated for implementation of a home program, pain management, posture retraining, orthotic training or following surgical stabilization.

What are the long-term effects of the patient's condition?

Prognosis for structural scoliosis is based on the age of onset and the severity of the curve. Early intervention results in the best possible outcome. Scoliosis does not usually progress significantly once bone growth is complete if the curvature remains below 40 degrees at the time of skeletal maturity. If the curvature is over 50 degrees there likely will be ongoing progression of the curve each year of life.

Comparison:

What are the distinguishing characteristics of a similar condition?

Torticollis is a deformity of the neck that is caused by shortened or spastic sternocleidomastoid muscles. The patient presents with a bending of the neck towards the affected side and rotation of the head towards the unaffected side. Causative factors include damage to the sternocleidomastoid muscle, malpositioning in utero, spasms secondary to central nervous system impairment or psychogenic origin. Conservative treatment for acquired torticollis includes heat, traction, massage, stretching, positioning, and bracing. Surgical intervention may be indicated if conservative management fails.

Clinical Scenarios:

Scenario One

An 11-year-old female is seen in physical therapy with diagnosis of a 30-degree right thoracic scoliosis. The physician has prescribed a spinal orthosis and physical therapy. The patient denies any pain, but states that she has soreness in her back. The patient is in the marching band and plays basketball. There is no past medical history and her parents are very supportive.

Scenario Two

A seven-year-old boy is referred to physical therapy with a 12-degree right thoracic scoliosis. The physical therapy prescription requests evaluation for a home exercise program. The patient has insulin-dependent diabetes and a low I.Q. The mother is present for the evaluation and appears to be supportive.

Spina Bifida – Myelomeningocele

Diagnosis:

What condition produces a patient's symptoms?

Spina bifida is a congenital neural tube defect that generally occurs in the lumbar spine but can also occur at the sacral, cervical, and thoracic levels. Spina bifida has three classifications that include spina bifida - occulta (incomplete fusion of the posterior vertebral arch with no neural tissue protruding), spina bifida - meningocele (incomplete fusion of the posterior vertebral arch with neural tissue/meninges protruding outside the neural arch), and spina bifida - myelomeningocele (incomplete fusion of the posterior vertebral arch with both meninges and spinal cord protruding outside the neural arch).

An injury was most likely sustained to which structure?

Spina bifida - myelomeningocele is characterized by a sac or cyst that protrudes outside the spine and contains a herniation of meninges, cerebrospinal fluid, and the spinal cord through the defect in the vertebrae. The cyst may or may not be covered by skin. Spina bifida results from failure of neural tube closure by day 28 of gestation when the spinal cord is expected to form. Approximately 75% of vertebral defects are found in the lumbar/sacral region, typically L5-S1 with injury to the structures at that level and below. Defects can also occur in the cervical or thoracic spine, however, this is rare.

Inference:

What is the most likely contributing factor in the development of this condition?

The Centers for Disease Control estimates the incidence for neural tube defects to be five per 10,000 live births within the United States. The incidence varies by socioeconomic status, geographic area, and ethnic background. The overall incidence is declining due to improved prenatal care. The exact etiology for spina bifida - myelomeningocele has not been identified; however, causative and risk factors include genetic predisposition, environmental influence (certain solvents, lead, herbicides, glycol ethers), insulin-dependent diabetes, low-levels of maternal folic acid, alcohol, maternal hyperthermia, and certain classifications of drugs (teratogenic exposure and vitamin A toxicity). Theories suggest that the cause is multifactorial rather than a single source of etiology. Prenatal care including recommended amounts of folic acid, especially in the first six weeks of pregnancy, appears to be the most effective way to prevent neural tube defects.

Confirmation:

What is the most likely clinical presentation?

Myelomeningocele is a severe condition that is characterized by a sac that is seen on an infant's back protruding from a specific area of the spinal cord. Impairments associated with myelomeningocele include motor and sensory loss below the vertebral defect, hydrocephalus, Arnold-Chiari Type II malformation, clubfoot, scoliosis, bowel and bladder dysfunction, and learning disabilities. The higher the neural lesion the worse the prognosis is for survival. The infant will require surgical intervention to close the lesion and in 90% of the cases a shunt is required for hydrocephalus. Approximately two-thirds of children with myelomeningocele and shunted hydrocephalus have normal intelligence and the other third demonstrate only mild retardation. Regardless of intelligence, children with myelomeningocele exhibit difficulties with perceptual abilities, attention, problem solving, and memory.

What laboratory or imaging studies would confirm the diagnosis?

Prior to birth a fetal ultrasound may identify the myelomeningocele defect in the spine. Prenatal testing of alpha-fetoprotein (AFP) in the blood will show an elevation in levels that indicate a probable neural tube defect at approximately week 16 of gestation. At birth an obvious sac will be present over the spinal defect. Spinal films and CT scan can evaluate for the presence of defects and hydrocephalus.

What additional information should be obtained to confirm the diagnosis?

Diagnosis is confirmed through prenatal testing or upon visual observation at birth. Past medical history of the mother, history of the pregnancy, and family history of neural tube defects may be noted.

Examination:

What history should be documented?

Important areas to explore with the parents include past medical history, current symptoms and health status, medications, past surgical procedures, living environment, and social support system.

What test/measures are most appropriate?

Aerobic capacity and endurance: assessment of vital signs at rest and with activity

Arousal, attention, and cognition: examine mental status, learning ability, memory, motivation

Assistive and adaptive devices: use of appropriate devices, analysis of components/safety of a device

Ergonomics and body mechanics: analysis of dexterity and coordination

Gait, locomotion, and balance: developmental milestones assessment, static/dynamic balance in prone and sitting, analysis of wheelchair management, standing with frame, gait with assistive device

Integumentary integrity: skin and sensation assessment

Motor function: equilibrium and righting reactions, motor assessment scales, balance in sitting

Muscle performance: assessment of active movement, muscle tone assessment

Orthotic, protective, and supportive devices: analysis of components of a device, analysis of movement while wearing a device

Range of motion: active and passive range of motion

Reflex integrity: assessment of deep tendon and pathological reflexes (e.g., Babinski, ATNR)

What additional findings are likely with this patient?

Immediately after birth, an infant with myelomeningocele has an increased risk of meningitis, hemorrhage, and hypoxia; however, surgical intervention may significantly reduce the risks. Ongoing additional findings with myelomeningocele include hydrocephalus, clubfoot, neuropathic fracture, visual problems, osteoporosis, kyphosis, hip dislocations, and latex allergy.

Management:

What is the most effective management of this patient?

Medical management of a patient with myelomeningocele begins with immediate surgical intervention to repair and close the defect and for placement of a shunt to alleviate hydrocephalus. Orthopedic surgical intervention may be warranted throughout a patient's life to correct deformities such as clubfoot, hip dysplasia, and scoliosis. Pharmacological intervention may include medications that assist in the management of bowel and bladder dysfunction. Physical and occupational therapies are important components in the management of myelomeningocele. Physical therapy is initiated immediately and focuses on family education regarding positioning, handling techniques, range of motion, and therapeutic play. Long-term physical therapy attempts to maximize functional capacity and may include range of motion, facilitation of developmental milestones, therapeutic exercise, skin care, strengthening, balance, and mobility training. Physical therapy will also assist with wheelchair prescription, assistive and adaptive device selection, and the use of orthotics and splinting.

What home care regimen should be recommended?

A home care regimen should include a formal exercise program, range of motion, and mobility training. Family and caregiver involvement are important in assisting a patient through their exercise program. The home program will require modification as the child matures and goals change.

Outcome:

What is the likely outcome of a course in physical therapy?

Physical therapy initially evaluates and documents the baseline information regarding the patient's motor and sensory function and level of ability. Physical therapy is ongoing through adolescence and is based on the severity of impairments and the needs of the child. Physical therapy is usually initiated based on symptoms, functional problems, and disability.

What are the long-term effects of the patient's condition?

A patient with myelomeningocele has a near normal life expectancy as long as the patient receives consistent and thorough health care. Functional outcome of the patient depends on the level of injury, the amount of associated impairments, and the caregiver support that is provided.

Comparison:

What are the distinguishing characteristics of a similar condition?

Anencephaly is a condition that is characterized by failed closure of the cranial end of the neural tube. The cerebral hemispheres do not form and some neural tissue may protrude through the defect. This type of neural tube defect cannot be repaired. Many infants with this condition are stillborn, while others only survive a short time after birth.

Clinical Scenarios:

Scenario One

A six-month-old boy is seen in physical therapy after revision of a ventriculoperitoneal shunt. The parents state that the child has been responsive at home and has been doing well. The child can position himself in prone on elbows and is able to sit with support.

Scenario Two

An 11-year-old girl with a T12 spinal cord lesion is seen in outpatient physical therapy. The patient presently uses a wheelchair for mobility; however, indicates that her goal is to walk in her home. The patient's upper body strength is good and intellect is normal.

Spinal Cord Injury – Complete C7 Tetraplegia

Diagnosis:

What condition produces a patient's symptoms?
The majority of traumatic spinal cord injuries result from compression, flexion or extension of the spine with or without rotation. Spinal cord injuries are classified as a concussion, contusion or laceration, and injury results in primary and secondary neural destruction. Traumatic injury to the spinal cord produces a physiological and biochemical chain of events that results in vascular impairment and permanent tissue and nerve damage.

An injury was most likely sustained to which structure?
A patient sustains primary damage to the spinal cord and surrounding tissues at the C7 level through disruption of the membrane, displacement or compression of the spinal cord, and subsequent hemorrhage and vascular damage. Secondary damage occurs beyond the level of injury due to biochemicals that are released as a result of the initial damage. This process destroys adjacent cells and neural tracts due to the acute inflammation and can last for days or even weeks. After injury, C7 is the most distal segment of the spinal cord that both the motor and sensory components remain intact.

Inference:

What is the most likely contributing factor in the development of this condition?
There is an estimated 190,000 to 230,000 persons living with SCI within the United States. Statistics from the National Spinal Cord Injury Database (NSCID) indicate that motor vehicle accidents, violence, and falls are the top causes of traumatic spinal cord injury. Statistics also indicate a higher ratio of injury in men (approximately 80%) and Caucasians. The highest incidence of age of injury (over 50%) occurs between 15 to 30 years of age.

Confirmation:

What is the most likely clinical presentation?
Spinal shock, which is the total depression of all nervous system function below the level of lesion, occurs immediately following injury and may last for days. Presentation includes total flaccid paralysis and loss of all reflexes and sensation. Surgical intervention may be required after injury in order to stabilize the spinal cord through decompression and fusion at the site of injury. A Halo device is commonly used with cervical injuries to stabilize the spine. As spinal shock subsides, a patient will experience an increase in muscle tone below the level of lesion and neurologic reflexes reappear. Spasticity will evolve and may become problematic. Autonomic dysreflexia and loss of thermoregulation are other impairments that occur secondary to autonomic nervous system dysfunction. A patient with C7 tetraplegia will also present with impaired cough and ability to clear secretions, altered breathing pattern, and poor endurance. The patient is at high risk for contractures and impaired skin integrity.

What laboratory or imaging studies would confirm the diagnosis?
X-rays of the cervical spine observe the positioning and damage of the involved vertebrae. The results of imaging determine subsequent medical intervention including stabilization of the spine. A myelogram or tomogram may be useful to confirm the extent of surrounding damage at the level of the injury.

What additional information should be obtained to confirm the diagnosis?
Other information commonly obtained in order to support the diagnosis includes physician conducted interviews regarding the mechanism of injury as well as a full neurological examination.

Examination:

What history should be documented?
Important areas to explore include past medical history, medications, mechanism of injury, precautions, current health status, social history and habits, occupation or school responsibilities, living environment, and social support system.

What test/measures are most appropriate?
Aerobic capacity and endurance: autonomic responses to positional changes, vital signs at rest/activity
Arousal, attention, and cognition: examine mental status, learning ability, memory, motivation
Assistive and adaptive devices: analysis of components and safety of a device, wheelchair prescription, adaptive devices, environmental controls
Integumentary integrity: skin assessment, American Spinal Injury Association (ASIA) - Standard Neurological Classification of Spinal Cord Injury Sensory Examination
Motor function: posture and balance in sitting
Muscle performance: ASIA - Standard Neurological Classification of Spinal Cord Injury Motor Examination, muscle tone assessment
Neuromotor development and sensory integration: analysis of reflex movement patterns
Pain: dysesthetic pain (deafferentation pain), nerve root pain, musculoskeletal pain

Posture: positioning, resting and dynamic posture
Range of motion: active and passive range of motion
Reflex integrity: assessment of deep tendon reflexes
and pathological reflexes
Sensory integrity: proprioception and kinesthesia
Ventilation, respiration, and circulation: assessment of
cough and clearance of secretions, breathing patterns,
respiratory muscle strength, accessory muscle
utilization, pulmonary function tests

What additional findings are likely with this patient?

There are many additional findings that can exist with a C7 injury, but the most common complications include orthostatic hypotension, pressure sores, spasticity, heterotopic ossification, and autonomic dysreflexia. Autonomic dysreflexia is considered a medical emergency and requires immediate attention to remove the noxious stimuli and lower the blood pressure or the patient will be at risk for subarachnoid hemorrhage. Other findings that require management include sexual dysfunction, respiratory complications, and pain management (neurogenic, central cord, peripheral nerve or musculoskeletal pain).

Management:

What is the most effective management of this patient?

Medical management of a SCI injury has both an acute and rehabilitation phase. The acute phase begins at injury and includes medically stabilizing the patient. Pharmacological intervention is started immediately using Methylprednisolone (corticosteroid), lipid peroxidation inhibitors, and drugs that block opiate receptors. These drugs appear to control the amount of secondary damage and improve the neurological damage. Once a patient is medically stable, inpatient rehabilitation, which is typically six to eight weeks, should initially focus on range of motion, positioning in bed, and respiratory management such as cough, clearance of secretions, bronchial drainage, and incentive spirometry. Compensatory techniques, strengthening, muscle substitution, the use of momentum, and the head-hips relationship should be utilized during all activities. Ongoing intervention should include mat and endurance activities, pressure relief training, wheelchair skills, self-range of motion, transfer skills, and community reintegration.

What home care regimen should be recommended?

A home care regimen should include breathing exercises, incentive spirometry, stretching, and mobility skills. Physical therapy intervention may be indicated for continuation of community skills and furthering the patient's independence within the boundaries of the physical limitations.

Outcome:

What is the likely outcome of a course in physical therapy?

A patient diagnosed with C7 tetraplegia will require extensive physical therapy with projected outcomes based upon the C7 level of motor and sensory innervation. Typical outcomes at this level include independence with feeding, grooming, and dressing, self-range of motion, independent manual wheelchair mobility, independent transfers, and independent driving with an adapted automobile. Independent living with adaptive equipment is possible.

What are the long-term effects of the patient's condition?

At this time there is no cure for a complete spinal cord injury, therefore a patient with a complete C7 injury will not regain innervation below this level. The triceps, extensor pollicis longus and brevis, extrinsic finger extensors, and flexor carpi radialis will remain the lowest innervated muscles. There will be ongoing musculoskeletal and cardiopulmonary deficits that can increase the risk for other health issues. The latest research suggests, however, that approximately 40% of the spinal cord injured population have a life expectancy over 45 years of age.

Comparison:

What are the distinguishing characteristics of a similar condition?

Brown-Sequard's syndrome is a condition that results from injury to one side of the spinal cord. Motor function, proprioception, and vibration are lost ipsilateral to the lesion and vibration, pain, and temperature are absent contralateral to the lesion.

Clinical Scenarios:

Scenario One

A patient is diagnosed with T12 paraplegia after a motor vehicle accident. Neurological examination reveals no active movement or sensation below T12. The patient is a chemistry teacher and coaches basketball. He is otherwise in good health.

Scenario Two

A 25-year-old male was injured when he was hit from behind. The blow produced cervical hyperextension and bleeding within the central gray matter of the spinal cord. The patient was diagnosed with central cord syndrome and referred to physical therapy. The patient resides alone in a second floor apartment and is a full-time graduate student.

Systemic Lupus Erythematosus

Diagnosis:

What condition produces a patient's symptoms?
Systemic lupus erythematosus (SLE) is a connective tissue disorder caused by an autoimmune reaction in the body. The primary manifestation of the condition is the production of destructive antibodies that are directed at the individual's own body. The chronic inflammatory disorder produces a variety of symptoms depending on the severity and extent of involvement.

An injury was most likely sustained to which structure?
SLE is an autoimmune disorder that creates high levels of autoantibodies (antinuclear antibodies) that attack various cells and tissues within the body. The autoantibodies form immune complexes that produce an inflammatory response and cause further tissue destruction. Proliferation of immune complexes precipitates inflammation responses that in turn destroy cells, tissues, and organs. Specific injury is organ or system dependent depending on which areas of the body are affected by SLE.

Inference:

What is the most likely contributing factor in the development of this condition?
The exact etiology of SLE is unknown; however, it is described as an immunoregulatory disturbance from genetic, environmental, viral, and hormonal contributing factors. Environmental factors associated with SLE include ultraviolet light exposure, infection, antibiotics (specifically penicillin and sulfa drugs), extreme stress, immunization, and pregnancy. SLE can occur at any age, but the most common age group is 15 to 40 years of age. The disorder is 10-15 times more common in women.

Confirmation:

What is the most likely clinical presentation?
There are an estimated 1.4 million individuals diagnosed with SLE in the United States. A patient with SLE will have diverse symptoms based on the involvement of the connective tissue throughout the body. Symptoms will appear with exacerbations and disappear with remissions throughout the course of the disease. Symptoms such as arthralgias, malaise, and fatigue may persist even during a remission period. A patient may initially see a physician for symptoms that include fever, malaise, rash, arthralgias, headache, and weight loss. Common clinical presentation throughout the course of SLE includes a red butterfly rash across the cheeks and nose, a red rash over light exposed areas, arthralgias, alopecia, pleurisy, kidney

involvement, seizures, depression, fibromyalgia, and cardiac involvement. SLE can affect the skin, joints, kidneys, lungs, heart, and other organs and tissues within the body. Patients can also have CNS involvement that can lead to neuropsychiatric manifestations that present with depression, irritability, emotional instability, and seizures.

What laboratory or imaging studies would confirm the diagnosis?
Microscopic fluorescent techniques are indicated to detect the presence of the antinuclear antibody (ANA) within the blood. A positive ANA test warrants an additional test for antideoxyribonucleic acid antibodies. These two tests in combination with the physical presentation support the presence of SLE. Other testing including erythrocyte sedimentation rate, complete blood count, and urinalysis.

What additional information should be obtained to confirm the diagnosis?
The American Rheumatism Association has designated criteria to confirm the diagnosis of SLE. A patient requires at least four of fourteen characteristics that occur during the same period of time. A patient evaluation including a thorough history and current symptoms assists with confirming a diagnosis of SLE.

Examination:

What history should be documented?
Important areas to explore include past medical and family history, medications, current symptoms and health status, living environment, social history and habits, occupation, and social support system.

What test/measures are most appropriate?
Aerobic capacity and endurance: assessment of vital signs at rest/activity, auscultation of the lungs/heart
Arousal, attention, and cognition: examine mental status, learning ability, memory, motivation
Assistive and adaptive devices: analysis of components and safety of a device
Community and work integration: analysis of community, work, and leisure activities
Environmental, home, and work barriers: analysis of current and potential barriers or hazards
Ergonomics and body mechanics: analysis of dexterity and coordination
Gait, locomotion, and balance: static/dynamic balance in sitting and standing, safety during gait, Tinetti Performance Oriented Mobility Assessment, Berg Balance Scale, Functional Ambulation Profile

Integumentary integrity: skin assessment, assessment of sensation, presence and assessment of rash
Joint integrity and mobility: soft tissue swelling and inflammation, presence of deformity
Motor function: posture and balance
Muscle performance: strength assessment
Neuromotor development and sensory integration: analysis of reflex movement patterns, sensory integration tests, gross and fine motor skills
Orthotic, protective, and supportive devices: potential utilization of bracing
Pain: pain perception assessment scale
Range of motion: active and passive range of motion
Self-care and home management: assessment of functional capacity

What additional findings are likely with this patient?

SLE can produce skeletal deformities such as ulnar deviation and subluxed interphalangeal joints. Kidney involvement and cardiovascular impairments such as endocarditis, myocarditis, and pericarditis can occur during an exacerbation. Patients that experience nephritis, myocarditis or neurological implications have a poor prognosis. Modifiable risk factors for exacerbation include high stress, limited emotional and social support, and psychological distress.

Management:

What is the most effective management of this patient?

Medical management of SLE focuses on reversing the autoimmune response in order to avoid complications and exacerbations of symptoms. Pharmacological intervention for a patient with mild SLE will include salicylates, Indomethacin or NSAIDs. Antimalarial medications, corticosteroids, and immunosuppressive therapy may be used. General management of SLE includes good nutrition, ongoing medical supervision, and avoidance of ultraviolet exposure. Physical therapy intervention is usually indicated after a period of exacerbation and includes a slow resumption of physical activity, energy conservation techniques, gradual endurance activities and significant patient education regarding skin care, pacing, exercise, and strengthening to tolerance.

What home care regimen should be recommended?

A home care regimen during an acute exacerbation of SLE should include relaxation and energy conservation techniques, stress reduction strategies, therapeutic exercise as tolerated, and pain management.

Outcome:

What is the likely outcome of a course in physical therapy?

Physical therapy cannot cease or alter the clinical course of SLE; however, it may assist in controlling the debilitating effects during an acute phase/exacerbation of the disease. Goals include focus on pain relief, relaxation, strengthening, and preventing deformity.

What are the long-term effects of the patient's condition?

The clinical course of SLE is highly unpredictable. A patient may only exhibit symptoms for skin and joint involvement or may exhibit multi-system involvement. Periods of remission may last years and the prognosis depends on the severity and the extent of the disease process. The overall prognosis for SLE is good, although in rare cases the disease process can remain acute and become fatal within a short period of time. There is a high ten-year survival rate with SLE. Death is usually attributed to kidney failure or secondary infections.

Comparison:

What are the distinguishing characteristics of a similar condition?

Scleroderma, also termed progressive systemic sclerosis, is a chronic disease that primarily affects the skin, but can involve articular structures and internal organs. There is long-term hardening and shrinking of the affected connective tissues. The two subtypes of this disease are systemic scleroderma and localized scleroderma. Etiology is unknown and the disease varies in course (months, years or a lifetime) and progression.

Clinical Scenarios:

Scenario One

A 25-year-old female is referred to physical therapy for a therapeutic exercise program. The patient was diagnosed last year with SLE and has not exercised since that time. The patient is currently taking corticosteroids and antimalarial medications to manage a recent exacerbation.

Scenario Two

A 43-year-old female was seen in outpatient physical therapy to assist with pain management. The patient was diagnosed five years ago with SLE and has recently experienced increased difficulty using her hands secondary to deformity and pain. The patient's goal is to reduce the pain in her hands.

Thoracic Outlet Syndrome

Diagnosis:

What condition produces a patient's symptoms?

Thoracic outlet syndrome is a term used to describe a group of disorders that presents with symptoms secondary to neurovascular compression of fibers of the brachial plexus. This usually occurs between the points of the interscalene triangle and the inferior border of the axilla. Compression of the nerves and blood supply can also occur as they pass over the first rib.

An injury was most likely sustained to which structure?

Thoracic outlet syndrome results from compression and damage to the brachial plexus nerve trunks, subclavian vascular supply, and/or the axillary artery. Nerve injury can result in neurapraxia with segmental degeneration and progress to axonotmesis due to continued and unrelieved compression.

Inference:

What is the most likely contributing factor in the development of this condition?

Contributing factors in the development of thoracic outlet syndrome include the presence of a cervical rib, an abnormal first rib, postural deviations or changes, body composition, chronic hyperabduction of the arm, hypertrophy or spasms of the scalene muscles, degenerative disorders, and an elongated cervical transverse process.

Confirmation:

What is the most likely clinical presentation?

A patient with thoracic outlet syndrome will present with symptoms based on nerve and/or vascular compression. Typical symptoms include diffuse pain in the arm most often at night, paresthesias in the fingers and through the upper extremities, weakness and muscle wasting, poor posture, edema, and discoloration. If the upper plexus is involved, pain will be reported in the neck that may radiate to the face and may follow the lateral aspect of the forearm into the hand. If the lower plexus is involved, pain is reported in the back of the neck and shoulder, which will radiate over the ulnar distribution to the hand. A patient's symptoms are usually enhanced with behaviors that aggravate the symptoms such as poor posture, lifting activities, and movements overhead.

What laboratory or imaging studies would confirm the diagnosis?

X-ray will confirm the presence of a cervical rib or other bony abnormality. Nerve conduction velocity testing may be valuable if a neuropathy exists.

Otherwise, diagnosis relies solely on a thorough history of patient symptoms, provocative testing, and a physical examination. Other testing should be used for differential diagnosis to rule out cervical radiculopathy, RSD, myofascial pain syndrome, tumor, carpal tunnel syndrome, brachial plexus injury, ulnar never compression, and angina.

What additional information should be obtained to confirm the diagnosis?

A patient can be diagnosed with thoracic outlet syndrome following a thorough history of symptoms, physical examination, and provocative testing that includes Adson's maneuver, Wright's maneuver, Roo's test, Halsted's test, Allen's test, and the costoclavicular and hyperabduction tests.

Examination:

What history should be documented?

Important areas to explore include past medical history, family history, medications, history of symptoms, current health status, living environment, social history and habits, occupation, and social support system.

What test/measures are most appropriate?

Anthropometric characteristics: upper extremity circumferential measurements

Arousal, attention, and cognition: examine mental status, learning ability, memory, motivation

Community and work integration: analysis of community, work, and leisure activities

Cranial nerve integrity: assessment of muscles innervation by the cranial nerves, dermatome assessment

Environmental, home, and work barriers: analysis of current and potential barriers or hazards

Ergonomics and body mechanics: analysis of dexterity and coordination

Integumentary integrity: skin assessment, assessment of sensation

Joint integrity and mobility: soft tissue swelling and inflammation, assessment of joint play, palpation of the joint

Motor function: posture and balance; upper quarter screening

Muscle performance: strength assessment

Pain: pain perception assessment scale, assessment of interscalene triangle point tenderness

Posture: analysis of resting and dynamic posture

Range of motion: active and passive range of motion

Reflex integrity: assessment of deep tendon and pathological reflexes (e.g., Babinski, ATNR)

Self-care and home management: assessment of functional capacity

What additional findings are likely with this patient?

A patient with thoracic outlet syndrome may have difficulty sleeping due to excessive pillows or malpositioning of the arm. The patient may have difficulty at work with carrying items on the affected side or with driving a car. Thoracic outlet most commonly affects the population between 30 and 40 years of age with women being affected two to three times more than men.

Management:

What is the most effective management of this patient?

Initial medical management of thoracic outlet syndrome takes a conservative approach. If conservative management fails, it is followed by surgical intervention. A patient with thoracic outlet syndrome requires physical therapy intervention to assist with modification of posture, breathing patterns, positioning in bed and at the work site, and gentle stretching. Physical therapy should focus on pain management, strengthening (especially the trapezius, levator scapulae, and rhomboids), joint mobilization, body mechanics, flexibility, and postural awareness. A therapist may utilize modalities such as transcutaneous nerve stimulation, ultrasound, and biofeedback to attain goals. Work site analysis and subsequent activity modification may be necessary to relieve the pain and other symptoms. A patient may benefit from anti-inflammatory agents in combination with physical therapy. If physical therapy management fails, the patient may require surgical decompression of bony or fibrotic abnormalities. The exact type of surgical intervention and approach is chosen by the surgeon based on symptoms and current damage.

What home care regimen should be recommended?

A home care regimen for a patient with thoracic outlet syndrome should include stretching, strengthening, and postural awareness. The patient should utilize these strategies on an ongoing basis at work and with recreational activities in order to promote pain free movement and limit undesirable symptoms associated with the condition.

Outcome:

What is the likely outcome of a course in physical therapy?

Most patients with thoracic outlet syndrome have positive results from physical therapy intervention and are able to return to their previous level of function within four to eight weeks.

What are the long-term effects of the patient's condition?

If a patient has positive results from physical therapy intervention, there will not be any long-term impairments; however, if the patient's symptoms persist for three to four months surgical intervention may be warranted. Approximately 75% of patients post surgery have a positive response; however, complications from surgery can include winging of the scapula, pneumothorax, and nerve compression. Research indicates no significant long-term difference between surgical resection of the first rib and successful conservative management.

Comparison:

What are the distinguishing characteristics of a similar condition?

A radial nerve lesion may be caused by direct trauma, excessive traction, entrapment or compression. A patient presents with an inability to extend the wrist, thumb, and fingers. The patient will also present with impaired grip strength and coordination. Splinting is recommended to maintain proper positioning. Passive range of motion is necessary to prevent secondary impairments such as contractures within the hand.

Clinical Scenarios:

Scenario One

A 35-year-old female is seen in physical therapy secondary to pain and paresthesias throughout the left upper extremity. The patient's work history reveals that she is employed as a telemarketer and is required to hold the phone between her ear and shoulder throughout her shift. The patient carries a five-pound brief case with a shoulder strap as she walks one-half mile to work. The patient has a one-year-old child.

Scenario Two

A 45-year-old female is referred to physical therapy secondary to pain when reaching overhead and carrying objects. The patient recently complains of waking up during the night with pain and paresthesias in the involved arm. The patient is very anxious and concerned because she is required to carry items and place them above her head as part of her job at a local production mill.

Temporomandibular Joint Dysfunction

Diagnosis:

What condition produces a patient's symptoms?
The temporomandibular joint (TMJ) is a complex joint that is classified as a condylar, hinge, and synovial joint. The TMJ contains fibrocartilaginous surfaces and articular discs. Temporomandibular joint dysfunction (TMD) occurs due to a change in the joint structure that can cause multiple symptoms and a limitation in function. In many instances inflammation and muscle spasm surrounding the joint produces symptoms for the patient with TMD.

An injury was most likely sustained to which structure?
TMD results from injury, derangement or incongruence of the TMJ itself, intraarticular disks, and/or supporting surrounding structures. Over time the meniscus of the TMJ becomes compressed and torn allowing for the bony portion of the joint (the ball and socket) to deteriorate secondary to the grinding of bone on bone.

Inference:

What is the most likely contributing factor in the development of this condition?
TMD can be classified by three primary etiological factors: predisposing factors; triggering factors; and perpetuating/sustaining factors. TMD can occur secondary to multiple causative factors including injury or trauma to the joint, congenital abnormalities, internal derangement of joint structure, arthritis, dislocation, disk degeneration, metabolic conditions or stress. Risk factors include chewing on one side, eating tough food, clenching, and grinding of teeth. Habits of gum chewing and nail biting may increase the incidence of injury to the TMJ. Patients are typically between 20 to 40 years of age with a greater incidence in women. Research indicates a possible link between gender-specific hormones and the risk for TMD.

Confirmation:

What is the most likely clinical presentation?
The National Institute of Dental and Craniofacial Research indicates that approximately 10.8 million individuals have TMD within the United States and 90% of the individuals that are seeking treatment are women in their childbearing years. A patient with TMD will present with symptoms that include pain (persistent or recurring), muscle spasm, abnormal or limited jaw motion, headache, and tinnitus. These symptoms can be unilateral or bilateral. The patient will often complain of feeling and hearing a "clicking or popping" sound with motion at the TMJ. Clinical manifestation of symptoms relates to the actual cause of the TMD.

What laboratory or imaging studies would confirm the diagnosis?
Procedures used in diagnosing TMD and its origin may include X-ray, CT scan, MRI, mandibular kinesiography, and a dental examination.

What additional information should be obtained to confirm the diagnosis?
A physical examination, upper quarter screening, TMJ loading, condyle-meniscus relationship, review of symptoms, and past medical history are all important components in the diagnosis of TMD. An occlusion examination may be indicated to evaluate a patient's bite.

Examination:

What history should be documented?
Important areas to explore include past medical history, medications, family history, current symptoms, current health status, diet, social history and habits, occupation, leisure activities, and social support system.

What test/measures are most appropriate?
Arousal, attention, and cognition: examine mental status, learning ability, memory, motivation
Community and work integration: analysis of community, work, and leisure activities
Cranial nerve integrity: assessment of muscle innervation by the cranial nerves, dermatome assessment
Integumentary integrity: skin assessment, assessment of sensation
Joint integrity and mobility: assessment of hyper- and hypomobility of a joint, soft tissue swelling and inflammation, joint play
Muscle performance: strength assessment including mastication, tongue, and lips; upper quarter screening
Pain: pain perception assessment scale, visual analog scale, assessment of muscle soreness
Posture: analysis of resting and dynamic posture
Range of motion: active and passive range of motion
Self-care and home management: assessment of functional capacity
Ventilation, respiration, and circulation: breathing patterns, respiratory muscle strength, accessory muscle utilization

What additional findings are likely with this patient?

TMD produces a general clinical presentation that includes pain, headache, muscle spasms, and tinnitus. Specific findings result from the specific cause of the TMD. Other findings can include popping and clicking when opening the mandible, locking of the TMJ, restriction of movement of the unaffected side, and/or pulling of the mandible towards the affected side. Common underlying causes include arthritis, fracture, congenital abnormalities, dislocations, and tension-relieving habits (chewing gum, bruxism, clenching or grinding the teeth).

Management:

What is the most effective management of this patient?

Medical management of TMD may include pharmacological intervention, the use of splinting, physical therapy treatment, and possible surgical intervention. Pharmacological treatment of TMD may include analgesics, NSAIDs, muscle relaxants, and antianxiety medications. A patient may also benefit from a splint to assist with realignment of the joint and a guard or bite plate to maintain proper positioning and avoid grinding of the teeth throughout the night. Specific physical therapy intervention is based on the exact etiology of the TMD. Generally, physical therapy intervention includes patient education regarding habits such as nail biting, posture retraining, the use of modalities such as moist heat, ice, biofeedback, ultrasound, electrostimulation, TENS, and massage. Soft tissue manipulation, joint mobilization, ROM, stretching, occlusal appliance prescription, and relaxation techniques are also appropriate. If conservative treatment fails or the exact etiology warrants surgical intervention, (approximately 5% of cases) the patient may require a condylectomy, osteotomy, arthrotomy, arthroscopy, reduction of subluxation or joint debridement.

What home care regimen should be recommended?

A home care regimen for a patient with TMD should include relaxation techniques, self-stretching, posture retraining exercises, and progressive ROM. A patient should avoid all foods and activities (such as gum chewing) that aggravate and stress the TMJ. The patient should continue with the proper use of an occlusal appliance if indicated. In order to maintain progress the patient must have ongoing consistency with the home program.

Outcome:

What is the likely outcome of a course in physical therapy?

Physical therapy intervention should improve a patient's condition and decrease the symptoms of the TMD. Physical therapy is usually conducted on an outpatient basis with focus on maximizing function and alleviating pain.

What are the long-term effects of the patient's condition?

A patient previously diagnosed with TMD is at an increased risk of recurrence; however, with successful management, ongoing compliance with the home program, and use of an indicated appliance, the patient may not have any long-term effects. If conservative management fails the patient may require surgical intervention for the underlying cause in order to alleviate the TMD.

Comparison:

What are the distinguishing characteristics of a similar condition?

Myofascial pain dysfunction (MPD) syndrome is a nonarticular disorder that affects the area surrounding the TMJ; however, symptoms are produced secondary to muscle spasm. MPD occurs more in females and can be of psychophysiologic origin. Habits such as grinding and jaw clenching increase tension in the muscles of mastication and create spasm. MPD can mimic the symptoms of TMD; however, differential diagnosis will rule out true TMJ involvement.

Clinical Scenarios:

Scenario One

A 12-year-old female is referred to physical therapy with a diagnosis of TMD secondary to condylar hyperplasia. The patient required a condylectomy with post-operative orders for physical therapy. The female is motivated and she has very supportive parents.

Scenario Two

A 30-year-old male is referred to physical therapy with a diagnosis of TMD. The physician referral notes inflammation, muscle spasm, and poor posture. The patient states that he will feel clicking when he eats certain foods. The patient has a history of childhood scoliosis that was controlled with exercise and short-term bracing. The patient is a stockbroker and spends a great deal of time talking on the phone.

Total Hip Arthroplasty

Diagnosis:

What condition produces a patient's symptoms?
A total hip arthroplasty (THA) may be warranted secondary to progressive and severe osteoarthritis or rheumatoid arthritis in the hip joint, developmental dysplasia of the hip, tumors, failed reconstruction of the hip or other hip conditions that produce incapacitating pain and disability. A THA may also be required secondary to trauma, avascular necrosis or a nonunion fracture.

An injury was most likely sustained to which structure?
Arthritis causes the hip joint to undergo a degenerative process including destruction of articular cartilage that results in bone-to-bone contact. Degenerative changes are usually apparent in both the acetabulum and the femoral head requiring a THA; however, if the acetabulum does not exhibit degenerative changes then only the femoral head will be replaced in a hemiarthroplasty procedure.

Inference:

What is the most likely contributing factor in the development of this condition?
Intra-articular disease or the destruction of articular cartilage may come from arthritis, repetitive microtrauma, obesity, nutritional imbalances, falls or abnormal joint mechanics. Indications for THA include osteoarthritis, rheumatoid arthritis, avascular necrosis, developmental dysplasia, osteomyelitis, failed fixation of a fracture, ankylosing spondylitis, and failed conservative management.

Confirmation:

What is the most likely clinical presentation?
A patient that requires a THA will present with decreased range of motion, impaired mobility skills, and persistent pain that increases with motion and weight bearing. The patient is usually over 55 years of age and has experienced consistent pain that is not relieved through conservative measures and limits the patient's functional mobility on a regular basis.

What laboratory or imaging studies would confirm the diagnosis?
X-ray, computed tomography, and magnetic resonance imaging procedures may be used to view the integrity of the joint. These procedures are also used to rule out a fracture or a tumor.

What additional information should be obtained to confirm the diagnosis?
Patient history, current functional status, and level of pain and disability are important factors in determining the need for surgical intervention. A standardized pain assessment scale and the Arthritis Impact Measurement tool may be used to establish an objective baseline. Relative or absolute contraindications must be considered prior to the recommendation for a THA. Contraindications may include but are not limited to active infection, severe obesity, arterial insufficiency, neuromuscular disease, and certain mental illness.

Examination:

What history should be documented?
Important areas to explore include past medical history, family history, medications, current symptoms, current health status, living environment, social history and habits, occupation, and social support system.

What test/measures are most appropriate?
Aerobic capacity and endurance: assessment of vital signs at rest and with activity, perceived exertion scale
Anthropometric characteristics: hip circumferential measurements, leg length measurements
Arousal, attention, and cognition: examine mental status, learning ability, memory, motivation
Assistive and adaptive devices: analysis of components and safety of a device
Environmental, home, and work barriers: analysis of current and potential barriers or hazards
Gait, locomotion, and balance: safety during gait with/without an assistive device, Functional Ambulation Profile
Joint integrity and mobility: soft tissue swelling and inflammation
Muscle performance: strength assessment, assessment of active movement
Pain: pain perception assessment scale
Range of motion: active and passive range of motion
Self-care and home assessment: assessment of functional capacity, Barthel Index
Sensory integrity: assessment of sensation

What additional findings are likely with this patient?
A patient that requires a THA may also have arthritis in other areas of the body. The patient may present with low endurance and may be deconditioned secondary to inactivity from the effects of arthritis. Post-surgical complications may include nerve injury, vascular damage, dislocation, pulmonary embolism, myocardial

infarction, and CVA. The prosthesis is also at risk for loosening, infection, heterotopic ossification, and fracture.

Management:

What is the most effective management of this patient?

Medical management includes choosing a surgical approach that meets the patient's needs and level of activity. A THA that utilizes a posterolateral approach allows the abductor muscles to remain intact; however, there may be a higher incidence of post-operative joint instability due to the interruption of the posterior capsule. This type of surgical approach requires a patient to avoid excessive hip flexion greater than 90 degrees, hip adduction, and hip medial rotation. A patient with a THA that utilizes an anterolateral approach should avoid hip flexion and lateral rotation. A direct lateral approach leaves the posterior portion of the gluteus medius attached to the greater trochanter and the posterior capsule left intact. This method is preferred for patients that may be noncompliant in order to avoid posterior dislocation. Pharmacological intervention status post THA will require anticoagulant therapy and pain medication. The patient's post-operative care includes hip precautions, use of an abduction pillow (with posterolateral approach), initiation of hip protocol exercises, and physical therapy intervention. The hip protocol exercises usually include ankle pumps, quadriceps sets, gluteal sets, heel slides, and isometric abduction. Physical therapy should emphasize patient education regarding hip precautions and weight bearing status, scar management, and soft tissue mobilization. At the time of hospital discharge the patient should be able to extend the hip to neutral and flex the hip to 90 degrees. A cemented hip replacement usually allows for partial weight bearing initially and a noncemented hip replacement requires toe touch weight bearing for up to six weeks. Physical therapy encourages early ambulation training in order to avoid deconditioning and the risk of deep vein thrombosis. A patient must practice all mobility skills using the proper hip precautions. Outpatient physical therapy may be indicated to assist with progression to a cane.

What home care regimen should be recommended?

The patient should be instructed in a home care regimen that includes range of motion, strengthening, and progressive ambulation. The patient must adhere to the hip precaution guidelines for a minimum of three months or until a physician determines that the hip demonstrates adequate stability.

Outcome:

What is the likely outcome of a course in physical therapy?

A patient status post THA will benefit from physical therapy and should attain an improved functional outcome. The patient should have diminished to no pain, increased strength and endurance, and improved mobility within six to eight weeks after surgery.

What are the long-term effects of the patient's condition?

A THA is a highly successful surgical procedure. The current life span of the prosthesis is less than 20 years and as a result some patients may require a subsequent replacement. Studies indicate pain relief and improved function with good to excellent results in 85-95% of the patients at 15 to 20 years post THA. Validated scoring systems such as the Harris Hip Scoring System or the Special Surgery Rating system are measures used to determine the quality of life after the THA.

Comparison:

What are the distinguishing characteristics of a similar condition?

A hemiarthroplasty of the hip is a replacement of the femoral head due to a subcapital fracture of the femur or degeneration of the femoral head. This type of surgical intervention is sometimes used as an alternative to a THA for elderly patients that sustain a hip fracture or patients that have a shortened expected life span.

Clinical Scenarios:

Scenario One

A patient is seen in physical therapy after THA surgery. The surgeon performed an anterolateral approach and used a noncemented prosthesis. The patient is mildly obese and has a lengthy cardiac history. The patient has osteoarthritis and had progressive pain and difficulty with mobility prior to surgery. The patient complains of soreness in the hip and is anxious to get home.

Scenario Two

A 75-year-old male is seen in physical therapy status post reduction of a dislocated right hip prosthesis. The patient had a THA three weeks ago and dislocated the hip two days ago while bending over to tie his shoes. The patient is currently using a walker for mobility and is toe touch weight bearing. The patient resides alone in a garden apartment and does not have any family in the area.

Total Knee Arthroplasty

Diagnosis:

What condition produces a patient's symptoms?
A total knee arthroplasty (TKA) may be warranted secondary to progressive and disabling pain within the knee joint. The pain is most often due to severe degenerative osteoarthritic destruction and deformity that can occur within the knee.

An injury was most likely sustained to which structure?
Arthritis causes the knee joint to undergo a degenerative process that includes destruction of articular cartilage and resultant bone-to-bone contact within the joint. The knee presents with decreased joint space and osteophyte formation. Injury occurs to the femoral condyles, tibial articulating surface, and the dorsal side of the patella.

Inference:

What is the most likely contributing factor in the development of this condition?
The destruction of articular cartilage secondary to osteoarthritis is the most common indication for a TKA. A patient with a history of participation in high-impact sports or has experienced trauma to the knee is at a higher risk for arthritis and subsequent TKA. Obesity, varus/valgus deformity, previous mechanical derangement, infection, rheumatoid arthritis, hemophilia, crystal deposition diseases, avascular necrosis or bone dysplasia at the knee are some other contributing factors that may warrant a TKA.

Confirmation:

What is the most likely clinical presentation?
Approximately 130,000 TKAs are performed each year within the United States. A patient that requires a TKA will present with severe knee pain that worsens with motion and weight bearing, impaired range of motion, possible deformity of the knee, and impaired mobility skills. Night pain is common and may include localized or diffuse pain. Other symptoms may include stiffness, swelling, locking, and giving way of the affected knee. Patients often attempt conservative treatment measures to address the condition with only limited success.

What laboratory or imaging studies would confirm the diagnosis?
X-ray, computed tomography, and magnetic resonance imaging are used to determine the extent of deterioration and bony abnormalities within the knee joint. Radiographic images can be utilized post-operatively to ensure proper fit and obtain baseline information.

What additional information should be obtained to confirm the diagnosis?
Patient history, current functional status, and level of pain and disability are important factors in determining the need for surgical intervention. A pain assessment scale and the Arthritis Impact Measurement tool may be used to establish an objective baseline.

Examination:

What history should be documented?
Important areas to explore include past medical history, family history, medications, current symptoms, living environment, social history and habits, occupation, current functional status, and social support system.

What test/measures are most appropriate?
Aerobic capacity and endurance: assessment of vital signs at rest and with activity, perceived exertion scale
Anthropometric characteristics: knee circumferential measurements
Arousal, attention, and cognition: examine mental status, learning ability, memory, motivation
Assistive and adaptive devices: analysis of components and safety of a device
Environmental, home, and work barriers: analysis of current and potential barriers or hazards
Gait, locomotion, and balance: safety during gait/stairs with device, Functional Ambulation Profile
Joint integrity and mobility: soft tissue swelling and inflammation
Muscle performance: strength/active movement assessment
Pain: pain perception assessment scale
Range of motion: active and passive range of motion
Self-care and home assessment: assessment of functional capacity, Barthel Index
Sensory integrity: assessment of sensation

What additional findings are likely with this patient?
A patient that requires TKA may have arthritis in other joints, previous replacement surgeries or previous trauma to the knee joint. Patients with significant osteoarthritis and severe pain may exhibit sleep disorders or depression due to the disease process. Relative or absolute contraindications must be considered prior to the recommendation for a TKA. Contraindications may include but are not limited to active infection of the knee, severe obesity, significant genu recurvatum, arterial insufficiency, neuropathic joint, and certain mental illnesses. Post-surgical complications after a TKA include infection, vascular

damage, fracture surrounding the prosthesis, patellofemoral instability, pulmonary embolism, nerve damage, loosening of the prosthesis, and arthrofibrosis.

Management:

What is the most effective management of this patient?

Medical management of a patient requiring a TKA includes choosing of the appropriate surgical procedure based on the patient's symptoms and level of activity. Pharmacological intervention status post TKA will require anticoagulant therapy and pain medications. The patient's post-operative care includes a knee immobilizer, elevation of the limb, cryotherapy, intermittent range of motion using a continuous passive motion (CPM) machine, and initiation of knee protocol exercises. A cemented knee prosthesis allows for either partial weight bearing or weight bearing as tolerated post surgery based on the individual physician's discretion. A noncemented knee prosthesis requires toe touch weight bearing for up to six weeks to allow for the bone to grow and affix to the prosthesis. Physical therapy should focus on mobility training with the proper weight bearing status using an appropriate assistive device. Early ambulation training is encouraged in order to avoid deconditioning and the risk of deep vein thrombosis. Physical therapy intervention should emphasize ankle pumps, quad sets, and hamstrings sets as well as range of motion and stretching. A goal of 90 degrees of knee flexion and 0 degrees knee extension is often established prior to discharge from the hospital or rehabilitation facility. The following precautions should be used for several months after surgery to avoid excessive stress to the knee: avoid squatting, avoid quick pivoting, do not use pillows under the knee while in bed, and avoid low seating. Outpatient therapy may be recommended to progress the patient from an assistive device. Once the physician progresses the patient to weight bearing as tolerated, physical therapy intervention should include strengthening with closed-chain exercises and functional activities.

What home care regimen should be recommended?

A home care regimen would typically include range of motion, strengthening, and progressive ambulation exercises. The patient must adhere to precautions, use of an immobilizer, and proper weight bearing status until a physician determines that the knee joint demonstrates adequate stability.

Outcome:

What is the likely outcome of a course in physical therapy?

A patient status post TKA will benefit from physical therapy and should attain an improved functional capacity. The patient should experience relief of pain that will allow for a full return to previous functional activities within eight to twelve weeks after surgery depending on a cemented or noncemented prosthesis and potential complications that were encountered.

What are the long-term effects of the patient's condition?

A TKA is a highly successful surgical procedure that should significantly reduce pain and increase function. After finishing a rehabilitation protocol, a patient may have only minor limitations in knee range of motion. A knee replacement may loosen over time and require revision; however, the life expectancy of the knee prosthesis is between 15 and 20 years.

Comparison:

What are the distinguishing characteristics of a similar condition?

A patellectomy (surgical removal of the patella) is a surgical procedure that is indicated for a comminuted facture of the patella that cannot be repaired with internal fixation. A patellectomy can include the entire patella or just the inferior or superior pole of the patella. The retinaculum and extensor mechanism are repaired with the surgical procedure and the patient is immobilized for six to eight weeks. Once rehabilitation is initiated the patient starts with range of motion and closed-chain exercises.

Clinical Scenarios:

Scenario One

An 80-year-old female in an acute care hospital is two days status post left TKA. The patient presents with partial hearing loss and moderate dementia. The patient's past medical history includes a right CVA with no residual impairment and hypertension that is controlled by medication. The patient resides with her sister in a ranch style home with three steps to enter.

Scenario Two

A 49-year-old male is referred to outpatient physical therapy seven weeks after surgery. The patient received a noncemented knee prosthesis and has recently advanced to weight bearing as tolerated. The patient's range of motion in the involved knee is 10-85 degrees. The patient is otherwise independent with axillary crutches. No significant past medical history is noted.

Total Shoulder Arthroplasty

Diagnosis:

What condition produces a patient's symptoms?
A patient that is a candidate for a total shoulder arthroplasty (TSA) will have severe pain and impaired shoulder motion due to deterioration of the glenohumeral joint. These candidates have undergone conservative treatment measures that have failed to improve their condition.

An injury was most likely sustained to which structure?
TSA candidates will have irreparable damage, deterioration, and destruction to the humeral head and the glenoid fossa within the shoulder complex. The joint surfaces are severely damaged or destroyed by wear and tear, inflammation, injury or previous surgery.

Inference:

What is the most likely contributing factor in the development of this condition?
Indications for a TSA include severe glenohumeral degenerative joint disease, pain and limited range of motion secondary to osteoarthritis, rheumatoid arthritis, avascular necrosis, fracture or rotator cuff arthropathy. Other patients that may require a TSA would include a patient with a bone tumor, Paget's disease or with recurrent dislocations. A patient will be considered for TSA if conservative treatment of the underlying cause fails.

Confirmation:

What is the most likely clinical presentation?
A patient will exhibit impaired range of motion at the shoulder, may lack independence with functional mobility and ADLs, and will experience severe pain. It is this unremitting pain (with failed conservative treatment) that is the primary indication for the TSA. A TSA performed secondary to arthritis is usually performed on patients between 55 and 70 years of age while TSA performed secondary to irreparable damage from dislocation or avascular necrosis is usually performed on patients between 40 and 50 years of age.

What laboratory or imaging studies would confirm the diagnosis?
X-ray will reveal the level of degeneration within the shoulder complex. MRI or CT scan will allow the physician to assess the integrity of the rotator cuff and deltoid muscles surrounding the joint as well as the overall integrity of the shoulder complex.

What additional information should be obtained to confirm the diagnosis?
A full medical history along with a physical examination is a key component that is required in determining if a patient is a candidate for a TSA. The patient must possess motivation, realistic expectations, and appropriate goals regarding outcome.

Examination:

What history should be documented?
Important areas to explore include past medical and family history, medication, current symptoms, surgical precautions/contraindications, rehabilitation protocol, social history and habits, occupation, leisure activities, and social support system.

What test/measures are most appropriate?
Aerobic capacity and endurance: assessment of vital signs at rest and with activity
Anthropometric characteristics: circumferential measurements of the affected upper extremity
Arousal, attention, and cognition: examine mental status, learning ability, memory, motivation
Community and work integration: analysis of community, work, and leisure activities
Environmental, home, and work barriers: analysis of current and potential barriers or hazards
Integumentary integrity: skin assessment, assessment of sensation
Joint integrity and mobility: assessment of hyper- and hypomobility of a joint, soft tissue swelling and inflammation
Muscle performance: strength assessment except for surgical extremity
Pain: pain perception assessment scale, visual analog scale, assessment of muscle soreness
Range of motion: passive range of motion within limits of physician protocol for involved shoulder, active and passive range of motion for all other extremities
Self-care and home management: assessment of functional capacity, Functional Independence Measure (FIM)
Sensory integrity: assessment of proprioception and kinesthesia

What additional findings are likely with this patient?
Surgical complications post TSA include mechanical loosening of the prosthesis, instability, rotator cuff tear, implant failure, heterotopic ossification and intraoperative fracture. Risk for complication is dependent on the type of prosthesis (unconstrained, semiconstrained, constrained), surgical skill in

reproducing proper alignment, use of cemented prosthesis versus press-fit prosthesis, and integrity of rotator cuff musculature.

Management:

What is the most effective management of this patient?

A patient status post TSA will remain hospitalized for an average of two to five days. Medical management of the patient will rely on a team approach including nursing, physician services, and rehabilitation therapies. The success of the TSA will rely on the style of the implant, the quality of the soft tissue, bone, and the rehabilitation program. A CPM may be prescribed by the surgeon for use during the patient's hospitalization. Pharmacological intervention includes anticoagulation and pain medications. Physical therapy is initiated the day after surgery and should follow the shoulder rehabilitation protocol designed by the surgeon. The shoulder usually remains immobilized using a sling during initial rehabilitation. The Neer shoulder protocol advocates initiating isometric shoulder exercises approximately three weeks after surgery and active shoulder exercises approximately six weeks after surgery. PROM and AAROM are indicated but AROM at the shoulder is contraindicated during the first phase of rehabilitation. Physical therapy intervention includes pain management, prevention of adhesions, functional activities, PROM/AAROM/AROM, therapeutic exercise, edema management, patient education in self-ROM and wand/pendulum exercises, and the use of modalities.

What home care regimen should be recommended?

The home care regimen should include a range of motion and therapeutic exercise program that follows the surgeon's shoulder rehabilitation protocol. During initial recovery, pendulum and wand exercises are appropriate as well as self-ROM. A patient must not perform any form of medial rotation or lateral rotation beyond 35 to 40 degrees during the first two to three weeks post surgery. Controlled motion and return to functional activity are incorporated into the home program as directed by the physician protocol. A patient must also continue to manage edema and follow other physician orders regarding precautions.

Outcome:

What is the likely outcome of a course in physical therapy?

The goal of a TSA is to relieve pain and regain functional motion. Physical therapy should assist the patient to meet these goals unless hindered by post-surgical or other complications.

What are the long-term effects of the patient's condition?

Since the shoulder is a non-weight bearing joint there is a longer life expectancy for the prosthesis than for the knee or hip. There is a high success rate for long-term results with a TSA. Patients should avoid activities such as heavy lifting, chopping wood or contact sports since these can increase the risk of fracture, loosening or rotator cuff tear.

Comparison:

What are the distinguishing characteristics of a similar condition?

A shoulder hemiarthroplasty is a similar surgery that involves the replacement of the head and neck of the humerus leaving the glenoid fossa of the scapula intact. This surgery is indicated when the humeral head has deteriorated or fractured without healing. This procedure may also be performed if the patient does not have enough bone density to support the glenoid component or when there are significant rotator cuff deficiencies that exist.

Clinical Scenarios:

Scenario One

A 60-year-old female is 14 days status post left TSA and is currently attending outpatient therapy three days per week. The patient's rehabilitation is complicated by right upper extremity paralysis secondary to a CVA two years ago. The patient is motivated, cooperative, and does not have any residual cognitive deficits.

Scenario Two

A 58-year-old male is one-month status post TSA and has been attending outpatient therapy three days per week. His wife states that he complains of significant pain during his home exercise program. He appears to be progressing otherwise. He has no significant medical history other than the rheumatoid arthritis that created the need for the TSA.

Transfemoral Amputation due to Osteosarcoma

Diagnosis:

What condition produces a patient's symptoms?
Osteosarcoma (osteogenic sarcoma) is the second most common primary bone tumor and accounts for 15-20% of bone tumors. Osteosarcoma is a highly malignant cancer that begins in the medullary cavity of a bone and leads to the formation of a mass. It usually affects bones with an active growth phase such as the femur or tibia and is often located in the metaphysis. Amputation may be necessary to remove the tumor and surrounding tissues to avoid metastatic disease.

An injury was most likely sustained to which structure?
The cancer cells are found in osteoblasts within the primitive mesenchymal cells of the medullary cavity of a bone. The cancer rapidly proliferates, replaces normal bone, and causes tissue destruction. Osteosarcoma will also metastasize to the lungs very early in the disease process.

Inference:

What is the most likely contributing factor in the development of this condition?
Osteosarcomas can occur as a primary or secondary cancer and the etiology remains unknown. This form of tumor primarily affects young children (especially males), adolescents, and young adults under 30 years of age. A peak time for incidence is during a growth spurt as an adolescent. Risk factors associated with secondary osteosarcoma include Paget's disease, osteoblastoma, giant cell tumor or chronic osteomyelitis. Environmental and genetic factors have been associated with the disease. In many instances amputation is required to cease the disease process.

Confirmation:

What is the most likely clinical presentation?
Osteosarcoma can be found most often in the long bones especially at the site of the most active epiphyseal growth plate, the distal femur, proximal tibia, proximal humerus and pelvis. The knee region accounts for approximately 50% of osteosarcomas. Patients that require amputation secondary to an osteosarcoma will present with a mass often found in the tibia or femur. The most common symptoms of osteosarcoma are pain and swelling within the extremity. Pain may worsen at night or with exercise and a lump may develop in the extremity sometime after the onset of pain. The osteosarcoma may weaken the involved extremity leading to a fracture. In some cases, a fracture may be the first sign of the osteosarcoma. Metastases appear in the lungs early in 90% of the cases.

What laboratory or imaging studies would confirm the diagnosis?
X-ray, MRI, and scintigraphy allow the physician to determine the presence, location, and size of a tumor. The "Codman's triangle" can be seen on x-ray indicating reactive bone at the site where the periosteum has been elevated by the neoplasm. Definitive diagnosis for an osteosarcoma is made through tissue biopsy of the tumor.

What additional information should be obtained to confirm the diagnosis?
Diagnosis of osteosarcoma is confirmed solely through biopsy. The course of treatment and the need for surgical amputation is determined by the size, location of the tumor, and progression of the malignancy.

Examination:

What history should be documented?
Important areas to explore include past medical history, medications, family history, current symptoms and health status, social history and habits, occupation, leisure activities, and social support system.

What test/measures are most appropriate?
Aerobic capacity and endurance: assessment of vital signs at rest and with activity, auscultation of the lungs, palpation of pulses
Anthropometric characteristics: residual limb circumferential measurements, length of limb
Arousal, attention, and cognition: examine mental status, learning ability, memory, motivation
Assistive and adaptive devices: analysis of components and safety of a device
Community and work integration: analysis of community, work, and leisure activities
Gait, locomotion, and balance: analysis of wheelchair mobility, static and dynamic balance in sitting and standing, safety during gait with an assistive device
Integumentary integrity: skin assessment, assessment of sensation, temperature of limb
Muscle performance: strength and tone assessment
Pain: phantom pain, pain perception assessment scale
Prosthetic requirements: analysis and safety of the prosthesis; alignment, efficiency, and fit of the prosthesis with the residual limb
Range of motion: active and passive range of motion

Self-care and home management: assessment of functional capacity, Barthel Index, Functional Independence Measure (FIM),
Sensory integrity: proprioception and kinesthesia

What additional findings are likely with this patient?

A patient status post transfemoral amputation secondary to an osteosarcoma may present with fatigue, loss of balance, phantom pain or sensation, hypersensitivity of the residual limb, and psychological issues regarding the loss of the limb. The patient may also have associated symptoms from chemotherapy that can include anemia, abnormal bleeding, infection, and kidney impairment. The presence of these findings can have a negative influence on a patient's ability to utilize a prosthesis.

Management:

What is the most effective management of this patient?

Medical management will focus on adjunctive therapies to treat the osteosarcoma. Pharmacological intervention may include pain medication and other medication to deter effects from cancer treatment. Physical and occupational therapies should begin immediately after the transfemoral amputation. Preprosthetic intervention should focus on range of motion, positioning, strengthening, desensitization, residual limb wrapping, functional mobility, gait training, and patient education for care of the residual limb. Patients with a transfemoral amputation should lie prone for a period of time each day to prevent a hip flexion contracture. Modalities may be used to improve range of motion and decrease pain. Serial casting may be indicated if a contracture develops. Without complication the patient should be able to return home with support and receive short-term physical therapy for prosthetic training.

What home care regimen should be recommended?

A home care regimen for a patient status post transfemoral amputation should include limb desensitization, stretching, proper positioning, and prone lying. The patient must be independent with residual limb care, skin inspection, and proper wrapping. Endurance activities, strengthening, and mobility with an assistive device are necessary as a precursor to prosthetic training.

Outcome:

What is the likely outcome of a course in physical therapy?

Physical therapy is necessary for both preprosthetic and prosthetic training. A patient should be able to achieve the established goals and function with a prosthesis for all mobility including: ambulation, balance, transfers, and stair activities. The general health, cognition, motivation, and social support system of the patient will influence the patient's functional outcome.

What are the long-term effects of the patient's condition?

The survival rate for a patient status post osteosarcoma has increased in recent years to a five-year cure rate of 70-80% with treatment that may include amputation, radiation, and chemotherapy. The transfemoral amputation should not permanently impair the patient's independence with mobility, self-care or ambulation using a prosthesis. The patient's long-term outcome is dependent on the status of the cancer.

Comparison:

What are the distinguishing characteristics of a similar condition?

Ewing's sarcoma is a malignant nonosteogenic primary bone tumor that infiltrates the bone marrow and usually affects children and adolescents under 20 years of age. A patient will present with pain of increasing severity, swelling, and fever. This tumor is not found consistently in a specific location within the bone and is extremely malignant with a high frequency of metastases. Ewing's sarcoma requires aggressive treatment that may include amputation and adjunctive chemotherapy. The five-year survival rate is approximately 70%.

Clinical Scenarios:

Scenario One

A 10-year-old female is seen in physical therapy after a right transfemoral amputation. The patient was diagnosed with osteosarcoma four months ago. The patient is in good spirits and is anxious to receive "a new leg" and begin walking. Her parents are supportive and are eager to assist her during rehabilitation.

Scenario Two

A 16-year-old male is seen for the first time in physical therapy since a left transfemoral amputation. The boy states that his leg had bothered him for a few weeks and the pain got worse everyday. He also stated that he was told that the cancer was now also found in his lungs. He wants to start an exercise program so that he will be ready for his prosthesis when his residual limb heals.

Transtibial Amputation due to Arteriosclerosis Obliterans

Diagnosis:

What condition produces a patient's symptoms?
Arteriosclerosis obliterans, also known as peripheral arterial disease (PAD), is a form of peripheral vascular disease that produces thickening, hardening, and eventual narrowing and occlusion of the arteries. Arteriosclerosis obliterans results in ischemia and subsequent ulceration of the affected tissues. The affected area may become necrotic, gangrenous, and require amputation.

An injury was most likely sustained to which structure?
Injury will occur to all structures that receive blood supply from vessels that have become occluded. Prolonged ischemia results in tissue death and infection. Arteriosclerosis obliterans is the most common arterial occlusive disease and accounts for approximately 95% of the cases of vascular disease.

Inference:

What is the most likely contributing factor in the development of this condition?
Risk factors associated with arteriosclerosis obliterans include age, diabetes, sex, hypertension, high serum cholesterol and low-density lipid levels, smoking, impaired glucose tolerance, obesity, and sedentary lifestyle. Unsuccessful management of peripheral vascular disease may ultimately lead to uncontrolled infection, gangrene, necrosis, and amputation. Males have an overall higher incidence of arteriosclerosis than female counterparts.

Confirmation:

What is the most likely clinical presentation?
The patient that requires a transtibial amputation secondary to arteriosclerosis obliterans is typically an individual over 45 years that smokes (75-90%) and will present with intermittent claudication that produces cramps and pain in the affected areas. Intermittent claudication will typically present in the gastrocnemius-soleus complex, secondary to its high oxygen demand. Other characteristics include resting pain, decreased pulses, ischemia, pallor skin, and decreased skin temperature.

What laboratory or imaging studies would confirm the diagnosis?
Arteriosclerosis obliterans can be diagnosed using Doppler ultrasonography, MRI or arteriography. These diagnostic tests examine the degree of blood flow throughout the extremities. A patient with arteriosclerosis obliterans would typically demonstrate poor results including blockage, tissue damage, and tissue death.

What additional information should be obtained to confirm the diagnosis?
The physician should examine the limb for temperature, skin condition, the presence of hair, sensation, and palpable pulses when determining the need for amputation. The physician may perform a selected non-invasive test such as a claudication test that examines the presence of intermittent claudication that can occur with prolonged ambulation. The ankle-brachial index, segmental limb pressures or pulse volume recordings may also be used to assist with the diagnosis.

Examination:

What history should be documented?
Important areas to explore include past medical history, medications, current health status, social history and habits, occupation, living environment, and social support system.

What test/measures are most appropriate?
Aerobic capacity and endurance: palpation of pulses, pulse oximetry, assessment of vital signs at rest and with activity
Anthropometric characteristics: residual limb circumferential measurements, length of limb
Arousal, attention, and cognition: examine mental status, learning ability, memory, motivation
Assistive and adaptive devices: analysis of components and safety of a device
Gait, locomotion, and balance: analysis of wheelchair mobility, static and dynamic balance in sitting and standing, safety during gait with an assistive device
Integumentary integrity: examine presence of hair growth, color, temperature, assessment of sensation
Muscle performance: strength assessment, muscle tone assessment
Pain: phantom pain, pain perception assessment scale
Prosthetic requirements: (when appropriate) analysis and safety of the prosthesis; assessment of alignment, efficiency, and fit of the prosthesis; assessment of residual limb with the prosthesis
Range of motion: active and passive range of motion
Self-care and home management: assessment of functional capacity, Barthel Index, Functional Independence Measure (FIM)
Sensory integrity: assessment of proprioception and kinesthesia

What additional findings are likely with this patient?

A patient status post transtibial amputation may have a decrease in cardiovascular status depending on the frequency of intermittent claudication the patient experienced prior to the amputation. The patient may initially experience diminished balance secondary to the loss of the limb. Other issues that directly affect the residual limb include phantom pain, decreased range of motion, poor skin integrity, and hypersensitivity. The presence of any of these findings can have a negative influence on a patient's ability to utilize a prosthesis.

Management:

What is the most effective management of this patient?

A patient should be a candidate for inpatient physical therapy services immediately after the transtibial amputation. Preprosthetic intervention should focus on strength, range of motion, functional mobility, use of assistive devices, desensitization, and patient education for care of the residual limb. Intervention should focus on proper positioning in order to avoid the risk of contractures, especially a knee flexion contracture. If the patient does not experience complications they should be able to return home either independently or with support. The patient may receive continued short-term physical therapy for prosthetic intervention once the residual limb has fully healed.

What home care regimen should be recommended?

A home care regimen for a patient status post transtibial amputation should include exercises, limb desensitization, proper positioning, and stretching. Since ambulation with a prosthesis increases the energy cost, the patient should be encouraged to perform cardiovascular activities on a frequent basis. In order to be successful, the patient will need to consistently monitor the residual limb and wrap the limb to ensure proper shaping until the prosthesis is tolerated.

Outcome:

What is the likely outcome of a course in physical therapy?

Physical therapy for both preprosthetic and prosthetic intervention is typically necessary. A patient should be able to achieve the established goals and function with a prosthesis and an assistive device if warranted. The general health, cognition, motivation, and social support system of the patient will influence the patient's functional outcome.

What are the long-term effects of the patient's condition?

Arteriosclerosis obliterans is a chronic disease that a patient should continue to manage. The current transtibial amputation should not permanently alter a patient's level of functional mobility. The patient should be able to manage all aspects of self-care and functional mobility after prosthetic training with the permanent prosthesis unless hindered by other ailments. Approximately 20% of all individuals with arteriosclerosis obliterans have a myocardial infarction or CVA at some point after diagnosis.

Comparison:

What are the distinguishing characteristics of a similar condition?

There will be many similar characteristics regardless of the level of amputation to the lower or upper extremity. Intervention will include desensitization, phantom pain education, proper compression and shaping, strength improvement, proper positioning, and self-care and mobility with all patients. In most cases patients and therapists share the common goal of functional prosthetic utilization.

Clinical Scenarios:

Scenario One

A two-year-old female born with congenital malformation of the ankle joint and without a foot is referred to physical therapy for a pre-operative evaluation. The child is in good health, active, and has no other past medical history. The child has become increasingly frustrated with her alternate means of mobility. Her parents are supportive and carry her for community mobility. She prefers to scoot and crawl around the house since she cannot bear weight through the affected lower extremity. She is scheduled for a Syme's amputation in one week.

Scenario Two

An 83-year-old male, status post right transtibial amputation secondary to insulin-dependent diabetes mellitus, is admitted to a skilled nursing facility for rehabilitation. The patient is obese and presents with cardiopulmonary insufficiency. The patient previously resided alone with intermittent home health care and requires two liters of oxygen with activity.

Traumatic Brain Injury

Diagnosis:

What condition produces a patient's symptoms?
Traumatic brain injury (TBI) occurs due to an open head injury where there is penetration through the skull or closed head injury where the brain makes contact with the skull secondary to a sudden, violent acceleration or deceleration impact. Traumatic brain injury can also occur secondary to anoxia as with cardiac arrest or near drowning.

An injury was most likely sustained to which structure?
Any structure within the brain is vulnerable to injury; however, primary damage will occur at the site of impact. Secondary damage occurs as a result of metabolic and physiologic reactions to the trauma. Brain injury may include swelling, axonal injury, hypoxia, hematoma, hemorrhage and changes in intracranial pressure (ICP).

Inference:

What is the most likely contributing factor in the development of this condition?
Statistics from the Brain Injury Association indicate that motor vehicle accidents (45-60%) and falls (25%) are the two leading causes of TBI. Statistics reveal that 92% of all children diagnosed with severe brain injuries were involved in motor vehicle accidents. Males between 15-24 years have the highest incidence of injury. Individuals over 65 years of age and children between 1-2 years of age are also in a higher risk group.

Confirmation:

What is the most likely clinical presentation?
The incidence of head injury is close to two million individuals per year with an estimated five million individuals living with a brain injury. The clinical presentation of a TBI varies due to the type, area, extent of injury, and secondary damage within the brain. Characteristics of a TBI may include altered consciousness (coma, obtundity, delirium), cognitive and behavioral deficits, changes in personality, motor impairments, alterations in tone, and speech and swallowing issues.

What laboratory or imaging studies would confirm the diagnosis?
Diagnostic imaging such as CT scan or MRI should be performed immediately in order to rule out hemorrhage, infarction, and swelling. X-rays taken of the cervical spine can be used to rule out fracture and potential for subluxation. An electroencephalogram (EEG), positron emission tomography (PET), and cerebral blood flow mapping (CBF) may also be utilized for diagnosis and baseline data.

What additional information should be obtained to confirm the diagnosis?
A full neurological evaluation by a physician should include a mental examination, cranial nerve assessment, tonal assessment and papillary reactivity assessment. The physician will classify the patient using the Glasgow Coma Scale and indicate severe (coma), moderate or mild brain injury. The Rancho Los Amigos Levels of Cognitive Functioning can also be used to classify injury and assist with developing an appropriate plan of care.

Examination:

What history should be documented?
Important areas to explore include past medical history, medications, family history, current symptoms, level of cognitive functioning, social history and habits, occupation, leisure activities, and social support system.

What test/measures are most appropriate?
Aerobic capacity and endurance: vital signs at rest/activity, pulse oximetry, auscultation of lungs
Arousal, attention, and cognition: using Rancho Los Amigos levels of cognitive functioning
Assistive and adaptive devices: analysis of components and safety of a device
Cranial nerve integrity: muscle innervation by the cranial nerves, dermatome assessment
Environmental, home, and work barriers: analysis of current and potential barriers or hazards
Gait, locomotion, and balance: static and dynamic balance in sitting and standing, safety during gait with/without an assistive device, Berg Balance Scale, Tinetti Performance Oriented Mobility Assessment, analysis of wheelchair management
Integumentary integrity: skin and sensation assessment
Joint integrity and mobility: assessment of hyper- and hypomobility of a joint
Motor function: equilibrium and righting reactions, motor assessment scales, coordination, posture and balance in sitting, assessment of sensorimotor integration, physical performance scales
Muscle performance: strength assessment, muscle tone assessment
Neuromotor development and sensory integration: analysis of reflex movement patterns, assessment of involuntary movements, sensory integration tests, gross and fine motor skills
Orthotic, protective, and supportive devices: analysis of components and movement while wearing a device

Pain: pain perception assessment scale, visual analog scale, assessment of muscle soreness
Posture: analysis of resting and dynamic posture
Range of motion: active and passive range of motion
Reflex integrity: assessment of deep tendon and pathological reflexes (e.g., Babinski, ATNR)
Self-care and home management: assessment of functional capacity, Functional Independence Measure (FIM), Barthel Index, Rankin Scale, Rivermead Motor Assessment

What additional findings are likely with this patient?

There are multiple impairments that can develop secondary to TBI. Intracranial pressure must be monitored initially since it is at risk to increase or develop hemorrhage. A patient can develop heterotopic ossification, contractures, skin breakdown, seizures, and deep vein thrombosis. A patient with a severe TBI may remain in a persistent vegetative state.

Management:

What is the most effective management of this patient?

Medical management is initiated at the site of injury or in the emergency room for life preserving measures. The initial goal is to stabilize the patient, control intracranial pressure, and prevent secondary complications. Surgical intervention may be required in attempt to regain homeostasis within the brain secondary to hemorrhage or fracture. Once a patient is medically stable, physical therapy rehabilitation is initiated. Treatment of a patient with TBI usually includes a team approach with goals based on the patient's level of injury. Pharmacological intervention may include cerebral vasoconstrictive agents, psychotropic agents, hypertensive agents, antispasticity agents and medication to assist with cognition and attention. Physical therapy will focus on sensory stimulation and PROM for a comatose patient or pathfinding and high-level balance activities for a patient with a mild injury. Physical therapy may include functional mobility training, behavior modification, serial casting, compensatory strategies, vestibular rehabilitation, task specific activities, wheelchair seating, and pulmonary intervention.

What home care regimen should be recommended?

A home care regimen should include ongoing therapeutic activities that focus on goals associated with the patient's current Rancho Los Amigos level. Consistency is vital to the success of a home program. The patient may also participate in a community

re-entry based program for the TBI population if warranted by their level of current function.

Outcome:

What is the likely outcome of a course in physical therapy?

A patient diagnosed with TBI does not have a specific projected outcome. Outcome is based on the degree of primary and secondary damage and the extent of cognitive and behavioral impairments. Physical therapy should continue in all settings until the patient has attained all realistic goals.

What are the long-term effects of the patient's condition?

TBI affects approximately two million Americans each year. Recent statistics state 80,000 Americans experience the onset of long-term disability secondary to TBI. Over 50,000 die each year as a result of TBI. Long-term effects are determined by the extent of injury and impairments resulting from the TBI. Many patients experience life long deficits that do not allow them to return to their pre-injury lifestyle.

Comparison:

What are the distinguishing characteristics of a similar condition?

Meningitis is a bacterial or viral infection that spreads through the cerebrospinal fluid to the brain. The meninges of the brain become inflamed as well as the meningeal membranes. The patient will have a headache and may complain of stiffness in the neck. The patient may also show symptoms of confusion, fatigue, and irritability. As the virus progresses the patient may experience seizures and may progress into a coma. Medical treatment varies based on the causative strain of the virus/bacteria. Mortality ranges from 5-25% and approximately 30% have some degree of permanent neurological impairment.

Clinical Scenarios:

Scenario One

A 22-year-old male with TBI is admitted to an inpatient rehabilitation hospital. The patient is presently classified as Rancho Los Amigos Level IV. The patient required surgical decompression after the TBI. The patient's parents are with the patient almost constantly.

Scenario Two

A 42-year-old female sustained a severe TBI in a motor vehicle accident and is presently classified as Rancho Los Amigos Level II. The accident was two weeks ago. Prior to admission the patient was healthy and worked full-time. She has a supportive husband.

Urinary Stress Incontinence

Diagnosis:

What condition produces a patient's symptoms?
Urinary incontinence is the involuntary loss of urine. There are four classifications that include functional incontinence, stress incontinence, urge incontinence, and overflow incontinence. Urinary stress incontinence may occur during activities when there is an increase in abdominal pressure through straining, sneezing, coughing or lifting.

An injury was most likely sustained to which structure?
Urinary stress incontinence usually occurs from loss of strength and/or integrity of the contractile and noncontractile tissues that maintain bladder control. Urinary stress incontinence is caused by weakness of the pelvic floor musculature (pubococcygeus muscle), damage of the pudendal nerve, weakness of the urogenital diaphragm muscles, malposition of the urethra and/or urethral sphincter incompetence.

Inference:

What is the most likely contributing factor in the development of this condition?
Risk factors for the development of urinary stress incontinence include pregnancy, vaginal delivery, episiotomy, prostate or pelvic surgery, aging, diabetes mellitus, central nervous system and peripheral system dysfunction, and recurrent urinary infection. A prolapsed bladder, uterus or bowel may contribute to leakage and is seen in women that have had multiple vaginal deliveries. Medications that treat other illnesses can sometimes contribute to incontinence especially with the older population. Obesity is another risk factor that is believed to increase the risk of stress incontinence due to increased intra-abdominal pressure and the effect of obesity on the neuromuscular function of the genitourinary tract.

Confirmation:

What is the most likely clinical presentation?
It is estimated that approximately 10 million adults experience some form of urinary incontinence. Urinary stress incontinence accounts for 50-60% of all incontinence cases and is manifested solely by the involuntary loss of urine with any form of exertion or increased abdominal pressure. The amount of urine that leaks is typically less than 50 milliliters with coughing, sneezing or straining. Physical activity or exercise can also produce leakage due to exertion with these activities. Other manifestations may include dribbling of urine, urgency, frequency, nocturia, and a weak stream while voiding.

What laboratory or imaging studies would confirm the diagnosis?
Cystometry is used to evaluate bladder capacity, control, contractility, and sensation. During this procedure provocative stress testing will be performed when stress incontinence is suspected. Urodynamic testing observes the stability of the bladder and electromyography observes bladder contractions. Urinalysis is used for differential diagnosis to rule out infection, diabetes, and other conditions.

What additional information should be obtained to confirm the diagnosis?
Urinary stress incontinence can be determined through history, pelvic examination, and noted loss of urine with straining activities. The Marshall-Marchetti test utilizes finger elevation of the paraurethral vaginal tissues at the neck of the bladder in order to stop the leakage of urine during coughing, sneezing or straining. Baseline exam should include the amount of time that a patient can hold urine, repetitions performed of a holding contraction, and the amount of pelvic floor contractions a patient can perform.

Examination:

What history should be documented?
Important areas to explore include past medical history, childbirth history, medications, current health status, fluid intake, social history, occupation, living environment, and social support system.

What test/measures are most appropriate?
Aerobic capacity and endurance: assessment of vital signs at rest and with activity, perceived exertion scale
Arousal, attention, and cognition: examine mental status, learning ability, memory, motivation, Urge Impact scale
Community and work integration: analysis of community, work, and leisure activities
Environmental, home, and work barriers: analysis of current and potential barriers or hazards
Ergonomics and body mechanics: analysis of dexterity and coordination, assessment of lifting techniques (intra-abdominal pressure)
Integumentary integrity: skin assessment, examination of the pelvic floor
Muscle performance: strength assessment of the pelvic floor muscles, muscle tone assessment
Pain: pain perception assessment scale
Posture: analysis of resting and dynamic posture
Range of motion: active and passive range of motion
Self-care and home management: assessment of functional capacity

What additional findings are likely with this patient?

A patient with urinary stress incontinence may be at increased risk for a urinary tract infection with subsequent skin breakdown. Pelvic floor weakness, uterine prolapse, and kidney infection may all relate to urinary stress incontinence. A patient that has poor diet and nutrition, constipation, and inadequate hydration will further promote incontinence.

Management:

What is the most effective management of this patient?

Medical management of urinary incontinence usually consists of conservative measures (physical therapy) as a first line of defense followed by pharmacological and surgical interventions depending on the underlying cause and response to conservative treatment. Physical therapy intervention for pelvic floor muscle weakness that is tested as 0/5 – 2/5 includes biofeedback, electrical stimulation, bladder retraining, and therapeutic exercise. Pelvic floor muscle strengthening at this level includes facilitation and tapping of the pelvic floor muscles, overflow exercises using the buttocks, adductors, and lower abdominals, and implementation of Kegel exercises. Physical therapy intervention for pelvic floor muscle weakness that is tested as 3/5 – 5/5 includes continued biofeedback and bladder retraining, weighted vaginal cones for resistance training, and implementation of pelvic floor muscle exercise during activities.

What home care regimen should be recommended?

A home care regimen for a patient with urinary stress incontinence should emphasize an active exercise program that includes pelvic floor strengthening in order to regain control of the flow of urine. Patients are encouraged to perform the recommended exercises throughout the day and integrate the pelvic exercises during activities that may trigger an increase in abdominal pressure within their daily routine.

Outcome:

What is the likely outcome of a course in physical therapy?

Outpatient physical therapy for urinary stress incontinence should alleviate pelvic floor weakness and involuntary leakage of urine within eight to twelve weeks. If a patient requires surgical intervention or presents with multiple impairments then physical therapy may be warranted for a longer period of time to assist with gaining bladder control.

What are the long-term effects of the patient's condition?

The long-term effects of urinary stress incontinence depend on the exact cause for the incontinence and the responsiveness to therapeutic intervention. Some patients do not have any long-term effects upon successful completion of physical therapy while other patients do not benefit from physical therapy intervention and require surgical intervention for the underlying cause. Compliance with the home exercise program is required when the underlying cause is weakness of the pelvic floor musculature. Research indicates that in an older population approximately 50% of all admissions to skilled nursing facilities have a direct relationship to unresolved urinary incontinence and impairments.

Comparison:

What are the distinguishing characteristics of a similar condition?

Bowel incontinence can occur from birth defects, trauma to the rectum, spinal cord injuries, fecal impaction, and tumor. Conservative treatment is preferred and includes diet, pharmacological agents, and strengthening of the sphincter muscles through exercise, electrical stimulation, and biofeedback. Surgical intervention may be warranted.

Clinical Scenarios:

Scenario One

A 32-year-old female is referred to physical therapy with a diagnosis of incontinence. The patient gave birth to her fourth child six weeks ago. The patient reports involuntary leakage of urine with exertion. The patient has no significant past medical history; however, reports that she is very anxious about participating in physical therapy.

Scenario Two

A 68-year-old female complains to her doctor during her annual examination that she has difficulty controlling her bladder since a kidney infection six months ago. The patient states that she is unable to hold her urine if she sneezes or coughs and cannot perform any activity of exertion without wearing feminine pads due to leakage. The physician referred the patient to physical therapy for Kegel exercises.

Unit Four
Content Outline

Perhaps the most valuable piece of information a candidate can utilize when preparing for the National Physical Therapy Examination is the content outline. The content outline provides a detailed analysis of each of the content areas of the National Physical Therapy Examination. A thorough understanding of each of the content areas and the corresponding categories and subcategories will streamline a candidate's preparation. Less time will be spent covering topics that are not clinically relevant to the actual examination and as a result, more time will be available for reviewing and relearning.

The information necessary to create each category is obtained after analyzing the responses of hundreds of physical therapists to a job analysis survey. The most recent job analysis survey was sent to over 8,153 physical therapists with between one and five years of clinical experience. The results obtained from the 1,359 returned surveys were used as the basis for the current content outline.

The chart below illustrates the four primary content areas of the current National Physical Therapy Examination and the percentage of examination items in each area.

Physical Therapist Examination Content Outline

Standards of Care (10.0%)
20 questions

Examination (26.0%)
52 questions

Intervention (41.5%)
83 questions

Evaluation, Diagnosis, Prognosis, and Outcomes (22.5%)
45 questions

Content Outline

Federation of State Boards of Physical Therapy

National Physical Therapist Examination

I. Examination - 52 questions

History and Systems Review

Tests and Measures Group I
1. Strength, ROM, Posture, Body Structures, Prosthetic & Orthotic Devices
2. Cognition, Nerve, Reflex and Sensory Integrity, Neurodevelopment

Tests and Measures Group II
1. Cardiovascular/Pulmonary System
2. Integumentary System
3. Functional Status/Community Integration

II. Evaluation, Diagnosis, Prognosis, and Outcomes – 45 questions

Evaluation and Diagnosis
Prognosis and Outcomes

III. Intervention – 83 questions

Non-Procedural Intervention
1. Coordination of care
2. Communication
3. Documentation
4. Patient/family/client-related instructions

Procedural Intervention
Group I: Exercise and manual therapy
Group II: Transfer and functional activities, gait training, assistive and adaptive devices, and modification of the environment
Group III: Physical agents and modalities, airway clearance techniques, wound care, promoting health and wellness

IV. Standards of Care – 20 questions

1. Maintaining patient autonomy, confidentiality, and obtaining informed consent
2. Recognizing scope of physical therapy practice, including limitations of the PT role that necessitate referral to other disciplines
3. Utilizing body mechanics/positioning
4. Considering the patient's cultural background, social history, home situation, and geographic barriers, etc.
5. Safety, CPR, emergency care, first aid, standard precautions

System Specific Specifications

The approximate number of questions on the examination according to the system specific specifications is illustrated in the following table. Although the percentage of items in each of the system specific areas will fluctuate slightly from examination to examination, the table provides candidates with a reasonable idea of which areas will be emphasized. This information can be extremely valuable when candidates are determining the weighting of their individual study plan.

System	Percent of the Exam
Musculoskeletal	24% +/- 5%
Neuromuscular	24% +/- 5%
Cardiovascular/Pulmonary	13% +/- 3%
Integumentary	7% +/- 2%
Non-System	32% +/- 5%

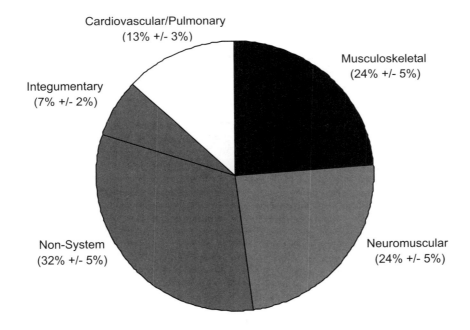

Since the four primary content areas vary significantly in their weighting, it is imperative that candidates also weight the study time dedicated to each area. A sample two-month, long-range schedule presented below is designed to illustrate this important concept. Detailed information on the specific weighting of each of the areas is discussed later in this unit.

Sample Two-Month Long-Range Schedule

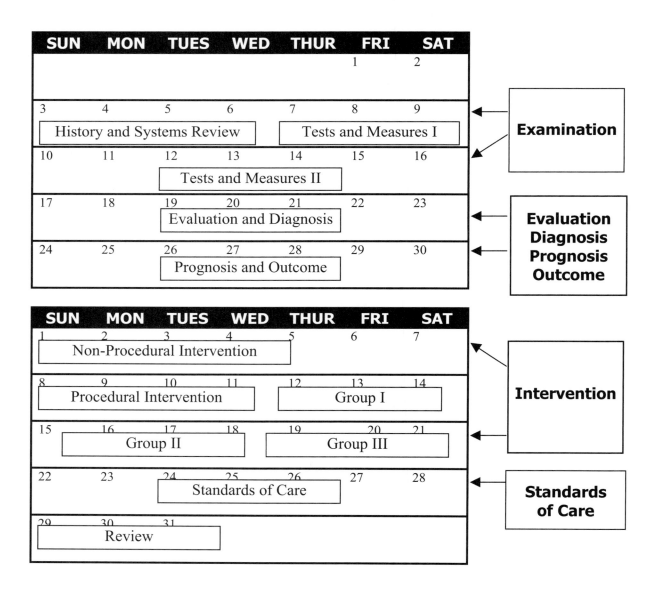

Examination: Content Outline

Directions

Candidates have the opportunity to take a 200 question sample examination consisting of 20 examination questions from each of the 10 content areas of the current Physical Therapist Content Outline. By exploring the different content areas candidates will gain a better appreciation of the breadth and depth of the current examination. Candidates should begin to assess their own strengths and weaknesses and gain an appreciation for the endurance necessary to complete a 200 question examination. Since there are an infinite number of possible questions in each category of the content outline, candidates should avoid familiarizing themselves with only the stated answers and instead use the presented information as a platform to explore a myriad of related topics. More specific indicators of examination performance will be discussed in future units.

Candidates should attempt to identify the best answer for each examination question. Candidates will have a maximum of four hours to complete the sample examination. The sample examination should be completed in a single session in order to more closely simulate the actual examination. A detailed answer key immediately follows the sample examination. The answer key includes the correct answer, an explanation supporting the correct answer, and a cited resource with page number. The resources utilized in the explanations were selected since they are often required textbooks in physical therapy academic programs. When consulting specific page numbers candidates should make sure that the edition of a given textbook they are using is consistent with the edition referenced in the bibliography.

Scoring can be calculated using the formula:

$$\frac{\%}{\text{Correct}} = \frac{\text{Number of Questions Correct}}{200} * 100$$

Important Information for all Sample Examinations

Candidate performance on the sample examination should be used only as a method to assess strengths and weaknesses and should not be utilized as a predictor of actual examination performance. Any similarity in the questions contained within the sample examinations in *PTEXAM: The Complete Study Guide* and questions on any version of the National Physical Therapy Examination is purely coincidental.

EXAM: CONTENT OUTLINE

Physical Therapist Examination Content Outline Analysis

I.   Examination

Examination (26%)
52 questions

Examination	
History and Systems Review	15
Tests and Measures Group I	22
Tests and Measures Group II	15
Total = 52	

History and Systems Review

History and Systems
Review (7.5%)
15 questions

History

Included are critical knowledge and skills related to obtaining past and current patient history information from medical records, and interviews with patients and others. Information includes demographics, general health status, chief complaint, medications, medical/surgical and social history, functional status/activity level, social/health habits, living environment, employment, and growth and development.

Systems Review

Included are critical knowledge and skills related to:

- Conducting a systems review of the cardiovascular/pulmonary system
- Conducting a systems review of the integumentary system
- Conducting a systems review of the musculoskeletal system
- Conducting a systems review of the neuromuscular system

Sample Questions

1. A physical therapist reviews the medical record of a patient with venous insufficiency. A recent entry in the medical record indicates that the physician ordered diagnostic testing in an attempt to rule out deep venous thrombosis. Which diagnostic test would be most beneficial to accomplish the physician's objective?

   1. Doppler ultrasonography
   2. hematocrit
   3. partial thromboplastin time
   4. pulmonary function tests

2. A physical therapist reviews the results of a complete blood count taken on a 65-year-old male recently admitted to the hospital. Which of the following lab values may be considered a precaution for therapeutic exercise?

   1. white blood cell count: $5,500 \times 10^3$ mm^3
   2. hematocrit: 46 mL/dL
   3. hemoglobin: 8 gm/dL
   4. platelet count: 250,000 mm^3

3. A patient diagnosed with low back pain is referred to physical therapy. During the examination the physical therapist asks if the patient had any formal diagnostic screening. The patient states that she had an x-ray and a test where dye was injected into the spinal canal. This description most closely resembles:

1. arthrography
2. myelography
3. computed tomography
4. magnetic resonance imaging

4. A physical therapist obtains the past medical history of a patient recently referred to physical therapy after being diagnosed with adhesive capsulitis. Which medical condition is associated with an increased incidence of adhesive capsulitis?

1. diabetes mellitus
2. hemophilia
3. peripheral vascular disease
4. osteomalacia

5. A physical therapist working on an oncology unit reviews the medical chart of a patient prior to initiating an exercise program. The patient's cell counts are as follows: hematocrit 24 mL/dL, white blood cells 2,500 x 10^3 mm^3, platelet 80,000 mm^3, hemoglobin levels 7 gm/dL. Based on the patient's blood counts, which of the following would be the most accurate statement regarding the patient's allowable exercise level?

1. no exercise is allowed
2. light exercise is allowed
3. active exercise is allowed
4. resistive exercise is allowed

6. A physical therapist receives a referral for a 48-year-old female diagnosed with lung cancer. The patient reports smoking three packs of cigarettes a day for the last 25 years. Assuming the patient was diagnosed with cancer two years ago, which of the following pieces of data would provide the therapist with the most valuable information when establishing the plan of care and the associated goals?

1. premorbid lifestyle
2. staging of cancer
3. past medical history
4. motivation level

7. A physical therapist employed in an outpatient clinic discusses the daily treatment program with a patient three weeks status post medial meniscectomy. During the discussion the patient indicates that she is able to exercise, however, did experience a low-grade temperature three days ago. Assuming the therapist measures and records the patient's temperature as 98.9 degrees Fahrenheit, the most appropriate therapist action would be to:

1. continue with treatment as planned
2. continue with treatment, however, avoid active exercise
3. refer the patient to her primary care physician
4. contact the patient's surgeon to discuss the situation

8. A physical therapist reviews the medical record of a 46-year-old female diagnosed with myasthenia gravis. A recent physician entry indicates that the patient is currently taking immunosuppressive medication. Which laboratory test should be the most frequently monitored based on the patient's medication?

1. hematocrit
2. hemoglobin
3. platelet count
4. white blood cell count

9. A physical therapist examines a 27-year-old female with lower leg pain. The patient was referred to physical therapy after diagnostic imaging ruled out the possibility of a stress fracture. Which imaging technique would be the most appropriate when attempting to identify a stress fracture?

1. arthrography
2. bone densiometry
3. bone scan
4. x-ray

10. A physical therapist examines a patient with an acute grade II lateral ankle sprain. The most common mechanism for an anterior talofibular ligament sprain is:

1. inversion and dorsiflexion
2. inversion and plantar flexion
3. inversion
4. eversion and dorsiflexion

11. A physical therapist reviews a laboratory report for a patient recently admitted to the hospital. The patient sustained burns over 25 percent of her body in a fire. Assuming the patient exhibits hypovolemia, which of the following laboratory values would be the most significantly affected?

    1. hematocrit
    2. hemoglobin
    3. oxygen saturation rate
    4. prothrombin time

12. A physical therapist participates in a community based screening program designed to identify individuals with osteoporosis. Which group would have the highest risk for developing osteoporosis?

    1. white females over the age of 60
    2. black females over the age of 60
    3. white females over the age of 40
    4. black females over the age of 40

13. A 46-year-old male with high blood pressure is placed on diuretics in an attempt to lower his blood pressure. What is the most serious complication of diuretic therapy?

    1. hypernatremia
    2. hypokalemia
    3. hypercalcemia
    4. hypocythemia

14. A physical therapist employed in an outpatient orthopedic clinic works with an 18-year-old female diagnosed with iliotibial band syndrome. After treating the patient for several weeks, the therapist suspects that the patient is bulimic. The most appropriate therapist action is to:

    1. discuss the situation with the patient
    2. request an immediate meeting with the patient's family
    3. schedule the patient for a dietary consultation
    4. continue to monitor the patient's behavior during scheduled therapy sessions

15. A patient with coronary artery disease is placed on antihypertensive medication in order to control severe hypertension. Which antihypertensive drug category functions by decreasing myocardial force and rate of contraction?

    1. diuretics
    2. vasodilators
    3. angiotensin-converting enzyme inhibitors
    4. calcium channel blockers

16. A patient employed in a machine shop is referred to physical therapy with a diagnosis of carpal tunnel syndrome. The patient indicates that he is scheduled for a diagnostic test that may help to confirm the diagnosis. Which of the following electrodiagnostic tests would be the most appropriate?

    1. electroencephalography
    2. evoked potentials
    3. nerve conduction velocity
    4. electromyography

17. A patient complains of sharp pain in the abdomen that has been present for at least eight hours. Physical examination reveals tenderness in the left upper quadrant of the abdomen. Which structure is located within this region?

    1. appendix
    2. gallbladder
    3. liver
    4. spleen

18. A physical therapist interviews a 21-year-old football player referred to physical therapy after sustaining a grade II acromioclavicular sprain. Which of the following patient descriptions best describes the injury mechanism associated with an acromioclavicular sprain?

    1. "I was being tackled and landed directly on my shoulder."
    2. "I fell with my arm extended and another player fell on top of me."
    3. "My arm was hit with a helmet while I was throwing the ball."
    4. "My arm was stepped on while I was lying on the ground."

19. A patient diagnosed with an anterior cruciate ligament injury is examined in physical therapy. During the examination, the patient asks the physical therapist why the physician would order x-rays after already diagnosing the ligament injury. The primary purpose for ordering the radiographs would be to:

    1. confirm the physician's diagnosis
    2. check for possible meniscal involvement
    3. examine the patient's skeletal maturity
    4. rule out the possibility of a fracture

20. A self-referred patient is examined in physical therapy. The physical therapist asks the patient a variety of questions in an attempt to rule out systemic involvement. Which of the following questions would provide the most direct information on the presence of a brain tumor?

    1. Have you had any unusual headaches or changes in your vision?
    2. Can you think of any time during the past week when you may have fallen or been injured?
    3. Have you had any sudden weight loss in the last three weeks without dieting?
    4. Have you noticed any change in your bowel movements or flow of urination?

Tests and Measures: Group I

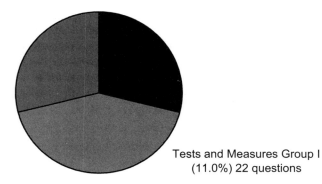

Tests and Measures Group I
(11.0%) 22 questions

Group I:

Strength, ROM, Posture, Body Structures, Prosthetic & Orthotic Devices
    Anthropometric characteristics
    Joint integrity and mobility
    Posture
    Prosthetic devices
    Range of motion/muscle length
    Muscle performance
    Orthotic, protective & supportive devices

Cognition, Nerve, Reflex and Sensory Integrity, Neurodevelopment
    Arousal, attention, and cognition
    Cranial and peripheral nerve integrity (motor and sensory)
    Motor function
    Neurodevelopment and sensory integration
    Reflex integrity
    Sensory integrity

Sample Questions

21. A physical therapist attempts to place a patient's hip in the resting position prior to assessing joint play. Which position would be most consistent with the therapist's objective?

    1. 10 degrees flexion, 15 degrees abduction, slight medial rotation
    2. 30 degrees flexion, 30 degrees abduction, slight lateral rotation
    3. 30 degrees flexion, 30 degrees adduction, 20 degrees lateral rotation
    4. 10 degrees extension, 20 degrees adduction, 20 degrees medial rotation

22. A physical therapist completes a manual muscle test on a patient that sustained a laceration to the anterior surface of the forearm. When performing a test on the flexor pollicis brevis, the therapist should direct the force:

    1. along the volar aspect of the proximal phalanx of the thumb
    2. along the volar aspect of the distal phalanx of the thumb
    3. along the dorsal aspect of the proximal phalanx of the thumb
    4. along the dorsal aspect of the distal phalanx of the thumb

23. A physical therapist examines a patient referred to physical therapy with sacroiliac pain. As part of the examination, the therapist assesses the position of the sacrum by palpating the inferior lateral angles. Which spinal level is most consistent with the inferior lateral angles?

    1. S2
    2. S3
    3. S4
    4. S5

24. A physical therapist performs a manual muscle test on a patient with bilateral upper extremity weakness. The therapist should test the patient's scapular adductors with the patient positioned in:

    1. prone
    2. sidelying
    3. standing
    4. supine

25. A physical therapist completes an upper extremity goniometric examination. The therapist records right elbow range of motion as 15-0-150 degrees. The total available range of motion for this patient is:

    1. 135 degrees
    2. 150 degrees
    3. 165 degrees
    4. 180 degrees

26. A physical therapist classifies a patient's end-feel as soft after completing a specific passive movement. Which of the following joint motions would typically produce a soft end-feel?

    1. hip flexion with the knee extended
    2. knee flexion
    3. elbow extension
    4. forearm supination

27. A physical therapist completes a series of special tests designed to examine the ligamentous integrity of a patient's knee. After completing the tests, the therapist is unsure if the laxity is normal or if it is indicative of a ligamentous injury. The most appropriate step to gather more information is to:

    1. attempt to quantify the millimeters of laxity and compare the values with established norms
    2. contact the physician and suggest a referral for magnetic resonance imaging
    3. directly compare the laxity in the involved knee to the laxity in the uninvolved knee
    4. attempt to identify other special tests that can offer more information on the ligamentous integrity of the knee

28. A physical therapist records grip strength measurements on a patient diagnosed with bilateral carpal tunnel syndrome. Which description does not accurately describe typical results when using a handheld dynamometer?

    1. a bell curve is seen when charting multiple recordings from adjustable hand spacings in consecutive order
    2. twenty to twenty-five percent differences in grip strength may be observed between the dominant and non-dominant hands
    3. discrepancies of more than twenty-five percent in a test-retest situation may indicate the patient is not exerting maximal force
    4. an individual who does not exert maximal force for each test will not show the typical bell curve

29. A physical therapist examines the motor component of the trigeminal nerve by observing a patient open and close his mouth repeatedly. Which clinical finding would be most indicative of weakness of the right pterygoid muscles?

    1. right deviation of the jaw during opening of the mouth
    2. left deviation of the jaw during opening of the mouth
    3. difficulty depressing the mandible during opening of the mouth
    4. audible crepitation during opening of the mouth

30. A physical therapist assesses kinesthesia in a 61-year-old male patient with Parkinson's disease. Which of the following patient responses would be the most appropriate during the testing?

1. my arm is moving up toward the ceiling
2. my arm is parallel with the floor
3. my arm just started moving
4. my arm is in approximately the same position as my other arm

31. A physical therapist performs a test to measure the strength of a patient's lower abdominal muscles. The most appropriate technique to examine the strength of the abdominals is:

1. partial sit-up
2. full sit-up with rotation
3. single leg lowering test
4. double leg lowering test

32. A physical therapist performs a manual muscle test of the peroneus tertius on a patient diagnosed with anterior compartment syndrome. When providing resistance to the peroneus tertius, the physical therapist should direct pressure towards:

1. dorsiflexion and eversion
2. dorsiflexion and inversion
3. plantar flexion and eversion
4. plantar flexion and inversion

33. A patient diagnosed with right bicipital tendonitis performs upper extremity resistance exercises using a piece of elastic tubing. What muscle is emphasized when laterally rotating the involved extremity against resistance?

1. teres minor
2. pectoralis major
3. teres major
4. subscapularis

34. A physical therapist examines a patient diagnosed with a C5 disk herniation. During the examination the therapist identifies a diminished deep tendon reflex response. The most likely reflexes affected would be the:

1. biceps and brachioradialis reflex
2. biceps and triceps reflex
3. brachioradialis and supinator reflex
4. triceps and brachioradialis reflex

35. A physical therapist examines a 40-year-old female referred to physical therapy after spraining her ankle playing volleyball. During the examination, the patient exhibits extreme tenderness to palpation over the sinus tarsi. What ligament is most often associated with tenderness in this area?

1. anterior talofibular
2. calcaneofibular
3. deltoid
4. posterior talofibular

36. A physical therapist completes a sensory examination on a patient with incomplete T7-T8 paraplegia. The therapist examines the patient's sensation using a piece of cotton. The therapist applies the cotton in a random fashion and the patient is asked to indicate when she feels the stimulus. This method of sensory testing is used to examine:

1. kinesthesia
2. light touch
3. proprioception
4. superficial pain

37. A physical therapist determines that a patient has a one half-inch leg length discrepancy. The therapist suspects the patient's leg length discrepancy may be due to tibial shortening. The most appropriate measurement to confirm the therapist's suspicions is from the:

1. anterior superior iliac spine to the medial malleolus
2. iliac crest to the lateral malleolus
3. medial knee joint line to the medial malleolus
4. lateral knee joint line to the medial malleolus

38. A physical therapist examines a patient with limited cervical range of motion. As part of the examination, the therapist attempts to screen the patient for possible vertebral artery involvement, but is unable to position the patient's head and neck in the recommended test position. The most appropriate action is to:

    1. complete the vertebral artery test with the head and neck positioned in approximately 50 percent of the available cervical range of motion
    2. complete the vertebral artery test as far into the available cervical range of motion as tolerated
    3. avoid completing the vertebral artery test until the patient has full cervical range of motion
    4. avoid all direct cervical treatment techniques until the vertebral artery test can be assessed at the limits of normal cervical range of motion

39. A physical therapist positions a patient in prone on a plinth and passively flexes her knee. As the knee flexes, the patient's hip on the same side also begins to flex. This clinical finding is most indicative of a:

    1. tight iliopsoas
    2. tight rectus femoris
    3. tight tensor fasciae latae
    4. tight hamstrings

40. A physical therapist assesses a patient's lower extremity deep tendon reflexes using a reflex hammer. Which of the following reflexes would provide the therapist with the most information on the L3-L4 neurologic level?

    1. patellar reflex
    2. lateral hamstrings reflex
    3. posterior tibial reflex
    4. Achilles reflex

Tests and Measures: Group II

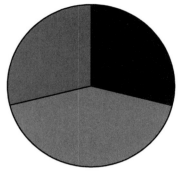

Tests and Measures Group II
(7.5%) 15 questions

Group II:
Cardiovascular/pulmonary System
    Aerobic capacity/endurance
    Circulation (arterial, venous, lymphatic)
    Ventilation and respiration/gas exchange

Integumentary System
    Integumentary integrity

Functional Status and Community Integration
    Self-care and home management, including activities of daily living and instrumental activities of
        daily living
    Work (job/school/play), community and leisure integration or
        reintegration, including instrumental activities of daily living
    Assistive and adaptive devices
    Gait, locomotion, and balance
    Pain
    Ergonomics and body mechanics

Sample Questions

41. A physical therapist monitors a patient's blood pressure using the brachial artery. What effect would you expect to see on the measured blood pressure value if the therapist selects a blood pressure cuff that is too narrow in relation to the circumference of the patient's arm?

    1. systolic values will be higher and diastolic values will be lower
    2. systolic values will be lower and diastolic values will be higher
    3. systolic and diastolic values will be higher
    4. systolic and diastolic values will be lower

42. A physical therapist assesses a one-month-old infant. During the treatment session the therapist strokes the cheek of the infant causing the infant to turn its mouth towards the stimulus. This action is utilized to assess the:

    1. Moro reflex
    2. rooting reflex
    3. startle reflex
    4. righting reflex

43. A patient with cardiac disease rates the intensity of exercise as a 12 using Borg's Original Rate of Perceived Exertion Scale. What percentage of the patient's age-adjusted maximum heart rate best corresponds to a rating of 12 on the exertion scale?

    1. 50
    2. 60
    3. 75
    4. 85

44. A physical therapist completes a gait analysis on a patient diagnosed with Parkinson's disease. As part of the examination the therapist measures the distance between right heel strike and the next consecutive left heel strike. This measurement is used to measure:

    1. left stride length
    2. right stride length
    3. left step length
    4. right step length

45. A physical therapist attempts to assess the dorsal pedal pulse of a patient diagnosed with peripheral vascular disease. To locate the dorsal pedal pulse the therapist should palpate:

    1. between the extensor hallucis longus and the extensor digitorum longus tendons on the dorsum of the foot
    2. between the flexor digitorum longus and the flexor hallucis longus tendons on the dorsum of the foot
    3. immediately posterior to the medial malleolus
    4. immediately posterior to the lateral malleolus

46. A patient with an irregular heart rate is monitored using a single lead electrocardiogram during exercise. Which of the following techniques would provide the physical therapist with the most accurate measurement of heart rate?

    1. count the number of QRS complexes that occur in sixty seconds
    2. count the number of R waves that occur in thirty seconds and multiply by two
    3. count the number of P waves that occur in fifteen seconds and multiply by four
    4. count the number of T waves that occur in six seconds and multiply by ten

47. A physical therapist examines a patient diagnosed with an acute posterior cruciate sprain. The most common mechanism of injury for the posterior cruciate is:

    1. a forceful landing on the anterior tibia with the knee hyperflexed
    2. an anteriorly directed force applied to the tibia when the foot is fixed
    3. a valgus force applied to the knee when the foot is fixed
    4. hyperextension and medial rotation of the leg with lateral rotation of the body

48. A 56-year-old female diagnosed with emphysema is referred to physical therapy. As part of the examination the physical therapist assesses tactile fremitus by asking the patient to repeat the term "ninety-nine" several times in succession. The most appropriate method when assessing tactile fremitus is:

    1. examine voice sounds through auscultation
    2. examine vibration using the ulnar border of the hand
    3. examine chest excursion with a tape measure
    4. examine the intensity and clarity of spoken words using a recording device

49. A physical therapist examines the viscosity and color of a sputum sample after completing postural drainage activities. The sputum is a yellowish-greenish color and is very thick. The therapist can best describe the sputum as:

    1. fetid
    2. frothy
    3. mucoid
    4. purulent

The following image should be used to answer question 50:

50. A physical therapist enters the room of a patient in an acute care hospital and observes that the patient is having a formal diagnostic test. The patient was admitted to the hospital three days ago after being diagnosed with peripheral arterial disease. Based on the supplied picture, the diagnostic testing was most likely being administered to determine the patient's:

   1. rate of arterial perfusion
   2. oxygen saturation rate
   3. prothrombin time
   4. maximum oxygen consumption

51. A physical therapist works with a patient status post stroke on a mat program. The therapist assists the patient in lateral weight shifting activities while positioned in prone on elbows. Which therapeutic exercise technique would allow the patient to improve dynamic stability with this activity?

   1. alternating isometrics
   2. approximation
   3. rhythmic initiation
   4. timing for emphasis

52. A physical therapist performs a capillary refill test on a patient diagnosed with bronchitis by applying direct pressure to the nailbeds of the fingers. Which finding would be most indicative of a normal response after releasing the direct pressure?

   1. blanching should appear in less than two seconds
   2. blanching should appear in less than four seconds
   3. blanching should resolve in less than two seconds
   4. blanching should resolve in less than four seconds

53. A physical therapist presents a community inservice on risk factors associated with coronary artery disease. Which of the following individuals would be at greatest risk?

   1. a 45-year-old male with a cholesterol level of 260 mg/dL
   2. a 39-year-old female with a cholesterol level of 180mg/dL and a family history of cardiac disease
   3. a 42-year-old male with a cholesterol level of 200 mg/dL and hypertension
   4. a 47-year-old female with a cholesterol level of 170 mg/dL, moderate hypotension, and a family history of cardiac disease

54. A physical therapist performs auscultation on a patient with known cardiac pathology. When attempting to assess the pulmonic valve the therapist should position the stethoscope:

   1. in the second right intercostal space at the right sternal margin
   2. in the second left intercostal space at the left sternal margin
   3. in the fifth left intercostal space in line with the middle of the clavicle
   4. in the fourth left intercostal space along the lower left sternal border

55. A patient with known cardiac involvement performs upper extremity active range of motion exercises on a tilt table. The patient's medical record indicates he is currently taking beta-blockers. Which of the following is the most appropriate subjective measure to monitor the patient's response to exercise?

    1. heart rate
    2. respiration rate
    3. blood pressure
    4. perceived exertion

56. A physical therapist assesses a patient's voice sounds as part of a respiratory examination. The therapist positions the stethoscope over the thorax and asks the patient to say "ninety nine." Which type of voice sound is assessed using this technique?

    1. bronchophony
    2. egophony
    3. pectoriloquy
    4. pneumophony

57. A physical therapist prepares to initiate an exercise program for a patient with diabetes mellitus. Which objective measure would be the most appropriate to examine in order to avoid significant complications from exercise?

    1. systolic blood pressure
    2. respiratory rate
    3. blood glucose values
    4. oxygen saturation rate

58. A physical therapist observes the electrocardiogram of a patient during exercise. Which of the following ECG changes would be considered abnormal during exercise?

    1. increase in amplitude of P wave
    2. shortening of PR interval
    3. ST segment depression of greater than 1 mm
    4. decrease in amplitude of T wave

59. A physical therapist reviews the medical record of a patient recently diagnosed with peripheral vascular disease. A note in the medical record indicates that the patient's ankle-brachial index (ABI) was within normal limits. The value most consistent with this measure is:

    1. .5
    2. .7
    3. 1.0
    4. 1.3

60. A 32-year-old female is admitted to the hospital after sustaining extensive burns to her trunk and right upper extremity. Which of the following burn classifications would most likely require the use of a graft?

    1. superficial burn
    2. superficial partial-thickness burn
    3. deep partial-thickness burn
    4. full-thickness burn

II. *Evaluation, Diagnosis, Prognosis, and Outcomes*

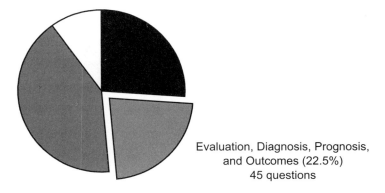

Evaluation, Diagnosis, Prognosis,
and Outcomes (22.5%)
45 questions

Evaluation, Diagnosis, Prognosis, and Outcomes	
Evaluation and Diagnosis	23
Prognosis and Outcome	22
Total = 45	

Evaluation and Diagnosis

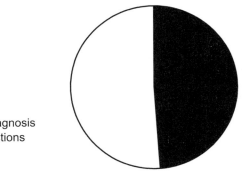

Evaluation and Diagnosis
(11.5%) 23 questions

Identifying and prioritizing impairments
Determining the dysfunction toward which the intervention will be directed

Sample Questions

61. A physical therapist reviews the medical record of a patient admitted to the hospital. A recent entry in the medical record indicates the patient has a lesion affecting the facial motor nucleus. Based on the patient's diagnosis, the most probable clinical presentation is:

    1. facial muscle weakness ipsilateral to the lesion
    2. facial muscle weakness contralateral to the lesion
    3. impaired facial sensation ipsilateral to the lesion
    4. impaired facial sensation contralateral to the lesion

62. A physical therapist completes an examination on a 14-year-old male with a genetic disorder caused by a chromosomal abnormality. The patient appears to be quite tall with a slender build and proportionately long arms. He is alert and oriented, however, appears to possess below average intelligence. This type of clinical presentation is most consistent with:

    1. Down syndrome
    2. Edward's syndrome
    3. Klinefelter's syndrome
    4. Turner's syndrome

63. A physical therapist is growing increasingly concerned about a patient that is demonstrating symptoms that are consistent with neoplastic activity. What is the most significant symptom of a rapidly growing neoplasm?

    1. fatigue
    2. swelling
    3. tenderness to palpation
    4. pain

64. A physical therapist employed in a rehabilitation hospital performs an examination on a 52-year-old male diagnosed with amyotrophic lateral sclerosis. Which of the following signs and symptoms is not consistent with this disease?

    1. mental deterioration
    2. hyperactive deep tendon reflexes
    3. weakness of the forearms and hands
    4. impaired speech

65. A physical therapist examines a patient with T1 paraplegia. As the therapist and patient perform balance activities in sitting, the patient begins to complain of a pounding headache. The patient exhibits profuse sweating above the T1 lesion, and blotching of the skin. The therapist should immediately identify this as:

    1. orthostatic hypotension
    2. autonomic dysreflexia
    3. Lowe's syndrome
    4. homonymous hemianopsia

66. A physical therapist reviews the results of a patient's arterial blood gases. The report indicates the following: $PaO_2 = 45$ mm Hg, $PaCO_2 = 55$ mm Hg, $HCO_3 = 24$ mEq/L, pH = 7.20. These values are most indicative of:

    1. respiratory acidosis
    2. respiratory alkalosis
    3. metabolic acidosis
    4. metabolic alkalosis

67. A physical therapist reviews the results of a pulmonary function test for a patient with chronic obstructive pulmonary disease. Which of the following results is typical with chronic obstructive pulmonary disease?

    1. decreased functional residual capacity
    2. increased vital capacity
    3. increased residual volume
    4. increased forced expiratory volume in one second

68. A physical therapist examines a 28-year-old male with burns covering 30 percent of his body. The patient sustained the burns approximately 24 hours earlier in a house fire. The medical record indicates an unremarkable medical history with the exception of a benign cardiac arrhythmia. Which of the following emergent conditions is the patient most susceptible to?

    1. aortic aneurysm
    2. autonomic dysreflexia
    3. diabetic coma
    4. shock

69. A physical therapist administers a series of cranial nerve tests to a patient with a confirmed lower motor neuron disease. Assuming the patient has a lesion impacting the left hypoglossal nerve, which clinical presentation would be most likely?

    1. right-sided tongue atrophy and deviation toward the left with tongue protrusion
    2. right-sided tongue atrophy and deviation toward the right with tongue protrusion
    3. left-sided tongue atrophy and deviation toward the left with tongue protrusion
    4. left-sided tongue atrophy and deviation toward the right with tongue protrusion

70. A physical therapist examines a five-year-old child's gait. The therapist notes that the child is unsteady and uses a wide base of support. The child appears to lurch at times with minimal truncal bobbing in an anterior and posterior direction. The child cannot maintain a standing position with the feet placed together for more than five seconds. The area of the brain most likely affected is the:

    1. corticospinal tracts
    2. basal ganglia
    3. substantia nigra
    4. cerebellum

71. A 28-year-old male diagnosed with a medial meniscus injury is referred to physical therapy following arthroscopic surgery. During the examination the physical therapist identifies decreased range of motion in the involved knee. This objective finding is best termed a/an:

    1. pathology
    2. impairment
    3. functional limitation
    4. disability

72. A physical therapist examines a patient with low back pain. Diagnostic imaging reveals the patient has a mild disk protrusion at the L4-L5 level. Physical examination reveals a diminished lumbar curve and the presence of a lateral shift. The most appropriate treatment intervention is:

    1. instruct the patient in active extension exercises
    2. instruct the patient in passive extension exercises
    3. attempt to correct the lateral shift
    4. apply palliative modalities

73. A 13-year-old boy is referred to physical therapy after being diagnosed with an injury to the proximal tibial epiphysis. The boy was hit by a car and sustained a severe hyperextension force applied to the left knee. What is the most serious complication of this injury?

    1. lesion of the common peroneal nerve
    2. tear of the posterior cruciate ligament
    3. damage to the popliteal artery
    4. patellar instability

74. A physical therapist examines the gait of a 62-year-old male with peripheral neuropathy. The therapist observes that the patient's right foot has a tendency to slap the ground during the loading response. The observation can best be explained by weakness of the:

    1. iliopsoas
    2. tibialis anterior
    3. tibialis posterior
    4. gastrocnemius

75. Documentation from an orthopedic surgeon's report indicates that a patient sustained damage to several structures that provide anterolateral stability to the knee. Which of the following structures would most likely be involved?

    1. anterior cruciate ligament, posterior oblique ligament, iliotibial band
    2. anterior cruciate ligament, medial collateral ligament, medial meniscus
    3. anterior cruciate ligament, lateral collateral ligament, iliotibial band
    4. posterior cruciate ligament, lateral collateral ligament, biceps femoris tendon

76. A patient rehabilitating from a CVA is referred to physical therapy. The medical record indicates the CVA primarily involved the right hemisphere of the brain. Which of the following objective findings would be least likely when examining the patient?

    1. diminished motor control of the left side of the body
    2. impaired awareness of the right side of the body
    3. impaired spatial ability
    4. diminished awareness of disability

77. A physical therapist discusses a patient care plan with a physical therapist assistant in preparation for treatment. The physical therapist indicates that the patient has ideomotor apraxia. This condition is most consistent with:

    1. difficulty performing sequenced motor acts
    2. inability to carry out purposeful movement on command
    3. failure to recognize familiar objects
    4. inability to respond to stimuli presented contralateral to the side of a brain lesion

78. A physical therapist examines a patient who complains of occasional difficulty maintaining her balance when walking and frequent episodes of vertigo. The most likely cause of the patient's difficulty is a disorder of the:

    1. visual system
    2. proprioceptive system
    3. auditory system
    4. vestibular system

79. A physical therapist determines that a patient has diminished calf sensation and an absent Achilles reflex on the right lower extremity. Earlier the patient had communicated to the therapist that she experienced difficulty controlling her bowel movements. The neurologic level of most concern is:

    1. L2
    2. L4
    3. L5
    4. S2

80. A physical therapist receives a referral for a patient who is one week status post CVA. When observing the patient lying in bed, the therapist notes that the patient's calf and foot are edematous. The patient reports that the area is somewhat painful. The therapist should:

    1. discontinue the examination and hope the patient's leg is better tomorrow
    2. consider ordering compression stockings for the patient
    3. continue with the examination and disregard the patient's condition
    4. inform the physician of the situation and discontinue the examination

Prognosis and Outcome

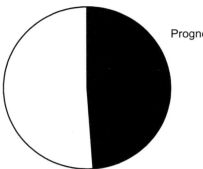

Prognosis and Outcomes (11%)
22 questions

Determining the predicted optimal level of improvement in function and the amount of time needed to reach that level

Determining the prognosis with consideration of modifying factors, e.g., age, medications, co-morbidities, cognitive status, nutrition, social support

Planning and sequencing patient interventions and progressing treatment based upon outcome

Determining outcomes

Collecting outcome data

Determining discharge criteria based upon patient goals and functional status

Differentiating between discharge of patient, discontinuation of service and transfer of care and re-evaluation

Modifying tests/measures and interventions when necessary

Recognizing effectiveness of PT interventions

Sample Questions

81. A physical therapist completes a family training session with a patient rehabilitating from a spinal cord injury. During the training the family asks a question regarding the functional ability of the patient following rehabilitation. The most appropriate therapist response is to:

1. explain to the family that it is difficult to predict since all patients progress differently
2. provide information on the expected prognosis based on the nature and severity of the injury
3. refer the family to the director of rehabilitation
4. refer the family to the patient's physiatrist

82. A 32-year-old male of Portuguese descent is referred to physical therapy for instruction in a home exercise program. The physician referral indicates that the patient is approved for one visit. What is the likelihood the patient will comprehend the home exercise program in the allotted time?

1. the patient will require external assistance such as the use of an interpreter to comprehend the home exercise program
2. the patient will comprehend the home exercise program
3. the patient will not be able to comprehend the home exercise program
4. the physical therapist cannot make a prediction based on the supplied information

83. A physical therapist determines that a patient rehabilitating from an anterior cruciate ligament reconstruction is not ready to return to athletic competition. Which of the following best supports the therapist's decision?

    1. a 20 percent quadriceps peak torque deficit at 60 degrees per second
    2. trace effusion in the knee after a therapy session
    3. a 5 degree limitation in knee flexion
    4. inability to complete a functional progression

84. A physical therapist develops a chart detailing expected functional outcomes for a variety of spinal cord injuries. Which is the highest spinal level at which independent transfers with a sliding board would be feasible?

    1. C4
    2. C6
    3. T1
    4. T3

85. A patient rehabilitating from a grade I medial collateral ligament injury questions a physical therapist about his expected functional activity level following rehabilitation. The most accurate predictor of the patient's expected functional activity level is the:

    1. patient's age and past medical history
    2. patient's previous functional activity level
    3. duration of physical therapy services
    4. patient's compliance with the established home exercise program

86. A patient with anterior cruciate ligament insufficiency, who elects not to have surgical reconstruction, could probably expect to reach which minimal functional level?

    1. able to participate in all sports
    2. able to participate in light recreational sports
    3. cannot play any type of sport
    4. problems with normal walking

87. A physical therapist treats a patient referred to physical therapy after sustaining a comminuted Colles' fracture. The fracture was stabilized with an external fixator device. Which post-operative time frame best represents the amount of time the external fixator device will be utilized?

    1. 2-4 weeks
    2. 6-8 weeks
    3. 10-12 weeks
    4. 14-16 weeks

88. A patient demonstrates dizziness and nausea during vertebral artery testing. The physical therapist should pay particular attention when treating the patient to avoid positioning the neck in:

    1. extension and extremes of rotation
    2. flexion and slight rotation
    3. flexion and extreme sidebending
    4. extension and slight sidebending

89. A physical therapist treats a patient status post surgical repair of the ulnar collateral ligament of the thumb. The patient injured the thumb approximately three weeks ago while skiing. Which of the following would be the most realistic post-operative time frame for the patient to resume unrestricted activity?

    1. 6 weeks
    2. 12 weeks
    3. 18 weeks
    4. 24 weeks

90. A physical therapist treats a patient rehabilitating from a chemical burn sustained in a work-related injury. The patient has been in the hospital for nearly a month and as a result the therapist is concerned about the patient's cardiovascular status. Which of the following would serve as the best indicator that the patient does not need to participate in a formal cardiovascular rehabilitation program?

    1. arterial blood gas analysis within normal limits
    2. functional capacity greater than 10 metabolic equivalents
    3. oxygen saturation rate greater than 90 percent
    4. resting heart rate of 58 beats per minute

91. A physical therapist treats a 32-year-old female rehabilitating from a closed head injury presently functioning at Rancho Los Amigos level IV. The therapist treats the patient in her home for 60 minute sessions, three times per week. Recently the therapist has noticed that the patient becomes increasingly combative as the session progresses and believes the deterioration in behavior is linked to the patient becoming fatigued. The most appropriate treatment modification is:

    1. reduce the treatment sessions to 30 minutes, three times per week
    2. reduce the frequency of the treatment sessions to two times per week
    3. increase the rest periods during existing treatment sessions
    4. increase the treatment sessions to 90 minutes, two times per week

92. A physical therapist reviews the medical record of a patient with Hodgkin's disease. The patient is a 45-year-old male who recently began chemotherapy treatment. What effect will chemotherapy have on the patient's ability to participate in a rehabilitation program?

    1. the patient may be susceptible to infection
    2. the patient may experience excessive fatigue
    3. the patient may demonstrate cardiac anomalies
    4. the patient may exhibit signs and symptoms of gastrointestinal distress

93. A physical therapist that recently returned from maternity leave reviews her daily patient schedule. Her first patient is a 46-year-old male that is referred to physical therapy for wound debridement. The patient's medical record indicates that he is HIV positive. The most appropriate therapist action is:

    1. have support personnel complete the treatment under direct supervision
    2. ask another therapist to treat the patient
    3. treat the patient
    4. contact the referring physician to discuss the treatment orders

94. A patient in a rehabilitation hospital returns to physical therapy after a meeting with his physiatrist. The patient indicates that during the meeting the physiatrist discussed the effect of his spinal cord injury on sexual function. Which of the following statements is typically not accurate for a male patient with complete T7 paraplegia?

    1. The patient will be able to achieve an erection.
    2. The patient will be able to ejaculate.
    3. The patient's fertility will be diminished.
    4. The patient's medications may affect his sexual function.

95. A patient diagnosed with peripheral vascular disease is examined in physical therapy. Which of the following objective findings would result in an ambulation exercise program being contraindicated?

    1. decreased peripheral pulses
    2. resting claudication
    3. increased resting systolic blood pressure
    4. decreased lower extremity strength

96. A physical therapist treats a patient rehabilitating from total hip replacement surgery. As part of the session, the therapist discusses the importance of preventing deep venous thrombosis. Which finding is the best indicator that the patient is at a reduced risk for acquiring a deep venous thrombosis?

    1. ability to perform ankle pumps and muscle setting exercises
    2. ability to achieve full hip range of motion within the allowable limits
    3. ability to utilize pneumatic compression devices and elastic stockings
    4. ability to ambulate on a frequent schedule

97. A physical therapist examines a 72-year-old female four weeks status post CVA. The therapist informs the patient that she could benefit from having physical therapy services to improve her ambulatory status. The patient explains that she is no longer able to drive and does not have access to any other form of transportation. The patient lives alone, however, is currently receiving some assistance from a neighbor. The most appropriate setting for continued therapy would be:

    1. outpatient rehabilitation
    2. skilled nursing facility
    3. home health services
    4. inpatient rehabilitation

98. A patient successfully advances through a series of short-term goals, but is unable to attain the associated long-term goal. The therapist's most appropriate response is to:

    1. develop another more attainable long-term goal
    2. develop additional short-term goals that facilitate achievement of the established long-term goal
    3. contact the referring physician to discuss the patient's lack of progress
    4. discharge the patient since he is no longer making progress toward the established long-term goal

99. A patient originally referred to physical therapy for six weeks of treatment has achieved all of the established short and long-term goals in less than three weeks. The patient is completely asymptomatic and has returned to all previously performed activities of daily living. The physical therapist's most appropriate action is to:

    1. continue to treat the patient three times a week for the remaining three weeks
    2. reduce the frequency of the patient's appointments to twice a week
    3. reduce the frequency of the patient's appointments to once a week
    4. discharge the patient and send a copy of the discharge summary to the referring physician

100. A physical therapist treats a patient with C5-C6 tetraplegia. During the treatment session the patient's spouse asks a question regarding the patient's ability to transfer independently following rehabilitation. The most appropriate therapist response is to:

    1. refer the spouse to the director of rehabilitation
    2. refer the spouse to the patient's primary physician
    3. refer the spouse to the patient's primary nurse
    4. answer the spouse's question

III. *Intervention*

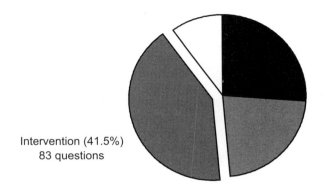

Intervention (41.5%)
83 questions

Intervention	
Non-procedural Intervention	14
Procedural Intervention	
Group I:	27
Group II:	20
Group III:	22
Total = 83	

Non-procedural Intervention

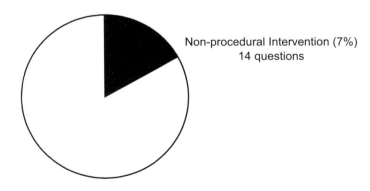

Non-procedural Intervention (7%)
14 questions

Coordination of Care, i.e., knowledge of resources and coordination with team members (PTA, RN, OT, SLHP, SW, Psychology, etc.), including appropriate referral or direction and supervision as indicated

Communication

Educating members of other health care disciplines regarding safe, effective patient handling techniques

Conferring with members of other health care disciplines about the physical therapy plan of care

Conferring with the patient/client and family regarding plan of care, interventions, and outcomes

Documentation

Documentation of objective, patient-centered, functional outcomes (goal statements)

Objective documentation of examination, evaluation, diagnosis, prognosis, interventions, and outcomes

Patient/Family/Client-related Instructions

Utilizing teaching strategies, theories, and techniques to achieve desired goals including consideration of variables that may require adjusting educational methods, e.g., learning styles, communication deficits, cultural/language style, motor learning principles

Educating the patient/family about patient's current condition/examination findings, plan of care and expected outcomes, utilizing their feedback to modify the plan as needed

Providing and modifying same according to the patient/family's needs

Sample Questions

101. A work site examination is scheduled for a patient rehabilitating from a closed head injury eight weeks ago. The patient presents with mild dysarthria and right-sided hemiparesis with moderate upper extremity involvement. The patient's job duties are secretarial including: answering phones, filing, and organizing the office. The most appropriate provider to participate in the work site examination is a/an:

    1. physical therapist
    2. occupational therapist
    3. speech therapist
    4. social worker

102. A physical therapist works on bed mobility exercises with a patient recently diagnosed with terminal cancer. The patient is extremely upset and tells the therapist, "I know I will never get better." The therapist's most appropriate response would be:

    1. Radiation treatments will make you feel much better.
    2. Many people have overcome larger obstacles.
    3. Having cancer must be very difficult for you to deal with.
    4. Physical therapy can improve your condition.

103. A physical therapist suspects a patient may be under the influence of alcohol during a treatment session. The therapist has been treating the patient for over five weeks and during that time has failed to recognize any signs or symptoms of substance abuse. The therapist's most immediate action would be to:

    1. contact the referring physician and discuss the patient's problem
    2. ask the patient if they have been drinking
    3. discharge the patient from physical therapy
    4. refer the patient to a local Alcoholics Anonymous group

104. A physical therapist prepares a presentation on preseason conditioning for a group of high school athletes. To maximize the effectiveness of the presentation the therapist should:

    1. develop specific learning objectives
    2. utilize a variety of audiovisual equipment
    3. assess the needs of the target audience
    4. provide an outline

105. A physical therapist treats a patient one day status post posterior hip dislocation. The injury was treated using closed reduction. As part of the treatment session the therapist educates the patient on hip precautions to avoid the recurrence of dislocation and implements an exercise program including gluteal sets, quadriceps sets, hamstrings sets, ankle pumps, upper extremity exercises, and bed mobility. Which activity would be the most essential for the physical therapy session the following day?

    1. review the exercise program
    2. initiate straight leg raises
    3. begin ambulation activities
    4. start active-assisted range of motion

106. A physical therapist treats a 61-year-old male at home following thoracic surgery. As part of treatment, the therapist designs a general exercise program for the patient. The patient is extremely eager to begin the exercise program, however, his spouse expresses serious doubt about the program's importance. The most appropriate therapist action is to:

    1. explain to the patient and spouse why the exercise program is an essential part of rehabilitation
    2. redesign the exercise program to address the spouse's concerns
    3. ask the spouse to leave the room during treatment sessions
    4. discharge the patient from physical therapy

107. An orthopedic surgeon instructs a patient to remain non-weight bearing for three weeks following a medial meniscus repair. During the examination it becomes obvious that the patient has not adhered to the prescribed weight bearing status. The most immediate physical therapist action is to:

    1. contact the orthopedic surgeon
    2. explain to the patient the potential consequences of ignoring the weight bearing restrictions
    3. draft a letter to the patient's third party payer
    4. complete an incident report

108. A physical therapist treats a five-year-old with cerebral palsy. Initially the therapist was frustrated by the child's poor participation in therapy and as a result developed a reward system that enables the child to earn a sticker for good behavior. Since the therapist initiated the reward system the child has earned a sticker in each of the last five treatment sessions. This type of associated learning is termed:

    1. classical conditioning
    2. operant conditioning
    3. procedural learning
    4. declarative learning

109. A five-year-old patient is examined in physical therapy. The patient seems very uncomfortable during the examination and offers little useful information concerning her injury. The most appropriate physical therapist action is to:

    1. speak loudly and directly to the patient
    2. request that the patient's parents come into the treatment room
    3. explain to the patient the importance of physical therapy
    4. inform the patient that effective communication involves more than one individual

110. A patient with osteoarthritis in the right knee is referred to physical therapy. Examination reveals moderate inflammation in the involved knee and significant muscle weakness particularly in the quadriceps. The patient rates the intensity of pain in the knee as a 4 on a scale of 0 to 10. The most appropriate activity to address the muscle impairment is:

    1. isometric quadriceps contraction
    2. straight leg raises with ankle weights
    3. limited range active knee extension in short sitting
    4. avoid strengthening exercises until the patient is pain free

111. A physical therapist treats a 15-year-old female of Spanish descent. The patient speaks only a few words of English and has significant difficulty understanding the therapist's instructions. The most appropriate therapist action is to:

     1. speak strongly and directly to the patient
     2. encourage frequent feedback from the patient
     3. utilize an interpreter
     4. emphasize nonverbal communication

112. A physical therapist employed in an acute care hospital returns to work after a brief vacation and finds a number of items that require her immediate attention. Which of the following items should be given the highest priority?

     1. a message to call a physician
     2. a patient referral from two days ago
     3. a laboratory test report
     4. a patient record that has not been completed

113. A physical therapist reviews the medical record of a patient rehabilitating from knee surgery. A recent entry in the medical record uses the term effusion. Which description most appropriately defines this term?

     1. increased volume of fluid
     2. increased volume of fluid within the joint capsule
     3. increased volume of fluid in the soft tissue external to the joint
     4. increased volume of fluid in the joint capsule and the soft tissue external to the joint

114. A patient diagnosed with impingement syndrome is referred to physical therapy. During the examination the physical therapist identifies several clinical findings that indicate the possibility of a small rotator cuff tear. The therapist's most appropriate action would be to:

     1. contact the referring physician to discuss the clinical findings
     2. treat the patient as diagnosed on the referral
     3. refer the patient back to the physician
     4. discharge the patient from physical therapy

115. A female diagnosed with a cervical spine injury reports to physical therapy for a scheduled treatment session. While walking with the patient to the treatment area the physical therapist notices that the patient's cervical orthosis is very loose. The most appropriate therapist action is:

     1. document the observation in the medical record
     2. reapply the orthosis correctly at the conclusion of the treatment session
     3. remind the patient of the donning instructions for the orthosis
     4. contact the referring physician

116. A physical therapist examines a 43-year-old female diagnosed with a nondisplaced fracture of the humerus. During the examination the patient tells the therapist she has kept her arm in a sling sporadically, but would like the therapist's permission to stop using it. An appropriate course of action would be to:

     1. instruct the patient to wear the sling at all times
     2. instruct the patient not to use the sling because it will inhibit her range of motion
     3. use their best judgment based on how the referring physician usually treats humerus fractures
     4. contact the physician and ask what instructions were given to the patient

117. A physical therapist prepares a presentation on proper body mechanics for a group of 100 autoworkers. Which of the following media would be most effective to maximize learning during the presentation?

     1. lecture, handouts
     2. lecture, charts, statistics
     3. lecture, handouts, demonstration
     4. lecture, statistics

118. A physical therapist prepares an inservice on repetitive use injuries for a group of administrative assistants. As part of the presentation, the therapist develops learning objectives. Which of the following objectives would be considered in the cognitive domain?

    1. List three potential consequences of an improperly designed workstation.
    2. Correctly adjust the level of a computer keyboard.
    3. Devote five minutes in the morning and afternoon for stretching exercises.
    4. Demonstrate proper posture when sitting at a desk.

119. A physical therapist receives an order to devise a home program for a nine-year-old boy diagnosed with chondromalacia patella. As the therapist starts to explain the exercise instructions, it becomes obvious that the boy is not interested. Which of the following would be the most appropriate action to improve compliance with the home exercise program?

    1. Tell the boy he can leave because it is very difficult to help someone who does not want to be helped.
    2. Continue with the instructions hoping that the boy is a better listener than he appears to be.
    3. Lecture the boy on the importance of compliance with the home program.
    4. Ask a family member to come into the room while you explain the home program.

120. A physical therapist transports a patient with a brain injury to the physical therapy gym. Each day after arriving in the gym, the patient asks the therapist, "Where am I?" Recognizing the patient has short-term memory loss, the therapist's most appropriate response should be:

    1. You know where you are.
    2. You are in the same place you were yesterday at this time.
    3. You are in the physical therapy gym for your treatment session.
    4. You are in the hospital because of your injury.

Procedural Intervention

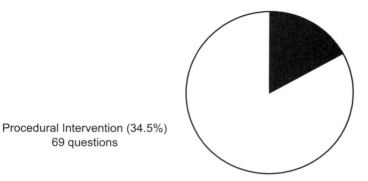

Procedural Intervention (34.5%)
69 questions

Procedural Intervention: Group I

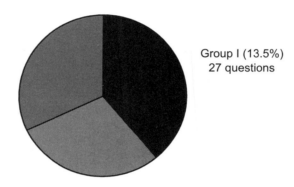

Group I (13.5%)
27 questions

Group I: Exercise and Manual Therapy
Exercise
> Aerobic capacity training/cardiovascular training
> Strengthening/muscular endurance
> Stretching/range of motion
> Neuromuscular re-education (including perceptual training)
> Balance/coordination
> Breathing
> Aquatic
> Postural
> Developmental

Manual therapy
> Techniques, including spinal & peripheral mobilization, manual traction
> Techniques of soft tissue mobilization

Sample Questions

121. A physical therapist treats a 47-year-old female with diminished lower extremity range of motion due to hamstrings tightness. As part of the treatment program, the therapist attempts to identify an appropriate active exercise technique to improve range of motion. Which objective finding would result in contract-relax being an undesirable treatment option?

1. the limitation of movement is accompanied by pain
2. the limitation of movement is greater than 50% of the normal available range
3. the limitation of movement involves multiple planes
4. the limitation of movement occurs in a non-capsular pattern

122. A physical therapist administers a submaximal exercise test using the YMCA Cycle Ergometry Protocol. The test consists of a variable number of three minute stages of continuous exercise and requires the examiner to raise the patient's steady state heart rate to 110-150 beats per minute for two consecutive stages. Which of the following would be the most accurate guideline for terminating a submaximal exercise test?

1. the subject reaches 75% of their age-predicted maximal heart rate
2. the subject reaches 80% of their age-predicted maximal heart rate
3. the subject reaches 85% of their age-predicted maximal heart rate
4. the subject reaches 90% of their age-predicted maximal heart rate

123. A patient diagnosed with right shoulder adhesive capsulitis is limited to 25 degrees of lateral rotation. Which mobilization technique would be indicated based on the patient's limitation?

1. lateral distraction and anterior glide
2. medial distraction and posterior glide
3. lateral distraction and posterior glide
4. medial distraction and inferior glide

124. A 12-year-old female that became anoxic in a near drowning performs dynamic activities in quadruped. The next posture to attain in the developmental sequence would be:

1. half kneeling
2. tall kneeling
3. plantigrade
4. standing

125. A physical therapist implements an aquatic program for a patient rehabilitating from a total hip replacement. During the treatment session the patient indicates how much easier it is to walk in the water compared to on land. What factor is responsible for the patient's ability to walk in water?

1. buoyancy
2. pressure
3. cohesion
4. viscosity

126. A patient is limited to 55 degrees in an active straight leg raise. When using the contract-relax technique to improve the patient's active range of motion, the therapist should emphasize contraction of the:

1. abductors and hip flexors
2. hamstrings and hip extensors
3. quadriceps and hip flexors
4. adductors and hip extensors

127. A physical therapist designs an exercise program for a patient rehabilitating from a prolonged illness. Which of the following exercises is indicated for coordination training?

1. Buerger-Allen exercises
2. Codman's exercises
3. DeLorme's exercises
4. Frenkel's exercises

The following image should be used to answer question 128:

128. A physical therapist prepares a home exercise program for a patient rehabilitating from a disk protrusion in the lumbar spine. Assuming the patient successfully completes the pictured exercise, which activity would be next to occur in the extension progression?

    1. single knee to chest
    2. double knee to chest
    3. prone on elbows
    4. extension exercises in standing

129. A physical therapist employed in a rehabilitation hospital works with a patient diagnosed with Parkinson's disease on preambulation activities. As part of the program the physical therapist focuses on improving the patient's lower trunk rotation. The most appropriate patient position to accomplish this goal is:

    1. bridging
    2. hooklying
    3. prone on elbows
    4. quadruped

130. A physical therapist discusses how to perform pelvic floor muscle strengthening exercises with a 36-year-old female diagnosed with stress incontinence. The patient describes involuntary leakage of urine when she coughs, sneezes or exercises. The most appropriate ratio of rest to hold time when initiating pelvic floor muscle strengthening is:

    1. 1:2
    2. 1:5
    3. 2:1
    4. 5:1

131. A physical therapist treats a patient status post CVA. Which action would be most likely to facilitate elbow extension in a patient with hemiplegia?

    1. turn the head to the affected side
    2. turn the head to the unaffected side
    3. extend the lower extremities
    4. flex the lower extremities

132. A physical therapist administers a submaximal exercise test using a cycle ergometer. The test consists of a warm-up followed by three stages of increasing increments of work each lasting three minutes, and a cool down. During the second stage of the exercise test the therapist records the patient's heart rate as 122 beats per minute after two minutes and 134 beats per minute after three minutes. Which of the following would be the most appropriate therapist action?

    1. administer a rating of perceived exertion scale
    2. maintain the present work rate for an additional minute
    3. progress to the specified work rate for the third stage
    4. discontinue the submaximal exercise test

133. A physical therapist administers a submaximal exercise test on a patient using a cycle ergometer. The test consists of four stages, each lasting three minutes in duration at increasing exercise intensities. The exercise intensities for the stages were recorded as 50, 75, 100, and 125 watts respectively. If the therapist elects to have the patient cool down using the cycle ergometer, which exercise intensity would be the most appropriate to select?

    1. 40 watts
    2. 60 watts
    3. 80 watts
    4. 100 watts

134. A patient two weeks status post anterior cruciate ligament reconstruction using a patellar tendon autograft is examined in physical therapy. When designing the patient's rehabilitation program the physical therapist focuses on avoiding activities that place shearing stress on the reconstructed ligament. Which exercise would be the least desirable to include in the exercise program?

    1. straight leg raises in supine from 0-60 degrees of hip flexion
    2. standing hamstrings curls from 0-90 degrees of knee flexion
    3. supine short arc quadriceps exercises using a bolster
    4. gravity assisted knee extension in supine

135. A patient with patellar tracking dysfunction is examined in physical therapy. Physical examination reveals diminished vastus medialis obliquus activity. The most appropriate method to selectively train the vastus medialis obliquus is:

    1. quadriceps setting exercises and biofeedback
    2. full arc terminal extension with manual resistance
    3. straight leg raises with leg weights
    4. multiple angle isometric exercises

136. A physical therapist employed in an acute care hospital prepares to perform suctioning on a patient that is intubated. What type of protective equipment would be necessary in order for the therapist to administer suctioning?

    1. non-sterile gloves
    2. sterile gloves
    3. sterile gloves, gown
    4. sterile gloves, gown, mask

137. Which of the following goals is not realistic upon discharge from a phase I cardiac rehabilitation program for a patient status post coronary artery bypass graft?

    1. ambulate 100 feet on level surfaces
    2. walk up and down a flight of stairs
    3. locate and recognize changes in pulse rate
    4. range of motion and exercise at 6 metabolic equivalents

138. A physical therapist is treating a patient with a diagnosis of chronic arterial insufficiency. Assuming the patient does not demonstrate pain at rest, which of the following treatment techniques would be contraindicated for this patient?

    1. ambulation with an assistive device
    2. patient education regarding proper skin care
    3. stationary cycling
    4. ankle pumps with legs elevated

139. A physical therapist determines that a patient is limited in right hip range of motion in a capsular pattern. If the therapist elects to focus on increasing hip flexion, which mobilization techniques would be indicated?

    1. anterior glide
    2. posterior glide
    3. lateral glide
    4. medial glide

140. A physical therapist utilizes joint mobilization techniques for pain control and muscle relaxation at the shoulder. If the therapist begins by mobilizing the glenohumeral joint in the resting position, the limb should be positioned in:

    1. 55 degrees of abduction, 30 degrees of horizontal adduction
    2. 30 degrees of abduction, 10 degrees of horizontal adduction
    3. 25 degrees of abduction, 5 degrees of horizontal abduction
    4. 10 degrees of adduction, 5 degrees of horizontal abduction

Procedural Intervention: Group II

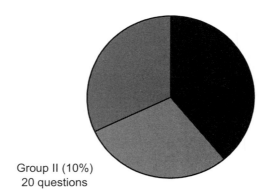

Group II (10%)
20 questions

Group II: Transfer and functional activities, gait training, assistive and adaptive devices, and modification of the environment

Transfer activities and functional activities, including safety related to transfers
    Performing transfers
    Performing functional activities

Gait training and use of gait assistive devices (normal/abnormal weight bearing status, common deviations, balance deficits, components of gait cycle)
    Performing gait-training techniques, including pre-gait activities
    Ensuring/facilitating proper weight bearing status

Prescription, application, and as appropriate, fabrication of devices, and equipment and environmental modification
    Adaptive devices
    Assistive devices
    Orthotic devices
    Prosthetic devices
    Protective devices
    Supportive devices
    Ensuring/facilitating proper weight bearing status
    Modification of environment for home/work/leisure activities

Sample Questions

141. A physical therapist orders a wheelchair for a patient with T9 paraplegia. Which wheelchair option would not be necessary for the patient?

    1. detachable legrests
    2. pneumatic tires
    3. removable arms
    4. wheel rim projections

142. A 58-year-old female diagnosed with peripheral neuropathy returns from an appointment with an orthotist wearing a posterior leaf spring ankle-foot orthosis. Which of the following clinical descriptions would most warrant the use of this particular type of orthosis?

    1. foot drop without medial or lateral instability
    2. weak plantar flexors during swing phase
    3. diminished knee stability
    4. foot drop with multi-plane instability

143. A patient rehabilitating from a tibial plateau fracture is referred to physical therapy for instruction in gait training. The patient has been cleared by his physician for weight bearing up to 40 lbs. Assuming the patient has no significant balance or coordination deficits, which gait pattern would be the most appropriate?

    1. two-point
    2. four-point
    3. three-point
    4. swing-through

144. A physical therapist examines a patient seated in a wheelchair. After completing the examination the therapist determines the wheelchair has inadequate seat width. Which of the following is the most likely consequence?

    1. excessive pressure under the distal thigh
    2. excessive pressure under the ischial tuberosities
    3. excessive pressure in the popliteal fossa
    4. excessive pressure on the greater trochanters

145. A patient five days status post anterior cruciate ligament reconstruction using a patellar tendon autograft is referred to physical therapy. The patient uses a postsurgical rehabilitative brace that consists of a metal offset hinge with medial and lateral plastic supports. It is applied directly over the skin and is secured using a series of velcro straps. The brace has a flexion and extension setting and comes in six different sizes based on a series of circumferential measurements. The primary purpose of the brace is to:

    1. reduce post-operative edema
    2. increase anterior and posterior stability
    3. enhance quadriceps activation time
    4. limit knee flexion and extension

146. A 26-year-old male involved in a motorcycle accident sustains a T10 vertebral fracture. The patient's physician attempts to restrict forward thoracic flexion by using an externally applied device. Which of the following would be the most appropriate selection?

    1. Minerva cervical-thoracic orthosis
    2. Philadelphia collar
    3. sternal-occipital-mandibular immobilizer
    4. thoraco-lumbar-sacral orthosis

147. A 50-year-old male rehabilitating from a recent stroke has good strength in the affected lower extremity with the exception of trace to poor strength in the right ankle joint. The patient's sensation is severely impaired for deep pressure, light touch, and sharp stimuli. The patient also has severe fluctuating edema at the ankle. The most appropriate orthosis for the patient is:

    1. metal upright ankle-foot orthosis
    2. polypropylene solid ankle-foot orthosis
    3. prefabricated posterior leaf orthosis
    4. metal upright knee-ankle-foot orthosis

148. A physical therapist receives orders for a patient that was recently injured in a motor vehicle accident. The patient's injuries include a Colles' fracture and a right tibial plateau fracture. The patient is mentally alert and does not exhibit any balance or coordination deficits. Assuming the patient is touchdown weight bearing, the most appropriate assistive device for the patient is:

    1. Lofstrand crutches
    2. rolling walker with platform attachments
    3. axillary crutch and a straight cane
    4. walker with a platform attachment

149. A physical therapist instructs a 62-year-old female rehabilitating from an ankle sprain in the use of a straight cane. The patient is confused as to why it is necessary to use the cane in the left hand since it is her right ankle that is injured. The most appropriate explanation would be:

    1. using the cane in the left hand will increase your base of support
    2. using the cane in the left hand will improve your coordination and balance
    3. using the cane in the left hand will reduce the pressure over your injured ankle
    4. using the cane in the left hand will allow more weight bearing on your injured ankle and will therefore accelerate your rehabilitation time

150. A physical therapist closely examines a small area of redness over the lateral portion of the lower leg of a patient diagnosed with peripheral neuropathy. The therapist is concerned that the skin irritation may have been caused by the leather calf band of the patient's metal upright ankle-foot orthosis. The most appropriate location for the calf band is:

    1. immediately inferior to the fibular head
    2. immediately superior to the fibular head
    3. immediately inferior to the tibial plateau
    4. immediately superior to the tibial plateau

151. A physical therapist employed in a rehabilitation hospital examines a patient prior to ordering a wheelchair. After completing the examination the therapist concludes that the patient would receive the greatest benefit from a tilt-in-space wheelchair. Which patient would be the best suited for this type of wheelchair?

    1. a 37-year-old male incapable of independent pressure relief
    2. a 42-year-old female with contractures at the hips and knees
    3. a 57-year-old male with poor upper extremity strength
    4. a 75-year-old female with significantly impaired sitting balance

152. A physical therapist selects an assistive device for a patient rehabilitating from an ankle injury. Which of the following would serve as the most significant obstacle to independent ambulation with axillary crutches?

    1. cognitive impairment
    2. weight bearing restrictions
    3. architectural barriers
    4. unilateral lower extremity weakness

153. A physical therapist observes a patient with a transfemoral amputation during gait training. The therapist identifies marked lateral rotation of the prosthesis at heel strike. Which of the following would not be a contributing factor to the patient's gait deviation?

    1. weak hip medial rotators
    2. inadequate suspension
    3. excessive toe-out built into the prosthesis
    4. prosthesis is too short

154. A patient diagnosed with T5 paraplegia is discharged from a rehabilitation hospital following 16 weeks of therapy. Assuming a normal recovery, which of the following most accurately describes the status of the patient's bathroom transfers?

    1. independent with the presence of an attendant
    2. independent with adaptive devices and a sliding board
    3. independent with bathroom adaptations
    4. independent

155. A physical therapist orders a wheelchair with anti-tip tubes for a patient in preparation for discharge from a rehabilitation hospital. Which patient would most significantly benefit from this option?

    1. a patient with Guillain-Barre syndrome
    2. a patient with C5 tetraplegia
    3. a patient with hemiparesis
    4. a patient with amyotrophic lateral sclerosis

156. A physical therapist instructs a patient who is unable to perform a standing transfer how to utilize a sliding board. When using the sliding board to transfer from a wheelchair to a bed, which wheelchair option is most desirable?

    1. swing-away detachable legrests
    2. elevating legrests
    3. full length, detachable armrests
    4. adjustable height armrests

157. A 16-year-old patient with a complete C5 spinal cord injury is two weeks status post injury. The patient presently tolerates only 30 degrees on the tilt table secondary to orthostatic hypotension. Which transfer would be the most appropriate to utilize when moving the patient from bed to the tilt table?

    1. hydraulic lift
    2. sliding transfer with draw sheet
    3. two person lift
    4. dependent standing pivot transfer

158. A physical therapist begins gait training with a patient who recently received an ankle-foot orthosis to assist with foot drop and sensory loss. A reddened area over the lateral malleolus persists after ambulating sixty feet. The most appropriate therapist response is to:

    1. direct the patient to wear the orthosis at all times because the body will eventually get used to it
    2. direct the patient to make an appointment with the orthotist and continue to wear the orthosis until that time
    3. direct the patient not to wear the orthosis until modifications are made
    4. direct the patient to make an appointment with the physician

159. A patient in a work hardening program is required to lift packages weighing approximately 30 pounds overhead to a conveyor belt. The patient can complete the task, but is unable to prevent excessive lumbar hyperextension while reaching for the conveyor belt. Which of the following assumptions is most accurate?

    1. additional weight should be added to the packages that will promote lumbar stability
    2. the patient should continue lifting the 30 pound packages because he will gradually become stronger
    3. the task is too easy for the patient
    4. the task is too difficult for the patient

160. A physical therapist instructs a patient how to rise from a chair before beginning ambulation activities with a walker. Which of the following instructions would be helpful to the patient?

    1. place both hands on the walker and pull yourself to a standing position
    2. push up on the chair with one hand and place the other hand on the edge of the walker for balance
    3. push up on the chair with both hands and reach for the walker once you are standing
    4. push up on the chair with both hands and reach for the walker while rising

Procedural Intervention: Group III

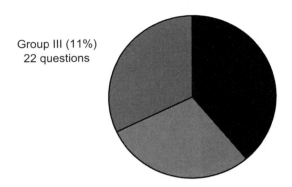

Group III (11%)
22 questions

Group III: Physical agents and modalities, airway clearance techniques, wound care, promoting health and wellness (includes some components of non-procedural intervention)

Physical agents and modalities
    Intermittent compression
    Superficial thermotherapy, e.g., hot packs, paraffin, and cryotherapy
    Ultrasound including phonophoresis
    Electrical stimulation including iontophoresis
    Biofeedback
    Mechanical modalities: traction, tilt table/standing frames, continuous passive motion
    Whirlpool/Hubbard tank

Airway clearance techniques
    Breathing strategies, e.g., coughing, huffing, and pacing
    Manual/mechanical techniques, e.g., percussion, vibration, suctioning
    Positioning

Wound care and skin integrity
    Skin status monitoring
    Patient positioning and use of adaptive/protective equipment for pressure relief
    Dressing application and removal
    Topical agent application
    Debridement technique
    Oxygen therapy

Promoting health and wellness and prevention, including instructions and intervention

Sample Questions

161. A physical therapist treats a patient with emphysema. As part of the treatment session the therapist teaches the patient to perform diaphragmatic breathing exercises. The primary goal for diaphragmatic breathing is to:

    1. decrease tidal ventilation
    2. increase respiration rate
    3. decrease accessory muscle use
    4. decrease oxygenation

162. A patient status post spinal fusion is referred for chest physical therapy. The physical therapist instructs the patient in diaphragmatic breathing exercises. Instructions are given to the patient to place his dominant hand over the midrectus abdominis area and his non-dominant hand over the midsternal area. As the patient inhales slowly through the nose the therapist encourages the patient to:

    1. direct air so that the non-dominant hand rises during inspiration
    2. direct air so that the dominant hand rises during inspiration
    3. direct air so that both hands rise equally during inspiration
    4. direct air so that both hands do not move during inspiration

163. A physician refers a patient rehabilitating from an intertrochanteric fracture to physical therapy. On the referral form the physician specifies the use of continuous ultrasound at 2.4 W/cm^2 over the fracture site. The most appropriate physical therapist action is to:

    1. treat the patient as indicated on the referral form
    2. request that the patient obtain a new referral from the physician
    3. use another more acceptable modality
    4. contact the referring physician

164. A 55-year-old female diagnosed with a right hip intertrochanteric fracture is eight weeks status post open reduction and internal fixation with a plate and pinning. The patient has pain with active hip flexion and abduction. Acceptable modalities for the patient include all of the following except:

    1. hot packs
    2. whirlpool
    3. pulsed ultrasound
    4. shortwave diathermy

165. A patient that sustained a lower extremity burn three months ago is treated in an outpatient physical therapy clinic. The patient's burns appear to be fully healed, however, the patient exhibits decreased knee flexion due to scar tissue. As part of the treatment program the physical therapist performs passive stretching activities in an attempt to promote collagen extensibility. Which thermal agent would be the most beneficial to enhance the effectiveness of the treatment session?

    1. pulsed ultrasound
    2. continuous ultrasound
    3. hydrotherapy
    4. fluidotherapy

166. An 18-year-old male six weeks status post open reduction of a Colles' fracture is referred to physical therapy. Examination reveals mild swelling on the dorsum of the hand and limited flexion of the metacarpophalangeal joints in all digits. The most appropriate heating agent for the patient is:

    1. paraffin
    2. hot packs
    3. vapocoolant sprays
    4. ultrasound

167. A physical therapist applies electrical stimulation to a patient rehabilitating from an Achilles tendon rupture. Which of the following types of current has the lowest total average current?

    1. low-volt
    2. high-volt
    3. Russian
    4. interferential

168. A physical therapist explains the benefits of using electrical stimulation for muscle re-education. The patient appears to understand the therapist's explanation, however, seems extremely frightened and asks the therapist not to use the electrical device. The most appropriate therapist action is to:

    1. reassure the patient that the electrical stimulation will not be harmful
    2. use only small amounts of current
    3. select another appropriate treatment technique
    4. discharge the patient from physical therapy

169. A physical therapist prepares to treat a patient using ultraviolet light by determining the patient's minimal erythemal dose. The most common location for testing is:

    1. on the posterior aspect of the upper arm
    2. on the anterior aspect of the forearm
    3. on the anterior aspect of the thigh
    4. on the posterior aspect of the lower leg

170. A physical therapist administers ultrasound to a patient rehabilitating from a burn in an attempt to increase range of motion and decrease joint stiffness in the foot. When applying ultrasound to the dorsum of the foot, the patient complains of significant discomfort from the soundhead contacting the skin. The most appropriate treatment modification is:

    1. decrease the intensity of the ultrasound beam
    2. reduce the size of the area being sonated
    3. utilize an underwater technique
    4. select another thermal agent

171. A patient with chronic obstructive pulmonary disease receives two liters per minute of supplemental oxygen using a nasal cannula. The most relevant indicator for the use of supplemental oxygen for the patient would be:

    1. arterial saturation = 85%
    2. partial pressure of arterial oxygen = 70 mm Hg
    3. partial pressure of carbon dioxide = 40 mm Hg
    4. pH = 7.40

172. A physical therapist positions a patient in prone with two pillows under the hips in preparation for bronchial drainage. If the therapist's goal is to perform bronchial drainage to the superior segments of the lower lobes, where should the therapist's force be directed?

    1. between the clavicle and nipple on each side
    2. over the area between the clavicle and top of the scapula on each side
    3. over the lower ribs on each side
    4. over the middle of the back at the tip of the scapula on each side

173. A 64-year-old male diagnosed with chronic bronchitis was admitted to the hospital three days ago after experiencing an acute exacerbation. While assessing the patient's vital signs the physical therapist determines the respiratory rate is 28 breaths per minute. Which breathing technique would be the most appropriate to decrease the patient's respiratory rate?

    1. glossopharyngeal breathing
    2. diaphragmatic breathing
    3. segmental breathing
    4. pursed-lip breathing

174. A patient with a low back injury rings a call bell and informs the physical therapist that the hot pack is too intense. Assuming the patient has had the hot pack on for three minutes, the most appropriate initial action is to:

    1. check the patient's skin
    2. add additional towel layers
    3. select another superficial heating agent
    4. document the incident in the medical record

175. A physical therapist administers neuromuscular electrical stimulation to the quadriceps using a bipolar electrode configuration. After observing the muscle contraction, the therapist decides to modify the treatment set up in order to increase the depth of current penetration. The most appropriate action is to:

    1. utilize carbon-rubber electrodes
    2. increase the size of the electrodes
    3. utilize additional electrodes using a bifurcated lead
    4. increase the distance between the electrodes

176. A home assessment is performed for a patient that will utilize a wheelchair. The patient's home presently does not possess a ramp and therefore is inaccessible. The distance from the ground to the front doorway is approximately three feet. In order for the patient to enter and exit the home safely and independently, the ramp should be at least:

    1. 27 feet long
    2. 30 feet long
    3. 36 feet long
    4. 45 feet long

177. A patient who is comatose due to a recent head injury receives chest physical therapy. When performing this treatment, the physical therapist should avoid placing the patient in:

    1. partial sitting using the head of the bed for support
    2. sidelying
    3. Trendelenburg position
    4. prone

178. A physical therapist receives a referral to instruct a patient diagnosed with peroneal tendonitis in a home exercise program. As part of the home exercise program, the therapist would like the patient to apply superficial heat to the injured area before beginning a stretching regimen. Which of the following modalities would be the most effective for the patient to incorporate into the program?

    1. diathermy
    2. paraffin
    3. pulsed ultrasound
    4. warm water bath

179. An order for chest physical therapy is received for an 82-year-old female. The patient recently underwent surgery for a hip fracture and has been taking Coumadin post-operatively. She has a history of multiple compression fractures of the thoracic vertebrae. The greatest amount of caution should be taken in the administration of:

    1. diaphragmatic breathing exercises
    2. postural drainage
    3. therapeutic percussion
    4. pursed-lip breathing

180. A patient who sustained a deep laceration in the antecubital fossa is treated in physical therapy. The patient's wound has been healing poorly secondary to motion occurring at the elbow joint. Which type of dressing would be the most appropriate to facilitate wound healing?

    1. wet
    2. dry
    3. occlusive
    4. rigid

IV. *Standards of Care*

Standards of Care (10%)
20 questions

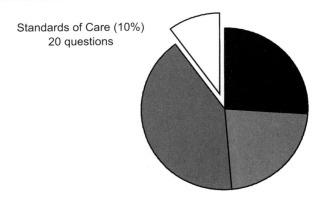

Standards of Care

Maintaining patient autonomy and obtaining consent for physical therapy and intervention

Maintaining patient confidentiality

Recognizing scope of physical therapy practice, including limitations of the PT role that necessitate referral to other disciplines

Recognizing implications of research on PT practice and modifying practice accordingly

Utilizing body mechanics/positioning
    Body mechanics (utilize, teach, reinforce, observe)
    Positioning, draping, and stabilization of patient

Considering the patient's cultural background, social history, home situation, and geographic barriers, etc.
    Safety, CPR, Emergency Care, First Aid
    Ensuring patient safety and safe application of patient care
    Performing first aid
    Performing emergency procedures
    Performing CPR

Standard precautions
    Sterile procedures
    Demonstrating appropriate sequencing of events related to universal precautions
    Demonstrating aseptic techniques
    Properly discarding soiled items
    Determining equipment to be used and assembling all materials, sterile and non-sterile

Sample Questions

181. A group of physical therapy students presents a research project entitled "Effects of Ultrasound on Blood Flow and Nerve Conduction Velocity." The dependent variables in the students' study is/are:

    1. ultrasound
    2. ultrasound and blood flow
    3. ultrasound and nerve conduction velocity
    4. blood flow and nerve conduction velocity

182. A physical therapist receives orders to design an exercise program for a 13-year-old boy recovering from thoracic surgery. The therapist explains the purpose and inherent risks of the exercise session as outlined in an informed consent form to the boy and his parents. After asking several additional questions the boy and his parents indicate that they would like to move forward with the session. The most appropriate therapist action is:

    1. ask the boy to sign the informed consent form
    2. ask one of the boy's parents to sign the informed consent form
    3. initiate the exercise program
    4. confirm the parameters of the exercise session with the referring physician

183. A patient in a rehabilitation hospital confides to a physical therapist that she has been physically abused by her husband in the past and is concerned about returning home following discharge. The most appropriate therapist action is to:

    1. report the findings to a law enforcement agency
    2. contact the patient's physiatrist
    3. ask the patient to leave her husband
    4. question the patient's spouse

184. A physical therapist observes a patient in the physical therapy waiting room that appears to be experiencing a heart attack. The most significant sign of a heart attack is:

    1. shortness of breath
    2. chest pain
    3. sweating
    4. nausea

185. A physical therapist working in an acute care hospital attempts to determine the effectiveness of treating psoriatic lesions with ultraviolet. The most appropriate initial action is to:

    1. design a research study which examines the effectiveness of treating psoriatic lesions with ultraviolet
    2. determine if the current patient population would allow for an adequate sample size for a research study
    3. submit a research proposal to the hospital's institutional review board
    4. conduct a literary search for research related to treating psoriatic lesions with ultraviolet

186. A physical therapist treating a patient overhears two of his colleagues discussing another patient's case in the charting area. The therapist is concerned that patients may overhear the same conversation. The most appropriate action is to:

    1. discuss the situation with the director of rehabilitation
    2. discuss confidentiality issues at the next department meeting
    3. move the patient away from the charting area
    4. inform the physical therapists that their conversation may be audible to patients

187. A patient completing an exercise program starts to demonstrate signs of an insulin reaction including dizziness, vision difficulties, and a change in the level of consciousness. The most appropriate response for a conscious victim would include:

    1. give the patient sugar, candy or juice
    2. monitor airway, breathing, and circulation
    3. treat the patient for shock
    4. continue to supervise the patient, however, do not intervene

188. While performing high-level balance activities, a patient falls into a piece of equipment that causes a deep laceration to the calf. Immediate first aid includes direct pressure to the area and elevation, however, the bleeding does not stop. The physical therapist should continue to administer first aid by providing:

    1. heat to the laceration site
    2. ice to the laceration site
    3. pressure to the dorsalis pedis artery pressure point
    4. pressure to the femoral artery pressure point

189. A physical therapy department designs a study examining rehabilitation outcomes in patients who have undergone anterior cruciate ligament reconstruction. The study will include a sample of patients from 25 orthopedic surgeons in the local region. If the physical therapists compile a list of all eligible patients and select every third patient to participate in the study, what type of sampling was used?

    1. simple random sampling
    2. stratified sampling
    3. systematic sampling
    4. cluster sampling

190. A physical therapist examines a six-month-old infant with spina bifida. The infant suddenly begins to act strangely at the conclusion of treatment. A primary survey reveals the infant is not breathing, but does have a pulse. The most immediate response would be to:

    1. begin chest compressions
    2. begin mouth to mouth breathing
    3. begin mouth to nose breathing
    4. begin mouth to mouth and nose breathing

191. A physical therapist prepares to administer a dressing change on a patient rehabilitating from a deep partial-thickness burn over the dorsal surface of the forearm and hand. The patient's current regimen consists of dressing changes twice daily and reapplication of a topical antibiotic. When sequencing the activities associated with the dressing change, which activity would occur second?

    1. gentle debridement in a hydrotherapy tank
    2. reapplication of the topical antibiotic
    3. application of gauze wraps in a distal to proximal pattern
    4. removal of current dressings

192. A patient begins to demonstrate signs and symptoms of a seizure including uncontrollable muscular movements, convulsions, and confused behavior. Appropriate intervention would include:

    1. attempt to check airway, breathing, and circulation
    2. place a soft object between the patient's teeth
    3. hold or restrain the patient
    4. protect the victim from injury, but do not restrain

193. A physical therapist conducts a home health visit for a patient status post transtibial amputation that lives in a two-room efficiency. The therapist treats the patient for a small wound on the anterior surface of the residual limb. After completing the treatment session, the therapist would like to wash her hands. Which of the following actions would be the most inappropriate?

    1. wash hands thoroughly in the kitchen sink
    2. utilize liquid soap instead of bar soap
    3. use paper towels to turn the faucets on and off
    4. rub hands together under flowing water with soap for at least 10 seconds

194. A patient that collapsed in the physical therapy gym fails to exhibit a pulse. Upon viewing the patient's mouth it becomes obvious that the patient has dentures. The physical therapist is hesitant to remove the dentures since they seem secure, however, does not want them to interfere with rescue breathing. The most appropriate action is to:

    1. leave the dentures in place
    2. loosen the dentures
    3. remove the dentures
    4. remove the dentures and utilize a mask to limit direct pressure on the patient's mouth

195. A patient who recently tested positive for hepatitis B has a one-inch diameter wound on the anterior surface of her forearm. Upon inspection, the borders of the wound are slightly raised and a small amount of drainage is visible. When changing the dressing on the wound the most appropriate protective equipment to utilize would be:

    1. gloves
    2. gloves, gown
    3. gloves, gown, mask
    4. gloves, gown, mask, protective eyewear

196. A physical therapist enters a remote storage area to retrieve a piece of equipment and observes flames and smoke throughout the room. The most appropriate immediate action is:

    1. attempt to extinguish the fire
    2. remove patients from the physical therapy area
    3. announce the code for fire over the facility's public address system
    4. attempt to contain the fire to the storage room

197. A physical therapist attempts to obtain consent to participate in a formal aquatic exercise program from a patient rehabilitating from multiple lower extremity injuries sustained in a motor vehicle accident. The therapist's action is most representative of the ethical principle termed:

    1. autonomy
    2. beneficence
    3. nonmaleficence
    4. justice

198. A physical therapist and a physical therapist assistant employed in an acute care hospital are responsible for providing weekend therapy coverage. After examining the patient treatment list, the therapists attempt to develop an action plan. Which of the following activities would be the least appropriate for the physical therapist assistant?

    1. instruct a patient in prosthetic donning and doffing
    2. assist a patient with ambulation activities
    3. examine a patient referred to physical therapy for instruction in a home exercise program
    4. perform goniometric measurements on a patient two days status post anterior cruciate ligament reconstruction

199. A patient rehabilitating from a fractured humerus has completed six weeks of physical therapy and is ready to be discharged with a home exercise program. The patient is extremely pleased with his progress in therapy and gives the physical therapist a check for $50.00 as a token of his appreciation. The most appropriate therapist action is to:

    1. accept the gift
    2. accept the gift and donate it to charity
    3. accept the gift and donate it to the department's general expense fund
    4. explain to the patient that you are not permitted to accept the gift

200. A physical therapist awaiting the arrival of her next patient observes another patient ambulating independently in the parallel bars. The patient appears to lack the necessary strength and coordination required to complete the activity independently. The therapist's most appropriate response would be to:

    1. inform the patient's therapist of her observations
    2. assist the patient back to a chair and contact the patient's therapist
    3. ask the patient if she is having difficulty or needs any assistance
    4. continue to observe the patient, but do not interfere

EXAM: CONTENT OUTLINE
Answer Key

1. Correct Answer: 1
    Explanation: Doppler ultrasonography is a diagnostic technique that uses ultrasound to produce an image or photograph of an organ or tissue. The non-invasive test is commonly used to evaluate blood flow in the major veins and arteries of the upper and lower extremities as well as in the extracranial cerebrovascular system. (Physical Therapist's Clinical Companion p. 134)

2. Correct Answer: 3
    Explanation: Hemoglobin refers to an iron based pigment that binds and transports oxygen in blood. The typical reference range for a male is 14-18 gm/dL, therefore a value of 8 gm/dL may result in decreased exercise tolerance, fatigue, and tachycardia. (Paz p. 381)

3. Correct Answer: 2
    Explanation: Myelography can be used to detect disk herniation, nerve root entrapment, spinal stenosis, and tumors of the spinal cord. (Magee p. 53)

4. Correct Answer: 1
    Explanation: Adhesive capsulitis refers to an inflammation and adherence of the articular capsule resulting in limited joint play and restricted active and passive movement. The condition is more common in women than in men and tends to appear in the fourth, fifth, and sixth decades of life. Patients with diabetes mellitus are particularly susceptible to this condition and often experience a longer duration of symptoms and greater limitation of motion. (Goodman – Pathology p. 349)

5. Correct Answer: 1
    Explanation: The patient's lab values for hematocrit, white blood cells, platelet, and hemoglobin are significantly below acceptable ranges. As a result exercise is not indicated. (Paz p. 380)

6. Correct Answer: 2
    Explanation: The TMN Classification System (T=tumor, M=metastasis, N=node) is a commonly used cancer classification system. This type of staging offers guidance to health care professionals when determining treatment options, life expectancy, and prognosis for complete resolution. The physical therapy plan of care may vary significantly based on the results of the staging. (Paz p. 336)

7. Correct Answer: 1
    Explanation: A temperature of 98.9 degrees Fahrenheit represents a slightly elevated temperature when compared to the average temperature of 98.6 degrees Fahrenheit. Since the patient reports being able to exercise and the elevated temperature is within the accepted normal range (96.8°F – 99.5°F), the most appropriate action is to continue with treatment as planned. (Pierson p. 48)

8. Correct Answer: 4
    Explanation: Immunosuppressive pharmacological agents are desirable when the body loses its ability to differentiate between the body's own tissues and pathogenic tissues. White blood cell count provides valuable information related to the degree of immunosuppression. (Ciccone p. 633)

9. Correct Answer: 3
    Explanation: A bone scan can identify bone disease or stress fractures with as little as 4-7% bone loss. Traditional radiographs are far less sensitive than bone scans, requiring 30-50% bone loss. (Magee p. 56)

10. Correct Answer: 2
    Explanation: The anterior talofibular ligament runs from the anterior portion of the lateral malleolus to the lateral aspect of the talar neck. The ligament is placed under stress with inversion and plantar flexion. The anterior talofibular, calcaneofibular, and posterior talofibular ligaments make up the lateral collateral ligaments of the ankle complex. (Magee p. 766)

11. Correct Answer: 1
Explanation: Hematocrit is the volume percentage of red blood cells in whole blood. The hematocrit rises immediately after a severe burn and gradually decreases with fluid replacement. (Paz p. 765)

12. Correct Answer: 1
Explanation: Osteoporosis is a metabolic bone disease characterized by increased bone resorption resulting in a reduction in bone mass. Osteoporosis is more prevalent in females than in males, in older more than younger individuals, and in whites more than in blacks. (Paz p. 689)

13. Correct Answer: 2
Explanation: Diuretics function by increasing the formation and excretion of urine and as a result serve to decrease the volume of fluid in the vascular system. Sodium depletion (hyponatremia) and potassium depletion (hypokalemia) are serious side effects of diuretics. (Ciccone p. 309)

14. Correct Answer: 1
Explanation: The patient is 18-years-old and is therefore considered to be an adult. As a result, the most appropriate physical therapist action would be to discuss the situation with the patient. It would be inappropriate to schedule a dietary consult prior to discussing the information with the patient and since the patient has been treated for "several weeks" it would be of little benefit to continue to monitor the patient. (Standards of Practice)

15. Correct Answer: 4
Explanation: Calcium channel blockers selectively block calcium entry into vascular smooth muscle. This action serves to inhibit the contractile process resulting in vasodilation and decreased peripheral resistance. (Ciccone p. 318)

16. Correct Answer: 3
Explanation: Carpal tunnel syndrome results from repetitive compression of the median nerve where it passes through the carpal tunnel at the wrist. Nerve conduction velocity can be extremely useful in diagnosing the condition. Less formal methods to assist in identifying carpal tunnel syndrome include Phalen's test and Tinel's sign. (Tan p. 44)

17. Correct Answer: 4
Explanation: The spleen is located in the left upper quadrant of the abdomen while the appendix, gallbladder, and liver are located on the right side of the body. (Magee p. 536)

18. Correct Answer: 1
Explanation: The injury mechanism associated with an acromioclavicular injury is a direct blow to the tip of the shoulder that serves to displace the acromion inferior to the clavicle. (Shamus p. 400)

19. Correct Answer: 4
Explanation: Although x-rays can be used to assess skeletal maturity, the primary purpose would be to rule out a fracture. (Magee p. 52)

20. Correct Answer: 1
Explanation: Headaches occur in 30% - 50% of patients with brain tumors. Visual changes can be caused by space occupying tumors. (Goodman – Differential Diagnosis p. 370)

21. Correct Answer: 2
Explanation: The hip is a ball and socket joint whose resting position is 30 degrees flexion, 30 degrees abduction, and slight lateral rotation. The close packed position is extension and medial rotation. (Magee p. 607)

22. Correct Answer: 1
Explanation: The flexor pollicis brevis inserts on the volar aspect of the base of the proximal phalanx of the thumb. The muscle flexes the metacarpophalangeal and carpometacarpal joints of the thumb and assists in opposition. (Kendall p. 241)

23. Correct Answer: 4
Explanation: The inferior lateral angles of the sacrum are formed by the transverse processes of S5. (Hertling p. 709)

24. Correct Answer: 1
Explanation: Scapular adductors including the rhomboids, middle trapezius, and the lower trapezius are tested with the patient in a prone position. (Kendall p. 282)

25. Correct Answer: 3
Explanation: Since the "15" is to the left of the "0", it is indicative of hyperextension. Therefore total available range of motion is determined as follows: 15 + 150 = 165. (Norkin p. 31)

26. Correct Answer: 2
Explanation: The end-feel associated with knee flexion is typically described as soft due to contact between the posterior calf and thigh or between the heel and buttocks. (Norkin p. 230)

27. Correct Answer: 3
Explanation: Performing ligamentous testing on an uninvolved joint provides a physical therapist with a valuable baseline that can then be compared to the involved joint. (Magee p. 12)

28. Correct Answer: 2
Explanation: Grip strength may vary by 5-10% when comparing the dominant and non-dominant hands. (Magee p. 380)

29. Correct Answer: 1
Explanation: The trigeminal nerve innervates the primary muscles of mastication including the pterygoids. The pterygoids on one side function to open the jaw and cause the jaw to deviate to the opposite side. As a result, if the right pterygoids are weak the jaw will deviate to the right with opening. (Clarkson p. 51)

30. Correct Answer: 1
Explanation: Kinesthesia refers to the ability to perceive the extent or direction of movement. An appropriate patient response must include an indication of the direction of movement while the physical therapist actively moves the patient's extremity. (O'Sullivan p. 145)

31. Correct Answer: 4
Explanation: The double leg lowering test assesses the strength of the lower abdominals. The test is performed by slowly lowering the legs from a vertical position with the knees extended. (Kendall p. 154)

32. Correct Answer: 4
Explanation: The peroneus tertius acts to dorsiflex the ankle joint and evert the foot. As a result, resistance should be applied against the lateral side of the dorsal surface of the foot in the direction of plantar flexion and inversion. The deep peroneal nerve innervates the peroneus tertius. (Kendall p. 198)

33. Correct Answer: 1
Explanation: The teres minor is a lateral rotator of the shoulder while the pectoralis major, teres major, and subscapularis are medial rotators of the shoulder. (Kendall p. 281)

34. Correct Answer: 1
Explanation: The biceps is innervated by the musculocutaneous nerve via C5-C6 and the brachioradialis reflex is innervated by the radial nerve via C5-C6. (Hoppenfeld p. 55)

35. Correct Answer: 1
Explanation: The sinus tarsi area is located immediately anterior to the lateral malleolus. The soft tissue depression consists of a tunnel between the calcaneus and talus. The anterior talofibular ligament is often the first ligament affected by an inversion ankle injury. (Hoppenfeld p. 216)

36. Correct Answer: 2
Explanation: Sensory testing for light touch is performed by applying the piece of cotton to selected dermatomes and asking the patient when the sensation is perceived. (Hertling p. 85)

37. Correct Answer: 3
Explanation: Measuring from the medial knee joint line to the medial malleolus allows for an independent assessment of tibial length and also avoids any potential asymmetries due to leg girth. (Magee p. 629)

38. Correct Answer: 2
Explanation: The therapist should perform the test and clear the patient's vertebral artery for their available range of motion. As the patient gains additional range of motion the test can be readministered. It is possible to observe findings such as nystagmus and slurring of speech prior to achieving full rotation, extension, and lateral flexion. (Gross p. 73)

39. Correct Answer: 2
Explanation: This scenario describes Ely's test which, if positive, is indicative of tightness of the rectus femoris (two-joint hip flexor). (Magee p. 632)

40. Correct Answer: 1
Explanation: Patellar L3-L4, lateral hamstrings S1-S2, posterior tibial L4-L5, Achilles S1-S2. (Magee p. 453)

41. Correct Answer: 3
Explanation: A blood pressure cuff that is too narrow in relation to a patient's arm will tend to artificially increase measured values. The width of the bladder should be 40% of the circumference of the midpoint of the limb. An average size adult requires a bladder that is 5-6 inches wide. (Pierson p. 57)

42. Correct Answer: 2
Explanation: The rooting reflex is a primitive reflex that is normally present from 28 weeks of gestation through three months of age. The reflex assists the mother when feeding an infant. (Ratliffe p. 26)

43. Correct Answer: 2
Explanation: Rating on a perceived exertion scale provides a subjective measure of exercise intensity. A rating of 12 on Borg's Rate of Perceived Exertion Scale corresponds to roughly 60 percent of the age-adjusted maximum heart rate. (Brannon p. 316)

44. Correct Answer: 3
Explanation: Step length is defined as the distance between two successive points of contact of opposite extremities. (Levangie p. 445)

45. Correct Answer: 1
Explanation: The dorsal pedal artery is located between the tendons of the extensor hallucis longus and the extensor digitorum longus. The pulse can be absent in up to 15% of the population. (Hoppenfeld p. 214)

46. Correct Answer: 1
Explanation: Measurement error decreases as the time associated with data collection increases. (Brannon p. 190)

47. Correct Answer: 1
Explanation: The posterior cruciate ligament is responsible for preventing posterior displacement of the tibia on the femur. The ligament is most often injured by a direct force on the tibia, which displaces it in a posterior direction in relation to the femur. (Hertling p. 324)

48. Correct Answer: 2
Explanation: Tactile fremitus is often examined by using a hand or portion of a hand to assess the vibration associated with spoken words. The examination technique can be used to provide information on the density of the lungs and thoracic cavity. (Frownfelter p. 225)

49. Correct Answer: 4
Explanation: A sputum sample classified as purulent is described as a viscous fluid exudate that is often yellow or green and may be associated with acute or chronic infection. (Rothstein p. 533)

50. Correct Answer: 1 *Item Includes Graphic*
Explanation: The ankle-brachial index (ABI) is a common diagnostic test used to assess the rate of vascular perfusion. The ABI is determined by dividing the systolic pressure of the lower extremity by the systolic pressure of the upper extremity. (Meyers p. 210)

51. Correct Answer: 2
Explanation: Approximation is a therapeutic exercise technique designed to facilitate contraction and stability through joint compression. (Sullivan p. 27)

52. Correct Answer: 3
Explanation: Blanching or whitening of the nailbeds occurs due to the interruption in circulation caused by the physical therapist's direct pressure. The capillary refill test is often used as a gross indicator of vascular perfusion. (Magee p. 934)

53. Correct Answer: 3
Explanation: Positive risk factors for coronary artery disease include age, male gender, family history, current cigarette smoking, hypertension, hypercholesterolemia, diabetes mellitus, and sedentary lifestyle. Hypertension combined with borderline cholesterol levels places the 42-year-old male at the greatest risk for coronary artery disease. (American College of Sports Medicine p. 24)

54. Correct Answer: 2
Explanation: The pulmonic valve is located between the right ventricle and the opening of the pulmonary artery. Auscultation should be performed in the second left intercostal space at the left sternal margin. (Hillegass p. 628)

55. Correct Answer: 4
Explanation: Heart rate and perceived exertion are the most appropriate measures to monitor the patient's response to exercise, however, perceived exertion is the only subjective measure. In addition, the patient's heart rate response would be diminished due to the effect of the beta-blockers. (Brannon p. 136)

56. Correct Answer: 1
Explanation: Bronchophony can be assessed by asking the patient to say "ninety-nine" while the therapist auscultates over the entire chest. Consolidated tissue will typically yield stronger, louder sounds while hyperinflation results in softer sounds. (Hillegass p. 626)

57. Correct Answer: 3
Explanation: Diabetes mellitus is a disorder of carbohydrate metabolism that results from inadequate production or uptake of insulin. Signs and symptoms of diabetes mellitus include polyuria, polydipsia, rapid weight loss, polyphagia, and elevation of blood glucose levels. A normal blood glucose level is 80–100 mg/dL. (Paz p. 677)

58. Correct Answer: 3
Explanation: ST segment depression of less than 1 mm may occur in a healthy individual during exercise, however, changes of greater than 1 mm would be considered abnormal. (Brannon p. 226)

59. Correct Answer: 3
Explanation: The ankle-brachial index (ABI) is a ratio that is calculated by dividing the lower extremity pressure by the upper extremity pressure. Normal values for the ABI are 1.0 or slightly higher. Values less than .50 are indicative of severe arterial disease. (Goodman – Pathology p. 455)

60. Correct Answer: 4
Explanation: Full-thickness burns are characterized by complete destruction of the epidermis and dermis with or without damage to the subcutaneous fat layer. Since new tissue is only generated from the periphery of the burn site, grafts are necessary. (Rothstein p. 1117)

61. Correct Answer: 1
Explanation: A lesion involving the motor component of the facial nerve from damage to the nucleus is considered a lower motor neuron lesion. The most likely clinical presentation is facial muscle weakness ipsilateral to the lesion. (Bickley p. 612)

62. Correct Answer: 3
Explanation: Klinefelter's syndrome is characterized by the presence of an extra X chromosome. Individuals with this syndrome are characterized by small testes, abnormally long limbs, and below average intelligence. The syndrome is estimated to occur in one of 700 live male births. (Ratliffe p. 230)

63. Correct Answer: 4
Explanation: A rapidly growing neoplasm often results in pain due to direct pressure or displacement of specific nerves. Pain can also occur due to interference with blood supply or from blockage within an organ. Symptoms are magnified as the neoplasm continues to grow. (Goodman – Differential Diagnosis p. 445)

64. Correct Answer: 1
Explanation: Amyotrophic lateral sclerosis is a progressive syndrome marked by muscular weakness and atrophy with spasticity and hyperreflexia due to degeneration of the motor neurons of the spinal cord, medulla, and cortex. The disease is commonly referred to as Lou Gehrig's disease and is not associated with mental deterioration. (Physical Therapist's Clinical Companion p. 207)

65. Correct Answer: 2
Explanation: Autonomic dysreflexia is a condition that occurs in patients with spinal cord injuries above the T6 level. The condition is triggered when a noxious stimuli is present followed by an increase in autonomic responses. Symptoms include headache, blotching of the skin, dilation of the pupils, nausea, and a dangerous increase in blood pressure. (Goodman - Pathology p. 1090)

66. Correct Answer: 1
Explanation: Respiratory acidosis is characterized by decreased pH, increased $PaCO_2$, and HCO_3 that is within normal limits. (Rothstein p. 529)

67. Correct Answer: 3
Explanation: Chronic obstructive pulmonary disease is characterized by a progressive reduction in expiratory flow rates. Hyperinflation of the lungs results in an increase in residual volume. (Brannon p. 115)

68. Correct Answer: 4
Explanation: The primary cause of shock related to burns is hypovolemia or loss of circulating fluid. Symptoms of shock include a drop in blood pressure, increased pulse rate, and decreased urine output. (Paz p. 441)

69. Correct Answer: 3
Explanation: The hypoglossal nerve innervates the primary muscles of the tongue. As a result, a lower motor neuron disease affecting the left hypoglossal nerve will cause weakness and resultant deviation of the tongue to the left (toward the side of weakness). Muscle atrophy is a common finding in lower motor neuron lesions. (Bickley p. 571)

70. Correct Answer: 4
Explanation: The cerebellum is the area of the brain responsible for modulation of movement. Lesions to the cerebellum may produce hypotonia, tremor, impaired reflexes, ataxic gait, and nystagmus. (Bennett p. 160)

71. Correct Answer: 2
Explanation: An impairment is defined as a loss or abnormality of physiological, psychological or anatomical structure or function. (Guide to Physical Therapist Practice p. 22)

72. Correct Answer: 3
Explanation: If possible, the lateral shift should be corrected prior to any form of active and passive exercise. (Kisner p. 619)

73. Correct Answer: 3
Explanation: Damage to an artery can create a life threatening emergency that requires immediate medical attention. The term epiphysis refers to a center for ossification at the end of a long bone. (Anemaet p. 567)

74. Correct Answer: 2
Explanation: The tibialis anterior acts to dorsiflex the ankle joint and invert the foot. Injury to the deep peroneal nerve (L4, L5, S1) may produce dramatic weakness in dorsiflexion and resultant foot drop. (Kendall p. 201)

75. Correct Answer: 3
Explanation: The anterior cruciate ligament, lateral collateral ligament, and iliotibial band provide anterolateral stability to the knee. (Magee p. 695)

76. Correct Answer: 2
Explanation: A patient rehabilitating from a CVA with right hemisphere involvement and resultant left hemiplegia would most likely exhibit impaired awareness of the left side of the body. Other characteristics of this patient may include poor attention span, left hemianopsia, and impulsive behaviors. (Umphred p. 755)

77. Correct Answer: 2
Explanation: Ideomotor apraxia refers to an inability to perform movements necessary to use objects properly on command, although in some instances automatic movement may occur. (Goodman - Pathology p. 988)

78. Correct Answer: 4
Explanation: Abnormalities of the vestibular system result in dizziness and impaired balance. The vestibular system itself is stimulated by the position of the head in space and changes in the direction of movement of the head. (Goodman - Pathology p. 1131)

79. Correct Answer: 4
Explanation: The Achilles reflex is from the S1 spinal level. Sensation on the posterior calf is from the S1-S2 level while the bowel is associated with the sacral segments of the spinal cord (S2-S4). (Hoppenfeld p. 254)

80. Correct Answer: 4
Explanation: The patient's signs and symptoms are consistent with the presence of a deep venous thrombosis. Referral for additional medical examination is necessary. (Paz p. 401)

81. Correct Answer: 2
Explanation: The physical therapist should answer questions asked by the family as long as they are within the therapist's scope of practice. A therapist should possess a basic understanding of expected functional outcomes of patients with spinal cord injuries. (Purtilo p. 30)

82. Correct Answer: 4
Explanation: The cultural background of a patient without additional information offers little indication as to the patient's ability to comprehend a home exercise program. (Purtilo p. 50)

83. Correct Answer: 4
Explanation: A functional progression is a series of progressive active movements designed to simulate a selected sport or activity. Failure to successfully complete a functional progression often indicates that a patient is not ready to return to competition. (Hall p. 449)

84. Correct Answer: 2
Explanation: Key muscles that are partially or fully innervated at the C6 level include the brachialis, biceps, trapezius, deltoids, rhomboids, latissimus dorsi, rotator cuff, serratus anterior, and extensor carpi radialis. (Rothstein p. 476)

85. Correct Answer: 2
Explanation: The patient should return to his previous functional activity level in a matter of weeks following a grade I medial collateral ligament sprain. (Magee p. 1)

86. Correct Answer: 2
Explanation: Although there is a wide range of outcomes with non-operative anterior cruciate ligament injuries, most individuals are able to return to a minimum level of light recreational sports. Therapeutic management of an anterior cruciate ligament injury includes range of motion, progressive resistive exercises, functional activities, and bracing. (Kisner p. 538)

87. Correct Answer: 2
Explanation: The rate and amount of bone healing as determined through radiographs determines the actual amount of time an external fixation device is applied. A general estimate of the necessary time would be 6-8 weeks. (Paz p. 229)

88. Correct Answer: 1
Explanation: Positioning the neck in extension and extremes of rotation places the vertebral artery in a compromised position. Extension, sidebending, and rotation are components of the vertebral artery test. (Hertling p. 535)

89. Correct Answer: 2
Explanation: Surgical repair of the ulnar collateral ligament of the thumb requires a pin to be inserted into the metacarpophalangeal joint of the thumb. The pin may remain in place for 3-6 weeks followed by the application of a wrist and thumb splint. Progressive strengthening typically commences at eight weeks and a return to unrestricted activity may occur at approximately 12 weeks. (Brotzman p. 58)

90. Correct Answer: 2
Explanation: Many patients on extended bed rest following a burn experience significant cardiovascular complications. A functional capacity of 10 or more metabolic equivalents is a good indication that a formal cardiovascular rehabilitation program is not necessary. An intensity of 10 METs corresponds to running at six miles per hour. (Paz p. 35)

91. Correct Answer: 3
Explanation: A patient functioning at Rancho Los Amigos level IV, confused-agitated, may be particularly susceptible to changes in behavior based on fatigue. Ideally the physical therapist should attempt to maintain the integrity of the current treatment regimen, however, if increased rest periods do not produce an observable change in the patient's behavior it may be appropriate to modify other parameters such as the frequency or length of treatment. (Campbell, M. p. 157)

92. Correct Answer: 2
Explanation: Chemotherapy uses toxic chemicals to destroy cancerous cells in an attempt to reduce the size of a tumor for resection or palliative care. Chemotherapy is a systemic intervention usually administered by an intravenous line. Excessive fatigue caused by chemotherapy can considerably limit the patient's ability to participate in a formal exercise program. (Paz p. 341)

93. Correct Answer: 3
Explanation: Therapists should treat all patients as if they have a potentially transmissible or infectious disease. Therapists have the responsibility to treat patients regardless of their particular medical diagnosis. (Pierson p. 27)

94. Correct Answer: 2
Explanation: A patient with complete paraplegia would likely be able to achieve a reflexogenic erection, but would be less likely to ejaculate. (O'Sullivan p. 882)

95. Correct Answer: 2
Explanation: A patient with peripheral vascular disease that presents with resting claudication is not a candidate for an ambulation exercise program. (Kisner p. 715)

96. Correct Answer: 4
Explanation: Activities requiring increased circulation through muscle pumping can significantly reduce the incidence for acquiring a deep venous thrombosis. Although ankle pumps and muscle setting exercises are commonly prescribed following surgery, higher level activities such as ambulation on a frequent schedule will be more effective to achieve the stated objective. Signs and symptoms of a deep venous thrombosis include a positive Homans' sign, swelling, redness, and warmth in the calf. Physical therapy treatment should not continue until a physician evaluates and clears the patient. (Kisner p. 717)

97. Correct Answer: 3
Explanation: Home health services are warranted based on the patient's homebound status and present functional level. (Anemaet p. 34)

98. Correct Answer: 2
Explanation: The patient appears to be making progress through the established short-term goals and by developing additional, perhaps more appropriate, short-term goals it may facilitate achievement of the established long-term goal. Not enough information is given to assume the long-term goal is unrealistic particularly since the patient is making progress. (Quinn p. 100)

99. Correct Answer: 4
Explanation: The patient has achieved all established short and long-term goals and has returned to his previous lifestyle. There is no longer a need for physical therapy services. (Standards of Practice)

100. Correct Answer: 4
Explanation: The question asked by the spouse falls within the therapist's scope of practice and should therefore be answered directly. (Guide for Professional Conduct)

101. Correct Answer: 2
Explanation: Occupational therapists focus on activities of daily living, work and leisure skills, and as a result may be best suited to address the obstacles that impact the patient's ability to return to work. (Anemaet p. 29)

102. Correct Answer: 3
Explanation: The statement "having cancer must be very difficult for you to deal with" acknowledges the patient's present condition without providing a false sense of hope. This type of approach is particularly important with patients who have recently been diagnosed with a terminal disease. (Purtilo p. 321)

103. Correct Answer: 2
Explanation: A physical therapist should attempt to determine if a patient is under the influence of alcohol. Alcohol consumption can significantly influence a patient's ability to tolerate treatment. Asking the patient directly is an immediate step that can be used to gather additional information. (Goodman - Differential Diagnosis p. 50)

104. Correct Answer: 3
Explanation: It is essential to assess the needs of the target audience prior to designing a formal or informal presentation. (Shepard p. XXIII)

105. Correct Answer: 1
Explanation: It is often advisable to review an exercise program with a patient. It is particularly essential in the given scenario since failure to perform the exercises correctly could have a detrimental effect on the patient's condition. Although some of the other presented options may be appropriate, they would not offer the same degree of benefit for the patient. (American College of Sports Medicine p. 242)

106. Correct Answer: 1
Explanation: A supportive spouse can be extremely helpful to a patient completing a home exercise program. In order for the spouse to be an asset, she must first recognize the value of the program. (Pierson p. 12)

107. Correct Answer: 2
Explanation: By addressing the issue directly with the patient, the physical therapist may improve compliance with the weight bearing restrictions and therefore promote a better environment for tissue healing. (Scott - Foundations p. 177)

108. Correct Answer: 2
Explanation: Operant conditioning is a form of learning where a particular action or behavior is followed by the administration of a reward (positive reinforcement). B.F. Skinner first publicized this learning approach. (Shepard p. 48)

109. Correct Answer: 2
Explanation: The presence of parents can often be reassuring to a young child when confronted with a new experience. (Purtilo p. 245)

110. Correct Answer: 1
Explanation: Isometric exercises are often the strengthening exercise of choice for patients with acute osteoarthritis. This form of exercise limits muscle atrophy while avoiding unnecessary stress on the joint. Avoiding strengthening exercises until the patient is pain-free is unrealistic given the diagnosis of osteoarthritis. (Hall p. 192)

111. Correct Answer: 3
Explanation: The patient's inability to communicate using the English language necessitates the use of an interpreter. (Purtilo p. 43)

112. Correct Answer: 2
Explanation: Although each of the options is a viable answer, the therapist's primary responsibility is direct patient care. Failure to provide physical therapy services to a patient for this period of time in an acute care environment could pose a serious problem. (Scott – Health Care Malpractice p. 16)

113. Correct Answer: 2
Explanation: Effusion is defined as an increased volume of fluid within the joint capsule. Edema is defined as an increased volume of fluid in the soft tissue external to the joint. (Kisner p. 222)

114. Correct Answer: 1
Explanation: The therapist's hypothesis necessitates contact with the referring physician, however, does not indicate the need to discontinue physical therapy services. (Guide for Professional Conduct)

115. Correct Answer: 3
Explanation: Reminding the patient of the donning instructions for the orthosis provides the patient with the best opportunity to learn the correct technique. Although reapplying the orthosis correctly at the conclusion of the treatment session is appropriate, the action does not provide any specific feedback to the patient. (Physical Therapist's Clinical Companion p. 315)

116. Correct Answer: 4
Explanation: The physician is responsible for determining when the sling can be discontinued. (Guide for Professional Conduct)

117. Correct Answer: 3
Explanation: Lecture, handouts, and demonstration provide not only verbal and written information, but provide the target audience with the opportunity to observe an actual demonstration. This multi-tiered approach accommodates for a variety of learning styles. (Shepard p. 138)

118. Correct Answer: 1
Explanation: Domains of learning include cognitive, affective, and psychomotor. Bloom's Taxonomy of Educational Objectives identifies six levels of the cognitive domain: knowledge, comprehension, application, analysis, synthesis, and evaluation. Listing potential complications of an improperly designed workstation requires knowledge and is therefore considered to be in the cognitive domain. (Shepard p. 53)

119. Correct Answer: 4
Explanation: Due to the patient's age it would be appropriate to ask a family member to come into the room. To reprimand the boy in any form may only serve to diminish compliance. (Davis p. 208)

120. Correct Answer: 3
Explanation: A patient's question should be answered in a direct and forthcoming manner whenever possible. Frequent repetition is a component of any treatment plan for patients with short-term memory loss. (O'Sullivan p. 802)

121. Correct Answer: 1
Explanation: In contract-relax the build up of tension is immediate and may therefore be problematic when the limitation in movement is accompanied by pain. In contrast, hold-relax requires a gradual buildup of tension over a period of several seconds and is therefore often the treatment of choice when pain is present. (Sullivan p. 66)

122. Correct Answer: 3
Explanation: Termination guidelines for submaximal exercise testing indicate that a subject should not exceed 85% of his/her age-predicted maximal heart rate. (American College of Sports Medicine p. 72)

123. Correct Answer: 1
Explanation: The glenohumeral joint is a ball and socket joint consisting of the convex head of the humerus articulating with the concave glenoid fossa of the scapula. Lateral distraction and anterior glide of the glenohumeral joint can be utilized to increase lateral rotation and extension. (Kisner p. 203)

124. Correct Answer: 2
Explanation: Tall kneeling follows the quadruped position in the developmental sequence. Tall kneeling emphasizes hip extension in combination with knee flexion and serves to promote stability. (O'Sullivan p. 382)

125. Correct Answer: 1
Explanation: Archimedes' principle of buoyancy states that a body immersed in a liquid experiences an upward force equal to the weight of the displaced liquid. In aquatic therapy, a patient may experience greater ease of movement due to the buoyant force of the water. (Belanger p. 341)

126. Correct Answer: 2
Explanation: Contract-relax is a therapeutic technique designed to increase range of motion to muscles on one side of a joint. Tightness of the hamstrings and hip extensors would serve to limit a straight leg raise. (Sullivan p. 66)

127. Correct Answer: 4
Explanation: Frenkel's exercises are designed to improve coordination by emphasizing the use of vision and hearing to compensate for altered or impaired proprioception. (Umphred p. 734)

128. Correct Answer: 4 **_Item Includes Graphic_**
Explanation: The traditional progression from lowest to highest level is: lie in prone on a firm surface, prone on elbows, prone press-up, extension exercises in standing. (Prentice – Techniques p. 649)

129. Correct Answer: 2
Explanation: Hooklying is a term used to describe a position where a patient is in supine with the hips and knees flexed and the feet in contact with the floor. In this position the physical therapist can facilitate lower trunk rotation by moving the lower extremities across the midline. (Sullivan p. 46)

130. Correct Answer: 3
Explanation: Since the pelvic floor muscles are weak and the patient is "initiating" the strengthening exercises, it is desirable for periods of rest to exceed the periods of exercise. Weak pelvic floor muscles generally require twice as much rest time as hold time. (Hall p. 363)

131. Correct Answer: 1
Explanation: The asymmetrical tonic neck reflex may produce extension of the affected upper extremity by turning the patient's head toward the affected side. (Sullivan p. 19)

132. Correct Answer: 2
Explanation: Submaximal exercise testing protocols usually consist of a number of three minute stages with increasing increments of work. Heart rate should be formally measured at least two times during each stage. Heart rate should reach "steady-state" (two heart rate measurements within 6 beats per minute) before the work rate is increased. (American College of Sports Medicine p. 72)

133. Correct Answer: 1
Explanation: A cool down or recovery period should occur at an intensity equal to or lower than the intensity of the first stage of the exercise test protocol. (American College of Sports Medicine p. 72)

134. Correct Answer: 3
Explanation: The amount of muscle force generated by short arc quadriceps exercises causes an anterior gliding force on the tibia and may place an undesirable amount of stress on the patient's reconstructed ligament given his post-operative status. (Kisner p. 540)

135. Correct Answer: 1
Explanation: Quadriceps setting exercises and biofeedback provide an excellent opportunity for the patient to selectively train the vastus medialis obliquus (VMO). Biofeedback can offer the patient auditory or visual feedback that can assist the patient to enhance VMO activity. (Kisner p. 525)

136. Correct Answer: 2
Explanation: Insertion of the catheter into the patient's trachea necessitates the use of sterile gloves. (Hillegass p. 653)

137. Correct Answer: 4
Explanation: Activities in a phase I cardiac rehabilitation program typically progress up to 3 METs. (Brannon p. 3)

138. Correct Answer: 4
Explanation: Patients with chronic arterial insufficiency typically have diminished blood flow and resultant ischemia. Positioning with the legs elevated will serve to exacerbate the patient's symptoms. (Kisner p. 710)

139. Correct Answer: 2
Explanation: A posterior glide of the femur on the acetabulum is indicated to increase hip flexion and medial rotation. (Kisner p. 245)

140. Correct Answer: 1
Explanation: The glenohumeral joint is a ball and socket joint that has three axes and three degrees of freedom. The close packed position is full abduction and lateral rotation, while the open packed or resting position is 55 degrees of abduction and 30 degrees of horizontal adduction. (Magee p. 208)

141. Correct Answer: 4
Explanation: A patient with paraplegia does not require the use of projection wheel rims due to full innervation of the upper extremities. Patients with C5-C6 tetraplegia utilize projection handrims in order to assist with manual wheelchair propulsion. (Rothstein p. 476)

142. Correct Answer: 1
Explanation: A posterior leaf spring ankle-foot orthosis is a plastic insert with a semirigid posterior upright that yields slightly at heel contact and recoils when the brace is unloaded during the swing phase. It is used to assist with dorsiflexion, however, does not promote medial or lateral stability. (Physical Therapist's Clinical Companion p. 313)

143. Correct Answer: 3
Explanation: The patient would likely utilize a three-point gait pattern using axillary crutches. A three-point gait pattern can accommodate different levels of weight bearing. (Pierson p. 223)

144. Correct Answer: 4
Explanation: Inadequate seat width results in difficulty changing positions, pressure on the greater trochanters, and difficulty wearing bulky clothing or orthoses. (Pierson p. 172)

145. Correct Answer: 4
Explanation: Rehabilitative braces with flexion and extension settings are designed to allow controlled motion within a specified range of motion. The braces function to protect the injured limb during the early phases of rehabilitation. (Paz p. 225)

146. Correct Answer: 4
Explanation: Thoraco-lumbar-sacral orthoses limit spinal motion of the lower thoracic and upper lumbar spine and are commonly used following surgery or as a result of an injury to the spine. (Seymour p. 438)

147. Correct Answer: 1
Explanation: Minimal contact with the skin allows a metal upright ankle-foot orthosis to accommodate for fluctuating edema while providing the appropriate support to the ankle joint. (Seymour p. 379)

148. Correct Answer: 4
Explanation: A walker provides the necessary stability for a patient that is touchdown weight bearing. The platform attachment permits weight bearing through the involved arm without placing undue stress on the distal radius. A rolling walker may not provide enough stability given the patient's weight bearing status. (Pierson p. 218)

149. Correct Answer: 3
Explanation: Using the cane in the left hand will allow the patient to shift her center of gravity away from the involved lower extremity and therefore reduce the pressure on the injured ankle. (Physical Therapist's Clinical Companion p. 297)

150. Correct Answer: 1
Explanation: The calf band of an ankle-foot orthosis should be placed immediately inferior to the fibular head. A calf band superior to the level of the fibular head may interfere with the normal function of the knee, while placement directly over the fibular head may result in impingement of the peroneal nerve. (Palmer p. 87)

151. Correct Answer: 1
Explanation: A tilt-in-space wheelchair is designed to provide pressure relief without shearing forces. The wheelchair has a fixed seat to back angle even when reclined and as a result is often able to accommodate customized seating systems. The wheelchair is commonly prescribed for patients unable to perform independent pressure relief. (Physical Therapist's Clinical Companion p. 324)

152. Correct Answer: 1
Explanation: A significant cognitive impairment may result in a patient being unable to safely use axillary crutches. (Pierson p. 214)

153. Correct Answer: 4
Explanation: A prosthesis with insufficient length would not be responsible for excessive lateral rotation of the prosthesis upon heel strike. The deviation may be caused by weak hip medial rotators, poor suspension of the prosthesis or excessive toe-out of the prosthesis. (Seymour p. 231)

154. Correct Answer: 3
Explanation: A patient with T5 paraplegia should be able to complete bathroom transfers using adaptive devices such as grab bars. The patient would possess full upper extremity innervation and limited trunk control. (Umphred p. 494)

155. Correct Answer: 2
Explanation: Anti-tip tubes are designed to prevent a patient from tipping over while in a wheelchair during activities of daily living. A patient with C5 tetraplegia would be the most likely candidate to benefit from this option based on the patient's expected level of function following discharge from the rehabilitation hospital. (O'Sullivan p. 907)

156. Correct Answer: 3
Explanation: Detachable armrests will make it easier for the patient to correctly position the sliding board and successfully transfer from the wheelchair to the bed. (Minor p. 248)

157. Correct Answer: 2
Explanation: A sliding transfer with draw sheet is the only transfer that will allow the patient to maintain a position of less than 30 degrees of upper body elevation. (Minor p. 228)

158. Correct Answer: 3
Explanation: Since the patient has a sensory alteration and ambulating a distance of only sixty feet created irritation, it is advisable to avoid utilizing the orthosis until modifications are made. (Seymour p. 393)

159. Correct Answer: 4
Explanation: The packages may be too heavy or the conveyor belt may be too high. In both cases the task is too difficult for the patient. (Kisner p. 673)

160. Correct Answer: 3
Explanation: Pushing up on the chair with both hands provides the most stable base to achieve a standing position. It is important not to reach for the walker while standing since the action may have a tendency to move the patient's center of gravity outside their base of support. (Pierson p. 236)

161. Correct Answer: 3
Explanation: Diaphragmatic breathing is often used as a method to increase activity of the diaphragm during inspiration, while diminishing the reliance on accessory muscles. (Hodgkin p. 236)

162. Correct Answer: 2
Explanation: In diaphragmatic breathing, the patient's hand placed over the midrectus area should rise during inspiration and fall during expiration. (Kisner p. 750)

163. Correct Answer: 4
Explanation: Continuous ultrasound at 2.4 W/cm^2 over a fracture site is excessive and can be potentially dangerous to the patient. (Cameron p. 206)

164. Correct Answer: 4
Explanation: Internal or external metallic objects, including surgical metal implants, are contraindications for shortwave diathermy. Failure to recognize the presence of a surgical metal implant may result in excessive heat production and subsequent tissue damage. (Michlovitz p. 233)

165. Correct Answer: 2
Explanation: Continuous ultrasound is commonly used to treat patients with healed burns due to its ability to increase the extensibility of collagen and decrease pain. (Cameron p. 194)

166. Correct Answer: 1
Explanation: Paraffin is a superficial heating agent that is commonly used to treat the distal extremities. Due to the number of joints involved, immersion in paraffin is an appropriate and practical selection. (Michlovitz p. 119)

167. Correct Answer: 2
Explanation: High-voltage current is characterized by a monophasic waveform usually delivered in spiked pulse pairs. High-voltage current utilizes an extremely short pulse duration and voltage greater than 150 volts; as a result the total average current is quite low. High-voltage current is most often used to provide sensory level stimulation. (Robinson p. 62)

168. Correct Answer: 3
Explanation: A physical therapist should not administer any form of treatment without patient consent. (Scott - Health Care Malpractice p. 44)

169. Correct Answer: 2
Explanation: The anterior aspect of the forearm is a common site utilized for determining the minimal erythemal dose since it is relatively easy to determine mild reddening of the skin in this area. It may at times, however, be more appropriate to determine the minimal erythemal dose on the area to be treated. (Michlovitz p. 270)

170. Correct Answer: 3
Explanation: Ultrasound using the underwater technique eliminates the need for contact between the soundhead and the area being sonated. (Cameron p. 207)

171. Correct Answer: 1
Explanation: Supplemental oxygen is often warranted when the partial pressure of arterial oxygen is less than 60 mm Hg or when arterial saturation is below 90%. A partial pressure of arterial oxygen of 70 mm Hg corresponds to arterial saturation of 92-93%. Normal pH is 7.35-7.45. (Paz p. 770)

172. Correct Answer: 4
Explanation: The supplied description accurately describes the position and technique associated with bronchial drainage to the superior segments of the lower lobes. (Rothstein p. 535)

173. Correct Answer: 4
Explanation: Pursed-lip breathing is a technique designed to improve ventilation and oxygenation. Studies indicate that pursed-lip breathing decreases respiratory rate, increases tidal volume, and improves exercise tolerance. (Kisner p. 754)

174. Correct Answer: 1
Explanation: A physical therapist should always check the patient's skin prior to adjusting the number of towel layers utilized with a hot pack. (Michlovitz p. 117)

175. Correct Answer: 4
Explanation: The greater the distance between the electrodes the deeper the current can penetrate. When electrodes are placed in close proximity the current will flow superficially and current density will be greatest to the skin between the electrodes. (Cameron p. 242)

176. Correct Answer: 3
Explanation: For each inch of vertical rise a properly constructed ramp will have 12 inches of length. (Rothstein p. 24)

177. Correct Answer: 3
Explanation: The Trendelenburg position is an inclined position in which the body and legs are elevated in relation to the head. This position is not recommended for patients with a known or suspected head injury secondary to an increase in intracranial pressure. (Frownfelter p. 607)

178. Correct Answer: 4
Explanation: A warm water bath is the most appropriate superficial heating agent to incorporate into the home program since it is readily available and easily applied to the lower leg and foot. (Michlovitz p. 142)

179. Correct Answer: 3
Explanation: Percussion is a technique that can be used to mobilize retained secretions. The technique involves direct contact over a given segment of the lung and should therefore be used with caution based on the patient's past medical history. (Frownfelter p. 331)

180. Correct Answer: 4
Explanation: A rigid dressing will serve to immobilize the injured area and offer protection from outside contaminants. (Trofino p. 43)

181. Correct Answer: 4
Explanation: The dependent variable is defined as the conditions or characteristics that appear, disappear or change as the experimenter introduces, removes or changes the independent variable. In this particular study ultrasound is the independent variable, while blood flow and nerve conduction velocity are the dependent variables. (Domholdt p. 63)

182. Correct Answer: 2
Explanation: A legal guardian or parent must sign the informed consent form for a minor. (American College of Sports Medicine p. 52)

183. Correct Answer: 1
Explanation: Physical therapists are required to report known or suspected abuse to enforcement agencies. These agencies include, but are not limited to, adult protective services and local or state law enforcement. (Scott – Legal Aspects p. 171)

184. Correct Answer: 2
Explanation: All of the presented options are signs of a heart attack, however, chest pain is considered the most significant. In addition to chest pain, patients may experience pain in the arm, neck, and shoulder. (Paz p. 42)

185. Correct Answer: 4
Explanation: It is essential to ascertain if research exists on the effectiveness of treating psoriatic lesions with ultraviolet prior to initiating a formal research project. (Portney p. 127)

186. Correct Answer: 4
Explanation: The physical therapist must take immediate action to resolve the situation by speaking directly to the involved therapists. Patient information should not be discussed in or around a public area. (Scott - Foundations p. 353)

187. Correct Answer: 1
Explanation: An insulin reaction is often associated with hypoglycemia or low blood sugar. Treatment for hypoglycemia includes the administration of food or drink containing sugar. (American College of Sports Medicine p. 212)

188. Correct Answer: 4
Explanation: Pressure applied to an artery proximal to an injury site may be helpful to control bleeding. (Anemaet p. 567)

189. Correct Answer: 3
Explanation: A systematic sample is often used in place of a random sample when a population can be accurately listed or is finite. Members of the sample are automatically selected once the first subject has been chosen. (Domholdt p. 98)

190. Correct Answer: 4
Explanation: Mouth to mouth and nose breathing is appropriate for an infant (less than one-year-old). (American Heart Association p. 148)

191. Correct Answer: 1
Explanation: The correct sequence is as follows: removal of current dressings, gentle debridement in a hydrotherapy tank, reapplication of the topical antibiotic, application of gauze wraps in a distal to proximal pattern. (Paz p. 483)

192. Correct Answer: 4
Explanation: A seizure occurs as a result of abnormal stimulation of brain cells. Intervention should be initially limited to protecting the patient from injury. A seizure typically lasts less than two minutes. (Physical Therapist's Clinical Companion p. 98)

193. Correct Answer: 1
Explanation: The kitchen sink is often the site for food preparation and other essential functions of daily living. As a result, it is an inappropriate site for hand washing due to the potential to spread infectious material. (Anemaet p. 21)

194. Correct Answer: 1
Explanation: Dentures that are not loose should not be removed during rescue breathing since they can assist the therapist to form an appropriate seal around the patient's mouth. (American Heart Association p. 67)

195. Correct Answer: 1
Explanation: The location and size of the wound combined with a limited amount of drainage make gloves the most appropriate form of medical asepsis when changing the dressing. (Minor p. 56)

196. Correct Answer: 3
Explanation: A physical therapist will be much more efficient and effective in responding to an emergency with the assistance of other trained professionals. The question provides little information on the number of patients within the treatment area or the size of the health care facility, as a result the most appropriate response is to seek assistance by using the public address system. Although attempting to contain the fire through a specific action such as closing the door is very appropriate, other methods of containment such as attempting to extinguish the fire could further jeopardize the safety of the therapist and patient. (Standards of Practice)

197. Correct Answer: 1
Explanation: Autonomy is defined as independent functioning. As an ethical term it refers to the patient's freedom to decide or freedom to act. (Davis p. 61)

198. Correct Answer: 3
Explanation: Physical therapist assistants perform procedures and related tasks that have been selected and delegated by the supervising physical therapist. It is not appropriate to delegate an examination. (Guide to Physical Therapist Practice p. S31)

199. Correct Answer: 4
Explanation: The Code of Ethics states that physical therapists seek reimbursement for their services that is deserved and reasonable. Accepting a check from a patient, regardless of its use, is unacceptable. (Guide for Professional Conduct)

200. Correct Answer: 2
Explanation: The therapist has made a judgment that the patient "lacks the necessary strength and coordination required to complete the activity independently." The only method to resolve the situation and be sure the patient is unharmed is to become directly involved. (Guide for Professional Conduct)

Unit Five

Paper and Pencil Examinations

The section contains two, 200 question sample examinations offered in a traditional paper and pencil format. Candidates who are exposed to sample examinations have several distinct opportunities that otherwise may not be available.

1. Candidates have the opportunity to refine their test taking skills with sample questions that are similar in design and format to actual examination questions.

2. Candidates have the opportunity to assess their current level of preparedness prior to the actual examination.

Candidates should attempt to identify the best answer for each examination question. Candidates will have a maximum of four hours to complete the sample examination. The sample examination should be completed in a single session in order to more closely simulate the actual examination. A detailed answer key follows each of the sample examinations. The answer key includes the correct answer, an explanation supporting the correct answer, and a cited resource with page number. The resources utilized in the explanations were selected since they are often required textbooks in physical therapy academic programs. When consulting specific page numbers candidates should make sure that the edition of a given textbook they are using is consistent with the edition referenced in the bibliography.

Scoring can be calculated using the formula:

$$\frac{\%}{\text{Correct}} = \frac{\text{Number of Questions Correct}}{200} *100$$

Candidates should record their score for the sample examination on the Sample Examination Scoring Summary located in the Appendix. The Sample Examination Scoring Summary serves as a valuable tool to assess examination performance as candidates are exposed to additional full-length sample examinations.

There are a number of indicators that must be closely examined after completing each sample examination in order to assess a candidate's performance. Perhaps the most obvious indicator is the number of questions a candidate answers correctly. Candidates should attempt to answer 80% or more of the questions correctly. Although this is a relatively lofty goal 80% was selected since the score is safely above even the highest established criterion-referenced score and therefore would always be considered a passing score. Candidates should use the number of questions answered correctly on the sample examinations only as a general indicator of their current level of preparedness.

There are a number of less obvious indicators that can offer candidates feedback as they prepare for the National Physical Therapy Examination. These indicators often are best examined by answering several specific questions.

- Were you able to maintain the same level of concentration throughout the entire examination?
- Did you have adequate time to complete the examination?
- Did you effectively incorporate test taking strategies?
- Did you misinterpret or fail to identify what selected questions were asking?
- Did the questions that were answered incorrectly exhibit any similar characteristics?
- Did you make any careless mistakes?

Candidates should avoid becoming overly excited or depressed based on the results of a given sample examination. Studying for the examination is much closer to running a marathon than running a sprint. By engaging in meaningful self-assessment activities candidates can gather valuable information to improve future examination performance.

EXAM ONE: PAPER AND PENCIL

Paper and Pencil Exam One – Section One

1. An eleven-month-old child with cerebral palsy attempts to maintain a quadruped position. Which reflex would interfere with this activity if it was not integrated?

   1. Galant reflex
   2. symmetrical tonic neck reflex
   3. plantar grasp reflex
   4. positive support reflex

2. A physical therapist attempts to schedule a patient for an additional therapy session after completing the examination. The physician referral indicates the patient is to be seen two times a week. The therapist suggests several possible times to the patient, but the patient insists she can only come in on Wednesday at 4:30. The therapist would like to accommodate the patient, but already has two patients scheduled at that time. The most appropriate action is to:

   1. schedule the patient on Wednesday at 4:30
   2. attempt to move one of the patient's scheduled on Wednesday at 4:30 to a different time
   3. schedule the patient with another therapist on Wednesday at 4:30
   4. inform the referring physician the patient will only be seen once this week in therapy

3. A physical therapist consults with an orthotist regarding the need for an ankle-foot orthosis for a patient status post CVA. The patient has difficulty moving from sitting to standing when wearing a prefabricated ankle-foot orthosis. The therapist indicates the patient has poor strength at the ankle, intact sensation, and does not have any edema or tonal influence. The most appropriate type of ankle-foot orthosis for the patient would incorporate:

   1. an articulation at the ankle joint
   2. tone reducing features
   3. metal uprights
   4. dorsiflexion assist spring

4. A physical therapist provides pre-operative instruction for a patient scheduled for anterior cruciate ligament reconstructive surgery. During the treatment session, the patient expresses to the therapist a sincere fear of dying during surgery. The therapist's most appropriate response would be:

   1. This surgery is done many times every day.
   2. I have never had a patient die yet.
   3. Surgery can be a very frightening thought.
   4. You will be back to athletics before you know it.

5. A physical therapist using an electrical stimulation device attempts to quantify several characteristics of a monophasic waveform. When measuring phase charge, the standard unit of measure is the:

   1. coulomb
   2. ampere
   3. ohm
   4. second

6. A physical therapist assesses the functional strength of a patient's hip extensors while observing the patient move from standing to sitting. What type of contraction occurs in the hip extensors during this activity?

   1. concentric
   2. eccentric
   3. isometric
   4. isotonic

7. A patient referred to physical therapy with chronic low back pain has failed to make any progress toward meeting established goals in over three weeks of treatment. The physical therapist has employed a variety of treatment techniques, but has yet to observe any sign of subjective or objective improvement in the patient's condition. The most appropriate action would be to:

1. transfer the patient to another therapist's schedule
2. re-examine the patient and establish new goals
3. continue to modify the patient's treatment plan
4. alert the referring physician to the patient's status

8. A patient with cardiopulmonary pathology is referred to physical therapy. The physical therapist documents the following clinical signs: pallor, cyanosis, and cool skin. These clinical signs are most consistent with:

1. cor pulmonale
2. anemia
3. atelectasis
4. diaphoresis

9. A physical therapist employed by a home health care agency knocks on the door of a patient that has a scheduled therapy session. After waiting several minutes, the therapist concludes the patient is not at home. The most appropriate therapist action is:

1. contact the patient and reschedule
2. notify the patient's insurance provider
3. notify the referring physician
4. discharge the patient from physical therapy

10. A pregnant patient in her third trimester completes a series of exercises in supine. In order to prevent vena cava compression during the exercise session the therapist should:

1. place a folded towel under the right side of the patient's pelvis
2. place a folded towel under the left side of the patient's pelvis
3. complete the exercises in sidelying
4. elevate the patient's feet 12 inches

11. A physical therapist receives a referral for a two-month-old infant diagnosed with osteogenesis imperfecta. After completing the examination, the therapist discusses the physical therapy plan of care with the infant's parents. The primary goal of therapy should be:

1. improve muscle strength and diminish tone
2. facilitate protected weight bearing
3. promote safe handling and positioning
4. diminish pulmonary secretions

12. A physical therapist elects to utilize the Six-Minute Walk Test as a means of quantifying endurance for a patient rehabilitating from a lengthy illness. Which variable would be the most appropriate to measure when determining the patient's endurance level with this objective test?

1. perceived exertion
2. heart rate response
3. elapsed time
4. distance walked

13. Communication and perceptual problems are extremely common in patients with hemiplegia. Which clinical problem would be characteristic of a patient status post right CVA?

1. inability to recognize symbols and perform basic math problems
2. inability to plan and perform serial steps in activities
3. distorted awareness of self-image
4. diminished functional speech

14. A physician orders an electrocardiogram for a patient diagnosed with congestive heart failure. The medical record indicates the patient is currently taking digitalis. What effect would you expect digitalis to have on the patient's ECG?

1. lengthened ventricular activation time
2. increased refractory period of AV node
3. lengthened QT interval
4. elevated ST segment

15. A physical therapist completes an examination on a five-year-old boy diagnosed with Duchenne muscular dystrophy. The referral indicates that the boy was diagnosed with the disease less than one year ago. Assuming a normal progression, which of the following findings would be the first to occur?

   1. distal muscle weakness
   2. proximal muscle weakness
   3. impaired respiratory function
   4. inability to perform activities of daily living

The following image should be used to answer question 16:

16. A physical therapist obtains an x-ray of a 14-year-old female recently referred to physical therapy after experiencing an increase in back pain following activity. The patient previously participated in competitive gymnastics, however, states that her back was unable to tolerate the intensity of training. Based on the presented x-ray the therapist would expect the patient's medical diagnosis to be:

   1. spondylitis
   2. spondylolysis
   3. spondylolisthesis
   4. spondyloptosis

17. A physical therapist completes a developmental assessment on a five-month-old infant. If the therapist elects to examine the infant's palmar grasp reflex, which of the following stimuli is the most appropriate?

   1. contact to the ball of the foot in upright standing
   2. maintained pressure to the palm of the hand
   3. noxious stimulus to the palm of the hand
   4. sudden change in the position of the hand

18. A physical therapist treats a 54-year-old male rehabilitating from a tibial plateau fracture. While completing a resistive exercise the patient indicates that lifting weights often causes him to void small amounts of urine. The most appropriate therapist action is:

   1. refer the patient to a support group
   2. instruct the patient in pelvic floor muscle strengthening exercises
   3. discontinue resistive exercises as part of the established plan of care
   4. educate the patient about incontinence

19. A physical therapist treats a nine-year-old child diagnosed with cystic fibrosis. As part of the treatment session the therapist attempts to improve the efficiency of the patient's breathing. The most appropriate technique to encourage full expansion at the base of the lungs is:

   1. manual percussion on the posterior portion of the ribs with the patient in prone
   2. manual contacts with pressure on the lateral borders of the ribs with the patient in supine
   3. manual vibration on the lateral portion of the ribs with the patient in sidelying
   4. manual cues on the epigastric area with the patient in supine

20. A physician discusses a patient's plan of care with a physical therapist. The patient is a 29-year-old male that sustained deep partial-thickness burns to the anterior surface of his upper legs. The physician discusses the possibility of discontinuing use of the topical antibiotic silver sulfadiazine after identifying an irregularity in the patient's laboratory results. Which finding could be most related to the use of silver sulfadiazine?

    1. leukopenia
    2. peripheral edema
    3. hypokalemia
    4. altered pH balance

21. A patient recently admitted to the hospital with an acute illness is referred to physical therapy. During a scheduled treatment session the patient asks what effect anemia will have on his ability to complete a formal exercise program. The most appropriate therapist response is:

    1. you may feel as though your muscles are weak
    2. you may experience frequent nausea
    3. your aerobic capacity may be reduced
    4. you may have a tendency to become fatigued

22. When performing range of motion exercises with a patient who sustained a head injury, a physical therapist notes that the patient lacks full elbow extension and classifies the end-feel as hard. The most likely cause is:

    1. heterotopic ossification
    2. spasticity of the biceps
    3. anterior capsular tightness
    4. triceps weakness

23. A physical therapist develops a problem list after examining a patient with a transtibial amputation. Which of the following would be the most appropriate entry in the patient problem list?

    1. donning and doffing prosthesis requires verbal cues
    2. donning and doffing prosthesis requires verbal cues and minimal assist of one
    3. dependence with donning and doffing prosthesis
    4. independent donning and doffing prosthesis in one week

24. A 42-year-old female status post abdominal surgery is unable to satisfactorily control the retention and release of urine. Which type of urinary catheter would not be appropriate for the patient?

    1. indwelling urinary catheter
    2. external urinary catheter
    3. Foley catheter
    4. suprapubic catheter

25. A physical therapist monitors a 6 foot 3 inch, 275 pound, male's blood pressure using the brachial artery. Which of the following is most important when selecting an appropriate size blood pressure cuff for the patient?

    1. patient age
    2. percent body fat
    3. somatotype
    4. extremity circumference

26. A patient informs a physical therapist that he has to use the bathroom immediately after being transported outside the hospital to practice car transfers. The physical therapist's most appropriate response to meet the patient's physical need is to:

    1. ask the patient if it is an emergency
    2. complete the transfer training as quickly as possible and allow the patient to use the bathroom
    3. transport the patient back into the hospital to use the bathroom
    4. instruct the patient that in the future he should use the bathroom before beginning physical therapy

27. A physical therapist examines a patient four days status post total hip replacement. The patient's medical record indicates the surgeon utilized an anterolateral surgical approach. Which of the following motions would be the most important to restrict during the initial phase of rehabilitation?

    1. knee extension
    2. knee flexion
    3. hip lateral rotation
    4. hip medial rotation

28. A patient informs a physical therapist how frustrated she feels after being examined by her physician. The patient explains that she becomes so nervous, she cannot ask any questions during scheduled office visits. The therapist's most appropriate response is to:

   1. offer to go with the patient to her next scheduled physician visit
   2. offer to call the physician and ask any relevant questions
   3. suggest that the patient write down questions for the physician and bring them with her to the next scheduled visit
   4. tell the patient it is a very normal response to be nervous in the presence of a physician

29. A physical therapist observes an electrocardiogram of a patient on beta-blockers. Which of the following ECG changes could be facilitated by beta-blockers?

   1. bradycardia
   2. tachycardia
   3. increased AV conduction time
   4. ST segment sagging

30. An athlete is forced to contemplate knee surgery after spraining the anterior cruciate ligament while playing soccer. Which situation would provide the most direct support for an anterior cruciate ligament reconstruction?

   1. grade III ACL and grade I PCL injury
   2. grade III ACL sprain with a lateral meniscus tear
   3. grade II ACL sprain with a medial meniscus tear
   4. functional instability

31. A physical therapist examines a patient that recently sustained a cervical hyperextension injury. Results of the examination reveal a loss of proprioception and two-point discrimination with intact motor function. This type of incomplete spinal cord injury is most appropriately termed:

   1. anterior cord syndrome
   2. Brown-Sequard's syndrome
   3. central cord syndrome
   4. posterior cord syndrome

32. A physical therapist employed in a long-term care setting attempts to identify a screening tool that examines a patient's ability to perform a variety of activities of daily living independently. The therapist would like to readminister the tool to assess patient progress. The most appropriate screening tool is the:

   1. Barthel Index
   2. Berg Balance Scale
   3. Health Status Profile
   4. Tinetti Performance Oriented Mobility Assessment

33. A patient rehabilitating from a lower extremity injury is referred to physical therapy for hydrotherapy treatments. The physical therapist would like the patient to fully extend the involved lower extremity while in the hydrotherapy tank. Which type of whirlpool would not allow the patient to extend the involved lower extremity?

   1. Hubbard tank
   2. highboy tank
   3. lowboy tank
   4. walk tank

34. A patient recovering in the hospital from a total knee replacement is examined by a physical therapist. Assuming an uncomplicated recovery, how much knee range of motion is anticipated prior to discharge?

   1. 0-50 degrees
   2. 0-90 degrees
   3. 15-90 degrees
   4. 15-105 degrees

The following image should be used to answer question 35:

35. A physical therapist inspects a wound over the sacrum of a 58-year-old female. The therapist would most accurately classify the presented wound as:

    1. stage I
    2. stage II
    3. stage III
    4. stage IV

36. A physical therapist observes a patient's breathing as part of a respiratory assessment. Which muscle of respiration is most active during forced expiration?

    1. diaphragm
    2. external intercostals
    3. internal intercostals
    4. upper trapezius

37. A physical therapist performs a manual muscle test on a patient with unilateral upper extremity weakness. The patient is able to complete 75% of the available range of motion with gravity-eliminated. The therapist should record the muscle grade as:

    1. poor plus
    2. poor
    3. poor minus
    4. trace plus

38. A physical therapist measures a patient for a straight cane prior to beginning ambulation activities. Which gross measurement method would provide the best estimate of cane length?

    1. measuring from the head of the fibula straight to the floor and multiplying by two
    2. measuring from the iliac crest straight to the floor
    3. measuring from the greater trochanter straight to the floor
    4. dividing the patient's height by two and adding three inches

39. A physical therapist recommends a wheelchair for a patient rehabilitating from a CVA with the goal of independent mobility. The left upper and lower extremities are flaccid and present with edema. There is normal strength on the right, however, the patient's trunk is hypotonic. The patient is cognitively intact. The most appropriate wheelchair for the patient is:

    1. solid seat, solid back, elevating legrests, and anti-tippers
    2. sling seat, sling back, arm board, and elevating legrests
    3. light weight, solid seat, solid back, arm board, and elevating legrests
    4. light weight, solid seat, solid back, arm board, and standard footrests

40. A physical therapist reviews the results of a pulmonary function test for a 58-year-old male patient recently admitted to the hospital. The therapist notes that the patient's total lung capacity is significantly increased when compared to established norms. Which medical condition would most likely produce this type of result?

    1. chronic bronchitis
    2. emphysema
    3. spinal cord injury
    4. pulmonary fibrosis

41. A physical therapist observes a patient's skin shortly after applying moist heat to the low back. The therapist identifies several signs of heat intolerance including uneven blotching and a surface rash. The most appropriate action is to:

    1. continue with the present treatment
    2. select an alternate superficial heating agent
    3. limit moist heat exposure to five minutes
    4. discontinue the moist heat and document the findings

42. A physical therapist works with a patient rehabilitating from a traumatic brain injury on a mat program. The program emphasizes various developmental positions to prepare the patient for ambulation activities. Which developmental position would be the most demanding?

    1. hooklying
    2. quadruped
    3. kneeling
    4. modified plantigrade

43. A physical therapist prepares a patient status post CVA with global aphasia for discharge from a rehabilitation hospital. The patient will be returning home with her husband and daughter. The most appropriate form of education to facilitate a safe discharge is to:

    1. perform hands-on training sessions with the patient and family members
    2. videotape the patient performing transfers and ADLs
    3. provide written instructions on all ADLs and functional tasks
    4. meet with family members to discuss the patient's present status and abilities

44. A physical therapist treats a 36-year-old male status post knee surgery. The therapist performs goniometric measurements to quantify the extent of the patient's extension lag. Which of the following would not provide a plausible rationale for the extension lag?

    1. muscle weakness
    2. bony obstruction
    3. inhibition by pain
    4. patient apprehension

45. A patient successfully completes ten anterior lunges. The physical therapist would like to modify the activity to maximally challenge the patient in the sagittal plane. Which of the following modifications would be the most appropriate?

    1. anterior lunge with concurrent bilateral elbow flexion to 45 degrees with five pound weights
    2. anterior lunge with concurrent bilateral shoulder flexion to 90 degrees with five pound weights
    3. anterior lunge with concurrent unilateral shoulder flexion to 90 degrees with a five pound weight
    4. anterior lunge with concurrent bilateral shoulder abduction to 45 degrees with five pound weights

46. A physical therapist teaches a patient positioned in supine to posteriorly rotate her pelvis. The patient has full active and passive range of motion in the upper extremities, but is unable to achieve full shoulder flexion while maintaining the posterior pelvic tilt. Which of the following could best explain these findings?

    1. capsular tightness
    2. latissimus dorsi tightness
    3. pectoralis minor tightness
    4. quadratus lumborum tightness

47. A patient with paraplegia is interested in learning how to perform a wheelie to assist with community mobility. The patient is independent with basic wheelchair propulsion. When instructing the patient to perform a wheelie, the physical therapist first should teach the patient to:

    1. make small adjustments (forward and backward) after being placed in the wheelie position
    2. move into the wheelie position
    3. perform turns while holding the wheelie position
    4. statically hold the wheelie position after being placed in it by the therapist

48. A physical therapist observes a burn on the dorsal surface of a patient's arm. The wound area is mottled red with a number of blisters. The therapist informs the patient that healing should take place in less than three weeks. This description is most indicative of a:

    1. superficial burn
    2. superficial partial-thickness burn
    3. deep partial-thickness burn
    4. full-thickness burn

49. A group of physical therapists develops a research project that examines the effect of increased abdominal muscle strength on forced vital capacity and forced expiratory volume. In order to conduct the study, the therapists are required to have the approval of the Hospital Institutional Review Board. The primary purpose of the committee is to:

    1. protect the hospital from unnecessary litigation
    2. ensure that established patient care standards are not compromised
    3. examine the design of the research project
    4. assess the financial ramifications of the research project

50. Members of a community health task force evaluate a proposal for a new adolescent screening program. Several members of the task force raise questions as to the validity of the screening instrument. Which measure of validity examines the instrument's ability to identify diseased persons by comparing true positives?

    1. adaptability
    2. selectivity
    3. sensitivity
    4. specificity

Please make sure all of the questions in the section have been answered prior to beginning the next section. When a new section is initiated candidates will be unable to return to previously completed sections.

Paper and Pencil Exam One – Section Two

51. A physical therapist attempts to quantify a patient's endurance level by administering a maximal exercise test. What is the primary limitation of a maximal exercise test?

1. Maximal exercise testing requires participants to exercise only to the point of volitional fatigue.
2. Maximal exercise testing does not typically allow a steady state heart rate at each work rate.
3. Maximal exercise testing is not useful in diagnosing coronary artery disease.
4. Maximal exercise testing requires progressive stages of increasing work intensities without rest intervals.

52. A physical therapist prepares to complete a formal sensory examination on a patient rehabilitating from a lower extremity burn. Which of the following would serve as the best predictor of altered sensation?

1. presence of a skin graft
2. depth of burn injury
3. percentage of body surface affected
4. extent of hypertrophic scarring

53. An 18-year-old male status post fractured right femur with open reduction and internal fixation is referred to physical therapy. After the initial session the patient states that therapy is a waste of time and he will not return for any additional appointments. The most immediate response would be to:

1. inform the referring physician of the patient's decision
2. instruct the patient to return for one additional treatment session
3. discuss the importance of physical therapy with the patient
4. discharge the patient from physical therapy

54. A physical therapist instructs a physical therapist assistant to begin gait training with a patient one day status post noncemented total hip replacement. Assuming the patient has not had any significant problems postoperatively, the most likely weight bearing status would be:

1. wheelchair use only
2. toe touch weight bearing
3. weight bearing as tolerated
4. full weight bearing

55. A physical therapist completes a manual muscle test on the right lower trapezius muscle. In order to properly assess the muscle, the therapist should position the patient in:

1. supine
2. prone
3. right sidelying
4. left sidelying

56. A physical therapist attempts to have a patient with right hemiplegia brush his teeth while working on standing tolerance. The therapist notices that the patient attempts to put the toothpaste directly in his mouth and hair. The therapist would document this finding as:

1. ideomotor apraxia
2. ideational apraxia
3. constructional apraxia
4. conduction aphasia

57. A physical therapist monitors the vital signs of a 52-year-old male during a graded exercise test. The patient was prompted to seek medical assistance two weeks ago after becoming short of breath on two separate occasions. When interpreting the data collected during the exercise test, which finding would serve as the best indicator that the patient had exerted a maximal effort?

1. failure of the heart rate to increase with further increases in intensity
2. rise in systolic blood pressure of 50 mm Hg when compared to the resting value
3. rating of 12 on a perceived exertion scale
4. decrease in diastolic blood pressure of 20 mm Hg when compared to the resting value

58. A physical therapist instructs a patient in residual limb wrapping. Which bandage would be the most appropriate to utilize for a patient with a transfemoral amputation?

    1. two-inch
    2. four-inch
    3. six-inch
    4. eight-inch

59. A physical therapist performs an examination on a patient with hip-knee-ankle-foot orthoses. The patient can ambulate independently with the orthoses and Lofstrand crutches, however, due to the high energy expenditure often becomes fatigued very rapidly. Which disorder would be most consistent with this scenario?

    1. amyotrophic lateral sclerosis
    2. peripheral neuritis
    3. neurogenic arthropathy
    4. spina bifida

60. A physical therapist examines a patient's hamstrings length using a passive straight leg raise. While raising the tested lower extremity, the physical therapist attempts to stabilize the contralateral limb. If the patient has tight hip flexors which result in an excessive anterior pelvic tilt, what can the physical therapist conclude about the patient's measured hamstrings length?

    1. actual length is greater than measured length
    2. actual length is less than measured length
    3. shortened hip flexors do not influence apparent hamstrings length
    4. the apparent length measured is the actual length

61. A physician orders electromyography for a patient with a brachial plexus injury to objectively determine the extent of pathology. Which of the following responses is most indicative of a normal muscle at rest?

    1. electrical silence
    2. spontaneous potentials
    3. polyphasic potentials
    4. occasional motor unit potentials

62. A physical therapist examines a patient diagnosed with acromioclavicular joint dysfunction. The therapist instructs the patient to abduct his arm in a coronal plane to 180 degrees. Which portion of the range of motion would you most expect to elicit pain in the acromioclavicular joint?

    1. 30-70 degrees
    2. 50-90 degrees
    3. 90-120 degrees
    4. 120-180 degrees

63. A physical therapist completes a quantitative gait analysis on a patient rehabilitating from a lower extremity injury. As part of the examination the therapist measures the number of steps taken by the patient in a 30 second period. This measurement technique can be used to measure:

    1. acceleration
    2. cadence
    3. velocity
    4. speed

64. Members of a health promotion task force design a program that annually will screen individuals in selected retirement communities for osteoporosis. Which screening tool would be the most cost effective and reliable to incorporate as part of the program?

    1. physical activity survey
    2. dietary analysis
    3. measuring height
    4. urinalysis screening

65. A cardiac patient undergoes a low-level symptom limited exercise treadmill test that begins at 1.5 METs and progresses to 4 METs. Which of the following activities would require an energy expenditure of approximately 4 METs?

    1. sitting quietly at rest
    2. level walking at 1 mph
    3. level walking at 3 mph
    4. level walking at 5 mph

66. A physical therapist prepares a patient for prosthetic training. Which of the following amputations would require the highest energy expenditure when using the appropriate prosthesis?

    1. bilateral transtibial amputations
    2. unilateral transtibial amputation
    3. unilateral transfemoral amputation
    4. Syme's amputation

67. A physical therapist positions a patient in prone with the knee flexed to 70 degrees prior to completing a manual muscle test of the hamstrings. To isolate the biceps femoris the therapist should:

    1. place the thigh in slight lateral rotation and the lower leg in slight lateral rotation on the thigh
    2. place the thigh in slight medial rotation and the lower leg in slight medial rotation on the thigh
    3. position the knee in 90 degrees of flexion
    4. position the knee in 110 degrees of flexion

68. A physical therapist reviews a patient's blood gas analysis. The therapist identifies that the $PaCO_2$ is elevated and the pH is below the normal level. These findings are most representative of:

    1. respiratory acidosis
    2. respiratory alkalosis
    3. metabolic acidosis
    4. metabolic alkalosis

69. A physical therapist strongly suspects a patient is intoxicated after arriving for his treatment session. When asked if he has been drinking, the patient indicates he consumed six or seven alcoholic beverages before driving to therapy. The therapist's most appropriate action is to:

    1. continue to treat the patient, assuming he can remain inoffensive to other patients
    2. modify the patient's present treatment program to minimize the effects of alcohol
    3. contact a member of the patient's family to take the patient home
    4. instruct the patient to leave the clinic

70. A physical therapist instructs a patient to complete a biceps strengthening exercise using a ten pound dumbbell in standing. The exercise requires the patient to maximally flex her elbow twelve times without moving the trunk. While observing the patient performing the exercise, it becomes apparent that the patient is unable to maintain her trunk in a stationary position. Which of the following modifications would be the most appropriate?

    1. decrease the number of repetitions to six
    2. decrease the dumbbell weight to five pounds
    3. instruct the patient to perform the exercise while sitting on a stool
    4. no modifications are necessary

71. A physical therapist receives a referral to instruct a patient in pelvic floor muscle strengthening exercises. Which of the following explanations would be the most effective to assist the patient to perform a pelvic floor contraction?

    1. tighten your muscles like you were trying to expel a large amount of urine in a very short amount of time
    2. pull your muscles up and in like when you have to go to the bathroom, but there is no toilet
    3. tighten your abdominal muscles and anteriorly rotate your pelvis
    4. gently push out as if you had to pass gas

72. A physical therapist orders a wheelchair with a reclining back for a patient in a rehabilitation hospital. Which type of legrests would be the most appropriate for the wheelchair?

    1. swing-away
    2. detachable
    3. elevating
    4. fixed

73. A physical therapy department attempts to establish a quality assurance program. The first step in developing the program should be to:

    1. identify important aspects of patient care provided by the department
    2. collect and analyze data for each established indicator
    3. identify quality indicators that will allow the department to monitor selected aspects of patient care
    4. determine a percentage of occurrence that will dictate a specified action

74. A patient rehabilitating from cardiac surgery is monitored using an arterial line. The primary purpose of an arterial line is to:

    1. measure right arterial pressure
    2. measure heart rate and oxygen saturation
    3. measure pulmonary artery pressure
    4. measure blood pressure

75. A patient with complete C5 tetraplegia works on a forward raise for pressure relief. The patient utilizes loops that are attached to the back of the wheelchair to assist with the forward raise. Which muscles need to be particularly strong in order for the patient to be successful with the forward raise?

    1. brachioradialis, brachialis
    2. rhomboids, levator scapulae
    3. biceps, deltoids
    4. triceps, flexor digitorum

76. A physical therapist uses rhythmic initiation to assist a patient in learning to roll from supine to prone. The therapist's initial command should be:

    1. "Slowly roll over by yourself"
    2. "Help me roll you over"
    3. "Stop me from rolling you over"
    4. "Relax and let me move you"

77. A physical therapist employed in an outpatient clinic treats a 58-year-old female diagnosed with a traumatic anterior shoulder dislocation. The patient has no past history of shoulder instability, however, has been treated for impingement syndrome. Upon reading the physician referral the therapist is surprised that the period of shoulder immobilization was less than two weeks. Which of the following variables would have been the most significant when determining the length of immobilization?

    1. age
    2. sex
    3. vocation
    4. social history

78. A physical therapist uses proprioceptive neuromuscular facilitation to increase joint range of motion using the hold-relax technique. Which type of contraction is utilized at the end point of the available range of motion?

    1. isotonic
    2. isometric
    3. isokinetic
    4. eccentric

79. A physical therapist prepares to select an assistive device for a patient rehabilitation from a lower extremity injury. Which of the following would be of least importance when selecting an assistive device?

    1. the patient's level of understanding
    2. the patient's height and weight
    3. the patient's upper and lower extremity strength
    4. the patient's level of coordination

80. A patient sustained a fracture of the acetabulum that was treated with open reduction and internal fixation. The injury occurred in a motor vehicle accident approximately seven weeks ago. Which objective measure would be the most influential variable when determining the patient's weight bearing status?

    1. visual analogue pain scale rating
    2. radiographic confirmation of bone healing
    3. lower extremity manual muscle testing
    4. balance and coordination assessment

81. A patient with hemiplegia ambulates with an ankle-foot orthosis. The physical therapist notes that the patient's involved foot frequently drags during the initial swing phase of gait. To treat this problem most effectively the therapist should emphasize:

    1. eccentric strengthening of the hamstrings
    2. eccentric strengthening of the gluteus medius
    3. concentric strengthening of the plantar flexors
    4. concentric strengthening of the iliopsoas/rectus femoris

82. A physical therapist using the upper extremity D1 extension proprioceptive neuromuscular facilitation pattern resists elbow extension with the goal of increasing the patient's ability to extend her wrist. This is an example of:

    1. reciprocal excitation
    2. successive induction
    3. irradiation
    4. quick stretch

83. A patient who has suffered a CVA four weeks ago is beginning to show the ability to produce movement patterns outside of limb synergies. According to Brunnstrom, this patient is in which stage of recovery?

    1. two
    2. three
    3. four
    4. six

84. A physical therapist works with a patient to improve bed mobility. Which of the following techniques would be the most effective to increase the patient's hip stability?

    1. lower trunk rotation in the hooklying position
    2. bridging
    3. assisted hip and knee flexion in supine
    4. hip abduction and adduction in the hooklying position

85. A physical therapist completes a posture screening and a gross range of motion test on a patient referred to therapy with patella tendonitis. The therapist determines that the patient has extremely limited lower extremity flexibility, most notably in the hip flexors. What common structural deformity is often associated with tight hip flexors?

    1. scoliosis
    2. kyphosis
    3. lordosis
    4. spondylosis

86. A patient two weeks status post transtibial amputation is instructed by his physician to remain at rest for two days after contracting bronchitis. The most appropriate position for the patient in bed is:

    1. supine with a pillow under the patient's knees
    2. supine with a pillow under the patient's thighs and knees
    3. supine with the legs extended
    4. sidelying in the fetal position

87. A physical therapist tests a small area of skin for hypersensitivity prior to using a cold immersion bath. The patient begins to demonstrate evidence of cold intolerance within 60 seconds after cold application. The most appropriate response is to:

    1. limit cold exposure to ten minutes or less
    2. select an alternative cryotherapeutic agent
    3. continue with the cold immersion bath
    4. discontinue cold application and document your findings

88. A 27-year-old female diagnosed with anterior compartment syndrome reports to an outpatient clinic for physical therapy services. While reviewing the physician referral supplied by the patient, the physical therapist identifies that the referral form is over 90 days old. The most appropriate therapist action is:

    1. continue with the session since the existing referral is acceptable
    2. attempt to contact the physician's office by telephone to receive verbal orders
    3. send the physician written correspondence requesting an updated referral
    4. discontinue the session until the patient secures an updated referral

89. A physical therapist assesses the deep tendon reflexes of a patient as part of a lower quarter screening examination. The therapist determines that the right and left patellar tendon reflex and the left Achilles tendon reflex is 2+, while the right Achilles tendon reflex is absent. The clinical condition that could best explain this finding is:

    1. cerebral palsy
    2. multiple sclerosis
    3. peripheral neuropathy
    4. vascular claudication

90. A physical therapist completes an examination on a patient diagnosed with facet impingement in the lumbar spine. The patient appears to be somewhat fixed in a position of sidebending to the right and rotation to the left. When assessing lumbar range of motion, which motions would you expect to be most restricted?

    1. sidebending to the right and rotation to the left
    2. sidebending to the right and rotation to the right
    3. sidebending to the left and rotation to the right
    4. sidebending to the left and rotation to the left

91. An employee with a disclosed disability informs her employer that she is unable to perform an essential function of her job unless her workstation is modified. Which of the following would provide the employer with a legitimate reason for not granting the employee's request?

    1. the accommodation would cost hundreds of dollars
    2. the accommodation would require an expansion of the employee's present workstation
    3. the accommodation would fundamentally alter the operation of the business
    4. the accommodation would not address the needs of other employees

92. A group of health care professionals participates in a family conference for a patient with a spinal cord injury. During the conference one of the participants summarizes the patient's progress with bathing and dressing activities. This type of information is typically conveyed by a/an:

    1. nurse
    2. physical therapist
    3. occupational therapist
    4. case manager

93. A physical therapist attempts to palpate the tibialis posterior tendon. To facilitate palpation of this structure the therapist should:

    1. ask the patient to invert and plantar flex the foot
    2. ask the patient to evert and dorsiflex the foot
    3. ask the patient to invert and dorsiflex the foot
    4. passively evert and plantar flex the foot

94. A patient diagnosed with spinal stenosis is referred to physical therapy three times a week for six weeks. During the examination the patient informs the physical therapist that the commute to therapy is over 90 miles. The most appropriate therapist action is to:

    1. schedule the patient once a week
    2. schedule the patient three times a week
    3. attempt to locate a physical therapy clinic closer to the patient's home
    4. discharge the patient with a home exercise program

95. During a balance assessment of a patient with left hemiplegia, it is noted that in sitting the patient requires minimal assistance to maintain the position and cannot accept any additional challenge. The physical therapist would appropriately document the patient's sitting balance as:

1. normal
2. good
3. fair
4. poor

96. A short-term goal for a patient with a neurological deficit is as follows: The patient will transfer from tall kneeling to half kneeling with supervision. This activity is an example of:

1. mobility
2. stability
3. controlled mobility
4. skill

97. A physical therapist is treating a patient with a head injury who begins to perseverate. In order to refocus the patient and achieve the desired therapeutic outcome, the therapist should:

1. focus on the topic of perseveration for a short period of time in order to appease the patient
2. guide the patient into an interesting new activity and reward successful completion of the task
3. take the patient back to his room for quiet time and attempt to resume therapy once he has stopped perseverating
4. continue with repetitive verbal cues to cease perseveration

98. The goals for a patient status post total knee replacement include general conditioning and independent household mobility. Which component of the patient's treatment would be the most appropriate to delegate to a physical therapy aide?

1. stair training
2. progressive gait training with a straight cane
3. patient education regarding the surgical procedure
4. ambulation with a walker for endurance

99. A complete medical history should be conducted on all patients prior to initiating treatment. Questions asked during the patient history should not lead the patient. Which of the following questions would not be considered leading?

1. Does this increase your pain?
2. Does this alter your pain in any way?
3. Does your pain increase at night?
4. Does your pain decrease with activity?

100. A physical therapist examines the heart sounds of a 48-year-old female status post coronary artery bypass graft. When auscultating, the therapist identifies the heart sound associated with closing of the mitral and tricuspid valves. This heart sound best describes:

1. S1
2. S2
3. S3
4. S4

Please make sure all of the questions in the section have been answered prior to beginning the next section. When a new section is initiated candidates will be unable to return to previously completed sections.

Paper and Pencil Exam One – Section Three

101. A physical therapist employed in a work hardening program performs an examination on a patient diagnosed with fibromyalgia. During the examination the therapist identifies an inconsistency between the measured lumbar range of motion and the amount of lumbar range of motion observed while lifting a milk crate from the floor to a table. The most appropriate therapist action is:

1. avoid discussing the identified inconsistency with the patient
2. confront the patient with the identified inconsistency
3. discuss the identified inconsistency with the referring physician
4. discharge the patient from physical therapy

102. A patient is referred to physical therapy diagnosed with right hip trochanteric bursitis. Which clinical finding is usually not associated with trochanteric bursitis?

1. resisted abduction reproduces symptoms
2. full hip active range of motion
3. positive Ober test
4. joint play motions are limited in a capsular pattern

103. A patient is referred to physical therapy after surgery to repair a large rotator cuff tear. Which of the following motions would you initially expect to be the most restricted?

1. extension
2. abduction
3. medial rotation
4. lateral rotation

104. A physical therapist attempts to select an appropriate intervention to treat a patient with a 10 degree limitation in knee extension. Which of the following mobilization techniques would be indicated?

1. lateral glide of the patella
2. caudal glide of the patella
3. posterior glide of the tibia
4. anterior glide of the tibia

105. A physical therapist performs passive range of motion on a patient with C7 tetraplegia. The patient's bilateral straight leg raise is measured passively to 90 degrees. What should the therapist conclude about the patient's ability to perform activities of daily living?

1. The patient requires a straight leg raise of 110-120 degrees in order to perform long sit and activities of daily living.
2. The patient is at a functional range to perform long sit and activities of daily living.
3. The patient's range of motion is beyond the expected limit for long sit and activities of daily living.
4. The patient requires a straight leg raise of 150 degrees in order to perform long sit and activities of daily living.

106. A note in a patient's medical record indicates a specific drug is taken through enteral administration. Which of the following is an example of enteral administration?

1. inhalation
2. injection
3. topical
4. oral

107. A patient is positioned in supine with the hips flexed to 90 degrees and the knees extended. As the patient slowly lowers her extended legs toward the horizontal, there is an increase in lordosis of the low back. This finding is indicative of weakness of the:

1. hip flexors
2. back extensors
3. hip extensors
4. abdominals

108. A patient with C4 tetraplegia requires a custom wheelchair upon discharge from the hospital. The patient's diaphragm is partially innervated. The most appropriate recommendation for proper seating is:

    1. light weight manual wheelchair, upright frame, seat and back cushions
    2. folding reclining wheelchair, power chin control, seat and back cushions
    3. non-folding reclining wheelchair, power tongue control, underslung tray for ventilator
    4. upright power wheelchair, joystick hand control, seat cushion

109. A therapist examines a patient with a C6 spinal cord injury. Which muscle would not be innervated based on the patient's level of injury?

    1. biceps
    2. deltoids
    3. triceps
    4. diaphragm

110. A physical therapist attempts to assess the integrity of the vestibulocochlear nerve by administering the Rinne test on a patient with a suspected upper motor neuron lesion. After striking the tine of the tuning fork to begin vibration, which bony prominence should the therapist utilize to position the stem of the tuning fork?

    1. apex of the skull
    2. occipital protuberance
    3. inion
    4. mastoid process

111. A physical therapist prepares to apply a topical antibiotic to a small portion of the upper arm of a patient with a deep partial-thickness burn. When applying the topical antibiotic the therapist should utilize which form of medical asepsis?

    1. gloves
    2. sterile gloves
    3. sterile gloves, gown
    4. sterile gloves, gown, mask

112. A physical therapist attempts to obtain information on a patient's endurance level by administering a low-level exercise test on a treadmill. Which of the following measurement methods would provide the therapist with an objective measurement of endurance?

    1. facial color
    2. facial expression
    3. rating on a perceived exertion scale
    4. respiration rate

113. A physical therapist examines a patient status post stroke with a flaccid left side. In order to facilitate muscular activity, the treatment plan should include:

    1. weight bearing, tapping, elevation
    2. vibration, tapping, prolonged stretch
    3. weight bearing, tapping, approximation
    4. approximation, elevation, prolonged stretch

114. A patient with a right radial head fracture is examined in physical therapy. The patient's involved elbow range of motion begins at 15 degrees of flexion and ends at 90 degrees of flexion. The physical therapist should record the patient's elbow range of motion as:

    1. 0 - 15 - 90
    2. 15 - 0 - 90
    3. 15 - 90
    4. 0 - 90

115. A physical therapist reviews the medical record of a patient with Broca's aphasia. This condition most often results from a CVA that affects the:

    1. anterior cerebral artery
    2. middle cerebral artery
    3. posterior cerebral artery
    4. basilar artery

116. A patient involved in a motor vehicle accident sustains a proximal fibula fracture. The fracture damages the motor component of the common peroneal nerve. Ankle dorsiflexion and eversion are tested as 2/5. The most appropriate intervention to assist the patient with activities of daily living would be:

    1. electrical stimulation
    2. orthosis
    3. exercise program
    4. aquatic program

117. A 72-year-old female involved in a motor vehicle accident fractures the middle third of her femoral shaft. The patient's physician is concerned about the effects of prolonged bed rest and would like the patient to begin walking as soon as possible. Which form of treatment would facilitate early weight bearing through the involved extremity?

    1. immobilization in a hip spica cast
    2. internal fixation with an intramedullary nail
    3. external mobilization
    4. skeletal traction

118. A physical therapist discusses the importance of a proper diet with a patient diagnosed with congestive heart failure. Which of the following substances would most likely be restricted in the patient's diet?

    1. high density lipoproteins
    2. low density lipoproteins
    3. sodium
    4. triglycerides

119. A physical therapist instructs a patient with a pulmonary disease in energy conservation techniques. Which of the following techniques would be the most effective when assisting a patient to complete a selected activity without dyspnea?

    1. diaphragmatic breathing
    2. pacing
    3. pursed-lip breathing
    4. ventilatory muscle training

120. A physical therapist attempts to assist a patient to clear secretions after performing postural drainage by coughing. What position would allow the patient to produce the most forceful cough?

    1. prone
    2. sidelying
    3. supine
    4. upright sitting

121. A physical therapist observes excessive knee flexion from heel strike to midstance while observing a patient with a transtibial amputation during gait training. A possible cause for the deviation is:

    1. the foot is set in neutral
    2. the socket is set posterior in relation to the foot
    3. the prosthesis is too short
    4. the socket is aligned in excessive flexion

122. A physical therapist attempts to improve a patient's lower extremity strength. Which proprioceptive neuromuscular facilitation technique would be the most appropriate to achieve the therapist's goals?

    1. contract-relax
    2. repeated contractions
    3. rhythmic stabilization
    4. hold-relax

123. A physical therapist instructs a patient diagnosed with rotator cuff tendonitis in transverse plane resistive exercises. Which motions would be appropriate based on the given information?

    1. abduction and adduction
    2. flexion and extension
    3. medial and lateral rotation
    4. pronation and supination

124. A patient is limited in passive ankle dorsiflexion when the knee is extended, but is not limited when the knee is flexed. The most logical explanation is:

    1. the gastrocnemius is responsible for the limitation
    2. the soleus is responsible for the limitation
    3. the popliteus is responsible for the limitation
    4. the gastrocnemius and soleus are both responsible for the limitation

125. A patient with a C6 spinal cord injury relies on tenodesis to assist with functional activities. Which condition will reduce the benefits of tenodesis?

    1. lengthening of the long finger flexors
    2. excessive hamstrings length
    3. insufficient hamstrings length
    4. transferring with the fingers flexed

126. A patient is treated in physical therapy after injuring his hamstrings. The medical chart describes the injury as an avulsion fracture of the ischial tuberosity. This injury usually results from:

    1. forceful extension of the hip with an extended knee
    2. forceful extension of the hip with a flexed knee
    3. forceful flexion of the hip with an extended knee
    4. forceful flexion of the hip with a flexed knee

127. A physical therapist attempts to gain information on the ligamentous integrity of the knee. Which of the following special tests would not provide the therapist with the desired information?

    1. anterior drawer test
    2. apprehension test
    3. Lachman test
    4. pivot shift test

128. A physical therapist reviews the medical record of a patient 24 hours status post total hip replacement. A recent entry in the medical record indicates that the patient was placed on anticoagulant medication. Which of the following laboratory values would be most affected based on the patient's current medication?

    1. hematocrit
    2. hemoglobin
    3. prothrombin time
    4. white blood cell count

129. A physical therapist discusses the plan of care for a 61-year-old male diagnosed with spinal stenosis with the referring physician. During the discussion the physician shows the therapist a picture of the patient's spine obtained through computed tomography. What color would vertebrae appear when using this imaging technique?

    1. black
    2. light gray
    3. dark gray
    4. white

130. A physical therapist performs the talar tilt test on a 22-year-old female rehabilitating from an inversion ankle sprain. Which ligament does the talar tilt test examine?

    1. anterior tibiofibular
    2. calcaneofibular
    3. deltoid
    4. posterior tibiofibular

131. A physical therapist completes a developmental assessment on a seven-month-old infant. Assuming normal development, which of the following reflexes would not be integrated?

    1. asymmetrical tonic neck reflex
    2. Moro reflex
    3. Landau reflex
    4. symmetrical tonic neck reflex

132. A patient is referred to physical therapy after being diagnosed with a partial tear of the ulnar collateral ligament of the thumb. Which objective finding would be most consistent with this type of injury?

    1. excessive angulation of the metacarpophalangeal joint of the thumb with valgus stress
    2. excessive angulation of the metacarpophalangeal joint of the thumb with varus stress
    3. excessive angulation of the carpometacarpal joint of the thumb with radially directed stress
    4. excessive angulation of the carpometacarpal joint of the thumb with ulnarly directed stress

133. A 42-year-old female is admitted to a rehabilitation hospital after sustaining a stroke. During the examination the physical therapist identifies significant sensory deficits in the anterolateral spinothalamic system. Which sensation would be most affected?

    1. barognosis
    2. kinesthesia
    3. graphesthesia
    4. temperature

134. A physical therapist identifies a number of substances that influence circulation. Which of the following substances is stimulated by decreased arterial pressure and acts as a vasoconstrictor?

    1. angiotensin
    2. histamine
    3. epinephrine
    4. norepinephrine

135. A physical therapist records the vital signs of individuals at a health and wellness fair designed to promote physical therapy week. Which age group should the therapist expect to have the highest resting pulse rate?

    1. infants
    2. children
    3. teenagers
    4. adults

136. A 13-year-old girl discusses the possibility of anterior cruciate ligament reconstruction with an orthopedic surgeon. The girl injured her knee while playing soccer and is concerned about the future impact of the injury on her athletic career. Which of the following factors would have the greatest influence on her candidacy for surgery?

    1. anthropometric measurements
    2. hamstrings/quadriceps strength ratio
    3. skeletal maturity
    4. somatotype

137. A patient diagnosed with C5 quadriplegia receives physical therapy services in a rehabilitation hospital. The patient has made good progress in therapy and is scheduled for discharge in one week. During a treatment session the patient informs the physical therapist that one day in the future he will walk again. The most appropriate therapist response is:

    1. Your level of injury makes walking unrealistic.
    2. Future advances in spinal cord research may make your goal a reality.
    3. You can have a rewarding life even if confined to a wheelchair.
    4. Completing your exercises on a regular basis will help you to walk.

The following image should be used to answer question 138:

138. A physical therapist performs several surface palpations on a patient diagnosed with an acromioclavicular injury. Which anatomical landmark is most consistent with the location of the therapist's finger?

    1. manubrium
    2. sternoclavicular joint
    3. suprasternal notch
    4. xiphoid process

139. A physical therapist discusses the plan of care for a patient rehabilitating from total hip replacement surgery with the patient's surgeon. During the discussion the surgeon indicates that he would like the patient to continue to wear a knee immobilizer in order to help prevent hip dislocation. The primary rationale for this action is:

1. The knee immobilizer serves as a constant reminder to the patient that the hip is susceptible to injury.
2. The knee immobilizer reduces hip flexion by maintaining knee extension.
3. The knee immobilizer facilitates quadriceps contraction during weight bearing activities.
4. The knee immobilizer limits post-operative edema and as a result promotes lower extremity stability.

140. A physical therapist treats a patient that is on a waiting list for a heart transplant. The patient has a lengthy history of cardiac pathology and recently received a right ventricular assistive device due to persistent ventricular failure. Which two structures would house the tubes for this device?

1. left atrium and aorta
2. left atrium and pulmonary artery
3. right atrium and aorta
4. right atrium and pulmonary artery

141. A physical therapist treats a 72-year-old female who fractured her leg two weeks ago after losing her balance and falling to the floor in a nursing home. The patient's spouse died three years ago and left her with no appreciable assets or regular income. The patient has been a resident of the nursing home for eight years. Which form of insurance is the most likely to pay for the patient's daily care?

1. private insurance
2. workers' compensation
3. Medicaid
4. Medicare

142. A physical therapist administers a submaximal exercise test to a patient in a cardiac rehabilitation program. The protocol requires the patient to ride a cycle ergometer for a predetermined amount of time using progressive workloads. In order to predict the patient's maximum oxygen uptake it is necessary to determine the relationship between:

1. heart rate and perceived exertion
2. heart rate and oxygen uptake
3. perceived exertion and blood pressure
4. blood pressure and oxygen uptake

143. A physician orders the nursing staff to administer digitalis to a patient diagnosed with congestive heart failure. The physician's primary goal using this medication is to:

1. increase cardiac pumping ability
2. increase cellular metabolism
3. regulate fluid and electrolyte levels
4. regulate glucose metabolism

144. A physical therapist identifies a bluish discoloration of the skin and nailbeds of a 55-year-old male referred to physical therapy for pulmonary rehabilitation. What does this objective finding indicate?

1. hyperoxemia
2. hyperoxia
3. hypokalemia
4. hypoxemia

145. A physical therapist employed in a large medical center reviews the chart of a 63-year-old male referred to physical therapy for pulmonary rehabilitation. The chart indicates the patient has smoked 1-2 packs of cigarettes a day since the age of 25. The admitting physician documented that the patient's thorax was enlarged with flaring of the costal margins and widening of the costochondral angle. Which pulmonary disease does the chart most accurately describe?

1. asthma
2. bronchiectasis
3. chronic bronchitis
4. emphysema

146. A physical therapist reviews the results of pulmonary function testing on a 44-year-old female diagnosed with emphysema. Assuming the patient's testing was classified as unremarkable, which of the following lung volumes would most likely approximate 10% of the patient's total lung capacity?

    1. tidal volume
    2. inspiratory reserve volume
    3. residual volume
    4. functional residual capacity

147. A 26-year-old female is referred to physical therapy after being diagnosed with impingement syndrome. The patient is a competitive swimmer who complains of shoulder pain when performing strokes that require overhead motion. Which of the following results would be the most typical during the examination of the shoulder?

    1. excessive medial rotation
    2. diminished cutaneous sensation
    3. restricted posterior capsule
    4. weakness in the deltoid muscle

148. A patient rehabilitating from a spinal cord injury works on self-range of motion activities in sitting. Suddenly, the patient begins to demonstrate signs and symptoms of autonomic dysreflexia. The most appropriate physical therapist action is to:

    1. keep the patient in sitting, monitor blood pressure, and check the bowel and bladder for impairment
    2. lie the patient flat, monitor blood pressure, and check the bowel and bladder for impairment
    3. lie the patient flat, monitor blood pressure, and give the patient fluids
    4. place the patient in sidelying, monitor blood pressure, wait for medical assistance

149. A physical therapist administers the Body Mass Index Scale to a patient as a means of assessing total body composition. The therapist determines the body mass index by dividing the body weight in kilograms by height in meters squared. Which of the following values would be the most representative of a healthy male or female?

    1. 14 kg/m^2
    2. 22 kg/m^2
    3. 28 kg/m^2
    4. 35 kg/m^2

150. A patient diagnosed with patellofemoral syndrome discusses his past medical history with a physical therapist. The patient reports having anterior cruciate ligament reconstructive surgery in his right knee two years ago, however, the therapist is not able to identify a scar over the anterior surface of the right knee. Assuming the surgeon utilized an autograft for the reconstruction, which of the following would be the most likely graft site?

    1. semitendinosus and semimembranosus
    2. semitendinosus and gracilis
    3. semimembranosus and gracilis
    4. semitendinosus and biceps femoris

Please make sure all of the questions in the section have been answered prior to beginning the next section. When a new section is initiated candidates will be unable to return to previously completed sections.

Paper and Pencil Exam One – Section Four

151. A patient four weeks status post arthroscopic medial meniscectomy is limited in knee flexion range of motion. Which mobilization technique would be the most beneficial to increase knee flexion?

    1. anterior glide of the tibia
    2. superior glide of the patella
    3. posterior glide of the tibia
    4. anterior glide of the fibula head

152. After examining the respiratory status of a patient with a C6 spinal cord injury, which of the following clinical findings would you expect to be the most accurate?

    1. partial innervation of the diaphragm
    2. full epigastric rise in supine
    3. a ventilator is required for assisted breathing
    4. normal ventilatory reserve

153. A physical therapist instructs a patient with tight calf muscles to complete a closed kinematic chain standing wall stretch. Prior to beginning the stretch the therapist positions a folded towel under the medial arch of the patient's foot. The primary purpose of this action is to limit:

    1. talocrural dorsiflexion
    2. talocrural plantar flexion
    3. subtalar supination
    4. subtalar pronation

154. A patient rehabilitating from a motor vehicle accident completes a series of closed kinetic chain exercises. One of the exercises requires the patient to perform a mini-squat in an erect position with the center of gravity placed directly over the knee joint. If the physical therapist modifies the activity by asking the patient to move the buttocks posteriorly in relation to the knees, what muscle group is the therapist attempting to emphasize?

    1. knee extensors
    2. knee flexors
    3. hip extensors
    4. hip flexors

155. A physical therapist reviews a physician referral form that includes only the patient's name and the referring physician's signature. The therapist asks an administrative assistant to contact the physician's office to secure additional information while he begins the examination. During the examination the patient indicates that she had knee surgery two weeks ago, however, is unable to provide more specific information. After completing the examination the therapist checks with the administrative assistant who indicates that she was unable to reach anyone at the physician's office. The most appropriate therapist action is:

    1. initiate treatment based on the results of the examination
    2. initiate treatment based on an established protocol following knee surgery
    3. initiate treatment, however, avoid resistive exercises and high-level functional activities
    4. delay treatment until orders are received from the referring physician

156. A physical therapist employed in an acute care hospital reviews the results of recent laboratory testing for one of his patients. A note in the medical record indicates that the patient was dehydrated at the time the blood sample was taken. Which finding would be most likely based on the patient's hydration status?

    1. increased coagulation time
    2. decreased hematocrit level
    3. increased blood urea nitrogen level
    4. decreased hemoglobin level

157. A treatment program is designed to include late morning sessions involving aggressive stretching, moderate exercise, energy conservation, and stress management techniques. This program would be most appropriate for which diagnosis?

    1. Guillain-Barre syndrome
    2. myasthenia gravis
    3. Osgood-Schlatter disease
    4. multiple sclerosis

158. A 28-year-old male referred to physical therapy by his primary physician complains of recurrent ankle pain. As part of the treatment program, the therapist uses ultrasound over the peroneus longus and brevis tendons. The most appropriate location for ultrasound application is:

    1. inferior to the sustentaculum tali
    2. over the sinus tarsi
    3. posterior to the lateral malleolus
    4. anterior to the lateral malleolus

159. A physical therapist positions a patient in supine prior to performing a manual muscle test of the supinator. To isolate the supinator and minimize the action of the biceps the therapist should position the patient's elbow in:

    1. 30 degrees of elbow flexion
    2. 60 degrees of elbow flexion
    3. 90 degrees of elbow flexion
    4. terminal elbow flexion

160. A physical therapist reviews the surgical report of a patient that sustained extensive burns in a fire. The report indicates that at the time of primary excision, cadaver skin was utilized to close the wound. This type of graft is termed:

    1. allograft
    2. autograft
    3. heterograft
    4. xenograft

161. A physician completes a physical examination on a 16-year-old male who injured his knee while playing in a soccer contest yesterday. The physician's preliminary diagnosis is a grade II anterior cruciate ligament injury with probable meniscal involvement. Which of the following diagnostic tools would be the most appropriate in the immediate medical management of the patient?

    1. bone scan
    2. computerized tomography
    3. magnetic resonance imaging
    4. x-rays

162. A physical therapist performs goniometric measurements on a 38-year-old female rehabilitating from an acromioplasty. The therapist attempts to stabilize the scapula while measuring glenohumeral abduction. Failure to stabilize the scapula will lead to:

    1. downward rotation and elevation of the scapula
    2. downward rotation and depression of the scapula
    3. upward rotation and elevation of the scapula
    4. upward rotation and depression of the scapula

163. A physical therapist measures a patient's shoulder medial rotation with the patient positioned in supine, glenohumeral joint in 90 degrees of abduction, and the elbow in 90 degrees of flexion. The therapist records the patient's shoulder medial rotation as 0 - 70 degrees and classifies the end-feel as firm. Which portion of the joint capsule is primarily responsible for the firm end-feel?

    1. anterior joint capsule
    2. posterior joint capsule
    3. inferior joint capsule
    4. superior joint capsule

164. A physician suspects a stress fracture in a 16-year-old distance runner after completing a physical examination. Assuming the physician's preliminary diagnosis is correct, which of the following diagnostic tests would be the most appropriate to identify the stress fracture?

    1. bone scan
    2. magnetic resonance imaging
    3. telethermography
    4. ultrasound scan

165. A physical therapist performs an examination on a 46-year-old male patient diagnosed with piriformis syndrome. The patient indicates he has experienced pain in his lower back and buttock region for the last three weeks. Which motions would you expect to be weak and painful during muscle testing based on the patient's diagnosis?

    1. abduction and lateral rotation of the thigh
    2. abduction and medial rotation of the thigh
    3. adduction and lateral rotation of the thigh
    4. adduction and medial rotation of the thigh

166. A physical therapist examines a patient with a dorsal scapular nerve injury. Which muscles would you expect to be most affected by this condition?

    1. serratus anterior, pectoralis minor
    2. levator scapulae, rhomboids
    3. latissimus dorsi, teres major
    4. supraspinatus, infraspinatus

167. A physical therapist positions a patient in prone to measure passive knee flexion. Range of motion may be limited in this position due to:

    1. active insufficiency of the knee extensors
    2. active insufficiency of the knee flexors
    3. passive insufficiency of the knee extensors
    4. passive insufficiency of the knee flexors

168. A physical therapist examines a four-month-old infant. During mat activities the infant suddenly becomes unconscious. The most appropriate location to check the infant's pulse is the:

    1. radial artery
    2. brachial artery
    3. popliteal artery
    4. carotid artery

169. A physical therapist observes a patient during gait training. The patient has normal strength and equal leg length. As the patient passes midstance he slightly vaults and has early toe off. The most likely cause of this deviation is:

    1. patient has excessive forefoot pronation
    2. patient has limited hamstrings length
    3. patient has limited plantar flexion
    4. patient has limited dorsiflexion

170. A patient status post CVA with abnormal tone on the right side lies supine in bed. The patient's physical therapist discourages her from lying supine for long periods of time because:

    1. the position can cause shoulder-hand syndrome
    2. the position increases inferior subluxation
    3. the position encourages tonic neck and labyrinthine reflexes
    4. the position increases tone in the pectoralis

171. A physical therapist conducts a goniometric assessment of a patient's upper extremities. Which of the following values is most indicative of normal passive glenohumeral abduction?

    1. 80 degrees
    2. 120 degrees
    3. 155 degrees
    4. 180 degrees

172. A physical therapist monitors a patient's respiration rate during exercise. Which of the following would be considered a normal response?

    1. the respiration rate declines during exercise as the intensity of exercise increases
    2. the respiration rate does not increase during exercise
    3. the rhythm of the respiration pattern becomes irregular during exercise
    4. the respiration rate decreases as the intensity of the exercise plateaus

173. A physical therapist reviews the results of a pulmonary function test. Assuming normal values, which of the following measurements would you expect to be the greatest?

    1. vital capacity
    2. tidal volume
    3. residual volume
    4. inspiratory reserve volume

174. A patient involved in a motor vehicle accident sustains an injury to the posterior cord of the brachial plexus. Which muscle would not be affected by the injury?

    1. infraspinatus
    2. subscapularis
    3. latissimus dorsi
    4. teres major

175. A physical therapist designs a training program for a patient without cardiovascular pathology. The therapist calculates the patient's age-predicted maximal heart rate as 175 beats per minute. Which of the following would be an acceptable target heart rate for the patient during cardiovascular exercise?

    1. 93 beats per minute
    2. 122 beats per minute
    3. 169 beats per minute
    4. 195 beats per minute

176. A 13-year-old female diagnosed with cerebral palsy is referred to physical therapy. The patient exhibits slow, involuntary, continuous writhing movements of the upper and lower extremities. This type of motor disturbance is most representative of:

    1. spasticity
    2. ataxia
    3. hypotonia
    4. athetosis

177. A physician refers a patient rehabilitating from a fractured femur to physical therapy for gait training. Which of the following would not be the responsibility of the physical therapist?

    1. assessing balance
    2. determining weight bearing status
    3. selecting an assistive device
    4. assessing endurance

178. A physical therapist instructs a 55-year-old patient with significant bilateral lower extremity paresis to transfer from a wheelchair to a mat table. The patient has normal upper extremity strength and has no other known medical problems. The most appropriate transfer technique is a:

    1. dependent standing pivot
    2. sliding board transfer
    3. two-person carry
    4. hydraulic lift

179. A physical therapist instructs a patient to make a fist. The patient can make a fist, but is unable to flex the distal phalanx of the ring finger. This clinical finding can best be explained by:

    1. a ruptured flexor carpi radialis tendon
    2. a ruptured flexor digitorum superficialis tendon
    3. a ruptured flexor digitorum profundus tendon
    4. a ruptured extensor digitorum communis tendon

180. A patient with a confirmed posterior cruciate ligament tear is able to return to full dynamic activities following rehabilitation. Which of the following does not serve as a secondary restraint to the posterior cruciate ligament?

    1. iliotibial band
    2. popliteus tendon
    3. lateral collateral ligament
    4. medial collateral ligament

181. A 67-year-old patient is examined in physical therapy after having sutures removed following a transtibial amputation. The patient resides in a retirement community and describes herself as socially active. She is presently using a temporary prosthesis consisting of a plastic socket, a pylon, and a solid ankle cushion heel foot. When discussing a permanent prosthesis with the physical therapist the patient expresses concern that the device will look awful and will be obvious to everyone in her retirement community. Which type of prosthetic components would be the most appropriate for the patient?

    1. endoskeletal shank and single-axis articulated foot-ankle assembly
    2. endoskeletal shank and solid ankle cushion heel foot
    3. exoskeletal shank and single-axis articulated foot-ankle assembly
    4. exoskeletal shank and solid ankle cushion heel foot

182. A physical therapist measures forearm supination range of motion on a patient rehabilitating from a radial head fracture. The patient is eager to show progress in therapy and as a result often attempts to substitute for his limited range of motion by manipulating his body. Which of the following motions would most often be used to substitute for a limitation in supination?

1. shoulder abduction and lateral rotation
2. shoulder abduction and medial rotation
3. shoulder adduction and lateral rotation
4. shoulder adduction and medial rotation

183. A physical therapist develops an aquatic therapy program for a patient diagnosed with a lower extremity injury. The therapist plans to monitor the patient's response to exercise using heart rate, however, is concerned about the influence of the water on the patient's heart rate response. Which of the following best describes the effect of immersion in water on heart rate response when compared to traditional land activities?

1. heart rate response is increased during low intensity exercise in water
2. heart rate response is decreased during low intensity exercise in water
3. heart rate response is increased during high intensity exercise in water
4. heart rate response is decreased during high intensity exercise in water

184. A physical therapist measures passive forearm pronation and concludes that the results are within normal limits. Which measurement would be classified as within normal limits?

1. 60 degrees
2. 80 degrees
3. 100 degrees
4. 120 degrees

185. A physical therapist treats a patient rehabilitating from a fracture at the distal end of the humerus. The therapist notes that the patient's elbow is grossly swollen. Which position of the elbow would best accommodate the increased fluid?

1. full extension
2. 15 degrees of flexion
3. 70 degrees of flexion
4. 120 degrees of flexion

186. A physical therapist discusses the importance of proper posture with a patient rehabilitating from back surgery. Which body position would place the most pressure on the lumbar spine?

1. standing in the anatomical position
2. standing with 45 degrees of hip flexion
3. sitting in a chair
4. sitting in a chair with reduced lumbar lordosis

187. A physical therapist works on transfer activities with a patient diagnosed with a complete C5 spinal cord injury. Which of the following muscles would the patient be able to utilize during the training session?

1. brachioradialis
2. pronator teres
3. extensor carpi radialis brevis
4. latissimus dorsi

188. A physical therapist treats a 32-year-old female diagnosed with thoracic outlet syndrome. While exercising the patient begins to complain of feeling lightheaded and dizzy. The therapist immediately ushers the patient to a nearby chair and begins to monitor her vital signs. The therapist measures the patient's respiration rate as 10 breaths per minute, pulse rate of 45 beats per minute, and blood pressure of 115/85 mm Hg. Which of the following statements is most accurate?

1. pulse rate and respiration rate are below normal levels
2. pulse rate and blood pressure are above normal levels
3. blood pressure and respiration rate are above normal levels
4. the patient's vital signs are within normal limits

189. A physical therapy treatment plan for a patient rehabilitating from an anterior shoulder dislocation includes progressive resistive exercises. Which muscle groups should be emphasized during rehabilitation?

    1. abductors, lateral rotators
    2. adductors, lateral rotators
    3. abductors, medial rotators
    4. adductors, medial rotators

190. A physical therapist works with a patient diagnosed with anterior cruciate ligament insufficiency. The physician referral specifies closed kinematic chain rehabilitation. Which exercise would not be appropriate based on the physician order?

    1. exercise on a stair machine
    2. limited squats to 45 degrees
    3. walking backwards on a treadmill
    4. isokinetic knee extension and flexion

191. A patient paralyzed from the waist down discusses accessibility issues with an employer in preparation for her return to work. The patient is concerned about her ability to navigate a wheelchair in certain areas of the building. What is the minimum space required to turn 180 degrees in a standard wheelchair?

    1. 32 inches
    2. 48 inches
    3. 60 inches
    4. 72 inches

192. A patient is referred to physical therapy following surgery to repair a torn rotator cuff. The physician referral does not include post-operative guidelines and also does not classify the extent or size of the tear. The physical therapist's most appropriate action is to:

    1. consult various medical resources that discuss physical therapy management of rotator cuff repairs
    2. consult various protocols of other surgeons in the area
    3. contact the referring physician and discuss the patient's care
    4. discuss the patient's care with other staff members who are more experienced in treating rotator cuff repairs

193. A 52-year-old, self-referred male is examined in physical therapy. The patient states that over the last three months he has experienced increasing neck stiffness and pain at night. He also communicates that within the past week he has had several episodes of dizziness. The patient has a family history of cancer and has smoked two packs of cigarettes a day for the last twenty years. The patient denies any other significant past medical history and lists the date of his last medical examination as ten years ago. The physical therapist's most appropriate action is to:

    1. treat the patient conservatively and document any changes in the patient's status
    2. inform the patient that he is not a candidate for physical therapy
    3. refer the patient to an oncologist
    4. refer the patient to his primary care physician

194. A patient is scheduled to undergo a transtibial amputation secondary to poor healing of an ulcer on his left foot. In addition, the patient is two months status post right knee replacement due to osteoarthritis. Given the patient's past and current medical history, the physical therapist can expect which of the following tasks to be the most difficult for the patient following his amputation?

    1. rolling from supine to sidelying
    2. moving from sitting to supine
    3. moving from sitting to standing
    4. ambulating in the parallel bars

195. A physical therapist wears sterile protective clothing while treating a patient. Which area of the protective clothing would not be considered sterile even before coming in contact with a non-sterile object?

    1. gloves
    2. sleeves of the gown
    3. front of the gown above waist level
    4. front of the gown below waist level

196. A patient two days status post transfemoral amputation demonstrates decreased strength and generalized deconditioning. Which of the following positions should be utilized when wrapping the patient's residual limb?

1. sidelying
2. standing
3. supine
4. prone

197. A physical therapist transports a patient with multiple sclerosis to the gym for her treatment session. The patient is wheelchair dependent and uses a urinary catheter. When transporting the patient, the most appropriate location to secure the collection bag is:

1. in the patient's lap
2. on the patient's lower abdomen
3. on the wheelchair armrest
4. on the wheelchair cross brace beneath the seat

198. A physical therapist employed by a home health agency visits a patient status post total knee replacement. The patient was discharged from the hospital yesterday and according to the medical record had an unremarkable recovery. The physician orders include the use of a continuous passive motion machine. The most appropriate rate of motion for the patient would be:

1. 2 cycles per minute
2. 4 cycles per minute
3. 6 cycles per minute
4. 8 cycles per minute

199. A physical therapist attempts to examine the extent of ataxia in a patient's upper extremities. The preferred method to examine and document ataxia is:

1. manual muscle test
2. sensory test for light touch
3. functional assessment for rolling in bed
4. finger to nose

200. A physical therapist treats a patient with Parkinson's disease. In order to improve the patient's motor control, the therapist should incorporate which of the following techniques into the treatment session?

1. alternating isometrics
2. rhythmic initiation
3. manual resisted exercise
4. lumbar stabilization exercises in quadruped

Please make sure all of the questions in the section have been answered prior to ending the examination. Since candidates are not permitted to return to previously completed sections, this should signify the end of the examination.

EXAM ONE: Paper and Pencil
Answer Key

Paper and Pencil Exam One – Section One

1. Correct Answer: 2
Explanation: Head positioning is the stimulus for the symmetrical tonic neck reflex. When the head is flexed, the upper extremities flex and the lower extremities extend. When the head extends the upper extremities extend and the lower extremities flex. The reaction of the extremities would not allow the infant to maintain a quadruped position. (Ratliffe p. 26)

2. Correct Answer: 3
Explanation: Scheduling with another therapist will allow the patient to be seen two times per week as indicated on the referral and will accommodate the patient's schedule. (Guide for Professional Conduct)

3. Correct Answer: 1
Explanation: An articulation at the ankle joint would allow the tibia to advance forward over the fixed foot. This would assist with weight shifting during the sit to stand transfer as well as during ambulation. (Seymour p. 382)

4. Correct Answer: 3
Explanation: The response "surgery can be a very frightening thought" is an empathetic response that demonstrates respect and acknowledgement for the patient's feelings. (Purtilo p. 170)

5. Correct Answer: 1
Explanation: Phase charge is represented by the area under a single phase waveform. The unit of measure is the coulomb. (Robinson p. 23)

6. Correct Answer: 2
Explanation: The gluteus maximus and the hamstrings function as primary hip extensors. These muscles function in an eccentric fashion when moving from standing to sitting. (Levangie p. 310)

7. Correct Answer: 4
Explanation: The physician should be informed about the patient's lack of progress. The patient may be discharged from physical therapy or referred back to the physician. (Standards of Practice)

8. Correct Answer: 2
Explanation: Anemia refers to a reduction in the number of circulating red blood cells. Symptoms may include pallor, cyanosis, cool skin, vertigo, weakness, headache, and general malaise. (Paz p. 405)

9. Correct Answer: 1
Explanation: The question does not present enough information to determine why the patient was not at home. As a result, the physical therapist should document the missed appointment and contact the patient to reschedule. (Standards of Practice)

10. Correct Answer: 1
Explanation: Turning the patient slightly to the left by placing a towel under the right side of the patient's pelvis will tend to lessen the effects of uterine compression on abdominal vessels and improve cardiac output. (Kisner p. 693)

11. Correct Answer: 3
Explanation: Osteogenesis imperfecta is an autosomal disorder of collagen synthesis that affects bone metabolism. As a result, an infant with this condition is extremely susceptible to fractures during even basic activities such as being carried or bathing. The most common characteristic of osteogenesis imperfecta is bone fragility resulting in fractures. (Ratliffe p. 254)

12. Correct Answer: 4
Explanation: The Six-Minute Walk Test provides an indirect measure of cardiovascular endurance by examining the distance a patient can walk in six minutes. Patients are instructed to walk as far and as fast as possible in six minutes. (Paz p. 915)

13. Correct Answer: 3
Explanation: Patients with right CVA and left hemiplegia commonly have a distorted awareness of self-image. (Rothstein p. 445)

14. Correct Answer: 2   *Item Includes Graphic*
Explanation: Digitalis is used to alleviate symptoms of congestive heart failure. The drug increases the force of myocardial contraction and increases the refractory period of the AV node. The refractory period is the time the AV node is incapable of responding to an action potential. By slowing down the rate of ventricular contraction, digitalis allows for increased filling time and improved cardiac output. (Brannon p. 277)

15. Correct Answer: 2
Explanation: A patient with Duchenne muscular dystrophy often exhibits significant proximal muscle weakness, particularly in the shoulders and pelvic girdle. As the condition advances, the muscular weakness encompasses the distal musculature and interferes with activities of daily living. (Ratliffe p. 241)

16. Correct Answer: 3
Explanation: Spondylolisthesis refers to the forward displacement of one vertebra over another. The x-ray involves spondylolisthesis at the L5-S1 level. Individuals involved in physical activities such as weightlifting, gymnastics or football are particularly susceptible to this condition. The severity of the spondylolisthesis is classified on a scale of 1-5 based on how much a given vertebral body has slipped forward over the vertebral body beneath it. (Magee p. 467)

17. Correct Answer: 2
Explanation: The palmar grasp reflex is elicited through maintained pressure to the palm of the hand resulting in finger flexion. The reflex begins at birth and is integrated at approximately four to six months. (Rothstein p. 689)

18. Correct Answer: 4
Explanation: Incontinence refers to an inability to control the release of urine, feces or gas. Education may include basic information related to incontinence as well as referral to the patient's primary care provider. A vast majority of patients with incontinence can be successfully treated with non-invasive techniques such as pelvic floor exercises, however, without more definitive medical information this action would be premature. (Kisner p. 616)

19. Correct Answer: 2
Explanation: Applying direct pressure with the hands on the lateral borders of the ribs with the patient in supine can promote a more efficient breathing pattern. Physical therapy management for a child with cystic fibrosis may include bronchial drainage techniques, chest percussion, vibration, and suctioning. (Frownfelter p. 484)

20. Correct Answer: 1
Explanation: Silver sulfadiazine is a sulfa drug that can produce a decrease in the number of circulating white blood cells (leukopenia). The topical antibiotic works by interfering with bacterial nucleic acid production by disrupting folic acid synthesis in susceptible bacteria. Additional problems encountered with sulfa drugs include gastrointestinal distress and allergic reactions. (Paz p. 460)

21. Correct Answer: 4
Explanation: Anemia is defined as a reduction in the number of circulating red blood cells per cubic millimeter. Symptoms of anemia include pallor of the skin, vertigo, and general malaise. Although a patient may sense that his muscles are weak, fatigue will have a greater impact on the patient's ability to complete a formal exercise program. (Goodman - Pathology p. 515)

22. Correct Answer: 1
Explanation: Heterotopic ossification refers to abnormal bone growth in tissue. Signs and symptoms include decreased range of motion, local swelling, and warmth. Heterotopic ossification often occurs in patients following a head injury. (Goodman - Pathology p. 1078)

23. Correct Answer: 3
Explanation: The problem list should summarize the significant findings from the examination. Since the problem list relates back to the subjective and objective portion of the note each entry should be described in broad terms. (Quinn p. 34)

24. Correct Answer: 2
Explanation: External urinary catheters are applied over the shaft of the penis and are therefore inappropriate for females. (Pierson p. 289)

25. Correct Answer: 4
Explanation: The width of a bladder should be approximately 40% of the circumference of the midpoint of the limb. Bladder width for an average size adult is 5-6 inches. (Pierson p. 57)

26. Correct Answer: 3
Explanation: The only viable solution to meet the patient's physical need is to allow him to use the bathroom. (Code of Ethics)

27. Correct Answer: 3
Explanation: A patient status post total hip replacement using an anterolateral surgical approach would be most restricted in lateral rotation. Failure to restrict lateral rotation may result in hip dislocation or subluxation. Hip medial rotation would be most restricted using a posterolateral surgical approach. (Pierson p. 130)

28. Correct Answer: 3
Explanation: Suggesting the patient write down questions for the physician is a practical and realistic option that will assist her in future interactions. (Davis p. 85)

29. Correct Answer: 1
Explanation: Beta-blockers decrease heart rate and the force associated with myocardial contraction. On an electrocardiogram beta-blockers may cause sinus bradycardia. (Brannon p. 134)

30. Correct Answer: 4
Explanation: Many individuals are able to continue to function at high levels despite a variety of ligamentous and meniscal injuries, therefore functional instability provides the most direct support for an anterior cruciate ligament reconstruction. (Kisner p. 535)

31. Correct Answer: 4
Explanation: Posterior cord syndrome is a relatively rare form of incomplete spinal cord injury that is characterized by a loss of proprioception, two-point discrimination, and stereognosis with preserved motor function. The injury is typically classified as a cervical hyperextension injury. (Physical Therapist's Clinical Companion p. 91)

32. Correct Answer: 1
Explanation: The Barthel Index consists of 10 activities of daily living and is often used as a screening tool in rehabilitation, long-term care settings, and home care. Scoring on the assessment ranges from 0-100 in increments of 5. A score of 100 indicates that the patient is independent with mobility and self-care activities in the home. Observation and scoring should take approximately one hour. (Physical Therapist's Clinical Companion p. 104)

33. Correct Answer: 2
Explanation: The length of a highboy tank does not permit a patient to fully extend the lower extremities, however, its depth permits immersion to the midthoracic region. (Michlovitz p. 144)

34. Correct Answer: 2
Explanation: Range of motion activities are performed almost immediately following a total knee replacement. The patient ideally would be able to attain full extension range of motion and up to 90 degrees of knee flexion prior to discharge. (Kisner p. 519)

35. Correct Answer: 3   *Item Includes Graphic*
Explanation: A stage III ulcer is characterized by full-thickness skin loss involving damage or necrosis of subcutaneous tissue that may extend down to, but not through, underlying fascia. The ulcer presents clinically as a deep crater with or without involvement of adjacent tissue. (Sussman p. 58)

36. Correct Answer: 3
Explanation: The internal intercostals act to depress the ribs during forceful expiration. (Kisner p. 740)

37. Correct Answer: 3
Explanation: The ability to move through partial range of motion in a gravity-eliminated position is consistent with a muscle grade of poor minus. (Kendall p. 187)

38. Correct Answer: 3
Explanation: The handgrip of a proper fitting cane should be at the level of the greater trochanter. (Pierson p. 219)

39. Correct Answer: 3
Explanation: Independent propulsion is facilitated by the use of a lightweight wheelchair, while a solid seating system assists with posture and transfer activities. An arm board allows the flaccid upper extremity to be supported and elevating legrests assist to decrease dependent edema. (O'Sullivan p. 1061)

40. Correct Answer: 2
Explanation: Emphysema is a chronic obstructive pulmonary disease characterized by an increase in the size of air spaces distal to the terminal bronchiole accompanied by destructive changes in their walls. As a result, the lungs become hyperinflated and the chest wall becomes fixed in a hyperinflated position. Total lung capacity and dead space in the lungs significantly increase. (Frownfelter p. 516)

41 Correct Answer: 4
Explanation: Treatment should be discontinued when there is any sign of heat intolerance. It is important to document the incident in order to alert other possible providers to the patient's reaction and to make the incident part of the permanent medical record. (Michlovitz p. 132)

42. Correct Answer: 4
Explanation: The modified plantigrade position requires patients to possess control of equilibrium and proprioceptive reactions. The position offers a small base of support and high center of gravity with weight bearing occurring through the lower extremities. (Sullivan p. 54)

43. Correct Answer: 1
Explanation: Hands-on training sessions provide unique opportunities for the therapist to assess the competence of family members in a structured environment. (O'Sullivan p. 8)

44. Correct Answer: 2
Explanation: Patients that demonstrate an extension lag have greater passive extension than active extension. The difference in the passive and active extension range of motion is used to quantify the amount of the lag. Bony obstruction would not produce an extension lag since passive range of motion and active range of motion would be equal. (Placzek p. 319)

45. Correct Answer: 2
Explanation: The sagittal plane divides the body into left and right halves. Motions in the sagittal plane include flexion and extension. Bilateral shoulder flexion would create the largest forward movement and would therefore provide the greatest challenge for the patient. (Norkin p. 4)

46. Correct Answer: 2
Explanation: Shortening of the latissimus dorsi often presents as a limitation of shoulder flexion or abduction due to the muscles origin on the external lip of the iliac crest and its insertion on the intertubercular groove of the humerus. (Kendall p. 279)

47. Correct Answer: 4
Explanation: Holding the wheelie position after being placed into it by the therapist requires the least skill and therefore provides the patient with the opportunity to gain a sense of balance before moving on to more difficult activities. (O'Sullivan p. 1086)

48. Correct Answer: 2
Explanation: A superficial partial-thickness burn involves the epidermis and a portion of the dermis. Healing typically occurs in approximately three weeks with little or no scarring. (Goodman - Pathology p. 302)

49. Correct Answer: 2
Explanation: Institutional review boards are responsible for assuring the welfare and safety of patients and establishing that ethical, moral, and legal standards are not compromised by proposed research activities. (Portney p. 39)

50. Correct Answer: 3
Explanation: Sensitivity is the percentage of individuals with a particular diagnosis who are correctly identified as positive by a test. (Domholdt p. 180)

Paper and Pencil Exam One – Section Two

51. Correct Answer: 1
Explanation: Physical therapists gain information on a patient's response to exercise through various subjective and objective measures, however, remain dependent on a patient's willingness to exert a maximal effort in order to collect meaningful data. (American College of Sports Medicine p. 69)

52. Correct Answer: 2
Explanation: Patients with burns often experience a number of sensory changes. These changes can include impaired sensation or increased sensitivity. Although many factors contribute to sensory alteration, the depth of the burn appears to be the best predictor. (Paz p. 446)

53.   Correct Answer: 3
Explanation: The physical therapist must determine whether the patient understands the importance of physical therapy. If the patient continues to refuse treatment, the therapist should inform him of the expected consequences. (Scott - Foundations p. 76)

54.   Correct Answer: 2
Explanation: Total hip replacement using noncemented fixation requires toe touch weight bearing for a minimum of six weeks in order to allow adequate time for tissue and bone growth around the prosthesis. (Brotzman p. 287)

55.   Correct Answer: 2
Explanation: To perform a manual muscle test of the lower trapezius, the patient should be positioned in prone with the shoulder abducted greater than 120 degrees. Pressure should be applied against the forearm in a direction towards the floor. (Kendall p. 286)

56.   Correct Answer: 2
Explanation: Ideational apraxia is most commonly due to a lesion in the patient's dominant parietal lobe of the cerebrum. The condition deals with errors in concepts and sequencing of tasks. (Bennett p. 147)

57.   Correct Answer: 1
Explanation: Failure of the heart rate to increase with further increases in intensity occurs when a patient is no longer able to meet the demands imposed by a given exercise intensity. This objective finding often signifies that the patient has produced a maximal effort. (American College of Sports Medicine p. 145)

58.   Correct Answer: 3
Explanation: A six-inch ace wrap is the most appropriate bandage for wrapping the residual limb of a patient with a transfemoral amputation. The six-inch wrap adequately covers the larger surface area of the residual limb. (O'Sullivan p. 630)

59.   Correct Answer: 4
Explanation: Spina bifida is a neural tube defect characterized by a defective closure of the vertebral column. Although the exact clinical presentation of spina bifida can vary considerably, hip-knee-ankle-foot orthoses (HKAFO) are often employed to assist pediatric patients with ambulation activities. The high energy cost of ambulating with the orthoses often makes community ambulation difficult. (Physical Therapist's Clinical Companion p. 314)

60.   Correct Answer: 1
Explanation: Tight hip flexors result in excessive anterior tilt of the pelvis, as a result actual hamstrings length will be greater than the measured length. (Kendall p. 42)

61.   Correct Answer: 1
Explanation: The process of electromyography involves asking a patient to utilize a particular muscle so that voluntary potentials can be recorded. There should not be any recorded electrical activity in a muscle at rest. (Nelson p. 547)

62.   Correct Answer: 4
Explanation: Acromioclavicular dysfunction often results in a painful arc from 120-180 degrees of abduction. A painful arc from 90-120 degrees may be indicative of subacromial bursitis, calcium deposits or tendonitis of the rotator cuff muscles. (Magee p. 208)

63.   Correct Answer: 2
Explanation: Cadence is defined as the number of steps taken by a person per unit of time. (Levangie p. 445)

64.   Correct Answer: 3
Explanation: Osteoporosis refers to a disease process that results in a reduction of bone mass. Measuring a person's height is an inexpensive method to screen for this disease process. (Goodman – Differential Diagnosis p. 323)

65.   Correct Answer: 3
Explanation: Walking at 3 mph, bicycling at 6 mph or playing golf while pulling a walking cart are activities that require 3-4 METs. (Brannon p. 317)

66. Correct Answer: 3
Explanation: A patient walking at a comfortable pace with a transfemoral prosthesis requires nearly 50% more oxygen than normal. This value is significantly higher than the other stated options. (O'Sullivan p. 669)

67. Correct Answer: 1
Explanation: The test for the lateral hamstrings is described with the knee in 50-70 degrees of flexion with the thigh in slight lateral rotation and the lower leg in slight lateral rotation on the thigh. Pressure should be applied against the lower leg proximal to the ankle in the direction of knee extension. (Kendall p. 209)

68. Correct Answer: 1
Explanation: Respiratory acidosis is caused by retention of carbon dioxide due to pulmonary insufficiency. Signs and symptoms include dizziness, tingling, and syncope. (Hillegass p. 441)

69. Correct Answer: 3
Explanation: The patient is likely to be intoxicated if he has consumed six or seven alcoholic beverages. Contacting a member of the family will prevent the possibility of the patient attempting to drive. (Guide for Professional Conduct)

70. Correct Answer: 2
Explanation: Reducing the weight to five pounds will allow the patient to maintain the integrity of the originally prescribed exercise, while allowing the patient to perform the exercise correctly. (Kisner p. 97)

71. Correct Answer: 2
Explanation: Correct technique includes pulling the muscles up and in. Placing a downward pressure on the pelvic floor serves to exacerbate the patient's condition. Research indicates that nearly 50% of patients who receive verbal instructions for pelvic floor contractions perform the exercises incorrectly. (Hall p. 365)

72. Correct Answer: 3
Explanation: Elevating legrests promote patient comfort and stability when the wheelchair is in a reclined position. (Pierson p. 181)

73. Correct Answer: 1
Explanation: Quality improvement programs are designed to assess the services provided and the outcomes achieved for the purpose of improving patient care. Prior to collecting, analyzing or interpreting specific data it is essential to identify the important aspects of patient care provided by the department. (Nosse p. 233)

74. Correct Answer: 4
Explanation: An arterial line is inserted directly into an artery and is used to continuously monitor blood pressure or to obtain blood samples. (Pierson p. 284)

75. Correct Answer: 3
Explanation: A forward raise for pressure relief requires adequate strength of the biceps for elbow flexion and the deltoids for movement at the shoulder in the directions of flexion and extension. (Rothstein p. 474)

76. Correct Answer: 4
Explanation: The rhythmic initiation technique should begin with passive movement of the patient by the physical therapist. Progression using this technique would include active-assistive movement, active movement, and finally resisted movement. (Sullivan p. 71)

77. Correct Answer: 1
Explanation: Patients over 40 years old are more susceptible to shoulder stiffness with prolonged immobilization and as a result physicians tend to limit the length of the immobilization period. In addition, the recurrence rate for dislocation is relatively low in this age group. Several of the other listed variables are relevant, however, would not typically be as significant as age when determining the length of immobilization. (Brotzman p. 118)

78. Correct Answer: 2
Explanation: The hold-relax technique utilizes an isometric contraction at the end of available range of motion. The patient is then told to relax as the physical therapist moves the extremity into newly gained range. (Sullivan p. 64)

79. Correct Answer: 2
Explanation: Assistive devices can easily be adjusted to accommodate individuals of various height and weight. (Minor p. 290)

80. Correct Answer: 2
Explanation: The status of bone healing as determined through a radiograph would provide the physician with the best information on the stability of the acetabulum. It is important to emphasize that the physician is the health care provider responsible for determining weight bearing status. (Brotzman p. 147)

81. Correct Answer: 4
Explanation: The hip is required to flex during initial swing to allow for proper clearance and advancement of the limb during gait. Normally, dorsiflexion also occurs. Without the use of the dorsiflexors the hip flexors need to be strengthened in order to attain proper clearance. (Seymour p. 106)

82. Correct Answer: 3
Explanation: When resistance is applied against a strong component of a pattern it can result in irradiation or overflow of impulses from the stronger muscle group to the weaker muscle group. (Sullivan p. 25)

83. Correct Answer: 3
Explanation: Stage four in Brunnstrom's stages of recovery for hemiplegia is signified by the development of movement outside of synergy patterns. (Brunnstrom p. 45)

84. Correct Answer: 2
Explanation: Bridging causes the muscles of the low back and the hip extensors to isometrically contract. This action promotes hip stability. (Sullivan p. 48)

85. Correct Answer: 3
Explanation: Patients with tight hip flexors often exhibit increased lordosis. Shortened hip flexors is often identified in standing as lumbar lordosis or through a special test such as the Thomas test. (Magee p. 631)

86. Correct Answer: 3
Explanation: It is extremely important for a patient with a transtibial amputation to keep the knee in an extended position in order to avoid a knee flexion contracture. (Seymour p. 145)

87. Correct Answer: 4
Explanation: Signs of cold intolerance include pain, cyanosis, wheals, mottling, increased pulse rate, and a significant drop in blood pressure. A physical therapist should immediately stop the application of cold when any sign of cold intolerance is observed. (Cameron p. 144)

88. Correct Answer: 2
Explanation: A physical therapist should attempt to secure an updated physician referral prior to administering formal treatment. Contacting the physicians office by telephone provides the fastest, most direct method to update the referral without further delaying treatment. (Scott – Legal Aspects p. 50)

89. Correct Answer: 3
Explanation: Peripheral neuropathy is a broad term that describes a lesion to a peripheral nerve. The condition can be caused by a multitude of factors including diabetes, compression, trauma or nutritional deficiencies. Patients with peripheral neuropathy may exhibit motor, sensory, and autonomic changes including extreme sensitivity to touch, loss of sensation, muscle weakness, and loss of vasomotor tone. Deep tendon reflexes may be asymmetrical based on the location of the involved peripheral nerve and usually present as diminished or absent. (Goodman - Pathology p. 1143)

90. Correct Answer: 3
Explanation: Facet impingement often results in a patient being locked in a selected position. In the thoracic and lumbar spine the position involves sidebending and rotation occurring in opposite directions. The patient will experience the greatest discomfort and restriction of movement when moving away from the locked position. (Magee p. 488)

91. Correct Answer: 3
Explanation: An accommodation that would fundamentally alter the operation of a business may not be considered reasonable. It is unlikely, however, that a modification to a workstation would fall into this category. (Pierson p. 348)

92. Correct Answer: 3
Explanation: Occupational therapy is described as the art and science of helping people perform day to day activities. Although professional boundaries differ from facility to facility, bathing and dressing activities are typically addressed by occupational therapists. (Van Deusen p. 303)

93. Correct Answer: 1
Explanation: The tendon of the tibialis posterior is most prominent when the foot is inverted and plantar flexed. The tendon can be palpated posterior and inferior to the medial malleolus. (Kendall p. 202)

94. Correct Answer: 3
Explanation: The distance to the clinic is excessive; particularly when sitting for prolonged periods of time may exacerbate the patient's condition. The patient should receive therapy services at a clinic closer to home. (Hall p. 343)

95. Correct Answer: 4
Explanation: Inability to sit unsupported without assistance is indicative of poor sitting balance. (O'Sullivan p. 381)

96. Correct Answer: 3
Explanation: Controlled mobility is the stage in motor control where a patient is able to have some mobility while maintaining postural stability. Tall kneeling represents static control, while the transfer to half kneeling requires the mobility to weight shift and change position. (Sullivan p. 7)

97. Correct Answer: 2
Explanation: Perseveration is the continued repetition of a word, phrase or movement. Initiating a new activity during therapy may allow the patient to redirect attention and subsequently receive positive reinforcement for attending to a selected task. (O'Sullivan p. 375)

98. Correct Answer: 4
Explanation: A physical therapy aide is a non-licensed worker, trained under the direction of a physical therapist, who requires continuous on-site supervision. A physical therapist may delegate ambulation activities to an aide if the physical therapist feels the aide's training is adequate to complete the activity. Ambulation for endurance implies that the patient may already possess some level of basic competence with the activity. (Guide to Physical Therapist Practice p. 42)

99. Correct Answer: 2
Explanation: Leading questions often bias a patient toward a specific response. The question "Does this alter your pain in any way?" provides the patient with the opportunity to provide additional insight into his/her present condition. (Goodman – Differential Diagnosis p. 38)

100. Correct Answer: 1
Explanation: S1=closing of the mitral and tricuspid valves. S2=closing of the aortic and pulmonic valves. S3=early ventricular filling; noncompliant left ventricle S4=rapid ventricular filling that occurs after atrial contraction. (Frownfelter p. 221)

Paper and Pencil Exam One – Section Three

101. Correct Answer: 1
Explanation: Symptom magnification is best identified by inconsistencies in the presentation of function. Although the physical therapist has identified a given inconsistency, it would be inappropriate to immediately confront the patient. The therapist would be better served by continuing the examination and gathering additional information during future treatment sessions. (O'Sullivan p. 937)

102. Correct Answer: 4
Explanation: Capsular patterns of restriction result from loss of mobility of the entire joint capsule. In trochanteric bursitis, passive and active range of motion are typically preserved, although there is often pain at end range with selected motions such as abduction. (Hertling p. 304)

103. Correct Answer: 4
Explanation: Post-operative care of a rotator cuff repair often includes immobilization in abduction and medial rotation using an abduction splint. Lateral rotation is often restricted during the initial stages of rehabilitation since the position tends to place the repaired structures on stretch. (Kisner p. 347)

104. Correct Answer: 4
Explanation: The tibiofemoral articulation consists of a concave tibial plateau articulating with the convex femoral condyles. An anterior glide of the tibia on the femur is indicated to increase knee extension. (Kisner p. 248)

105. Correct Answer: 1
Explanation: A patient with C7 tetraplegia will not be able to independently perform activities of daily living secondary to inadequate hamstrings length. A patient requires between 110-120 degrees of straight leg raise in order to reach forward and don clothing. (O'Sullivan p. 895)

106. Correct Answer: 4
Explanation: A drug that enters the body through the alimentary canal is defined as enteral administration; therefore taking medication orally would fall into this category. (Ciccone p. 15)

107. Correct Answer: 4
Explanation: The supplied description is a standard method to assess the strength of the lower abdominal muscles. Failure to maintain the low back flat on the treatment table as the legs are lowered is indicative of muscle weakness. (Kendall p. 154)

108. Correct Answer: 2
Explanation: A patient with C4 tetraplegia is appropriate for a power reclining wheelchair with chin controls since the neck muscles are innervated. Back and seat cushions are necessary due to paralysis and inability to perform pressure relief. (O'Sullivan p. 875)

109. Correct Answer: 3
Explanation: The triceps muscle is innervated by the radial nerve (C7-C8). (Somers p. 82)

110. Correct Answer: 4
Explanation: The Rinne test is performed by placing the stem of the tuning fork on the mastoid process. The test is designed to compare bone conduction hearing with air conduction hearing. (Magee p. 107)

111. Correct Answer: 2
Explanation: Topical antibiotics are often utilized in the treatment of burns. They serve to reduce bacterial count, provide a covering for the wound, reduce stiffness, and reduce evaporative loss. Since topical antibiotics are applied directly to the affected area sterile gloves should be worn. Due to the limited size of the wound additional medical asepsis would not be necessary. (Paz p. 452)

112. Correct Answer: 4
Explanation: Respiratory rate is an objective measure that is used to assess endurance. Respiratory rate typically increases as a patient becomes fatigued. (Pierson p. 60)

113. Correct Answer: 3
Explanation: Normalization of tone is a priority in stroke rehabilitation. Facilitation techniques are utilized when hypotonia exists. Facilitation techniques include vibration, weight bearing, approximation, tapping, and quick stretch. (Bennett p. 72)

114. Correct Answer: 3
Explanation: Since the patient's elbow range of motion begins at 15 degrees of flexion and ends at 90 degrees of flexion, the measurement should be recorded as 15-90 degrees of right elbow flexion. The amount of available range of motion is considered hypomobile. (Norkin p. 31)

115. Correct Answer: 2
Explanation: Broca's area, located in the left hemisphere, receives its blood supply from the middle cerebral artery. Damage to Broca's area may result in expressive aphasia. (Umphred p. 745)

116. Correct Answer: 2
Explanation: The use of an orthosis would ensure adequate foot clearance and stability during activities of daily living. (Seymour p. 31)

117. Correct Answer: 2
Explanation: Internal fixation provides the fracture site with the necessary stability to allow early protected weight bearing. (Kisner p. 486)

118. Correct Answer: 3
Explanation: Patients with congestive heart failure tend to have excessive fluid retention in the pulmonary and systemic circulation. As a result a diet high in potassium is prescribed, while items high in sodium are restricted. (Goodman - Pathology p. 409)

119. Correct Answer: 2
Explanation: Pacing is a technique that can allow patients to complete functional activities without shortness of breath or dyspnea. (Kisner p. 755)

120. Correct Answer: 4
Explanation: Upright sitting in a forward leaning posture with the neck flexed and arms supported is the optimal position to produce a forceful cough. (Tan p. 694)

121. Correct Answer: 4
Explanation: When the socket of a transtibial prosthesis is aligned in excessive flexion it may cause exaggerated knee flexion during stance phase resulting in instability. (Seymour p. 204)

122. Correct Answer: 2
Explanation: Repeated contractions is a technique that focuses on movement on one side of the joint. The technique is facilitated by quick stretch and utilizes an isotonic contraction. Providing resistance at the point of weakness can enhance repeated contractions. (Sullivan p. 71)

123. Correct Answer: 3
Explanation: Shoulder medial and lateral rotation occur in a transverse plane around a longitudinal axis. (Kendall p. 15)

124. Correct Answer: 1
Explanation: By flexing the knee, the two joint gastrocnemius muscle is placed on slack. Since active ankle dorsiflexion is normal when the knee is flexed and is limited when the knee is extended, the gastrocnemius is likely responsible for the limitation. (Kendall p. 206)

125. Correct Answer: 1
Explanation: A patient with C6 tetraplegia relies on grasp through tenodesis. The grasp occurs through tension of the finger flexors when the wrist is extended. Tenodesis cannot occur if the finger flexors are stretched or lengthened. (O'Sullivan p. 895)

126. Correct Answer: 3
Explanation: The medial and lateral hamstrings originate on the ischial tuberosity. Forceful hip flexion and knee extension places significant stress on the ischial tuberosity and can result in an avulsion fracture. (Kendall p. 208)

127. Correct Answer: 2
Explanation: Apprehension tests are provocative tests that attempt to simulate the mechanism of injury associated with a selected injury. The primary indication for an apprehension test is to assist with diagnosis. Common apprehension tests include anterior shoulder dislocation and patellar dislocation. (Magee p. 732)

128. Correct Answer: 3
Explanation: Anticoagulant drugs are often prescribed post-operatively for patients at risk of acquiring deep venous thrombosis. Prothrombin time is often used as a screening procedure to examine extrinsic coagulation factors and to determine the effectiveness of oral anticoagulant therapy. (Physical Therapist's Clinical Companion p. 145)

129. Correct Answer: 4
Explanation: Computed tomography produces cross-sectional images based on x-ray attenuation. Since vertebrae are made of bone and are extremely dense, they appear to be white. Soft tissue structures appear in various shades of gray, while cerebrospinal fluid is black. (Magee p. 54)

130. Correct Answer: 2
Explanation: The talar tilt test can be used to identify the presence of a calcaneofibular ligament sprain. (Magee p. 802)

131. Correct Answer: 3
Explanation: The Landau reflex is an equilibrium response that occurs when a child responds to prone suspension by aligning his/her head and extremities in line with the plane of the body. Although this response begins around three months of age, it is not fully integrated until the child's second year. (Ratliffe p. 30)

132. Correct Answer: 1
Explanation: A complete tear of the ulnar collateral ligament of the thumb is often termed "gamekeeper's thumb" or "skier's thumb." The function of the ligament is to limit valgus stress at the metacarpophalangeal joint of the thumb. (Brotzman p. 57)

133. Correct Answer: 4
Explanation: The anterolateral spinothalamic system is involved with the transmission of discriminative sensations such as pain and temperature. The system is activated by mechanoreceptors, thermoreceptors, and nociceptors. (O'Sullivan p. 139)

134. Correct Answer: 1
Explanation: Angiotensin is a polypeptide in the blood that causes vasoconstriction, increased blood pressure, and the release of aldosterone from the adrenal cortex. Release of angiotensin is stimulated by decreased arterial pressure. (Paz p. 11)

135. Correct Answer: 1
Explanation: Infants have resting pulse rates of approximately 125-135 beats per minute. (Kisner p. 167)

136. Correct Answer: 3
Explanation: Due to the potential impact on future bone growth, lack of skeletal maturity can be a contraindication to anterior cruciate ligament reconstruction surgery. (Magee p. 52)

137. Correct Answer: 2
Explanation: The patient is making a general statement about his desire to walk again in the future. Although ambulation would not currently be realistic due to the level of injury, it would be inappropriate to dismiss the future chances of the patient being able to walk. (Umphred p. 512)

138. Correct Answer: 3   *Item Includes Graphic*
Explanation: The suprasternal notch refers to the "V" shaped notch at the top of the sternum. (Hoppenfeld p. 6)

139. Correct Answer: 2
Explanation: Hip flexion greater than 90 degrees is often considered a contraindication following total hip replacement surgery. The knee immobilizer limits hip flexion by maintaining the knee in an extended position. (Paz p. 195)

140. Correct Answer: 4
Explanation: A right ventricular assistive device is designed to pump a percentage of the pulmonic blood flow around the right ventricle in order to decrease the workload on the myocardium. The right atrium would house one tube because it functions as a primer for the right ventricle and the other tube would be located in the pulmonary artery since its function is to deliver blood from the right ventricle to the lungs. (Paz p. 832)

141. Correct Answer: 3
Explanation: Medicaid is the largest insurer of long-term care in the United States covering over two-thirds of nursing home residents. (Nosse p. 168)

142. Correct Answer: 2
Explanation: The purpose of submaximal exercise testing is to determine the relationship between heart rate and oxygen uptake in order to predict maximum oxygen uptake. In order to do this it is necessary to determine the relationship between heart rate and oxygen uptake at two or more different submaximal exercise intensities. (American College of Sports Medicine p. 68)

143. Correct Answer: 1
Explanation: Digitalis is utilized in the treatment of congestive heart failure. Digitalis works directly on electrolytes to improve the force and contractility of the heart. (Hillegass p. 554)

144. Correct Answer: 4
Explanation: Hypoxemia refers to a deficiency of oxygen in arterial blood. (Goodman – Differential Diagnosis p. 152)

145. Correct Answer: 4
Explanation: Emphysema is an obstructive pulmonary disease characterized by overinflation and destructive changes in alveolar walls. Although closely related to other obstructive pulmonary diseases, the presence of a barrel chest is most characteristic of emphysema. (Kisner p. 766)

146. Correct Answer: 1
Explanation: Tidal volume is defined as the amount of air inspired and expired per breath and is approximately 450-600 mL in an adult. This value represents approximately 10% of the total lung capacity. (Frownfelter p. 150)

147. Correct Answer: 3
Explanation: Athletes performing repetitive overhead activities are often subject to adaptive changes such as acquired anterior laxity, and a loss of flexibility in the posterior capsule and posterior muscles. (Brotzman p. 94)

148. Correct Answer: 1
Explanation: The most immediate response in treating autonomic dysreflexia is to support the patient in a sitting position in an attempt to lower blood pressure. The patient's bowel and bladder should be assessed and vital signs should be monitored. (Umphred p. 496)

149. Correct Answer: 2
Explanation: A desirable range for men and women according to the Body Mass Index is $20 – 24.9$ kg/m^2. (American College of Sports Medicine p. 63)

150. Correct Answer: 2
Explanation: The semitendinosus and gracilis are acceptable grafts for anterior cruciate ligament reconstruction surgery. The grafts result in a decreased incidence of post-operative patellofemoral knee pain, however, provide weaker initial fixation. (Brotzman p. 185)

Paper and Pencil Exam One – Section Four

151. Correct Answer: 3
Explanation: The tibiofemoral articulation consists of a concave tibial plateau articulating with the convex femoral condyles. A posterior glide of the tibia on the femur is indicated to increase knee flexion. (Kisner p. 247)

152. Correct Answer: 2
Explanation: A patient with C6 tetraplegia should demonstrate full epigastric rise secondary to complete innervation of the diaphragm. (Rothstein p. 476)

153. Correct Answer: 4
Explanation: Supporting the subtalar joint in a neutral or slightly supinated position limits subtalar pronation and promotes optimal stretching of the calf muscles. (Hall p. 258)

154. Correct Answer: 3
Explanation: Moving the buttocks posteriorly in relation to the knees causes the patient's center of gravity to move behind the knees. As a result, the patient relies on eccentric contraction of the hip extensors to control the movement. (Hall p. 257)

155. Correct Answer: 4
Explanation: Treating a patient following surgery without having specific information from the referring physician could be considered a negligent act. In this particular instance the physical therapist knows only that the patient had knee surgery two weeks ago. (Standards of Practice)

156. Correct Answer: 3
Explanation: Urea is the metabolic byproduct of the breakdown of amino acids used for energy production. The level of urea in the blood provides a gross estimate of kidney function. An increased blood urea nitrogen level can be indicative of dehydration, pre-renal failure or renal failure. Normal blood urea nitrogen levels for adults are 10-20 mg/dL. (Goodman - Pathology p. 1183)

157. Correct Answer: 4
Explanation: Multiple sclerosis is a progressive central nervous system disease marked by intermittent damage to the myelin sheath. Patients with multiple sclerosis tend to fatigue in the afternoon and as a result morning sessions are optimal. Stretching, exercise, energy conservation, and stress management are valuable components of a comprehensive plan of care for a patient with multiple sclerosis. (Umphred p. 607)

158. Correct Answer: 3
Explanation: The peroneus longus and brevis tendons pass posterior to the lateral malleolus. The longus inserts on the lateral side of the base of the first metatarsal and first cuneiform, while the brevis inserts on the tuberosity of the fifth metatarsal. (Kendall p. 203)

159. Correct Answer: 4
Explanation: Placing the biceps in a maximally shortened position significantly limits the muscle's ability to function as a supinator. (Kendall p. 265)

160. Correct Answer: 1
Explanation: An allograft refers to a graft or tissue between two genetically dissimilar individuals of the same species. (Paz p. 456)

161. Correct Answer: 4
Explanation: Immediate medical management should focus on identifying potential complications such as a fracture. X-rays are a cost effective diagnostic tool commonly utilized with orthopedic injuries. (Magee p. 40)

162. Correct Answer: 3
Explanation: Failure to stabilize the scapula when measuring glenohumeral abduction will result in upward rotation and elevation of the scapula. When measuring shoulder complex abduction the thorax should be stabilized to prevent lateral flexion of the trunk. (Norkin p. 78)

163. Correct Answer: 2
Explanation: The humeral head slides posteriorly on the glenoid fossa during shoulder complex medial rotation and as a result places pressure on the posterior capsule. (Norkin p. 84)

164. Correct Answer: 1
Explanation: A bone scan is a diagnostic test that utilizes radioactive isotopes to identify areas of bone that are hypervascular or have an increased rate of bone mineral turnover. Bone scans can demonstrate bone disease or stress fractures with as little as 4-7% bone loss. (Magee p. 56)

165. Correct Answer: 1
Explanation: Piriformis syndrome is caused by hypertrophy or spasm of the piriformis muscle causing pressure on the sciatic nerve. Abduction and lateral rotation would likely be weak and painful since the motions serve as the prime function of the piriformis. The piriformis originates on the anterior surface of the sacrum and the sacrotuberous ligament and inserts on the greater trochanter of the femur. The muscle is innervated by sacral nerves I and II. (Starkey p. 296)

166. Correct Answer: 2
Explanation: The dorsal scapular nerve innervates the levator scapulae and rhomboids. The levator scapulae function to elevate the scapula while the rhomboids adduct the scapula. (Kendall p. 282)

167. Correct Answer: 3
Explanation: Passive insufficiency occurs when a two joint muscle is stretched across two joints at the same time. When performing passive knee flexion the two joint knee extensors are placed on stretch and therefore in the presence of insufficient length may contribute to a limitation in knee flexion. (Kisner p. 34)

168. Correct Answer: 2
Explanation: An infant's pulse is often assessed at the brachial artery, while the radial artery is utilized for an older child. (American Heart Association p. 153)

169. Correct Answer: 4
Explanation: A patient with limited dorsiflexion may present with a vault or bounce through mid to late stance. Ten to twenty degrees of dorsiflexion is required for late stance through toe off. (Hall p. 492)

170. Correct Answer: 3
Explanation: A patient status post CVA should avoid prolonged supine positioning in bed. A supine position encourages abnormal reflexes including asymmetrical tonic neck reflex, symmetrical tonic neck reflex, and labyrinthine reflexes. (Bennett p. 72)

171. Correct Answer: 2
Explanation: Passive shoulder complex abduction is approximately 180 degrees, however, glenohumeral abduction is 120 degrees with approximately 60 degrees of motion occurring at the scapulothoracic articulation. (Magee p. 225)

172. Correct Answer: 4
Explanation: As the intensity of exercise plateaus, a patient will accommodate to the level of exercise and his/her respiration rate will tend to decrease. (Pierson p. 61)

173. Correct Answer: 1
Explanation: Vital capacity is defined as the amount of air that can be exhaled following a maximal inspiratory effort. Vital capacity varies directly with height and indirectly with age. (Brannon p. 50)

174. Correct Answer: 1
Explanation: The infraspinatus muscle is innervated by the suprascapular nerve (C4, C5, C6) that extends from the superior trunk of the brachial plexus. (Kendall p. 385)

175. Correct Answer: 2
Explanation: The American College of Sports Medicine recommends prescribing the intensity of exercise as 60 to 90% of maximum heart rate or 50-85% of $VO_{2\,max}$ or heart rate reserve. (American College of Sports Medicine p. 145)

176. Correct Answer: 4
Explanation: Athetosis refers to involuntary movements characterized as slow, irregular, and twisting. This type of motor disturbance makes it extremely difficult to maintain a static body position. (Tecklin p. 110)

177. Correct Answer: 2
Explanation: Determining weight bearing status is the responsibility of the referring physician. (Guide for Professional Conduct)

178. Correct Answer: 2
Explanation: A sliding board transfer is possible based on the patient's upper extremity strength. The transfer will allow the patient to maintain a high level of independence. (Pierson p. 146)

179. Correct Answer: 3
Explanation: The flexor digitorum profundus is responsible for flexing the distal interphalangeal joint of the four fingers and assisting with flexion of the proximal interphalangeal and metacarpophalangeal joints. (Hoppenfeld p. 101)

180. Correct Answer: 1
Explanation: The iliotibial band serves as a secondary restraint to the anterior cruciate ligament, not the posterior cruciate ligament. (Magee p. 691)

181. Correct Answer: 2
Explanation: An endoskeleton or modular shank is designed to incorporate a synthetic foam cover shaped like the opposite leg. As a result the device is more cosmetically attractive and would likely make the patient more comfortable in her social setting. A solid ankle cushion heel is the most frequently prescribed foot-ankle assembly. It is considered to be a nonarticulated foot since it does not incorporate a mechanical joint at the ankle. (Tan p. 232)

182. Correct Answer: 3
Explanation: In order to secure valid measurements of available range of motion physical therapists should not permit any type of substitution. In addition to shoulder adduction and lateral rotation, patients can also attempt to substitute for limited supination by ipsilateral trunk sidebending. (Clarkson p. 172)

183. Correct Answer: 4
Explanation: Heart rate response when immersed in water appears to be similar to the response expected for land activities during periods of rest and during periods of low intensity exercise, however, during periods of high intensity exercise the response is diminished. (Kisner p. 277)

184. Correct Answer: 2
Explanation: According to the American Academy of Orthopedic Surgeons, normal pronation of the forearm is 80 degrees. (Norkin p. 375)

185. Correct Answer: 3
Explanation: A position of 70 degrees of elbow flexion allows the elbow to reach its maximum volume and therefore accommodates the swelling with less discomfort. The degree of elbow flexion is consistent with the amount of flexion present in the resting position of the ulnohumeral joint. (Magee p. 325)

186. Correct Answer: 4
Explanation: According to a study performed by Nachemson, intradiskal pressure is greatest when sitting in a chair with reduced lumbar lordosis. (Hertling p. 658)

187. Correct Answer: 1
Explanation: A patient with C5 quadriplegia would be able to utilize muscles innervated at or above the C5 spinal level. The patient should be able to utilize the brachioradialis to flex the elbow since the muscle is innervated at the C5-C6 spinal level. (Kendall p. 266)

188. Correct Answer: 1
Explanation: Normal range for pulse rate is 60-100 beats per minute, while respiration rate is 12-18 breaths per minute. (Pierson p. 52)

189. Correct Answer: 4
Explanation: The shoulder medial rotators and adductors provide support for the anterior joint capsule and as a result strengthening of these muscles is an essential component of a rehabilitation program following anterior shoulder dislocation. (Kisner p. 352)

190. Correct Answer: 4
Explanation: Isokinetic knee extension and flexion require the distal segment to move freely in space, as a result the exercise is considered to be an open kinematic chain exercise. (Kisner p. 91)

191. Correct Answer: 3
Explanation: According to the Americans with Disabilities Act Accessibility Guidelines the space necessary for a 180 degree turn using a wheelchair is 60 inches. (Rothstein p. 17)

192. Correct Answer: 3
Explanation: Direct personal contact with the referring physician is necessary to plan an effective care plan for the patient. (Standards of Practice)

193. Correct Answer: 4
Explanation: The self-referred patient offers a medical history that presents several significant issues including episodes of dizziness, neck stiffness with pain at night, and a family history of cancer. Based on the history and the date of the last medical examination, the patient should be referred to a physician. (Magee p. 2)

194. Correct Answer: 3
   Explanation: All of the listed tasks are reasonable expectations for the patient, however, moving from sitting to standing would be the most difficult due to the potential limitation in right knee range of motion as well as inadequate lower extremity strength. (Paz p. 196)

195. Correct Answer: 4
   Explanation: Due to the probability associated with incidental contact, the front of a sterile gown below waist level is considered to be non-sterile. (Pierson p. 297)

196. Correct Answer: 3
   Explanation: A supine position will ensure patient safety and allow the therapist full access to the residual limb. (Seymour p. 124)

197. Correct Answer: 4
   Explanation: Positioning the collection bag on the cross brace beneath the seat will allow for it to be below the level of the bladder. (Pierson p. 288)

198. Correct Answer: 1
   Explanation: The patient's post-operative status would require a rate of motion of one to two cycles per minute. Intermittent passive range of motion at a more rapid rate may cause discomfort, guarding or splinting. (Kisner p. 54)

199. Correct Answer: 4
   Explanation: Ataxia refers to defective muscular coordination with active movement. A gross measurement of upper extremity ataxia can be assessed through a finger to nose test. (Umphred p. 724)

200. Correct Answer: 2
   Explanation: Rhythmic initiation is a particularly effective technique to improve motor control in patients with Parkinson's disease since they often have difficulty initiating movement. (Sullivan p. 71)

Score

200 - 66 = 134

67%

Fail!

EXAM TWO: PAPER AND PENCIL

Paper and Pencil Exam Two – Section One

1. A patient prepares for discharge from a rehabilitation hospital after completing three months of therapy. The patient has made significant progress in his rehabilitation, however, expresses concern that his previous employer may not want him to return to work due to his injury. The most appropriate action is to:

   1. explain to the patient that to return to work after a serious injury is very difficult
   2. inform the patient of his rights according to the Americans with Disabilities Act
   3. request that the patient consider vocational retraining
   4. refer the patient to a psychologist to assist with the transition back to work

2. A physical therapist employed in an acute care hospital attempts to identify a standardized instrument that measures level of consciousness. The most appropriate standardized instrument is the:

   1. Glasgow Coma Scale
   2. Rankin Scale
   3. Barthel Index
   4. Sickness Impact Profile

3. A physical therapist reviews the medical chart of a patient with a history of recurrent dysrhythmias. The therapist is concerned about the patient's past medical history and would like to monitor the patient during selected formal exercise activities. Which of the following monitoring devices would be the most beneficial?

   1. pulmonary artery catheter
   2. electrocardiogram
   3. intracranial pressure monitor
   4. pulse oximeter

4. A physical therapist attempts to reduce a child's genu recurvatum using an ankle-foot orthosis. Which ankle setting would be the most effective to achieve the therapist's objective?

   1. 5-10 degrees of dorsiflexion
   2. neutral
   3. 5-10 degrees of plantar flexion
   4. 15-20 degrees of plantar flexion

5. A physical therapist completes an examination on a patient diagnosed with complete C7 tetraplegia. The patient problem list includes the following: inability to complete an independent bed to wheelchair transfer, decreased passive lower extremity range of motion, tissue breakdown over the ischial tuberosities, and decreased upper extremity strength. Which of the following treatment activities should be given the highest priority?

   1. pressure relief activities
   2. transfer training using a sliding board
   3. self range of motion activities
   4. upper extremity strengthening exercises

6. A physical therapist critically analyzes the methodology used in a published research study. Which type of sampling procedure would result in the greatest degree of sampling error?

   1. simple random sample
   2. systematic sample
   3. cluster sample
   4. stratified random sample

7. A physical therapy program designs a study that uses performance on the Scholastic Aptitude Test as a predictor of grade point average in a physical therapy academic program. The results of the study identify that the overall correlation between the variables is r =.87. Which statement is most accurate based on the results of the study?

   1. grade point average in a physical therapy program is a function of performance on the scholastic aptitude test
   2. a student that performs well on the scholastic aptitude test is likely to have a high grade point average in a physical therapy academic program
   3. there is no relationship between grade point average in a physical therapy program and performance on the scholastic aptitude test
   4. there is an inverse relationship between grade point average in a physical therapy program and performance on the scholastic aptitude test

8. A patient is referred to physical therapy with a C6 nerve root injury. Which of the following clinical findings would not be expected with this type of injury?

   1. diminished sensation on the anterior arm and the index finger
   2. weakness in the biceps and supinator
   3. diminished brachioradialis reflex
   4. paresthesias of the long and ring fingers

9. A physical therapist completes a vertebral artery test on a patient diagnosed with a cervical strain. Which component of the vertebral artery test is most likely to assess the patency of the intervertebral foramen?

   1. rotation
   2. lateral flexion
   3. flexion
   4. extension

10. A 22-year-old male status post traumatic brain injury receives physical therapy services in a rehabilitation hospital. The patient is presently functioning at Rancho Los Amigos level VI. The patient has progressed well in therapy, however, has been bothered by diplopia. Which treatment strategy would be the most appropriate to address diplopia?

    1. provide verbal and non-verbal instructions within the patient's direct line of sight
    2. place a patch over one of the patient's eyes
    3. ask the patient to turn his head to one side when he experiences diplopia
    4. instruct the patient to carefully focus on a single object

11. A physical therapist completes an upper extremity manual muscle test on a patient diagnosed with rotator cuff tendonitis. Assuming the patient has the ability to move the upper extremities against gravity, which of the following muscles would not be tested with the patient in a supine position?

    1. pronator teres
    2. pectoralis major
    3. lateral rotators of the shoulder
    4. middle trapezius

12. A two-year-old with T10 spina bifida receives physical therapy for gait training. The preferred method to initially teach a child how to maintain standing is with the use of:

    1. bilateral hip-knee-ankle-foot orthoses and forearm crutches
    2. parapodium and the parallel bars
    3. bilateral knee-ankle-foot orthoses and the parallel bars
    4. bilateral ankle-foot orthoses and the parallel bars

13. A physical therapist prepares a patient education program for an individual with chronic venous insufficiency. Which of the following would not be appropriate to include in the patient education program?

    1. wear shoes that accommodate to the size and shape of your feet
    2. observe your skin daily for breakdown
    3. wear your compression stockings only at night
    4. keep your feet elevated as much as possible throughout the day

14. A 72-year-old female six weeks status post CVA is scheduled for discharge from an acute rehabilitation hospital in one week. At the present time the patient is unable to ambulate and requires maximal assistance to complete most transfers. Prior to her CVA the patient lived alone in an apartment on the first floor. The most appropriate discharge plan would be:

    1. home without support services
    2. home with a home health aide during the day
    3. home with physical therapy three times per week
    4. a nursing facility

15. A physical therapist prepares to perform manual vibration as a means of airway clearance with a patient diagnosed with chronic obstructive pulmonary disease. When performing vibration the most appropriate form of manual contact over the affected lung segment is:

    1. contact with a cupped hand
    2. contact with the entire palmar surface of the hand
    3. contact with the ulnar border of the hand
    4. contact with the distal phalanx of the middle finger

16. A physical therapist examines a 72-year-old female recently admitted to an acute care hospital following complications from elective surgery. The patient is moderately obese and has a lengthy medical history including diabetes mellitus. The following day the therapist notices that the patient's breath has a very distinctive fruity odor. The patient complains of feeling nauseous and very weak. An entry in the medical record indicates that the patient had diarrhea during the night. This type of scenario is most consistent with:

    1. respiratory acidosis
    2. respiratory alkalosis
    3. metabolic acidosis
    4. metabolic alkalosis

17. A physical therapist determines that a patient rehabilitating from ankle surgery has consistent difficulty with functional activities that emphasize the frontal plane. Which of the following would be the most difficult for the patient?

    1. anterior lunge
    2. six-inch lateral step down
    3. six-inch posterior step up
    4. eight-inch posterior step down

18. A patient rehabilitating from a radial head fracture is examined in physical therapy. During the examination, the physical therapist notes that the patient appears to have an elbow flexion contracture. Which of the following would not serve as an appropriate active exercise technique to increase range of motion?

    1. contract-relax
    2. hold-relax
    3. maintained pressure
    4. rhythmic stabilization

19. A physical therapist positions a patient in sitting prior to administering bronchial drainage. Which lung segment would require the patient to be in this position?

    1. anterior basal segments of the lower lobes
    2. posterior apical segments of the upper lobes
    3. posterior basal segments of the lower lobes
    4. right middle lobe

20. When examining a patient for a wheelchair, a physical therapist determines that the patient's hip width in sitting and the measurement from the back of the buttocks to the popliteal space are each 16 inches. Given these measurements, which of the following wheelchair sizes would best fit this patient?

    1. seat width 16 inches, seat depth 14 inches
    2. seat width 18 inches, seat depth 18 inches
    3. seat width 16 inches, seat depth 18 inches
    4. seat width 18 inches, seat depth 14 inches

21. A patient with a lengthy history of substance abuse is referred to physical therapy after sustaining multiple injuries in a motor vehicle accident. Which of the following controlled substances would not typically foster physical dependence?

    1. depressants
    2. hallucinogens
    3. narcotics
    4. stimulants

22. A physical therapist employed in an acute care hospital conducts an initial interview with a patient referred to physical therapy. During the interview the therapist asks the patient if he feels dependent on coffee, tea or soft drinks. Which clinical scenario would most appropriately warrant this type of question?

    1. a 27-year-old female status post arthroscopic medial meniscectomy
    2. a 42-year-old male with premature ventricular contractions
    3. a 37-year-old female with restrictive pulmonary disease
    4. a 57-year-old male with respiratory alkalosis

23. A nurse takes the temperature of a patient before a scheduled physical therapy session. Which of the following temperature values would be classified as normal?

    1. 35 degrees Celsius
    2. 36 degrees Celsius
    3. 37 degrees Celsius
    4. 38 degrees Celsius

24. A patient with a lengthy medical history of cardiac pathology is referred to a phase II cardiac rehabilitation program. During the first session the physical therapist prepares to measure the patient's blood pressure by inflating the cuff 20 mm Hg above the patient's estimated systolic value. Which of the following values best describes the most appropriate rate to release the pressure when obtaining the blood pressure measurement?

    1. 2-3 mm Hg per second
    2. 3-5 mm Hg per second
    3. 5-7 mm Hg per second
    4. 8-10 mm Hg per second

25. A physical therapist performs goniometric measurements on a patient rehabilitating from injuries sustained in a motor vehicle accident. When measuring rotation of the cervical spine, which of the following landmarks would be the most appropriate for the axis of the goniometer?

    1. centered over the external auditory meatus
    2. centered over the center of the cranial aspect of the head
    3. centered over the C7 spinous process
    4. centered over the midline of the occiput

26. A physical therapist performs girth measurements on a patient rehabilitating from knee surgery. The therapist takes the measurements 5 cm and 10 cm above the superior pole of the patella with the patient in supine. The girth measurements are recorded as 32 cm and 37 cm on the right and 34 cm and 40 cm on the left. Which of the following conclusions can be made regarding the strength of the patient's quadriceps?

    1. The right quadriceps will be capable of producing a greater force than the left.
    2. The left quadriceps will be capable of producing a greater force than the right.
    3. The right and left quadriceps will be capable of producing equal force.
    4. Not enough information is given to form a conclusion.

27. A physical therapist instructs a patient to expire maximally after taking a maximal inspiration. The therapist can use these instructions to measure the patient's:

    1. expiratory reserve volume
    2. inspiratory reserve volume
    3. total lung capacity
    4. vital capacity

28. A patient diagnosed with an acute cervical strain is referred to physical therapy. During the examination the physical therapist asks the patient to bend his head to the right and then proceeds to apply a downward compressive force to the patient's head. Which of the following subjective findings would be indicative of a positive test?

    1. pain radiates into the right arm
    2. pain radiates into the left arm
    3. pain radiates into the arms bilaterally
    4. pain radiates into the arms and legs bilaterally

29. A physical therapist volunteers to assist participants at the finish line in a 10K road race. The race takes place on a hot and humid day and some of the race organizers are concerned about the potential for heat related disorders. The most significant variables to differentiate between heat exhaustion and heat stroke are:

    1. blood pressure and pulse rate
    2. coordination and level of fatigue
    3. mental status and skin temperature
    4. pupil dilation and blood pressure

30. A physical therapist monitors a patient's vital signs while exercising in a phase I cardiac rehabilitation program. The patient is status post myocardial infarction and has progressed without difficulty while involved in the program. Which of the following vital sign recordings would exceed the typical limits of a phase I program?

    1. heart rate elevated 18 beats per minute above resting level
    2. respiration rate of 25 breaths per minute
    3. systolic blood pressure decreases by 20 mm Hg from resting level
    4. diastolic blood pressure less than 100 mm Hg

31. A physical therapist asks a patient who has been inconsistent with his attendance in physical therapy, why he is having difficulty keeping scheduled appointments. The patient responds that it is difficult to understand the scheduling card that lists the appointments. The therapist's most appropriate action would be to:

    1. contact the referring physician to discuss the patient's poor attendance in therapy
    2. make sure the patient is given a scheduling card at the conclusion of each session
    3. write down the patient's appointments on a piece of paper in a manner that the patient can understand
    4. discharge the patient from physical therapy

32. A physical therapist reviews the medical chart of a patient diagnosed with a fracture of the lower thoracic spine. The chart indicates the patient has worn an anterior control thoracolumbar-sacral-orthosis (TLSO) for eight weeks. What is the primary purpose of the anterior control TLSO?

    1. prevent thoracic flexion
    2. prevent thoracic extension
    3. prevent lumbar flexion
    4. prevent lumbar extension

33. A physical therapist establishes the following short-term goal for a patient rehabilitating from total knee replacement surgery: Patient will ambulate with walker 50% weight bearing and moderate assist of 1 for 20 feet within one week. Three days later, the patient successfully achieves the established goal. Which of the following would be the most appropriate revision of the short-term goal?

    1. ambulate with walker 25% weight bearing and moderate assist of 1 for 30 feet within one week
    2. ambulate with walker 50% weight bearing and moderate assist of 2 for 30 feet within one week
    3. ambulate with walker 50% weight bearing and minimal assist of 1 for 30 feet within one week
    4. ambulate with the walker 25% weight bearing and minimal assist of 1 for 10 feet within one week

34. A physician orders a nasogastric tube for a patient on an acute rehabilitation unit. Which of the following does not accurately describe a potential use of the nasogastric tube?

   1. administer medications directly into the gastrointestinal tract
   2. obtain gastric specimens
   3. remove fluid or gas from the stomach
   4. obtain venous blood samples from the stomach

35. A physical therapist conducts a goniometric assessment of the wrist and hand. When determining the available range of motion for thumb flexion, the therapist should align the axis of the goniometer over the:

   1. dorsal aspect of the first interphalangeal joint
   2. palmar aspect of the first carpometacarpal joint
   3. midway between the dorsal aspect of the first and second carpometacarpal joints
   4. midway between the palmar aspect of the first and second carpometacarpal joints

36. A physical therapist examines a patient diagnosed with post-polio syndrome. Which of the following areas is the least likely to be affected based on the patient's diagnosis?

   1. strength
   2. sensation
   3. endurance
   4. functional mobility

37. When observing a patient ambulating, a physical therapist notes that the patient's gait has the following characteristics: narrow base of support, short bilateral step length, and decreased trunk rotation. This gait pattern is often observed in patients with a diagnosis of:

   1. CVA
   2. Parkinson's disease
   3. post-polio syndrome
   4. multiple sclerosis

38. A physical therapist prepares to complete an assisted standing pivot transfer with a patient that requires moderate assistance. In order to increase a patient's independence with the transfer, which of the following instructions would be the most appropriate?

   1. I want you to help me perform the transfer.
   2. Try to utilize your own strength to complete the transfer.
   3. Only grab onto me if it is absolutely necessary.
   4. Pretend you were home alone and needed to complete the transfer.

39. A physical therapist instructs a patient with a lower extremity amputation to wrap her residual limb. Which of the following would be the least acceptable method of securing the bandage?

   1. clips
   2. safety pins
   3. tape
   4. velcro

40. A patient uses transcutaneous electrical neuromuscular stimulation for pain modulation. Which set of parameters best describes conventional TENS?

   1. 50-100 pps, short phase duration, low intensity
   2. 100-150 pps, short phase duration, high intensity
   3. 150-200 pps, long phase duration, low intensity
   4. 200-250 pps, short phase duration, low intensity

41. A physical therapist notices a small area of skin irritation under the chin of a patient wearing a cervical orthosis. The patient expresses that the area is not painful, but is becoming increasingly itchy. The most appropriate therapist action is:

   1. instruct the patient to apply 1% hydrocortisone cream to the area twice daily
   2. apply powder to the area and instruct the patient to avoid scratching
   3. provide the patient with a liner to use as a barrier between the skin and the orthosis
   4. discontinue use of the orthosis until the skin has become less irritated

42. A physical therapist attempts to identify a patient's coronary artery disease risk factors as part of a health screening. The patient's heart rate is recorded as 78 beats per minute and blood pressure as 130/85 mm Hg. A recent laboratory report indicates a total cholesterol level of 170 mg/dL with high-density lipoproteins reported as 20 mg/dL and low-density lipoproteins as 150 mg/dL. Which of the following values would be considered atypical?

1. heart rate
2. blood pressure
3. high-density lipoproteins
4. low-density lipoproteins

43. A physical therapist performs palpation with a patient positioned in standing as part of a respiratory assessment. Which structure would be the most appropriate to assess with the therapist positioned behind the patient?

1. mediastinum
2. upper lobes
3. right middle lobe
4. lower lobes

44. While examining a patient diagnosed with Achilles tendonitis, a physical therapist notes that the foot and ankle appear to be pronated in standing. Which motions combine to create pronation?

1. abduction, dorsiflexion, eversion
2. adduction, dorsiflexion, inversion
3. abduction, plantar flexion, eversion
4. adduction, plantar flexion, inversion

45. A patient eight weeks status post right total hip replacement loses his balance and falls to the ground during a physical therapy session. The patient is visibly shaken by the fall, but insists that he is uninjured. The physical therapist examines the right hip and although active motion elicits pain, all other findings are inconclusive. The therapist should:

1. continue with the current treatment so the patient does not focus on the incident
2. notify the supervisor about the incident
3. document the incident and contact a physician to examine the patient before resuming treatment
4. document the incident and gradually resume prior treatment

46. A physical therapist measures body composition using skinfold measurements prior to initiating an exercise program. When measuring the abdominal skinfold the most appropriate method is:

1. utilize a vertical fold approximately 2 cm to the right of the umbilicus
2. utilize a horizontal fold approximately 2 cm to the right of the umbilicus
3. utilize a vertical fold approximately 2 cm to the left of the umbilicus
4. utilize a horizontal fold approximately 2 cm to the left of the umbilicus

47. A patient diagnosed with shoulder pain of unknown etiology is referred by his physician for magnetic resonance imaging. Results of the test reveal a partial tear of the infraspinatus muscle. Which muscle group would be the most seriously affected by the injury?

1. shoulder lateral rotators
2. shoulder medial rotators
3. shoulder abductors
4. shoulder adductors

The following image should be used to answer question 48:

48. A physical therapist assesses the strength of selected lower extremity muscles on a patient rehabilitating from a knee injury. The pictured test would be most effective to examine the strength of the:

1. hip abductors
2. hip adductors
3. hip medial rotators
4. hip lateral rotators

49. A seven-year-old patient sustains a deep partial-thickness burn to his heel. When teaching the patient a stretching program the greatest emphasis should be placed in the direction of:

1. plantar flexion
2. dorsiflexion
3. inversion
4. eversion

50. A physical therapist employed in an acute care hospital treats a patient who receives health care insurance through Medicaid. From a patient perspective, what is the primary problem with this type of insurance?

1. large copayments and deductibles
2. limited reimbursement for specific levels of care
3. limited access to primary care providers
4. no prescription drug benefit

Please make sure all of the questions in the section have been answered prior to beginning the next section. When a new section is initiated candidates will be unable to return to previously completed sections.

Paper and Pencil Exam Two – Section Two

51. A physical therapist discusses the importance of proper skin care with a patient and his family. Which of the following sites is least likely to develop a pressure ulcer in a patient that is wheelchair dependent?

1. scapula
2. ischium
3. heel
4. elbow

52. A group of physical therapists conducts scoliosis screenings on adolescents as part of physical therapy week. The most appropriate action after identifying an adolescent with a moderate scoliotic curve is to:

1. refer the adolescent for further orthopedic assessment
2. educate the adolescent as to the cause of the scoliosis
3. devise an exercise program for the adolescent
4. instruct the adolescent in the importance of proper posture

53. A physical therapist designs a treatment program for a patient with a traumatic brain injury. The patient currently is classified as confused-agitated using the Rancho Los Amigos Levels of Cognitive Functioning Scale. Which of the following guidelines would be the least beneficial when developing the treatment program?

1. The therapist should emphasize previously learned skills and avoid teaching only new skills.
2. The therapist should maintain a calm and focused affect.
3. The therapist should concentrate on one specific activity for each treatment session.
4. The therapist should schedule the patient at the same time and same place each day.

54. A physical therapist checks the water temperature of the hot pack machine after several patients report the heat being very strong. Which of the following temperatures would be acceptable?

1. 71 degrees Celsius
2. 88 degrees Celsius
3. 130 degrees Fahrenheit
4. 190 degrees Fahrenheit

55. A physical therapist employed in an outpatient physical therapy clinic attempts to obtain informed consent from a 17-year-old male prior to initiating a formal exercise test. The patient signs the informed consent form, however, the patient's parents dropped him off at the clinic and are now unavailable to sign the form. The most appropriate therapist action is:

1. complete the exercise test
2. secure another physical therapist to witness the exercise test
3. contact the referring physician and request approval to complete the exercise test
4. reschedule the exercise test

56. A physical therapist examines a 22-year-old female athlete who sustained an ankle sprain three days ago playing soccer. The patient is currently full weight bearing, however, walks with an antalgic gait. In order to assess the ligamentous integrity of the ankle, the therapist prepares to administer the anterior drawer test. The therapist positions the patient in supine and stabilizes the tibia and fibula. The most appropriate method for performing the anterior drawer test is:

1. maintain the foot in neutral and draw the talus forward
2. maintain the foot in 20 degrees of plantar flexion and draw the talus forward
3. maintain the foot in neutral and draw the calcaneus forward
4. maintain the foot in 20 degrees of plantar flexion and draw the calcaneus forward

57. A patient who has completed six months of therapy receives a referral for eight additional weeks of physical therapy. The physical therapist feels the patient has reached a plateau and is not a realistic candidate for continued therapy. The therapist's most appropriate action is to:

    1. continue the patient in physical therapy for eight additional weeks
    2. re-examine the patient and develop new short and long-term goals
    3. conduct a four week trial to determine if the patient can make objective progress
    4. contact the referring physician and discuss the concerns regarding the patient's rehabilitation potential

58. A physical therapist attempts to identify an appropriate standardized assessment tool to examine developmental gross and fine motor skills in a pediatric population ranging from six to ten years of age. The most appropriate assessment tool is the:

    1. Peabody Developmental Motor Scale
    2. Bruininks-Oseretsky Motor Development Scale
    3. Erhardt Developmental Prehension Assessment
    4. Gross Motor Function Measure

59. A physical therapist attempts to obtain a general assessment of a patient's cognitive status. The patient is a 62-year-old female three days status post total hip replacement. The most appropriate action is:

    1. review the patient's medical record
    2. conduct a patient interview
    3. conduct a physical examination
    4. consult with family members

60. A patient suffers a chemical burn on the cubital area of the elbow. Which position would be the most appropriate for splinting of the involved upper extremity?

    1. elbow flexion and forearm pronation
    2. elbow flexion and forearm supination
    3. elbow extension and forearm pronation
    4. elbow extension and forearm supination

61. A physical therapist attempts to secure a wheelchair for a patient with an incomplete spinal cord injury. The patient is a 28-year-old female that is very active and relies on a wheelchair as her primary mode of transportation. Which type of wheelchair design would be the most appropriate for the patient?

    1. standard chair with a rigid frame
    2. lightweight chair with a rigid frame
    3. standard chair with a folding frame
    4. lightweight chair with a folding frame

62. A physical therapist attempts to select an assistive device for a patient rehabilitating from a traumatic brain injury. The patient is occasionally impulsive, however, has fair standing balance and good upper and lower extremity strength. Which of the following would be the most appropriate assistive device?

    1. cane
    2. axillary crutches
    3. Lofstrand crutches
    4. walker

63. A health care provider negotiates with an insurance company to provide health care services. As part of the agreement, the insurance company agrees to pay the health care provider a predetermined amount for each member in the plan on an annual basis. This type of arrangement is best termed:

    1. capitation
    2. fee for service
    3. case pricing
    4. negotiated compensation

64. A physical therapist examines a 16-year-old male diagnosed with left knee anterior cruciate ligament insufficiency. During the examination a Lachman test is performed. Ideally, the therapist should perform the test with the knee in:

    1. complete extension
    2. 20-30 degrees flexion
    3. 30-40 degrees flexion
    4. 40-50 degrees flexion

65. A physical therapist observes that a patient has an exaggerated heel strike on the left during ambulation activities. Which term is most consistent with heel strike using Rancho Los Amigos nomenclature?

1. terminal swing
2. loading response
3. initial contact
4. midstance

66. A patient with cerebellar dysfunction exhibits signs of dysmetria. Which of the following activities would be the most difficult for the patient?

1. rapid alternating pronation and supination of the forearm
2. placing feet on floor markers while walking
3. walking at varying speeds
4. marching in place

67. A physical therapist examines a 22-year-old baseball pitcher diagnosed with impingement syndrome. The athlete was prompted to see his physician after not being able to generate his usual velocity when throwing. Examination reveals positive impingement signs, mild anterior shoulder laxity, and limited flexibility in the posterior muscles and posterior capsule. The most appropriate treatment intervention is:

1. active abduction exercises using dumbbell weights in the frontal plane
2. medial and lateral rotation exercises with the arm at the side using elastic tubing
3. posterior capsule stretching
4. high voltage galvanic stimulation and ice

68. A physical therapist examines a patient referred to physical therapy diagnosed with a medial collateral ligament sprain. During the examination the patient appears to be relaxed and comfortable, however, is extremely withdrawn. Which of the following questions would be the most appropriate to further engage the patient?

1. Is this the first time you have injured your knee?
2. Have you ever been to physical therapy before?
3. How long after your injury did you see a physician?
4. What do you hope to achieve in physical therapy?

69. A physical therapist conducts a pre-operative training session for a patient scheduled for surgery to repair a large rotator cuff tear. The patient is a 54-year-old male who is employed as an insurance agent. During the pre-operative training session the patient inquires as to the amount of time before he is able to return to recreational activities such as tennis and golf. The most appropriate time frame is typically:

1. 6–8 weeks
2. 12-14 weeks
3. 24-28 weeks
4. 36-40 weeks

70. A physical therapist determines a patient's heart rate by counting the number of QRS complexes in a six second electrocardiogram strip. Assuming the therapist identifies eight QRS complexes in the strip, the patient's heart rate should be recorded as:

1. 40 bpm
2. 60 bpm
3. 80 bpm
4. 100 bpm

71. A physical therapist prepares to apply a sterile dressing to a wound after debridement. The therapist begins the process by drying the wound using a towel. The therapist applies medication to the wound using a gauze pad and then applies a series of dressings that are secured using a bandage. Which step would not warrant the use of sterile technique?

   1. bandage
   2. dressings
   3. medication
   4. towel

72. A physical therapist interviews a patient in an attempt to gather information to assist with discharge planning. The patient is rehabilitating from an intertrochanteric fracture sustained six weeks ago after a fall. The patient has moderate dementia, but has no other significant past medical history. Which of the following situations would present the patient with the largest barrier toward living independently?

   1. The patient resides alone and has no outside support from family or friends.
   2. The patient is no longer able to drive and relies on a neighbor for all cooking, cleaning, and shopping.
   3. The patient has a two-story home.
   4. The patient resides with a woman who has rheumatoid arthritis.

73. A physical therapist examines a patient diagnosed with Guillain-Barre syndrome. Which of the following signs or symptoms is not typically associated with this condition?

   1. difficulty breathing
   2. areflexia
   3. weakness
   4. absent sensation

74. A physical therapist listens to the lung sounds of a 56-year-old male with chronic bronchitis. The patient was admitted to the hospital two days ago after complaining of shortness of breath and difficulty breathing. While performing auscultation the therapist identifies distinct lung sounds with a relatively high constant pitch during exhalation. This type of sound is most consistent with:

   1. crackles
   2. rales
   3. rhonchi
   4. wheezes

75. A physical therapist administers iontophoresis to a patient with a lower extremity injury in an attempt to decrease the patient's soft tissue pain through the use of a local anesthetic. Which pharmacological agent would best meet the stated objective?

   1. acetic acid
   2. dexamethasone
   3. lidocaine
   4. zinc oxide

76. A patient with muscle weakness and compromised balance uses a four-point gait pattern with two canes. The physical therapist would like to instruct the patient to ascend and descend the stairs according to the normal flow of traffic. When ascending stairs the most practical method is to:

   1. use the handrail with the right hand and place the two canes in the left hand
   2. use the handrail with the left hand and place the two canes in the right hand
   3. place one cane in each hand and avoid using the handrail
   4. place the two canes in the left hand and avoid using the handrail

77. A physical therapist receives a referral for a patient who is one week status post head injury. In the patient's medical record it notes that the patient demonstrates decorticate posturing. This type of posturing is characterized by:

1. upper extremity extension and lower extremity flexion
2. upper extremity flexion and lower extremity flexion
3. upper extremity extension and lower extremity extension
4. upper extremity flexion and lower extremity extension

78. A twelve-month-old child with cerebral palsy demonstrates an abnormal persistence of the positive support reflex. During therapy this would most likely interfere with:

1. sitting activities
2. standing activities
3. prone on elbows activities
4. supine activities

79. A physical therapist treats a patient with limited shoulder range of motion. The therapist hypothesizes that the patient's range of motion limitation is due to pain and not a specific tissue restriction. Which mobilization grades would be most appropriate to treat this patient?

1. Grades I, II
2. Grades II, III
3. Grades III, IV
4. Grades IV, V

80. A patient diagnosed with lateral epicondylitis is referred to physical therapy. The therapist elects to use iontophoresis over the lateral epicondyle. Which type of current would the physical therapist use to administer the treatment?

1. direct
2. alternating
3. pulsatile
4. interferential

81. A physical therapist designs an exercise program for a patient rehabilitating from anterior cruciate ligament reconstruction. Which of the following treatment options would place the least amount of stress on the reconstructed ligament?

1. stationary cycling
2. walking
3. slow running on a level surface
4. fast running on a level surface

82. A physical therapist designs an exercise program for a patient rehabilitating from cardiac surgery. During the treatment session the therapist monitors the patient's oxygen saturation rate. Which of the following would be most representative of a normal oxygen saturation rate?

1. 82%
2. 87%
3. 92%
4. 97%

83. A patient rehabilitating from a total hip replacement receives home physical therapy services. The patient is currently full weight bearing and is able to ascend and descend stairs independently. The patient expresses that her goal following rehabilitation is to walk one mile each day. The most appropriate plan to accomplish the patient's goal is to:

1. continue home physical therapy services until the patient's goal is attained
2. refer the patient to an outpatient orthopedic physical therapy clinic
3. design a home exercise program that emphasizes progressive ambulation
4. admit the patient to a rehabilitation hospital

84. A physical therapist attempts to assess the integrity of the L4 spinal level. Which deep tendon reflex would provide the therapist with the most useful information?

1. lateral hamstrings
2. medial hamstrings
3. patellar reflex
4. Achilles reflex

85. A patient is scheduled to receive occupational and physical therapy services in his home. During the physical therapy examination the therapist determines that the patient requires assistance with tub transfers using a tub bench. The physical therapist is scheduled to treat the patient three times a week, however, the occupational therapist cannot examine the patient for six days. The most appropriate physical therapist action is:

1. practice tub transfers during physical therapy treatment sessions
2. wait until an occupational therapist can examine the patient
3. provide the patient with written information on tub transfers
4. call another agency and request immediate occupational therapy services

86. A patient completes a D1 extension pattern for the upper extremity. The prime movers of the scapula during this pattern are the:

1. trapezius and middle deltoid
2. pectoralis minor and pectoralis major
3. serratus anterior, pectoralis major, and anterior deltoid
4. rhomboids, pectoralis minor, and levator scapulae

87. A physical therapist examines a patient diagnosed with rotator cuff tendonitis in physical therapy. The physician referral indicates the patient should be seen three times a week, however after examining the patient the therapist feels once a week is adequate. The most appropriate therapist action is to:

1. schedule the patient once a week and notify the referring physician of your rationale
2. schedule the patient as indicated on the physician referral
3. ask the patient how often they would like to be seen in physical therapy
4. attempt to determine if the patient's insurance will cover physical therapy visits three times a week

88. A patient receiving physical therapy services in an outpatient clinic explains that he has felt nauseous since having his methotrexate medication level altered. The most appropriate physical therapist action is to:

1. explain to the patient that nausea is very common when altering medication levels
2. ask the patient to stop taking the prescribed medication
3. request that the patient make an appointment with the physician
4. request that the patient contact the physician's office

89. A physical therapist treats a 26-year-old male with complete C6 tetraplegia. During treatment the patient makes a culturally insensitive remark that the therapist feels is offensive. The most appropriate therapist action is to:

1. document the incident in the medical record
2. transfer the patient to another physical therapist's schedule
3. discharge the patient from physical therapy
4. inform the patient that the remark was offensive and continue with treatment

90. A physical therapist completes a fitness screening on a 34-year-old male prior to prescribing an aerobic exercise program. Which value is most representative of the patient's age-predicted maximal heart rate?

1. 168
2. 174
3. 186
4. 196

91. A physical therapist observes a patient ambulating in the clinic. The therapist notes that the patient's pelvis drops on the left during left swing phase. This deviation is usually caused by weakness of the:

1. left gluteus medius
2. right gluteus medius
3. left gluteus minimus
4. right gluteus minimus

92. A physical therapist examines a patient diagnosed with cerebellar degeneration. Which of the following clinical findings is not typically associated with this condition?

    1. athetosis
    2. dysmetria
    3. nystagmus
    4. dysdiadochokinesia

93. A physical therapist examines the reflex status of a patient. The therapist should use which technique to assess the patient's superficial reflexes?

    1. brushing the skin with a light feathery object
    2. percussing a muscle over the musculotendinous junction
    3. stroking the skin with a non-cutting, but pointed object
    4. tapping a tendon or bony prominence

94. A patient referred to physical therapy with cervical rib syndrome reports tingling and numbness throughout the upper extremity when carrying heavy objects at their side. Which structures are commonly affected by the cervical rib?

    1. common carotid artery and inferior trunk of the brachial plexus
    2. common carotid artery and superior trunk of the brachial plexus
    3. subclavian artery and inferior trunk of the brachial plexus
    4. subclavian artery and superior trunk of the brachial plexus

95. A patient status post CVA exercises in supine. As the physical therapist resists adduction of the unaffected leg, the affected leg begins to adduct. This should be documented as:

    1. Souque's phenomenon
    2. overextension phenomenon
    3. Schunkel reflex
    4. Raimiste's phenomenon

96. A physical therapist is employed at a physician owned physical therapy clinic that charges for treatment by the modality. One of the physicians, who is an owner of the practice, requests that all of his patients receive a minimum of heat, ultrasound, and electrical stimulation during each treatment session. The therapist feels that the majority of patients receive little clinical benefit from the proposed treatment regime. The most appropriate immediate response would be to:

    1. ignore the physician's request and treat each patient as you feel is indicated
    2. discuss with the physician the rationale for requesting modalities on each patient
    3. report the physician's conduct to the American Medical Association
    4. inform the physician that he is abusing the health care system

97. A physical therapist completes a developmental assessment on an infant. At what age should an infant begin to sit with hand support for an extended period of time?

    1. 6-7 months
    2. 8-9 months
    3. 10-11 months
    4. 12 months

98. A physical therapist is required to train a 71-year-old patient to ascend and descend a flight of stairs. The patient presents with a fractured left tibia and is weight bearing as tolerated. There is moderate weakness in the involved lower extremity secondary to the fracture. The most appropriate instructions are:

    1. "One step at a time, right foot first to ascend and to descend the stairs."
    2. "One step at a time, right foot first to ascend the stairs and left foot first to descend the stairs."
    3. "Step over step slowly."
    4. "One step at a time, left foot first to ascend and to descend the stairs."

99. A physical therapist examines a 36-year-old female referred to physical therapy after experiencing back pain two weeks ago. The patient identifies the majority of pain in the buttock and lateral thigh and denies any referred pain down the posterior leg. Presently she rates the pain as a "3" on a 0-10 scale, however, indicates that the pain is a "6" or a "7" during activity or at night. This description most closely resembles:

1. sacroilitis
2. iliolumbar syndrome
3. piriformis syndrome
4. trochanteric bursitis

100. A physical therapist completes a sensory assessment on a 61-year-old female diagnosed with multiple sclerosis. As part of the assessment the therapist examines stereognosis, kinesthesia, and two-point discrimination. What type of receptor is primarily responsible for generating the necessary information?

1. deep sensory receptors
2. mechanoreceptors
3. nociceptors
4. thermoreceptors

Please make sure all of the questions in the section have been answered prior to beginning the next section. When a new section is initiated candidates will be unable to return to previously completed sections.

Paper and Pencil Exam Two – Section Three

101. During an examination a physical therapist attempts to determine a patient's general willingness to use an affected body part. What objective information would provide the most useful information?

1. bony palpation
2. active movement
3. passive movement
4. sensory testing

102. A male physical therapist examines a female diagnosed with subacromial bursitis. After taking a thorough history, the therapist asks the patient to change into a gown. The patient seems very uneasy about this suggestion, but finally agrees to use the gown. The most appropriate course of action would be to:

1. continue with treatment as planned
2. attempt to treat the patient without using the gown
3. bring a female staff member into the treatment room and continue with treatment
4. offer to transfer the patient to a female physical therapist

103. A physical therapist attends an inservice on risk management. During the presentation the speaker describes guidelines to decrease the incidence of lawsuits. Which of the following would be considered the most essential action?

1. conduct a thorough initial examination
2. instruct patients carefully in all exercise activities
3. keep the referring physician informed
4. maintain accurate and timely documentation

104. A former patient calls to ask for advice after injuring his lower back in a work related accident. The patient explains that he cannot bend down and touch his toes without severe pain and has muscle spasms throughout the entire lower back. The physical therapist works in a state without direct access, but would like to help the former patient. The most appropriate response would be:

1. explain to the patient that you would be happy to treat him, however, since you have not completed a formal examination it would be unfair to prescribe treatment over the phone
2. arrange a time for the patient to come into your clinic for immediate treatment
3. prescribe flexion exercises and ice every three hours
4. refer the patient to a qualified physician

105. A therapist examines a patient diagnosed with patellar femoral syndrome. As part of the examination the therapist elects to measure the patient's Q angle. Which three bony landmarks are used to measure the Q angle?

1. anterior superior iliac spine, superior border of the patella, tibial tubercle
2. anterior superior iliac spine, midpoint of the patella, tibial tubercle
3. anterior superior iliac spine, inferior border of the patella, midpoint of the patella tendon
4. greater trochanter, midpoint of the patella, superior border of the patella tendon

106. A patient with an acute burn is referred to physical therapy. The patient's burns range from superficial partial-thickness to deep partial-thickness and encompass approximately 35 percent of the patient's body. Which of the following findings would be most predictable based on the patient's injury?

1. increased oxygen consumption
2. decreased minute ventilation
3. increased intravascular fluid
4. decreased core temperature

107. A patient rehabilitating from congestive heart failure is examined in physical therapy. During the examination the patient begins to complain of pain. The most immediate physical therapist action is to:

    1. notify the nursing staff to administer pain medication
    2. contact the referring physician
    3. discontinue the treatment session
    4. ask the patient to describe the location and severity of the pain

108. A physical therapist reviews the medical record of a patient diagnosed with chronic obstructive pulmonary disease. The medical record indicates that the patient's current condition is consistent with chronic respiratory acidosis. Which testing procedure was likely used to identify this condition?

    1. arterial blood gas analysis
    2. pulmonary function testing
    3. graded exercise testing
    4. pulse oximetry

109. A physical therapist designs an exercise program for a patient rehabilitating from a lower extremity injury. The single most important factor in an exercise program designed to increase muscular strength is:

    1. the recovery time between exercise sets
    2. the number of repetitions per set
    3. the duration of the exercise session
    4. the intensity of the exercise

110. An order is received to perform chest physical therapy on a patient status post abdominal surgery. A chart review identifies right atelectasis. The most appropriate exercise to teach the patient is:

    1. reflex cough technique
    2. Codman's pendulum exercises
    3. segmental breathing
    4. quick paced shallow breathing

111. A patient with right hemiplegia is observed during gait training. The patient performs sidestepping towards the hemiplegic side. The physical therapist may expect the patient to compensate for weakened abductors by:

    1. hip hiking of the unaffected side
    2. lateral trunk flexion towards the affected side
    3. lateral trunk flexion towards the unaffected side
    4. hip extension of the affected side

112. A patient in a pulmonary rehabilitation program is positioned in supine with a pillow under the knees. The physical therapist claps between the clavicle and nipple bilaterally. This technique is utilized for postural drainage of the:

    1. anterior segments of the upper lobes
    2. anterior basal segments of the lower lobes
    3. superior segments of the lower lobes
    4. posterior basal segments of the lower lobes

113. A patient reports to a scheduled physical therapy session 25 minutes late. The patient has not been seen previously in physical therapy and was scheduled in a 45 minute block of time. The patient referral indicates the patient is 10 days status post arthroscopic medial meniscectomy. The most appropriate therapist action is:

    1. begin the examination
    2. design a home exercise program
    3. consult with the patient's physician
    4. ask the patient to reschedule

114. A patient with an ankle-foot orthosis demonstrates genu recurvatum during the stance phase of gait. Which action would be the most appropriate to decrease the recurvatum?

    1. increase the plantar flexion stop
    2. increase the dorsiflexion stop
    3. allow full range of motion at the ankle
    4. ankle joint position does not affect recurvatum

115. A physical therapist treats a patient with superficial partial-thickness burns to the anterior surface of his lower legs. In an attempt to assist the patient to control the pain associated with the burns, the therapist rewards the patient with a lengthy rest period after successfully completing an exercise sequence. This type of psychological approach is most representative of:

1. distraction
2. extinction
3. classical conditioning
4. operant conditioning

116. A physical therapist identifies that an infant is unable to roll from prone to supine. Which reflex could interfere with the infant's ability to roll?

1. asymmetrical tonic neck reflex
2. Moro reflex
3. Galant reflex
4. symmetrical tonic neck reflex

117. A physical therapist reviews a laboratory report for a 41-year-old male diagnosed with chronic obstructive pulmonary disease. Which of the following would be considered a normal hemoglobin value?

1. 10 gm/dL
2. 15 gm/dL
3. 20 gm/dL
4. 25 gm/dL

118. A patient diagnosed with an incomplete spinal cord lesion presents with muscle paralysis on the ipsilateral side of the lesion and a loss of pain, temperature, and sensitivity on the contralateral side of the lesion. This presentation best describes:

1. Steinert's disease
2. central cord syndrome
3. anterior spinal artery syndrome
4. Brown-Sequard's syndrome

119. A physical therapist reviews the medical record of a patient rehabilitating from a stroke. The patient exhibits paralysis and numbness on the side of the body contralateral to the vascular accident. Which descending pathway is most likely damaged based on the patient's clinical presentation?

1. corticospinal tract
2. vestibulospinal tract
3. tectospinal tract
4. rubrospinal tract

120. A patient diagnosed with emphysema is referred to physical therapy. Physical examination reveals increased accessory muscle use during normal breathing and a forward head posture. The primary goal for the patient is:

1. eliminate accessory muscle activity and decrease respiratory rate with pursed-lip breathing
2. optimize accessory muscle strength to promote alveolar ventilation
3. utilize the accessory muscles to balance the activity of the upper and lower chest
4. diminish accessory muscle use and emphasize diaphragmatic breathing

121. A patient returns to an outpatient physical therapy clinic two hours after completing a treatment session complaining of increased back pain. The patient has been seen in physical therapy for three previous visits and has had little difficulty with a program consisting of palliative modalities and pelvic stabilization exercises. The patient was referred to physical therapy after straining his back two weeks ago while lifting his daughter out of a car seat. The most appropriate physical therapist action is:

1. contact the referring physician to discuss the patient's care plan
2. instruct the patient to discontinue the pelvic stabilization exercises and re-examine the patient at his next visit
3. refer the patient to the emergency room of a local hospital
4. instruct the patient to cancel existing physical therapy visits and schedule an appointment with the physician

122. A physical therapist prepares to treat a patient in isolation. In what order should the protective clothing be applied?

    1. gloves, gown, mask
    2. gown, gloves, mask
    3. mask, gown, gloves
    4. gloves, mask, gown

123. A physical therapist reviews a physician's examination of a patient scheduled for physical therapy. The examination identifies excessive medial displacement of the elbow during ligamentous testing. Which ligament is typically involved with medial instability of the elbow?

    1. annular
    2. radial collateral
    3. ulnar collateral
    4. volar radioulnar

124. A physical therapist treating a patient in a special care unit notices a marked increase in fluid on the dorsum of a patient's hand around an intravenous site. The therapist, recognizing the possibility that the intravenous line has become dislodged, should immediately:

    1. continue with the present treatment
    2. contact the primary physician
    3. turn off the intravenous system
    4. reposition the peripheral intravenous line

125. A patient rehabilitating from a radial head fracture performs progressive resistive exercises designed to strengthen the forearm supinators. Which muscle would be of particular importance to achieve the desired outcome?

    1. brachialis
    2. brachioradialis
    3. biceps brachii
    4. anconeus

126. A physical therapist reviews the medical chart of a patient admitted to the hospital two days ago after being burned in a house fire. The chart specifies that the epidermal and dermal layers were completely destroyed and some of the subcutaneous tissue was damaged. Which type of burn does this best describe?

    1. superficial partial-thickness
    2. deep partial-thickness
    3. full-thickness
    4. subdermal

127. A patient is unable to take in an adequate supply of nutrients by mouth due to the side effects of radiation therapy. As a result the patient's physician orders the implementation of tube feeding. What type of tube is most commonly used for short-term feeding?

    1. endobronchial
    2. nasogastric
    3. otopharyngeal
    4. tracheostomy

128. A physical therapist employed in an acute care hospital prepares to work on standing balance with a patient rehabilitating from abdominal surgery. The patient has been on extended bed rest following the surgical procedure and has only been out of bed a few times with the assistance of the nursing staff. The most important objective measure to assess after assisting the patient from supine to sitting is:

    1. systolic blood pressure
    2. diastolic blood pressure
    3. perceived exertion
    4. oxygen saturation rate

129. A physical therapist treats a patient who sustained several orthopedic injures in a mountain climbing accident. Assuming the patient's upper extremity injuries include a partial tear of the ulnar collateral ligament, which of the following methods would most likely be used in the medical management of this injury?

    1. short-arm thumb spica cast
    2. long-arm thumb spica cast
    3. short-arm thumb spica splint
    4. long-arm thumb spica splint

130. A therapist attempts to quantify the amount of assistance a patient needs to complete a selected activity. Categories of assistance include maximal, moderate, minimal, stand-by or independent. This type of measurement scale is best classified as:

    1. interval
    2. nominal
    3. ordinal
    4. ratio

131. A physical therapist attempts to palpate the lunate by moving his finger immediately distal to Lister's tubercle. Which wrist motion will allow the therapist to facilitate palpation of the lunate?

    1. extension
    2. flexion
    3. radial deviation
    4. ulnar deviation

132. A physician indicates that a patient rehabilitating from a cerebrovascular accident has significant perceptual deficits. Which anatomical region would most likely be affected by the stroke?

    1. primary motor cortex
    2. sensory cortex
    3. basal ganglia
    4. cerebellum

133. A physical therapist reviews a research study that examines knee flexion range of motion two weeks following arthroscopic surgery. Assuming a normal distribution, what percentage of patients participating in the study would you expect to achieve a goniometric measurement value between the mean and one standard deviation above the mean?

    1. 25%
    2. 34%
    3. 46%
    4. 68%

134. A physical therapist treats a patient referred to physical therapy with incontinence. The patient describes her difficulty beginning after the birth of her son. After completing an examination the therapist concludes that the patient has extremely weak pelvic floor muscles. When instructing the patient in a pelvic floor muscle strengthening program, the most appropriate position to initiate treatment is:

    1. sidelying
    2. sitting
    3. standing
    4. supine

135. A physical therapist prepares to administer the Berg Balance Scale to a patient rehabilitating from a cerebrovascular accident. Which of the following tools is considered a necessary piece of equipment when administering this outcome measure?

    1. reflex hammer
    2. goniometer
    3. stopwatch
    4. stethoscope

136. A physical therapist employed in a school setting observes a 10-year-old boy attempt to move from the floor to a standing position. During the activity, the boy has to push on his legs with his hands in order to attain an upright position. This type of finding is most commonly associated with:

    1. cystic fibrosis
    2. Down syndrome
    3. Duchenne muscular dystrophy
    4. spinal muscular atrophy

137. A physical therapist performs a respiratory assessment on a patient with restrictive lung disease. If the therapist records the respiration rate as 22 breaths per minute, which term is most appropriate to classify the patient's respiration rate?

    1. eupnea
    2. tachypnea
    3. bradypnea
    4. hyperpnea

138. A physical therapist uses a spirometer to administer a pulmonary function test to a patient with suspected pulmonary dysfunction. Which of the following measurements would the therapist be able to obtain directly without utilizing the results of other pulmonary function tests?

    1. expiratory reserve volume
    2. total lung cacity
    3. minute volume
    4. residual volume

139. A physical therapist palpates the bony structures of the wrist and hand. Which of the following structures would not be identified in the distal row of carpals?

    1. capitate
    2. hamate
    3. triquetrum
    4. trapezoid

140. A physical therapist examines the electrocardiogram of a patient during exercise. What change in the electrocardiogram would be indicative of myocardial ischemia?

    1. P wave changes
    2. PR interval changes
    3. QRS changes
    4. ST segment changes

141. A physical therapist uses repeated contractions to strengthen the quadriceps of a patient that fails to exhibit the desired muscular response throughout a portion of the range of motion. This proprioceptive neuromuscular facilitation technique should be applied:

    1. at the initiation of movement
    2. at the point where the desired muscular response begins to diminish
    3. at the end of the available range of motion
    4. only after a manual stretch to the hamstrings

142. A patient is referred to physical therapy with a twenty degree restriction in wrist extension. Which mobilization technique would be the most appropriate based on the restriction?

    1. dorsal glide of the carpals
    2. stabilize lunate, volar glide radius
    3. stabilize capitate, volar glide lunate
    4. stabilize radius, volar glide scaphoid

143. A patient rehabilitating from extensive burns to the right upper extremity often complains of severe pain in the arm during physical therapy treatment sessions. The present plan of care emphasizes range of motion, stretching, and positioning. The most appropriate action to address the patient's complaint is to:

    1. reduce the frequency and duration of the treatment sessions
    2. schedule treatment sessions when the patient's pain medication is most effective
    3. avoid treatment activities that are uncomfortable for the patient
    4. request that the referring physician increase the dosage of the patient's pain medication

144. A physical therapist treats a patient diagnosed with chronic arteriosclerotic vascular disease. The patient exhibits cool skin, decreased sensitivity to temperature changes, and intermittent claudication with activity. The primary treatment goal is to increase the patient's ambulation distance. The most appropriate ambulation parameters to facilitate achievement of the goal are:

    1. short duration, frequent intervals
    2. short duration, infrequent intervals
    3. long duration, frequent intervals
    4. long duration, infrequent intervals

145. A patient rehabilitating from a bone marrow transplant is referred to physical therapy for instruction in an exercise program. The physical therapist plans to use oxygen saturation measurements to gain additional objective data related to the patient's exercise tolerance. Assuming the patient's oxygen saturation rate was measured as 95% at rest, which of the following guidelines would be the most appropriate?

    1. discontinue exercise if the patient's oxygen saturation rate is below 95%
    2. discontinue exercise if the patient's oxygen saturation rate is below 90%
    3. discontinue exercise if the patient's oxygen saturation rate is below 85%
    4. discontinue exercise if the patient's oxygen saturation rate is below 80%

146. A patient exhibits pain and sensory loss in the posterior thigh, lateral calf, and dorsal foot. Extension of the hallux is poor, however, the Achilles reflex is normal. What spinal level would you expect to be involved?

    1. L4
    2. L5
    3. S1
    4. S2

147. A physical therapist employed in a rehabilitation hospital completes an examination on a patient diagnosed with Parkinson's disease. Results of the examination include 4/5 strength in the lower extremities, 10 degree flexion contractures at the hips, and exaggerated forward standing posture. The patient has significant difficulty initiating movement and requires manual assistance for gait on level surfaces. The most appropriate activity to incorporate into a home program is:

    1. prone lying
    2. progressive relaxation exercises
    3. lower extremity resistive exercises with ankle weights
    4. postural awareness exercises in standing

148. A physical therapist examines a patient's hip range of motion. Which pattern of limitation is typically considered to be a capsular pattern at the hip?

    1. limitation of flexion, abduction, and medial rotation
    2. limitation of flexion, adduction, and lateral rotation
    3. limitation of extension, abduction, and lateral rotation
    4. limitation of extension, adduction, and medial rotation

149. A 62-year-old female is restricted from physical therapy for two days following surgical insertion of a urinary catheter. This type of procedure is most commonly performed with a:

    1. condom catheter
    2. Foley catheter
    3. suprapubic catheter
    4. Swan-Ganz catheter

150. A patient in the intensive care unit rehabilitating from a serious infection is connected to a series of lines and tubes. Which lower extremity intravenous infusion site would be the most appropriate to administer an intravenous line?

    1. antecubital vein
    2. basilic vein
    3. cephalic vein
    4. saphenous vein

 Please make sure all of the questions in the section have been answered prior to beginning the next section. When a new section is initiated candidates will be unable to return to previously completed sections.

Only 8 arrows for 75%

Paper and Pencil Exam Two – Section Four

151. A physical therapist orders a wheelchair for a patient with C5 tetraplegia. Which type of wheelchair would be the most appropriate for the patient?

1. electric wheelchair
2. manual wheelchair with handrim projections
3. manual wheelchair with friction surface handrims
4. manual wheelchair with standard handrims

152. A patient is instructed by the nursing staff to increase dietary consumption of food sources that are rich in vitamin A. Which of the following food groups would be the most appropriate to meet this goal?

1. green leaves, nuts, seafood
2. egg yolks, butter, yellow vegetables
3. milk, beef, grain
4. vegetable oil, wheat germ, dried yeast

153. A physical therapist reviews a medical chart to determine when a patient was last medicated. The chart indicates the patient received medication at 2300 hours. Assuming it is now 8:00 AM, how long ago did the patient receive the medication?

1. 5 hours
2. 9 hours
3. 15 hours
4. 18 hours

154. A physical therapist attempts to auscultate over the aortic valve. Which of the following areas is the most appropriate to isolate the desired valve?

1. second left intercostal space at the left sternal border
2. second right intercostal space at the right sternal border
3. fourth left intercostal space along the lower left sternal border
4. fifth left intercostal space at the midclavicular line

155. A physical therapist positions a patient for bronchial drainage to the anterior segments of the upper lobes. The most appropriate patient position is:

1. supine with a pillow under the knees
2. supine with the head of the bed elevated 16 inches
3. supine with the foot of the bed elevated 16 inches
4. prone with the head of the bed elevated 12 inches

156. A physical therapist attempts to estimate the energy expenditure in calories for a patient performing a selected activity for 15 minutes. Assuming the therapist has a metabolic equivalent value for the activity, what other variables are necessary in order to obtain an estimate of the patient's energy expenditure?

1. patient's height and weight
2. patient's weight and oxygen consumption
3. patient's stroke volume and heart rate
4. patient's residual volume and heart rate

157. A physical therapist examines the foot of a 17-year-old female referred to physical therapy with lower leg pain. After placing the foot in subtalar neutral the therapist determines that the medial border of the foot along the first metatarsal is higher than the lateral border of the foot along the fifth metatarsal. This position would most appropriately be documented as:

1. forefoot varus
2. forefoot valgus
3. rearfoot varus
4. rearfoot valgus

158. A physical therapist reviews the medical record of a patient recently admitted to an inpatient rehabilitation hospital. The patient sustained a traumatic head injury in a motor vehicle accident five weeks ago. The medical record indicates that the patient is often disoriented and can frequently become agitated with little provocation. The most appropriate location for the therapist to make initial contact with the patient is:

1. in the patient's room
2. in the physical therapy gym
3. in a private treatment room
4. in the physical therapy waiting room

The following image should be used to answer question 159:

159. A physical therapist instructs a patient positioned in supine to bring her left leg toward her chest and maintain the position using her left arm. Assuming the therapist observes the reaction shown in the picture, what muscle would most likely have insufficient length?

1. iliopsoas
2. quadratus lumborum
3. rectus femoris
4. sartorius

160. A physical therapist monitors the blood pressure of a 28-year-old male during increasing levels of physical exertion. Assuming a normal physiologic response, which of the following best describes the patient's blood pressure response to exercise?

1. systolic pressure decreases, diastolic pressure increases
2. systolic pressure remains the same, diastolic pressure decreases
3. systolic pressure and diastolic pressure remain the same
4. systolic pressure increases, diastolic pressure remains the same

161. A physical therapist employed in a rehabilitation hospital treats a patient status post traumatic brain injury. During the treatment session the therapist notices that the patient's toes are discolored below a bivalved lower extremity cast. The cast was applied approximately five hours ago in an attempt to reduce a plantar flexion contracture. The most appropriate therapist action is to:

1. document the observation in the medical record and continue to monitor the patient's circulation
2. contact the staff nurse and request that the cast is removed
3. refer the patient to an orthotist
4. remove the cast

162. A physical therapist examines a patient rehabilitating from a traumatic brain injury. The therapist makes the following entry in the medical record: The patient is able to respond to simple commands fairly consistently, however, has difficulty with increasingly complex commands. Responses are non-purposeful, random, and fragmented. According to the Rancho Los Amigos Cognitive Functioning Scale the patient is most representative of level:

1. III - localized responses
2. IV - confused-agitated
3. V - confused-inappropriate
4. VI - confused-appropriate

163. A physical therapist examines a 25-year-old male rehabilitating from a meniscus repair. The physician orders indicate the patient is non-weight bearing on the involved lower extremity. The most appropriate gait pattern for the patient is:

    1. two-point
    2. three-point
    3. four-point
    4. swing-to

164. A physical therapist examines a patient referred to physical therapy with olecranon bursitis. During the initial examination the therapist identifies diffuse swelling in the elbow joint. Which of the following joints would be affected with swelling in the elbow complex?

    1. ulnohumeral joint
    2. ulnohumeral and radiohumeral joints
    3. radiohumeral and proximal radioulnar joints
    4. ulnohumeral, radiohumeral, and proximal radioulnar joints

165. A physical therapist treats a patient status post right cerebrovascular accident with resultant left hemiplegia for a colleague on vacation. A note left by the primary therapist indicates that the patient exhibits "pusher syndrome." When examining the patient's sitting posture, which of the following findings would be most likely?

    1. increased lean to the left with increased weight bearing on the left buttock
    2. increased lean to the right with increased weight bearing on the right buttock
    3. increased forward lean with increased weight bearing on the right buttock
    4. increased forward lean with increased weight bearing on the left buttock

166. A physical therapist performs goniometric measurements for elbow flexion with a patient in supine. In order to isolate elbow flexion the therapist should stabilize the:

    1. distal end of the humerus
    2. proximal end of the humerus
    3. distal end of the ulna
    4. proximal end of the radius

167. A physical therapist observes that a number of aides appear to be unfamiliar with appropriate guarding techniques. The most appropriate remedial strategy to improve their performance is to:

    1. offer assistance to the aides when the inappropriate behavior is observed
    2. refer the aides to text books that explain proper guarding technique
    3. develop a mandatory inservice on guarding techniques for the aides
    4. inform the director of rehabilitation that the aides are incompetent

168. A physical therapist attempts to obtain information on the ability of noncontractile tissue to allow motion at a specific joint. Which selective tissue tension assessment would provide the therapist with the most valuable information?

    1. active range of motion
    2. active-assistive range of motion
    3. passive range of motion
    4. resisted isometrics

169. A physical therapist instructs a patient rehabilitating from a tibial plateau fracture to ascend a curb using axillary crutches. The patient is partial weight bearing and uses a three-point gait pattern when ambulating. When ascending a curb the therapist should instruct the patient to lead with the:

    1. uninvolved lower extremity
    2. involved lower extremity
    3. axillary crutches
    4. axillary crutch and uninvolved lower extremity

170. A physical therapist attempts to transfer a dependent patient from a wheelchair to a bed. The therapist is concerned about the size of the patient, but is unable to secure another staff member to assist with the transfer. Which type of transfer would allow the therapist to move the patient with the greatest ease?

    1. dependent standing pivot
    2. hydraulic lift
    3. sliding board
    4. assisted standing pivot

171. A physical therapist completes a manual muscle test where resistance is applied toward plantar flexion and eversion. This description best describes a manual muscle test of the:

    1. tibialis anterior
    2. tibialis posterior
    3. peroneus longus
    4. peroneus brevis

172. A physical therapist performs an examination on a 27-year-old male diagnosed with iliotibial band syndrome. The patient is an avid distance runner who routinely ran between 45-60 miles per week before experiencing pain in his knee. Standing posture reveals a varus position at the knee and a cavus foot. When palpating the lateral portion of the lower extremity, which area would you most likely identify marked tenderness?

    1. lateral femoral condyle
    2. lateral joint line
    3. lateral tibial condyle
    4. fibular head

173. A 24-year-old soccer player is referred to physical therapy after being diagnosed with Achilles tendonitis. Which of the following actions would place the greatest stress on the Achilles tendon?

    1. concentric contraction of the gastrocnemius
    2. eccentric contraction of the gastrocnemius
    3. concentric contraction of the gastrocnemius and soleus complex
    4. eccentric contraction of the gastrocnemius and soleus complex

174. A physical therapist employed in a rehabilitation hospital discusses the merits of several different outcome assessment measures with a colleague. When discussing the Barthel Index, which of the following would be considered a valid limitation of the outcome measure?

    1. limited sensitivity for individuals with mild disabilities
    2. requires specialized equipment
    3. necessitates fasting for 12 hours
    4. may take 6-8 hours to administer

175. A physical therapist examines the forefoot position of a 36-year-old male referred to physical therapy with ankle pain of unknown etiology. After placing the foot in subtalar neutral the therapist determines that the patient has a forefoot varus. What compensatory finding is most likely at the rearfoot based on the alignment of the forefoot?

    1. subtalar eversion
    2. subtalar inversion
    3. talocrural dorsiflexion
    4. talocrural plantar flexion

176. A 36-year-old female is limited to 30 degrees of lateral rotation at the right shoulder. Which shoulder mobilization technique would be the most appropriate to address the limitation?

    1. anterior glide of the humeral head
    2. posterior glide of the humeral head
    3. inferior glide of the humeral head
    4. superior glide of the humeral head

177. A patient waiting for a scheduled therapy session in the gym suddenly begins to scream. The patient sustained a traumatic brain injury in a motor vehicle accident and is currently functioning at the confused-appropriate stage. The most appropriate therapist action is:

    1. ask the patient if he needs assistance
    2. seek assistance from other health care professionals
    3. request that the patient is transported back to his room
    4. contact a physician and request that the patient's medication dosage is increased

178. A physical therapist transfers a patient in a wheelchair down a curb with a forward approach. Which of the following actions would be the most appropriate?

    1. have the patient lean forward
    2. have the wheelchair brakes locked
    3. tilt the wheelchair backwards
    4. position yourself in front of the patient

179. A physical therapist positions a patient in supine in order to perform passive stretching of the rectus femoris on the right. In order to effectively stabilize the pelvis in a supine position, the therapist should:

    1. passively flex the right hip to the patient's chest
    2. passively flex the right hip and knee to the patient's chest
    3. passively flex the left hip to the patient's chest
    4. passively flex the left hip and knee to the patient's chest

180. A physical therapist treats a patient with a fractured left hip. The patient is weight bearing as tolerated and uses a large base quad cane for gait activities. Correct use of the quad cane would include:

    1. using the quad cane on the left with the longer legs positioned away from the patient
    2. using the quad cane on the right with the longer legs positioned away from the patient
    3. using the quad cane on the left with the longer legs positioned toward the patient
    4. using the quad cane on the right with the longer legs positioned toward the patient

181. A physical therapist working in a school system develops long-term goals as part of an Individualized Educational Plan for a child with Down Syndrome. The most appropriate time frame for these goals is:

    1. one month
    2. four months
    3. six months
    4. one year

182. A physical therapist administers ultrasound over a patient's anterior thigh. After one minute of treatment, the patient reports feeling a slight burning sensation under the soundhead. The therapist's most appropriate action is to:

    1. explain to the patient that what she feels is not out of the ordinary when using ultrasound
    2. temporarily discontinue treatment and examine the amount of coupling agent utilized
    3. discontinue treatment and contact the referring physician
    4. continue with treatment utilizing the current parameters

183. A patient eight weeks status post myocardial infarction is involved in a phase II cardiac rehabilitation program at a local hospital. What event usually signifies the completion of a phase II program?

    1. echocardiogram
    2. initiation of a high-level aerobic exercise program
    3. low-level treadmill test
    4. maximal treadmill test

184. A 66-year-old female is referred to physical therapy with rheumatoid arthritis. During the initial examination the physical therapist notes increased flexion at the proximal interphalangeal joints and hyperextension at the metacarpophalangeal and distal interphalangeal joints. This deformity is most representative of:

    1. boutonniere deformity
    2. mallet finger
    3. swan neck deformity
    4. ulnar drift

185. A physician reduces a comminuted tibia fracture using an external fixation device. Which stage of bone healing is associated with the termination of external fixation?

    1. hematoma formation
    2. cellular proliferation
    3. callus formation
    4. clinical union

186. A 62-year-old male diagnosed with ankylosing spondylitis is referred to physical therapy. The patient's referral is for instruction in a home exercise program. Which of the following exercises would you expect to be the most appropriate for the patient?

    1. partial sit-ups
    2. posterior pelvic tilts
    3. spinal extension
    4. straight leg raises

187. A patient diagnosed with piriformis syndrome is referred to physical therapy for one visit for instruction in a home exercise program. After examining the patient, the physical therapist feels the patient's rehabilitation potential is excellent, but is concerned that one visit will not be sufficient to meet the patient's needs. The most appropriate action is to:

    1. schedule the patient for treatment sessions, as warranted by the results of the examination
    2. explain to the patient that recent health care reforms have drastically reduced the frequency of physical therapy visits covered by third party payers
    3. explain to the patient that she can continue with physical therapy beyond the initial session, but will be liable for all expenses not covered by her insurance
    4. contact the referring physician and request approval for additional physical therapy visits

188. A male patient with limited shoulder range of motion explains that he has difficulty wiping himself after going to the bathroom. How much shoulder range of motion is required to successfully complete toileting activities using a posterior approach?

    1. 50 degrees horizontal abduction, 30 degrees abduction, 45 degrees medial rotation
    2. 30 degrees horizontal abduction, 45 degrees adduction, 65 degrees medial rotation
    3. 80 degrees horizontal abduction, 40 degrees abduction, 90 degrees medial rotation
    4. 90 degrees horizontal adduction, 75 degrees abduction, 60 degrees medial rotation

189. A physical therapist completes lower extremity range of motion activities with a patient status post spinal cord injury. While performing passive range of motion, the therapist notices that the patient's urine is extremely dark and has a distinctive foul smelling odor. Which of the following is the most appropriate action?

    1. verbally report the observation to the patient's physician
    2. verbally report the observation to the patient's nurse
    3. document and verbally report the observation to the patient's nurse
    4. document and verbally report the observation to the director of rehabilitation

190. A rehabilitation manager designs a system to monitor the productivity of staff physical therapists. Which piece of data would be the least beneficial to accomplish the manager's objective?

    1. number of generated timed treatment units
    2. results of patient satisfaction survey data
    3. total hours of direct patient treatment time
    4. number of regular payroll hours

191. A physical therapist performs a manual muscle test on a patient's hip flexors. The therapist attempts to complete the test in supine, but the patient has difficulty holding the limb in the test position. What alternate test position would be appropriate to test the patient's hip flexors?

    1. prone
    2. sidelying
    3. sitting
    4. standing

192. A physical therapist palpates along the lateral portion of the hamstrings musculature to the tendinous attachment on the fibular head. The muscle should be identified as the:

    1. biceps femoris
    2. gracilis
    3. sartorius
    4. semitendinosus

The following image should be used to answer question 193:

193. A physical therapist observing a patient complete a leg curl exercise notices two prominent tendons visible on the posterior surface of the patient's left knee. The visible tendons are most likely associated with the:

1. semimembranosus and semitendinosus muscles
2. semitendinosus and biceps femoris muscles
3. popliteus and semitendinosus muscles
4. semimembranosus and biceps femoris muscles

194. A physical therapist examines a patient diagnosed with a wrist sprain. During the examination the therapist has difficulty identifying the scaphoid and attempts to use the tendinous radial and ulnar boundaries of the anatomical snuff box to assist him. Which of the following active motions would be the most helpful when locating the anatomical snuff box?

1. abduction of the thumb
2. adduction of the thumb
3. extension of the thumb
4. flexion of the thumb

195. A physical therapist uses proprioceptive neuromuscular facilitation techniques to increase muscular strength. The therapist instructs the patient to actively perform a pattern of hip extension, abduction, and medial rotation. This pattern emphasizes strengthening of the:

1. psoas major, psoas minor, iliacus
2. tensor fasciae latae, biceps femoris
3. gluteus maximus, gluteus medius, gluteus minimus
4. gluteus maximus, piriformis, adductor magnus

196. A physical therapist employed in an ambulatory care center prepares to apply a hot pack to the low back of a patient diagnosed with degenerative disk disease. When examining the patient the therapist identifies several blisters on the patient's right side. The patient indicates that the blisters were caused by heat from a hot pack applied during the previous treatment session. The patient blames himself for the incident because he was hesitant to tell the therapist that the heat was too intense. The most appropriate therapist action is to:

1. complete an incident report
2. contact the referring physician
3. modify the documentation from the previous treatment session
4. avoid documenting the event since it occurred during the previous treatment session

197. A physical therapist attempts to calculate the target heart rate range for a 32-year-old female with no significant past medical history. The patient's resting heart rate is recorded as 60 beats per minute and the maximal heart rate is 180 beats per minute. Using the heart rate reserve method (Karvonen formula) the patient's target heart rate range should be recorded as:

1. 96 – 120 beats per minute
2. 132 – 162 beats per minute
3. 144 – 174 beats per minute
4. 164 – 185 beats per minute

198. A patient in a work hardening program completes a training program consisting of ten different exercises requiring upper and lower extremity strength and endurance. The patient indicates that he is frustrated since he has been unable to increase the weight on a selected carrying activity in over two weeks. The most appropriate therapist action is:

1. provide the patient with verbal encouragement
2. attempt to substitute a different exercise for the carrying activity
3. vary the order of the exercises
4. decrease the number of repetitions

199. A 47-year-old patient with a diagnosis of CVA with left hemiplegia is referred for orthotic examination. Significant results of manual muscle testing include: hip flexion 3+/5, hip extension 3/5, knee flexion 3+/5, knee extension 3+/5, ankle dorsiflexion 2/5, and ankle inversion and eversion 1/5. Sensation is intact and no abnormal tone is noted. The most appropriate orthosis for this patient is a:

1. knee-ankle-foot orthosis with a locked knee
2. plastic articulating ankle-foot orthosis
3. metal upright ankle-foot orthosis locked in neutral
4. prefabricated posterior leaf orthosis

200. A physical therapist treats a patient diagnosed with Parkinson's disease. When working on controlled mobility, which of the following would best describe the physical therapist's objective?

1. facilitate postural muscle control
2. promote weight shifting and rotational trunk control
3. emphasize reciprocal extremity movement
4. facilitate tone and rigidity

Please make sure all of the questions in the section have been answered prior to ending the examination. Since candidates are not permitted to return to previously completed sections, this should signify the end of the examination.

58 wrong

EXAM TWO: Paper and Pencil
Answer Key

Paper and Pencil Exam Two – Section One

1. Correct Answer: 2
Explanation: The Americans with Disabilities Act (ADA) is federal legislation designed to eliminate discrimination against individuals with disabilities. Physical therapists have an ethical obligation to make patients aware of their rights according to the ADA. (Minor p. 466)

2. Correct Answer: 1
Explanation: The Glasgow Coma Scale provides a quick and practical method for assessing the degree of conscious impairment in the critically ill patient. The scale utilizes eye opening, verbal responses, and motor responses to determine the level of consciousness and degree of dysfunction. (Rothstein p. 426)

3. Correct Answer: 2
Explanation: An electrocardiogram is a common monitoring device for patients with known or suspected cardiac abnormalities. The electrocardiogram measures the electrical activity of the heart as well as heart rate, blood pressure, and respiration rate. (Pierson p. 273)

4. Correct Answer: 1
Explanation: Setting an ankle-foot orthosis in 5-10 degrees of dorsiflexion may serve to reduce genu recurvatum by inhibiting full extension of the knee during midstance. (Long p. 219)

5. Correct Answer: 1
Explanation: A physical therapist should give the highest priority to educating the patient on appropriate skin care including pressure relief activities. A patient with C7 tetraplegia can perform lateral and forward weight shifting in the wheelchair to assist with pressure relief. (Umphred p. 490)

6. Correct Answer: 3
Explanation: Cluster sampling is defined as successive random sampling of a series of units in the population. Cluster sampling is often utilized when a researcher is unable to obtain a complete listing of an identified population. Since the technique requires two or more samples to be drawn, sampling error is increased. (Portney p. 146)

7. Correct Answer: 2
Explanation: A correlation coefficient of r =.87 is classified as high to very high. As a result, performance on the Scholastic Aptitude Test and grade point average in a physical therapy academic program are strongly related. (Portney p. 493)

8. Correct Answer: 4
Explanation: Paresthesias of the long and ring fingers are commonly associated with the C7 nerve root, while the thumb and index finger are associated with C6. (Magee p. 12)

9. Correct Answer: 4
Explanation: Lateral flexion, extension, and rotation are all components of the vertebral artery test. Extension is the most likely motion to assess the integrity of the intervertebral foramen, while lateral flexion and rotation have a greater effect on the vertebral artery. (Magee p. 154)

10. Correct Answer: 2
Explanation: Diplopia refers to double vision caused by defective function of the extraocular muscles. Often times a patient with diplopia is instructed to wear a patch alternately over one of his/her eyes. Specific strengthening exercises of the extraocular muscles can serve to improve the patient's vision. (O'Sullivan p. 969)

11. Correct Answer: 4
Explanation: Muscle testing of the middle trapezius should occur with the patient in a prone position. (Kendall p. 284)

12. Correct Answer: 2
Explanation: For thoracic and high-level lumbar lesions the parapodium provides the necessary amount of support and is optimal to assist with standing activities. The parallel bars are the most stable assistive device to initiate standing and utilize during gait training. (Tecklin p. 194)

13. Correct Answer: 3
Explanation: Patients with chronic venous insufficiency must wear compression stockings during periods of activity, such as ambulation, in order to promote return to the heart and avoid venous stasis. (Kisner p. 718)

14. Correct Answer: 4
Explanation: The patient's dependence with ambulation and transfers eliminates home care as a viable option at this time. (O'Sullivan p. 540)

15. Correct Answer: 2
Explanation: The palmar aspect of the therapist's hands should be in full contact over the affected lung segment. The therapist may elect to partially or fully overlap the hands during manual vibration. (Hillegass p. 651)

16. Correct Answer: 3
Explanation: Metabolic acidosis usually results from an excess accumulation of acids in the blood. Patients with uncontrolled diabetes may be particularly susceptible to ketoacidosis, which is characterized by a fruity breath odor resulting from a build up of acids. The condition warrants immediate medical intervention. (Goodman – Pathology p. 116)

17. Correct Answer: 2
Explanation: The frontal plane divides the body into front and back halves. Movements in the frontal plane occur as side to side movements such as abduction or adduction. Rotary motion in the frontal plane occurs around an anterior-posterior axis. (Norkin p. 4)

18. Correct Answer: 3
Explanation: Maintained pressure is an effective technique that can be used to increase range of motion by facilitating local muscle relaxation, however, it is a passive technique. (Sullivan p. 64)

19. Correct Answer: 2
Explanation: Postural drainage to the posterior apical segments of the upper lobes is performed with the patient in sitting, leaning over a pillow at a 30 degree angle. (Hillegass p. 650)

20. Correct Answer: 4
Explanation: Seat width = hip width + 2 inches; Seat depth = posterior buttock to the popliteal space - 2 inches. (Pierson p. 168)

21. Correct Answer: 2
Explanation: Hallucinogens may cause distortion of senses, altered perception, severe hallucinations, panic, and psychotic reactions. Physical dependence is not characteristic of hallucinogens. (Ciccone p. 606)

22. Correct Answer: 2
Explanation: Premature ventricular contractions are premature beats arising from ectopic foci in the ventricle. Premature ventricular contractions are the most common form of arrhythmia and may be precipitated by caffeine, anxiety, alcohol, and tobacco. (Brannon p. 206)

23. Correct Answer: 3
Explanation: 98.6 degrees Fahrenheit or 37 degrees Celsius is considered normal body temperature. (Pierson p. 48)

24. Correct Answer: 1
Explanation: A rate of 2-3 mm Hg per second will enable the physical therapist to identify normal Korotkoff's sounds and obtain a valid measure of the patient's blood pressure. Rates faster than 2-3 mm Hg will tend to increase the measurement error of the obtained readings. (Pierson p. 59)

25. Correct Answer: 2
Explanation: The axis of the goniometer should be positioned over the center of the cranial aspect of the head. The stationary arm should be parallel to an imaginary line between the two acromial processes, while the moving arm should be aligned with the tip of the nose. (Norkin p. 324)

26. Correct Answer: 4
Explanation: Anthropometric measurements can be used to quantify muscle atrophy and edema, however, are not used to examine strength. (Guide to Physical Therapist Practice p. 50)

27. Correct Answer: 4
Explanation: Vital capacity equals the sum of inspiratory reserve volume, tidal volume, and expiratory reserve volume. (Brannon p. 293)

28. Correct Answer: 1
Explanation: A foraminal compression test or Spurling's test is considered to be positive if pain radiates into the arm toward the side of head flexion during compression. The provocative test can be administered in progressive stages. (Magee p. 145)

29. Correct Answer: 3
Explanation: Altered mental status and elevated skin temperature are classic signs associated with heat stroke. Heat stroke is a medical emergency that can result in death. Treatment should focus on attempting to rapidly cool the victim. (Anderson p. 540)

30. Correct Answer: 3
Explanation: A decrease in systolic pressure of greater than or equal to 15 mm Hg exceeds the typical limits associated with a phase I cardiac rehabilitation program. Since the patient's systolic blood pressure decreased by 20 mm Hg, this would be the correct response. (Brannon p. 4)

31. Correct Answer: 3
Explanation: In order to determine if the patient's poor attendance in therapy is due to difficulty understanding the scheduling card, the information must be presented in a manner the patient can understand. (Shepard p. 426)

32. Correct Answer: 1
Explanation: TLSOs limit mobility in the thoracolumbar spine. The orthosis is aimed at forcing the spine into a slightly hyperextended alignment, thereby unloading the vertebral bodies. Limiting thoracic flexion would be the most critical since the patient's fracture is in the lower thoracic spine. TLSOs are sometimes referred to as a "Jewett brace." (Seymour p. 438)

33. Correct Answer: 3
Explanation: The therapist should not alter the patient's weight bearing status without prior physician approval. (Guide for Professional Conduct)

34. Correct Answer: 4
Explanation: A nasogastric tube is a plastic tube that enters the body through a nostril and terminates in a patient's stomach. As a result the tube is not used for obtaining venous samples. (Pierson p. 286)

35. Correct Answer: 2
Explanation: Carpometacarpal flexion occurs in a frontal plane around an anterior-posterior axis with the patient in the anatomical position. (Norkin p. 160)

36. Correct Answer: 2
Explanation: Post-polio syndrome is a term used to describe symptoms that occur years after the onset of poliomyelitis. The condition is believed to result as remaining motor units become more dysfunctional. Sensation is typically not affected by post-polio syndrome. (Goodman - Pathology p. 1161)

37. Correct Answer: 2
Explanation: Patients with Parkinson's disease often exhibit gait abnormalities due to difficulty initiating movement, rigidity, absence of equilibrium responses, and diminished associated reactions. (Paz p. 321)

38. Correct Answer: 2
Explanation: "Try to utilize your own strength to complete the transfer" is a direct statement that expresses the therapist's desire for the patient to demonstrate greater independence with the transfer. The statement provides the patient with clear expectations surrounding the desired outcome without creating a fictitious scenario. (Purtilo p. 167)

39. Correct Answer: 1
Explanation: Clips often provide poor anchors and can cut the skin. Safety pins are also of questionable value, however, are not as dangerous as clips. Tape is the preferred method of securing the bandage. (Seymour p. 132)

40. Correct Answer: 1
Explanation: Conventional TENS utilizes a pulse rate of 50-150 pps, short pulse or phase duration, and low intensity to deliver sensory-level stimulation. (Robinson p. 285)

41. Correct Answer: 3
Explanation: Patients can experience itching or skin irritation as a result of a reaction to a liner of an orthosis. Since an orthosis is applied directly over the skin it is imperative to utilize a liner that maximizes patient comfort, promotes cleanliness, limits moisture, and reduces skin irritation. Failure to select an appropriate liner may result in skin breakdown or voluntary discontinuance of the orthosis. (Physical Therapist's Clinical Companion p. 316)

42. Correct Answer: 3
Explanation: Approximate normal ranges for cholesterol are as follows: cholesterol < 200 mg/dL, high-density lipoproteins = 30-80 mg/dL, low-density lipoproteins = 60-180 mg/dL. (American Heart Association p. 54)

43. Correct Answer: 4
Explanation: The lower lobes should be examined with the patient's back towards the physical therapist. The therapist positions their hands around the anterior axillary fold and draws the skin medially until the thumbs meet. The patient should be instructed to inspire once. The hand movement during inspiration is examined and recorded. (Frownfelter p. 224)

44. Correct Answer: 1
Explanation: Pronation of the foot consists of eversion of the heel, abduction of the forefoot, and dorsiflexion of the subtalar and midtarsal joints. (Anderson p. 494)

45. Correct Answer: 3
Explanation: Failure to have a patient examined by a physician after a fall can be considered a negligent act. In many facilities an incident report is required when a patient comes in contact with the floor. (Scott - Promoting Legal Awareness p. 88)

46. Correct Answer: 1
Explanation: All skinfold measurements should be taken on the right side of the body. Acceptable skinfold sites include the abdominal, biceps, chest/pectoral, medial calf, midaxillary, subscapular, suprailiac, and thigh. The abdominal skinfold site requires the therapist to utilize a vertical fold. (American College of Sports Medicine p. 65)

47. Correct Answer: 1
Explanation: The infraspinatus functions as a lateral rotator of the shoulder and is innervated by the suprascapular nerve. (Kendall p. 281)

48. Correct Answer: 4   *Item Includes Graphic*
Explanation: In order to assess the strength of the lateral rotators the physical therapist should apply pressure to the medial side of the leg above the ankle, pushing the leg outward in an attempt to rotate the thigh medially. The hip lateral rotators include the gluteus maximus, obturator internus, obturator externus, quadratus femoris, piriformis, gemellus superior, gemellus inferior, sartorius, and posterior portion of the gluteus medius. (Magee p. 219)

49. Correct Answer: 2
Explanation: A burn to the area surrounding the heel often results in a plantar flexion contracture. Special care must be taken to stretch the ankle into dorsiflexion to avoid a plantar flexion contracture. (O'Sullivan p. 861)

50. Correct Answer: 3
Explanation: Medicaid is a program that provides medical and health related services to qualifying individuals and families with low income and resources. Medicaid is a joint venture between the Federal and State governments. Medicaid offers a broad range of services, however, low product reimbursement rates makes it difficult for many Medicaid recipients to secure a primary care provider. (Nosse p. 168)

Paper and Pencil Exam Two – Section Two

51. Correct Answer: 4
Explanation: The elbow is not typically in direct contact with a given component of a wheelchair and is therefore not likely to be the site of a pressure ulcer. (Pierson p. 89)

52. Correct Answer: 1
Explanation: An adolescent with a moderate scoliotic curve should be referred to a physician for further assessment. (Guide for Professional Conduct)

53. Correct Answer: 3
Explanation: Patients in the confused-agitated stage have a short attention span and therefore require numerous activities. (O'Sullivan p. 800)

54. Correct Answer: 1
Explanation: Hot packs should be stored in water that is approximately 160 degrees Fahrenheit or 71 degrees Celsius. (Michlovitz p. 116)

55. Correct Answer: 4
Explanation: Therapists have an obligation to obtain informed consent from patients prior to initiating intervention activities. If a patient is under the age of 18 the therapist is required to obtain informed consent from the patient and a parent or legal guardian. (Scott - Foundations p. 188)

56. Correct Answer: 2
Explanation: By maintaining the foot in a plantar flexed position the anterior talofibular ligament is positioned perpendicular to the long axis of the tibia. The therapist should stabilize the tibia and fibula while maintaining the test position and draw the talus forward in the ankle mortise. (Magee p. 801)

57. Correct Answer: 4
Explanation: The therapist should not provide additional services when he/she believes the patient will no longer benefit from therapy. (Guide for Professional Conduct)

58. Correct Answer: 2
Explanation: The Bruininks-Oseretsky Motor Development Scale is a standardized test of developmental gross and fine motor skills. The test is designed to be administered to children 4.5 - 14.5 years of age who appear to have motor problems not related to obvious dysfunction. The test takes approximately 45 minutes to administer. (Van Deusen p. 381)

59. Correct Answer: 2
Explanation: A patient interview provides a physical therapist with an opportunity to assess patient cognition. This approach is often more appropriate than relying on a previous entry in the medical record, particularly with a patient status post surgery. (Bickley p. 23)

60. Correct Answer: 4
Explanation: Splinting in the position of elbow extension and slight forearm supination will effectively limit contractures and maximize functional use of the upper extremity. (O'Sullivan p. 861)

61. Correct Answer: 2
Explanation: A lightweight wheelchair will be significantly easier for the patient to propel and maneuver, while a rigid frame provides the necessary durability and strength required for an active individual. (Physical Therapist's Clinical Companion p. 324)

62. Correct Answer: 4
Explanation: A walker would be the most appropriate assistive device to use since the patient can stand without support, however, has only fair standing balance and is impulsive at times. A walker does not require a great deal of coordination. (Pierson p. 217)

63. Correct Answer: 1
Explanation: Capitation is defined as a fixed payment to a provider per enrollee. Managed care organizations utilize capitation to shift some of the financial risk toward individual providers. (Nosse p. 134)

64. Correct Answer: 2
Explanation: The Lachman test is perhaps the most common ligamentous instability test designed to assess the integrity of the anterior cruciate ligament. It is most commonly performed with the patient in a supine position and the knee flexed 20-30 degrees. (Magee p. 699)

65. Correct Answer: 3
Explanation: Initial contact refers to the instant the foot of the leading extremity hits the ground. (Levangie p. 443)

66. Correct Answer: 2
Explanation: Dysmetria is an inability to modulate movement where patients will either overestimate or underestimate their targets. Dysmetria is a common clinical finding with cerebellar dysfunction. (Umphred p. 722)

67. Correct Answer: 3
Explanation: A restriction in the posterior capsule may lead to anterior and superior translation of the humeral head. As a result, it is often advisable to incorporate posterior capsule stretching into the treatment program. (Brotzman p. 94)

68. Correct Answer: 4
Explanation: The question "What do you hope to achieve in physical therapy?" is an open-ended question that presents the patient with a myriad of possible responses. (Goodman – Differential Diagnosis p. 38)

69. Correct Answer: 3
Explanation: The majority of rotator cuff tears occurs in individuals greater than 40 years of age with a history of recurrent shoulder symptoms. A large tear is typically considered to be between 3-5 cm in diameter and most often requires 24-28 weeks of rehabilitation before a patient is allowed to return to full activity without restrictions. (Brotzman p. 100)

70. Correct Answer: 3
Explanation: The QRS complex reflects the electrical activity of the ventricles during the cardiac cycle. If the physical therapist identifies eight QRS complexes in a six second interval, the therapist should multiply the number by ten to determine the patient's heart rate. (Brannon p. 193)

71. Correct Answer: 1
Explanation: A bandage is used to secure the underlying dressing and therefore does not come in direct contact with the wound. (Pierson p. 306)

72. Correct Answer: 1
Explanation: A patient with moderate dementia cannot live independently without assistance and frequent supervision. Without adequate support the patient's safety is jeopardized. (Bickley p. 552)

73. Correct Answer: 4
Explanation: Guillain-Barre is an acute polyneuropathy causing rapid, progressive loss of motor function. Although mild sensory loss can be evident, absent sensation is extremely rare. (Paz p. 320)

74. Correct Answer: 4
Explanation: During expiration wheezes are often indicative of narrowed airways or an airway obstruction. This condition is most commonly associated with asthma or bronchitis. (Bickley p. 228)

75. Correct Answer: 3
Explanation: Lidocaine is a local anesthetic that can be utilized with iontophoresis. The primary treatment objective when utilizing lidocaine is to decrease pain and inflammation. (Ciccone p. 157)

76. Correct Answer: 1
Explanation: Since the patient does not have unilateral weakness it is most appropriate to ascend the stairs on the right. In addition, the normal flow of traffic assumes ascending on the right and descending on the left. This necessitates holding the canes with the left hand and grasping the handrail with the right. (Minor p. 308)

77. Correct Answer: 4
Explanation: Decorticate posturing is characterized by abnormal flexor responses in the upper extremity and extensor responses in the lower extremities. The posture is usually indicative of a lesion at or above the upper brainstem. (Goodman - Pathology p. 1078)

78. Correct Answer: 2
Explanation: The positive support reflex promotes extension of the lower extremities and trunk with weight bearing through the balls of the feet. The reflex normally integrates at two months of age. (Ratliffe p. 27)

79. Correct Answer: 1
Explanation: Grade I or II oscillation or slow intermittent grade I or II sustained joint distraction are primarily utilized for pain. (Kisner p. 224)

80. Correct Answer: 1
Explanation: Direct current is necessary to ensure a unidirectional flow of ions. (Robinson p. 340)

81. Correct Answer: 1
Explanation: A study performed by Henning et al. examined anterior cruciate stresses and elongation during functional and rehabilitative activities. The researchers concluded that the proper order of a rehabilitation program with regard to anterior cruciate ligament stress should be the following: crutch walking, stationary cycling, walking, slow running on level surface, faster running on level surface. (Brotzman p. 188)

82. Correct Answer: 4
Explanation: Oxygen saturation rate refers to the percentage of oxygen bound to hemoglobin in the blood. Normal oxygen saturation rates range from 95-98%. (Brannon p. 64)

83. Correct Answer: 3
Explanation: The patient's goal of walking one mile each day does not warrant continued physical therapy services. Physical therapists should avoid overutilization of physical therapy services, however, should assist patients to achieve individual goals through activities such as a home exercise program. (Guide for Professional Conduct)

84. Correct Answer: 3
Explanation: Lateral hamstrings reflex (S1-S2), medial hamstrings reflex (L5-S1), patellar reflex (L3-L4), Achilles reflex (S1-S2). (Magee p. 529)

85. Correct Answer: 1
Explanation: A physical therapist is qualified to instruct and assist a patient with transfers to all surfaces. The therapist should perform tub transfers with the patient so that independence is attained as soon as possible. (Guide to Physical Therapist Practice p. 34)

86. Correct Answer: 4
Explanation: During a D1 extension pattern there is scapular depression, adduction, and downward rotation. The pectoralis minor assists with both depression and downward rotation. The rhomboids assist with adduction and downward rotation, while the levator scapulae assists with downward rotation. (Kisner p. 114)

87. Correct Answer: 1
Explanation: The frequency of physical therapy visits should be based on the results of the patient examination, and not solely on the physician referral. (Guide for Professional Conduct)

88. Correct Answer: 4
Explanation: Methotrexate is used as a disease-modifying agent in the treatment of rheumatoid arthritis. Adverse effects include nausea, gastrointestinal distress and/or hemorrhage, cough, shortness of breath, and lower extremity edema. Although nausea is not a medical emergency, it is appropriate for the patient to inform the physician of any persistent side effects as soon as possible. (Ciccone p. 236)

89. Correct Answer: 4
Explanation: A physical therapist must make a patient aware of behavior that is unacceptable. Failure to address the issue directly with the patient may serve to reinforce the behavior. (Purtilo p. 230)

90. Correct Answer: 3
Explanation: Age-predicted maximal heart rate can be determined as follows: 220 – patient's age (34) = 186. (Minor p. 39)

91. Correct Answer: 2
Explanation: A drop in the pelvis on the left during right stance phase is often indicative of right gluteus medius weakness. This type of deviation is termed a Trendelenburg gait pattern. (Hertling p. 292)

92. Correct Answer: 1
Explanation: Athetosis is a term used to describe slow, writhing, and involuntary movements that may occur with damage to the basal ganglia. (Goodman - Pathology p. 1047)

93. Correct Answer: 3
Explanation: Superficial reflexes are tested with some form of noxious stimuli. An example of this is the method of testing for the Babinski reflex. (O'Sullivan p. 185)

94. Correct Answer: 3
Explanation: A cervical rib that arises from the seventh cervical vertebra often compresses the inferior trunk of the brachial plexus and the subclavian artery. Adson's test may be useful in confirming the diagnosis of cervical rib syndrome. Additional findings include weakness and atrophy of intrinsic hand muscles and sensory alterations in the hand and forearm. (Anderson p. 302)

95. Correct Answer: 4
Explanation: Raimiste's phenomenon is an associated reaction that is considered a form of overflow or irradiation. (O'Sullivan p. 532)

96. Correct Answer: 2
Explanation: The Guide for Professional Conduct states that physical therapists seek remuneration for their services that is deserved and reasonable. Despite the fact the presented information indicates the physician may be inappropriate with his/her referrals, the most appropriate immediate response should be to discuss the situation directly with the physician. (Guide for Professional Conduct)

97. Correct Answer: 1
Explanation: Infants develop the stability necessary to sit with hand support for extended periods of time in the sixth or seventh month. (Ratliffe p. 46)

98. Correct Answer: 2
    Explanation: The uninvolved extremity leads when ascending stairs and the involved extremity leads when descending. (Pierson p. 256)

99. Correct Answer: 4
    Explanation: Trochanteric bursitis refers to inflammation of the trochanteric bursa, which is a pad-like sac that protects the soft tissue structures that cross the posterior portion of the greater trochanter. The condition can be differentiated from piriformis syndrome due to the lateral thigh pain and absence of radiating pain down the leg. (Goodman – Differential Diagnosis p. 438)

100. Correct Answer: 2
    Explanation: Mechanoreceptors generate information related to discriminative sensations. The information is then mediated through the dorsal column-medial lemniscal system. Examples of mechanoreceptors include free nerve endings, Merkel's disks, Ruffini endings, and Pacinian corpuscles. (O'Sullivan p. 139)

Paper and Pencil Exam Two – Section Three

101. Correct Answer: 2
    Explanation: Active movement requires direct patient participation. (Magee p. 23)

102. Correct Answer: 3
    Explanation: The physical therapist should utilize a female to serve as an observer. This type of action is a form of risk management in order to prevent allegations of alleged misconduct. (Scott - Promoting Legal Awareness p. 104)

103. Correct Answer: 4
    Explanation: Although each of the presented options is important, maintaining accurate and timely documentation is the most important. Documentation often provides the primary evidence of what transpired during a given treatment session. The information is often utilized during litigation to determine if patient care standards were compromised. (Scott - Promoting Legal Awareness p. 66)

104. Correct Answer: 4
    Explanation: The most appropriate response is to refer the patient to a qualified physician. This action will allow the patient to receive a thorough examination, and if indicated, a referral to physical therapy. (Guide for Professional Conduct)

105. Correct Answer: 2
    Explanation: The Q angle is defined as the angle between the quadriceps muscles and the patellar tendon. Normal Q angle values are 13 degrees for males and 18 degrees for females. (Hertling p. 328)

106. Correct Answer: 1
    Explanation: An acute burn produces hypermetabolism and therefore results in increased oxygen consumption, increased minute ventilation, and increased core temperature. Intravascular, interstitial, and intracellular fluids are all diminished. (Paz p. 465)

107. Correct Answer: 4
    Explanation: In order to adequately address the patient's subjective report of pain, it is essential to gather additional information. (Magee p. 3)

108. Correct Answer: 1
    Explanation: Respiratory acidosis is characterized by elevated $PaCO_2$ and below normal pH due to hypoventilation. An arterial blood gas analysis includes the following:
    PaO_2 = partial pressure of oxygen in arterial blood
    $PaCO_2$ = partial pressure of carbon dioxide in arterial blood
    pH = the degree of acidity or alkalinity in arterial blood
    HCO_3 = the level of bicarbonate in arterial blood.
    (Paz p. 111)

109. Correct Answer: 4
    Explanation: Gains in strength are greatest when a muscle is exercised against resistance at maximal intensity. (Kisner p. 59)

110. Correct Answer: 3
    Explanation: Atelectasis refers to a collapsed or airless condition of a lobe or segment of a lung. Segmental breathing is a technique that can be used to direct inspired air to a selected area. (Goodman - Pathology p. 599)

111. Correct Answer: 3
    Explanation: A patient with right hemiplegia can compensate for weak hip abductors while side-stepping towards the right by leaning towards the left. This action unweights the right lower extremity and utilizes momentum along with the abductor muscles to perform sidestepping. (O'Sullivan p. 559)

112. Correct Answer: 1
Explanation: The supplied description is the classic position for the anterior segments of the upper lobes. (Rothstein p. 535)

113. Correct Answer: 1
Explanation: The physical therapist should utilize the remaining time to begin the examination. Although the patient may benefit from a home exercise program, it would be inappropriate to design a home exercise program without first completing a thorough examination. (Standards of Practice)

114. Correct Answer: 1
Explanation: A patient that presents with genu recurvatum while ambulating would benefit from increasing the plantar flexion stop of the ankle-foot orthosis. This would serve to prevent plantar flexion after heel strike and subsequently inhibit full extension of the knee during midstance. (Seymour p. 418)

115. Correct Answer: 4
Explanation: Operant conditioning is learning that takes place when the learner recognizes the connection between the behavior (completing an exercise progression) and its consequences (lengthy rest period). (Richard p. 486)

116. Correct Answer: 1
Explanation: Asymmetrical tonic neck reflex interferes with rolling due to the tonal influence of flexion to one side of the body and concurrent extension to the other. (Ratliffe p. 25)

117. Correct Answer: 2
Explanation: Normal hemoglobin values for a male range from 14-18 gm/dL. (American College of Sports Medicine p. 48)

118. Correct Answer: 4
Explanation: Brown-Sequard's syndrome is a spinal cord injury due to a partial or full hemisection of the cord. The syndrome is frequently observed in stab wound victims. (Pauls p. 168)

119. Correct Answer: 1
Explanation: The corticospinal tract carries information from the cerebral cortex to the spinal nerves. The tract's projections are primarily contralateral and have a strong influence on spinal motor neurons that innervate distal muscles. (Bennett p. 20)

120. Correct Answer: 4
Explanation: Emphysema is a disease of the alveoli with associated irreversible lung damage. Breathing exercises directed at increasing the activity of the diaphragm and decreasing the activity of the accessory muscles may influence the efficiency of the patient's breathing pattern. (Frownfelter p. 517)

121. Correct Answer: 2
Explanation: It is not unusual for a patient to experience increased pain at various points during a rehabilitation program. As a result, it is not necessary to discontinue formal treatment or to refer the patient to another health care professional at this time. (Standards of Practice)

122. Correct Answer: 3
Explanation: Although the order of application of the gown and mask may vary, gloves must be the last item to be applied. (Pierson p. 34)

123. Correct Answer: 3
Explanation: The medial collateral ligament, also termed the ulnar collateral ligament, is a fan shaped ligament that serves to restrict medial angulation of the ulna on the humerus. The ligament extends from the medial epicondyle to the medial margin of the ulna's trochlear notch and is assessed for potential instability by applying valgus force to the distal forearm. (Hertling p. 220)

124. Correct Answer: 3
Explanation: When an intravenous line becomes dislodged from a vein it is appropriate to immediately turn off the I.V. in order to prevent further accumulation of fluid. (Pierson p. 287)

125. Correct Answer: 3
Explanation: In addition to flexing the elbow the biceps brachii acts to supinate the forearm. The musculocutaneous nerve innervates the biceps brachii. (Kendall p. 268)

126. Correct Answer: 3
Explanation: A full-thickness burn is characterized by complete destruction of the epidermal and dermal layers of the skin. In addition, some of the subcutaneous tissue is damaged. Grafts are required with full-thickness burns. (Paz p. 449)

127. Correct Answer: 2
Explanation: Short-term tube feeding is often accomplished through the use of a nasogastric tube. A nasogastric tube is inserted through a nostril and terminates in the stomach. (Pierson p. 286)

128. Correct Answer: 1
Explanation: Patients on extended bed rest may experience a significant decrease in systolic blood pressure with vertical positioning. A decrease in systolic blood pressure of 20 mm Hg or more is indicative of orthostatic hypotension. (Pierson p. 336)

129. Correct Answer: 1
Explanation: A partial tear of the ulnar collateral ligament is most often treated with a short-arm thumb spica cast. A long-arm thumb spica cast may be more appropriate for an injury such as a nondisplaced fracture of the scaphoid. (Brotzman p. 57)

130. Correct Answer: 3
Explanation: An ordinal measurement scale allows for the ranking of items or individuals from highest to lowest. The amount of difference between rankings may not be equal. (Domholdt p. 222)

131. Correct Answer: 2
Explanation: The lunate lies in the proximal row immediately distal to Lister's tubercle and proximal to the capitate. Wrist flexion acts to facilitate palpation of the lunate. (Hoppenfeld p. 69)

132. Correct Answer: 2
Explanation: A lesion affecting the sensory cortex often results in numerous impairments including loss of sensation, perception, proprioception, and diminished motor control. (Bennett p. 33)

133. Correct Answer: 2
Explanation: In a normal distribution a known percentage of the population falls between specific standard deviation units. Therefore 68% of the population will fall between plus one and minus one standard deviation units which means that 34% would fall between the mean and one standard deviation above the mean. The question does not require formal computation beyond what is described. (Domholdt p. 287)

134. Correct Answer: 4
Explanation: Patients with very weak pelvic floor muscles should initiate strengthening exercises in a horizontal plane in order to avoid gravity exerting a downward force on the pelvic floor. Although sidelying would be an acceptable position, it is more awkward than the supine position for most patients. Patients should move to more challenging positions as their strength increases. (Hall p. 364)

135. Correct Answer: 3
Explanation: The Berg Balance Scale is used for assessing a patient's risk of falling. The Berg consists of 14 tasks of every day life that are scored according to a 0-4 scale. The maximum total score possible is 56, with a score of less than 45 indicating the patient is at risk for multiple falls. Necessary equipment to administer the Berg includes a stopwatch, two chairs, a ruler, and a step stool. Observation and scoring should take approximately 15-20 minutes. (Physical Therapist's Clinical Companion p. 105)

136. Correct Answer: 3
Explanation: Duchenne muscular dystrophy is a sex-linked disorder characterized by progressive muscular weakness beginning between the ages of two and five. Individuals typically lose the ability to ambulate and are dependent on a wheelchair by age 16. The majority of patients with Duchenne muscular dystrophy die by the end of their teenage years due to respiratory or cardiac failure. The described method of standing upright is termed Gowers' sign. (Ratliffe p. 242)

137. Correct Answer: 2
Explanation: Tachypnea refers to a respiratory rate of greater than 20 breaths per minute. (Paz p. 101)

138. Correct Answer: 1
Explanation: Expiratory reserve volume is defined as the maximal amount of air that can be expired after a normal exhalation. As a result, the measure can be obtained with relative ease using a spirometer. (Physical Therapist's Clinical Companion p. 147)

139. Correct Answer: 3
Explanation: The distal row of carpal bones consists of the trapezium, trapezoid, capitate, and hamate. (Hoppenfeld p. 65)

140. Correct Answer: 4
Explanation: ST segment depression of greater than 1 mm is indicative of ischemia and is often used to confirm the diagnosis of coronary artery disease. (Brannon p. 183)

141. Correct Answer: 2
Explanation: Repeated contractions should be applied at the point where the contraction begins to diminish. The technique utilizes an isometric contraction followed by subsequent manual stretching and resisted isotonic movement. Repeated contractions assist with enhancing motor neuron recruitment and strengthening of a muscle or group of muscles. (Sullivan p. 71)

142. Correct Answer: 4
Explanation: To increase wrist extension, stabilize the radius and glide the scaphoid in a volar direction. The radius is considered to be the concave joint partner and the scaphoid is considered convex. (Kisner p. 241)

143. Correct Answer: 2
Explanation: Rehabilitation following a burn can be extremely painful. Scheduling treatment sessions to coincide with the patient's pain medication schedule may reduce the patient's pain without compromising the established plan of care. (Paz p. 463)

144. Correct Answer: 1
Explanation: Intermittent claudication occurs as a result of insufficient blood supply and ischemia in active muscles. The condition occurs with activity and subsides during periods of rest and as a result can serve to limit the duration of exercise activities. Symptoms most commonly include pain and cramping distal to the occluded vessel. (Kisner p. 710)

145. Correct Answer: 2
Explanation: Oxygen saturation at rest is considered to be within normal limits between 95-98%. A rate of 90% or less is often used as a guideline to discontinue exercise activities. Supplemental oxygen may be indicated if oxygen saturation is 90% or less. (Paz p. 770)

146. Correct Answer: 2
Explanation: L5 nerve root:
    dermatome - buttock, posterior and lateral thigh, lateral aspect of leg, dorsum of foot, medial half of sole, first, second, and third toes
    myotome - extensor hallucis, peroneals, gluteus medius, dorsiflexors, hamstrings, soleus, plantaris
    reflexes - medial hamstrings, posterior tibial
(Magee p. 16)

147. Correct Answer: 1
Explanation: Prone lying is a commonly employed positional technique designed to stretch the hip flexors. Increased flexibility of the hip flexors will improve standing posture and enable the body's center of gravity to remain within the base of support. Although some of the other options are appropriate, they would not provide the same degree of benefit for the patient. (Umphred p. 675)

148. Correct Answer: 1
Explanation: The hip is a ball and socket joint whose capsular pattern is represented by a restriction in flexion, abduction, and medial rotation. (Magee p. 607)

149. Correct Answer: 3
Explanation: A suprapubic catheter is an indwelling urinary catheter that is surgically inserted directly into the patient's bladder. (Pierson p. 289)

150. Correct Answer: 4
Explanation: The saphenous vein is a superficial vein that extends from the foot to the saphenous opening. The antecubital, basilic, and cephalic vein are located in the upper extremity. (Pierson p. 287)

Paper and Pencil Exam Two – Section Four

151. Correct Answer: 2
Explanation: The appropriate wheelchair for a patient with C5 tetraplegia is a manual chair with handrim projections. The projections should be angled at 30 degrees during the training period to assist with propulsion. (Rothstein p. 475)

152. Correct Answer: 2
Explanation: Vitamin A is a fat soluble vitamin essential for functions such as bone growth, maintenance of body linings, and vision. Vitamin A is found in animal products such as butter, milk, liver, egg yolks, and in dark green, deep orange, and yellow vegetables. (Hamilton p. 224)

153. Correct Answer: 2
Explanation: Military time operates on the premise that 2400 hours is equivalent to 12:00 AM and 1200 hours is equivalent to 12:00 PM. 8:00 AM or 0800 is nine hours after 11:00 PM or 2300 hours. (Scott-Legal Aspects p. 1666)

154. Correct Answer: 2
Explanation: The aortic valve is located at the junction of the left ventricle and the ascending aorta. The aortic valve prevents regurgitation at the entrance of the aorta to the heart. (Rothstein p. 621)

155. Correct Answer: 1
Explanation: To perform bronchial drainage to the anterior segments of the upper lobes the physical therapist should clap between the clavicle and nipple on each side with the patient positioned in supine. (Rothstein p. 535)

156. Correct Answer: 2
Explanation: Energy expenditure expressed in the form of calories can be estimated using weight and oxygen consumption. (Rothstein p. 664)

157. Correct Answer: 1
Explanation: Forefoot varus refers to an inverted position of the forefoot in relationship to the rearfoot with the subtalar joint in a neutral position. (Brotzman p. 354)

158. Correct Answer: 1
Explanation: A patient with a traumatic brain injury that is disoriented will benefit from establishing contact with the physical therapist in familiar surroundings. Although the private treatment room would eliminate external stimuli, the patient is likely to be unfamiliar with the environment and therefore may become further disoriented or agitated. (Campbell, M. p. 210)

159. Correct Answer: 3   ***Item Includes Graphic***
Explanation: Extension of the right knee is an indication that the patient has tightness in the two-joint rectus femoris muscle. A patient without tightness in the rectus femoris would typically present with the knee in 90 degrees of flexion while maintaining the position. (Magee p. 631)

160. Correct Answer: 4
Explanation: Systolic pressure gradually increases as exercise intensity increases, however, diastolic pressure remains relatively stable. (Pierson p. 57)

161. Correct Answer: 4
Explanation: Discoloration of the patient's toes may be an indication that the cast is too tight and may be impeding the patient's circulation. Since the cast is bivalved, the cast can be easily removed by the physical therapist. (O'Sullivan p. 806)

162. Correct Answer: 3
Explanation: A patient at the confused-inappropriate level often exhibits inappropriate verbal output, poor memory, and difficulty performing new tasks. Physical therapy intervention may focus on following directions and goal-oriented tasks. (Rothstein p. 450)

163. Correct Answer: 2
Explanation: A three-point gait pattern can be used when a patient is able to bear weight on one lower extremity, but is non-weight bearing on the other. The gait pattern requires good upper extremity strength and the use of crutches or a walker. A swing-to gait pattern infers bilateral lower extremity weakness requiring the extremities to be advanced simultaneously. (Pierson p. 233)

164. Correct Answer: 4
Explanation: The elbow complex consists of the ulnohumeral, radiohumeral, and proximal radioulnar joint. Each of the joints is affected by swelling in the elbow complex. (Gross p. 182)

165. Correct Answer: 1
Explanation: Pusher syndrome is characterized by a significant lateral deviation toward the hemiplegic side in all positions. A patient with left hemiplegia would exhibit a lateral lean to the left in sitting with increased weight bearing on the left buttock. Pusher syndrome is most common in patients with right cerebrovascular accidents and left hemiplegia. (O'Sullivan p. 535)

166. Correct Answer: 1
Explanation: The distal end of the humerus should be stabilized when measuring elbow flexion. Failure to adequately stabilize the humerus permits shoulder flexion. (Norkin p. 72)

167. Correct Answer: 3
Explanation: A mandatory inservice would enable the physical therapists to provide a formal educational session on guarding techniques for the aides. (Scott – Legal Aspects p. 6)

168. Correct Answer: 3
Explanation: Passive range of motion provides a physical therapist with information on the integrity of the articular surfaces and the extensibility of the joint capsule and associated ligaments. Passive range of motion is independent of a patient's strength. (Norkin p. 7)

169. Correct Answer: 1
Explanation: When ascending a curb a patient should lead with the uninvolved lower extremity in order to avoid placing unnecessary force on the involved extremity. (Minor p. 309)

170. Correct Answer: 2
Explanation: A hydraulic lift can be a safe and efficient mode to transfer large and/or dependent patients with little physical exertion. (Pierson p. 156)

171. Correct Answer: 1
Explanation: The tibialis anterior acts to dorsiflex the ankle joint and assists in inversion of the foot. During muscle testing, pressure should be applied against the medial side of the dorsal surface of the foot, in the direction of plantar flexion of the ankle joint and eversion of the foot. (Kendall p. 201)

172. Correct Answer: 1
Explanation: The iliotibial band is a thickened strip of fascia that extends from the iliac crest to the lateral tibial tubercle. Activities requiring frequent flexion of the knee can produce an inflammatory reaction that occurs due to excessive contact between the iliotibial band and the lateral femoral condyle. Management of the condition often requires techniques for reducing inflammation and iliotibial band stretching. (Brotzman p. 225)

173. Correct Answer: 4
Explanation: Eccentric contraction of the gastrocnemius and soleus complex places the greatest amount of stress on the Achilles tendon. Running on an incline or pushing off to accelerate while weight bearing are two examples of activities that produces this type of contraction. Although these activities place a significant amount of stress on the Achilles tendon, they are a necessary component of a rehabilitation program designed to return an individual to athletic competition. (Brotzman p. 267)

174. Correct Answer: 1
Explanation: The Barthel Index demonstrates limited sensitivity for individuals with mild disabilities since it does not record improvement in a patient's functional status until he/she reaches a specified level of independence. (Physical Therapist's Clinical Companion p. 104)

175. Correct Answer: 1
Explanation: Subtalar eversion is a common compensatory finding in patients with forefoot varus. This position of the rearfoot allows the medial forefoot to come in contact with the ground, however, can lead to hypermobility in the foot and a loss of the necessary rigid lever from midstance through toe off. (Brotzman p. 354)

176. Correct Answer: 1
Explanation: The glenohumeral joint consists of the concave glenoid fossa and the convex humeral head. An anterior glide of the humeral head is indicated to increase lateral rotation. (Kisner p. 232)

177. Correct Answer: 1
Explanation: A patient with a traumatic brain injury functioning at Rancho Los Amigos level VI confused-appropriate typically demonstrates goal-directed behavior and is able to follow simple commands fairly consistently. Since the patient is no longer agitated, the verbal outburst would be considered an atypical event and therefore warrants direct contact with the physical therapist. (O'Sullivan p. 802)

178. Correct Answer: 3
Explanation: When descending a curb using a forward approach, the wheelchair must remain tipped backward until the rear wheels are in contact with the surface below the curb. (Pierson p. 193)

179. Correct Answer: 4
Explanation: The rectus femoris is a two-joint muscle that acts to flex the hip and extend the knee. Passively flexing the hip and knee of the contralateral lower extremity effectively serves to stabilize the pelvis. (Kisner p. 207)

180. Correct Answer: 2
Explanation: A quad cane should be utilized in the upper extremity that is opposite from the affected lower extremity. The device is designed so that the longer legs are positioned away from the patient. (Minor p. 405)

181. Correct Answer: 4
Explanation: An Individualized Education Plan articulates the goals and objectives of special education services for a given school aged child. The plan is for a one year period. (Tecklin p. 564)

182. Correct Answer: 2
Explanation: A patient report of a slight burning sensation under the soundhead can be due to inadequate coupling, loosening of the crystal or hot spots due to a high beam nonuniformity ratio. (Michlovitz p. 198)

183. Correct Answer: 4
Explanation: A phase II cardiac rehabilitation program begins with the completion of a low-level treadmill test and ends with a maximal treadmill test. (Hillegass p. 701)

184. Correct Answer: 1
Explanation: Boutonniere deformity is most frequently encountered in patients with rheumatoid arthritis or status post trauma. It is caused by damage to the central tendinous slip of the extensor hood. (Magee p. 364)

185. Correct Answer: 4
Explanation: Clinical union provides the necessary bony support to terminate external fixation. Callus formation represents the first stage in which bony union occurs, however, does not offer adequate support. (Brotzman p. 176)

186. Correct Answer: 3
Explanation: Ankylosing spondylitis is a form of rheumatic disease characterized by inflammation of the spine resulting in back pain. Patients with ankylosing spondylitis often exhibit postural changes such as forward head, increased thoracic kyphosis, and loss of lumbar curvature. Spinal extension exercises are a common component of a therapeutic exercise program for patients with this condition. (Goodman - Pathology p. 959)

187. Correct Answer: 4
Explanation: It is an appropriate action to request additional physical therapy visits from a referring physician. (Standards of Practice)

188. Correct Answer: 3
Explanation: Full shoulder medial rotation is necessary to reach the perineum. (Magee p. 237)

189. Correct Answer: 3
Explanation: Any change in the color or odor of urine is significant and should therefore be reported and documented. A nurse would be the most logical health care professional to initially receive this information. (Pierson p. 289)

190. Correct Answer: 2
Explanation: Productivity is a term used to describe the efficiency of a given worker or group of workers. Although measures of quality are often examined concurrently they are not used to determine productivity. (Nosse p. 62)

191. Correct Answer: 2
Explanation: Gravity eliminated testing positions are indicated when a patient cannot maintain the test position against the resistance of gravity. The gravity eliminated position for the hip flexors is sidelying. (Kendall p. 215)

192. Correct Answer: 1
Explanation: The biceps femoris muscle acts to flex and laterally rotate the knee joint and is innervated by the peroneal and tibial portions of the sciatic nerve. (Kendall p. 209)

193. Correct Answer: 2   *Item Includes Graphic*
Explanation: The semitendinosus and biceps femoris are hamstrings muscles whose tendons become prominent when performing a leg curl. The biceps femoris is the lateral tendon, while the semitendinosus is the medial tendon. The semimembranosus is also a medial hamstrings muscle, however, the muscle's tendon is not nearly as prominent. (Kendall p. 208)

194. Correct Answer: 3
Explanation: Extension of the thumb causes the borders of the anatomical snuffbox to become more prominent and as a result can be used as a method to identify the exact location of the scaphoid. Extension of the thumb occurs in a frontal plane around an anterior-posterior axis. Passive ulnar deviation of the wrist can also be utilized to facilitate palpation since the action serves to move the scaphoid out from under the radial styloid process. (Hoppenfeld p. 66)

195. Correct Answer: 3
Explanation: The gluteus maximus extends the hip. The medius and minimus are responsible for abduction and medial rotation of the hip. (Hall p. 391)

196. Correct Answer: 1
Explanation: An incident report is a factual written summary of an adverse event designed to memorialize specific details of the event and to limit future liability of the organization. Information obtained from the incident report is often used to guide risk management initiatives. Since the physical therapist directly observed the blistered skin and heard the patient relate the cause of the burn to the hot pack it is essential to complete an incident report. (Scott – Promoting Legal Awareness p. 69)

197. Correct Answer: 2
Explanation: The American College of Sports Medicine recommends prescribing the intensity of exercise as 60 to 90% of maximum heart rate or 50-85% of $VO_{2\,max}$ or heart rate reserve. The heart rate reserve method (Karvonen formula) is determined as follows:

Target heart rate range = $[(HR_{max} - HR_{rest}) * 0.60$ and $0.85] + HR_{rest}$

(American College of Sports Medicine p. 189)

198. Correct Answer: 3
Explanation: Varying the order of an exercise program is a common technique to avoid stagnation. Other listed options may change the focus of the exercise program or fail to address the patient's frustration in an appropriate manner. (Prentice-Techniques p. 379)

199. Correct Answer: 2
Explanation: Intact sensation along with the absence of tone allows for a plastic orthosis with an articulating ankle joint. This type of orthosis allows for a more normal gait pattern. Despite significant strength deficits in the ankle an articulating ankle-foot orthosis would still restrict motion into plantar flexion while allowing movement into dorsiflexion. (Seymour p. 382)

200. Correct Answer: 2
Explanation: Controlled mobility activities should emphasize weight shifting and trunk control with rotation. This type of activity may serve to decrease rigidity and improve the fluidity of gait in a patient with Parkinson's disease. (O'Sullivan p. 164)

Unit Six

Computer-Based Examinations

The section contains two, 200 question sample examinations located on a CD-ROM attached to the inside of the back cover of the text. The sample examinations provide candidates with additional opportunities for self-assessment and allow candidates to gain confidence when using a computer-based testing format. The sample examinations on the CD-ROM are weighted according to selected specifications of the current Physical Therapy Content Outline.

A sophisticated performance analysis section enables candidates to view their performance according to specific content outline and clinical practice areas. The performance analysis summary offers candidates detailed feedback on their examination performance according to nine clinical practice and four content outline areas.

Clinical Practice
Musculoskeletal
Neuromuscular
Cardiopulmonary
Integumentary
Patient Care Skills
Physical Agents
Education
Administration
Research

Content Outline
Examination
Evaluation, Diagnosis, Prognosis, and Outcomes
Intervention
Standards of Care

An answer key located in this section includes the correct answer, an explanation supporting the correct answer, a cited resource with page number, and the clinical practice and content outline area. Candidates should attempt to integrate this information in conjunction with the performance analysis summary to accurately identify current strengths and weaknesses and develop appropriate remedial strategies. The computer-based examinations include a number of helpful tools to assist candidates to integrate this information including an option to print the specific questions that were answered incorrectly.

Candidates should closely examine their scores on each of the full-length sample examinations in order to assess their preparedness for the actual examination. If candidates have been diligent in addressing identified deficits and implementing remedial strategies from previous sample examinations it is anticipated that their examination scores should exhibit an upward trend. Ideally, candidates should answer 80% or more of the questions correctly on each of the computer-based sample examinations.

EXAM ONE: COMPUTER-BASED
Answer Key

Computer-Based Exam One – Section One

Question Number: 1

A physical therapist reviews the medical record of a patient with a spinal cord injury. A note recently entered by the physician indicates that the patient contracted a respiratory infection. Which patient would be most susceptible to this condition?

1. **a patient with complete C4 tetraplegia**
2. a patient with a cauda equina lesion
3. a patient with Brown-Sequard's syndrome
4. a patient with posterior cord syndrome

Correct Answer: 1
Explanation: A patient with complete C4 tetraplegia will have a reduced ventilatory capacity due to muscle paralysis. This patient will have limited ability to clear secretions, impaired chest mobility, and alveolar hypoventilation. Patients with complete tetraplegia are at the highest risk for respiratory infection. (Umphred p. 499)

Clinical Practice: Neuromuscular System
Content Outline: Evaluation, Diagnosis, Prognosis, and Outcomes

Question Number: 2   *Item Includes Graphic*

A patient rehabilitating from an upper extremity injury uses a latissimus pull-down machine. The therapist specifically instructs the patient to pull the bar down behind their head. This action emphasizes strengthening of the:

1. **rhomboids and middle trapezius**
2. biceps and pectoralis major
3. teres minor and middle trapezius
4. pectoralis major and rhomboids

Correct Answer: 1
Explanation: The rhomboids and middle trapezius both function as strong adductors of the scapula. Adduction of the scapula (retraction) is required in order to complete the latissimus pull-down exercise with the bar positioned behind the subject's head. (Kendall p. 282)

Clinical Practice: Musculoskeletal System
Content Outline: Intervention

Question Number: 3

A physically active 27-year-old male receives pre-operative instruction prior to anterior cruciate ligament reconstruction. The patient's past medical history includes a medial meniscectomy of the contralateral knee eight months ago. The most likely functional level of the patient following rehabilitation is:

1. able to participate in light recreational activities
2. able to participate in all recreational activities
3. able to return to recreational and competitive athletic activities with a derotation brace
4. **able to return to previous functional level**

Correct Answer: 4
Explanation: A physically active, young patient should be expected to return to his previous functional level within 4-6 months following anterior cruciate ligament reconstruction. (Kisner p. 536)

Clinical Practice: Musculoskeletal System
Content Outline: Evaluation, Diagnosis, Prognosis, and Outcomes

Question Number: 4

A physical therapist adjusts the on/off time on an electrical stimulation unit prior to beginning treatment. When using the unit for muscle re-education the most appropriate on:off time ratio is:

1. 5:1
2. 15:1
3. **1:5**
4. 1:15

Correct Answer: 3
Explanation: A duty cycle of 1:5 prevents premature muscle fatigue and allows for adequate periods of muscle stimulation. "On" times are most commonly set at 6-10 seconds, while "off" times are approximately 50-60 seconds. (Robinson p. 142)

Clinical Practice: Physical Agents
Content Outline: Intervention

Question Number: 5
A physical therapist elects to begin a trial of mechanical lumbar traction on a 165 pound male diagnosed with suspected nerve root impingement. The most appropriate amount of force to initiate the session is:

1. 20 lbs.
2. 35 lbs.
3. 60 lbs.
4. 80 lbs.

Correct Answer: 2
Explanation: A traction force of 25-50 lbs. is recommended when initiating mechanical lumbar traction. A force of 50% of the patient's actual body weight may be necessary for mechanical separation of vertebrae in the lumbar spine. (Cameron p. 235)

Clinical Practice: Physical Agents
Content Outline: Intervention

Question Number: 6
A patient in the physical therapy gym suddenly grasps his throat and begins to cough. The physical therapist, recognizing the signs of an airway obstruction should:

1. attempt to ventilate
2. administer abdominal thrusts
3. perform a quick finger sweep of the mouth
4. continue to observe the patient, but do not interfere

Correct Answer: 4
Explanation: Coughing indicates that the airway is not completely obstructed. As a result the physical therapist should continue to monitor the patient, however, should not formally intervene. Usually a patient that is coughing will independently dislodge the object causing the obstruction. (American Heart Association p. 161)

Clinical Practice: Cardiopulmonary System
Content Outline: Standards of Care

Question Number: 7
A physical therapist designs a research study that examines body composition as a function of aerobic exercise and diet. Which method of data collection would provide the therapist with the most valid measurement of body composition?

1. anthropometric measurements
2. bioelectrical impedance
3. hydrostatic weighing
4. skinfold measurements

Correct Answer: 3
Explanation: Hydrostatic weighing is an underwater weighing technique designed to determine the specific gravity of an individual. The technique is considered the most valid measure of body composition. (Anderson p. 33)

Clinical Practice: Musculoskeletal System
Content Outline: Examination

Question Number: 8
A physical therapist prepares for gait training with a patient diagnosed with L3 paraplegia. What type of equipment would be the most appropriate for the treatment session?

1. bilateral hip-knee-ankle-foot orthoses and crutches
2. bilateral knee-ankle-foot orthoses and crutches
3. bilateral ankle-foot orthoses and crutches
4. crutches

Correct Answer: 2
Explanation: A patient with L3 paraplegia would require bilateral knee-ankle-foot orthoses in order to ambulate with crutches. This patient would possess trunk control, hip flexor innervation, and partial quadriceps innervation. Ankle-foot orthoses are indicated for patients with lesions below the level of L3. (Umphred p. 523)

Clinical Practice: Patient Care Skills
Content Outline: Intervention

Question Number: 9

A physical therapist completes a positional assessment of the sacrum with a patient lying in prone. Results of the examination reveal a deep sacral sulcus on the left and a posterior and caudal inferior lateral angle on the left when the patient moves into a prone on elbows position. This finding is most indicative of:

1. bilateral sacral flexion dysfunction
2. bilateral sacral extension dysfunction
3. **unilateral left flexed sacrum**
4. unilateral left extended sacrum

Correct Answer: 3

Explanation: If the inferior lateral angle on the same side as the deep sacral sulcus becomes more caudal in prone on elbows, it may be indicative of a unilateral flexed sacrum. (Hertling p. 710)

Clinical Practice: Musculoskeletal System
Content Outline: Examination

Question Number: 10

A physical therapist instructs a patient that is partial weight bearing on the right lower extremity to ascend stairs using axillary crutches. The therapist's first command should be:

1. place your right leg on the first step
2. place your right leg and left crutch on the first step
3. **place your left leg on the first step**
4. place your left leg and right crutch on the first step

Correct Answer: 3

Explanation: The physical therapist should instruct the patient to step up onto the stair with the uninvolved extremity since it will be used to propel the body upward. (Pierson p. 261)

Clinical Practice: Patient Care Skills
Content Outline: Intervention

Question Number: 11

A physical therapist examines a patient diagnosed with carpal tunnel syndrome. As part of the examination the therapist assesses end-feel. The therapist classifies the end-feel associated with wrist extension as firm. The most logical explanation is:

1. tension in the dorsal radiocarpal ligament and the dorsal joint capsule
2. contact between the ulna and the carpal bones
3. contact between the radius and the carpal bones
4. **tension in the palmar radiocarpal ligament and the palmar joint capsule**

Correct Answer: 4

Explanation: A firm end-feel with wrist extension can result from tension in the palmar radiocarpal ligament and palmar joint capsule, while a hard end-feel results from contact between the radius and the carpal bones. (Norkin p. 122)

Clinical Practice: Musculoskeletal System
Content Outline: Examination

Question Number: 12

A physical therapist is scheduled to administer a whirlpool treatment to a patient that is HIV positive. The therapist is concerned about her ability to complete the treatment since she sustained a small paper cut on her fourth digit approximately three hours ago. The most appropriate therapist action is:

1. refuse to treat the patient and document the rationale in the medical record
2. **treat the patient using appropriate medical asepsis**
3. ask the patient to reschedule their appointment
4. select another appropriate treatment procedure

Correct Answer: 2

Explanation: A physical therapist should always take precautions to prevent the possible transmission of blood or body fluids. By using appropriate medical asepsis the therapist does not place herself or the patient at any significant risk. (Pierson p. 26)

Clinical Practice: Integumentary System
Content Outline: Standards of Care

Question Number: 13
A physical therapist employed in an acute care hospital reviews the medical record of a seven-year-old child. The child has a lengthy medical history that includes a selective dorsal rhizotomy. This surgical procedure is most associated with:

1. **cerebral palsy**
2. Down syndrome
3. muscular dystrophy
4. spina bifida

Correct Answer: 1
Explanation: Selective dorsal rhizotomy is a surgical procedure designed to reduce spasticity in children with cerebral palsy. The surgery selects and divides a number of dorsal rootlets, usually across segments L2-S2, to reduce the influence on spasticity and abnormal movement patterns. (Tecklin p. 140)

Clinical Practice: Neuromuscular System
Content Outline: Examination

Question Number: 14
A physical therapist conducts a test for lower extremity muscle tightness by positioning a patient in supine with his knees bent over the edge of a treatment plinth. The patient is then asked to flex one knee to the chest and hold it. Which clinical finding would be most indicative of shortness in both the one-joint and two-joint hip flexors when assessing the test leg?

1. **25 degrees of hip flexion, 30 degrees of knee flexion**
2. 15 degrees of hip flexion, 40 degrees of knee flexion
3. 20 degrees of hip flexion, 70 degrees of knee flexion
4. 10 degrees of hip flexion, 90 degrees of knee flexion

Correct Answer: 1
Explanation: The amount of hip flexion correlates with tightness of the one-joint hip flexors, while limited knee flexion corresponds to tightness of the two-joint hip flexors. (Magee p. 631)

Clinical Practice: Musculoskeletal System
Content Outline: Examination

Question Number: 15
A group of patients with arthritis completes an established aquatic exercise program. Which member of the health care team would be the most appropriate to supervise the exercise session?

1. a physical therapist with six years of clinical experience
2. a physical therapy aide with continuing education in aquatic exercise
3. a recreational therapist with first aid and cardiopulmonary resuscitation training
4. **a physical therapist assistant certified in water safety instruction**

Correct Answer: 4
Explanation: Physical therapist assistants routinely supervise patients performing "established" exercise programs. In addition, the physical therapist assistant's certification in water safety instruction makes them the most logical candidate to supervise the exercise session. (Guide to Physical Therapist Practice p. 42)

Clinical Practice: Administration
Content Outline: Intervention

Question Number: 16
A physical therapist asks a physical therapist assistant to complete an upper extremity isokinetic test. The assistant is willing to complete the examination, however, indicates it has been quite some time since she has set up the machine. The most appropriate physical therapist action is:

1. provide verbal cueing for the assistant prior to beginning the set up
2. instruct the assistant to refer to the owner's manual
3. **observe the assistant complete the set up**
4. ask another assistant to complete the set up

Correct Answer: 3
Explanation: The most appropriate action would be to observe the assistant complete the set up. This option allows the physical therapist to help the physical therapist assistant as needed and at the same time ensure the set up is performed correctly. By having the physical therapist assistant perform the set up with supervision, it is likely they will be able to perform the activity independently in the future. (Scott - Foundations p. 19)

Clinical Practice: Administration
Content Outline: Intervention

Question Number: 17

A physical therapist examines a patient referred to physical therapy diagnosed with anterior compartment syndrome. The patient presents with an inability to dorsiflex the foot and a mild sensory disturbance between the first and second toes. The nerve most likely involved is the:

1. **deep peroneal nerve**
2. medial plantar nerve
3. tibial nerve
4. lateral plantar nerve

Correct Answer: 1

Explanation: Anterior compartment syndrome often affects the deep peroneal nerve as it passes under the extensor retinaculum. The result of the nerve compression ranges from a mild sensory disturbance to an inability to dorsiflex the foot. (Magee p. 811)

Clinical Practice: Neuromuscular System
Content Outline: Examination

Question Number: 18

A physical therapist examines a patient three days following shoulder surgery. The patient complains of general malaise and reports a slightly elevated body temperature during the last twenty-four hours. Physical examination reveals an edematous shoulder that is warm to the touch. A small amount of yellow fluid is observed seeping from the incision. The most appropriate therapist action is:

1. send the patient to the emergency room
2. **communicate the information to the referring physician**
3. document the findings in the medical record
4. ask the patient to make an appointment with the referring physician

Correct Answer: 2

Explanation: Signs of infection include elevated body temperature, purulent exudate, swelling, edema, and redness. The possibility of infection in a patient three days status post surgery warrants immediate consultation with the referring physician. (Anemaet p. 547)

Clinical Practice: Education/Communication
Content Outline: Intervention

Question Number: 19

A 35-year-old female is admitted to the hospital following a recent illness. Laboratory testing reveals a markedly high platelet count. This finding is typical with:

1. emphysema
2. metabolic acidosis
3. renal failure
4. **malignancy**

Correct Answer: 4

Explanation: Thrombocytosis refers to an increased number of blood platelets. This condition is usually temporary and can occur as a compensatory measure after severe hemorrhage, surgery, iron deficiency, and as a manifestation of an occult neoplasm. (Goodman - Differential Diagnosis p. 188)

Clinical Practice: Cardiopulmonary System
Content Outline: Evaluation, Diagnosis, Prognosis, and Outcomes

Question Number: 20

A physical therapist inspects a patient's wound prior to applying a dressing. When documenting the findings in the medical record the therapist classifies the exudate from the wound as serous. Based on the documentation, the most likely color of the exudate is:

1. **clear**
2. pink
3. red
4. yellow

Correct Answer: 1

Explanation: Serous exudate is described as clear or light color fluid with a thin, watery consistency. This particular type of exudate is normal during the inflammatory and proliferative phases of healing. (Sussman p. 218)

Clinical Practice: Integumentary System
Content Outline: Examination

Question Number: 21
A physical therapist reads in the medical record that a wound located near a patient's ischial tuberosity was classified as "black" using the Red-Yellow-Black system. The most relevant finding associated with a "black" classification would be the presence of:

1. granulation tissue
2. exudate
3. slough
4. **eschar**

Correct Answer: 4
Explanation: Eschar describes a particular type of necrosis, usually presenting as brown or black with a hard or soft appearance. Eschar is indicative of full-thickness tissue destruction and is most consistent with the label "black" using the Red-Yellow-Black system. (Sussman p. 199)

Clinical Practice: Integumentary System
Content Outline: Evaluation, Diagnosis, Prognosis, and Outcomes

Question Number: 22
A physical therapist discusses the importance of the cool-down period following an exercise session with a patient participating in a cardiac rehabilitation program. The patient is four weeks status post myocardial infarction and has had an uncomplicated recovery. Which of the following best describes the purpose of the cool-down period?

1. **prevent pooling of the blood in the extremities**
2. minimize ventricular arrhythmias
3. diminish patient nausea and vertigo
4. provide an opportunity to monitor vital signs following exercise termination

Correct Answer: 1
Explanation: Cessation of exercise without an adequate cool-down period may result in pooling of blood in the extremities. This condition may lead to insufficient blood supply to the heart and brain, vertigo, arrhythmias, and syncope. (Brannon p. 347)

Clinical Practice: Cardiopulmonary System
Content Outline: Intervention

Question Number: 23
A physical therapist interviews a patient referred to physical therapy with a diagnosis of chronic bronchitis. What finding obtained during the patient interview is most closely associated with the patient's medical diagnosis?

1. **patient is a smoker**
2. patient has a sedentary lifestyle
3. patient has numerous allergies
4. patient has severe scoliosis

Correct Answer: 1
Explanation: Chronic bronchitis is characterized by increased mucus secretion sufficient to produce a productive cough for at least three months during two consecutive years. Cigarette smoking is the most commonly cited causal factor in the development of chronic bronchitis. (Hillegass p. 275)

Clinical Practice: Cardiopulmonary System
Content Outline: Examination

Question Number: 24
A physical therapist inspects the skin of a patient with a recent spinal cord injury. The therapist identifies several areas that appear to be susceptible to tissue breakdown. The most appropriate health care member to discuss this information with is:

1. physician
2. **nurse**
3. case manager
4. occupational therapist

Correct Answer: 2
Explanation: Nursing has continual direct contact with the patient and is therefore the most appropriate health discipline to assist the patient with a proper positioning program. (O'Sullivan p. 883)

Clinical Practice: Education/Communication
Content Outline: Intervention

Question Number: 25

A patient begins to cry in the middle of a treatment session. The physical therapist attempts to comfort the patient, however, eventually has to discontinue treatment. Which section of a S.O.A.P. note would be the most appropriate to document the incident?

1. subjective
2. objective
3. **assessment**
4. plan

Correct Answer: 3

Explanation: Inability to continue treatment due to a patient's emotional state should be documented in the assessment portion of the S.O.A.P. note. This type of entry serves to justify the decision to terminate treatment. (Quinn p. 124)

Clinical Practice: Education/Communication
Content Outline: Intervention

Question Number: 26

A physical therapist employs a neuromuscular electrical stimulation (NMES) strengthening program for a patient with quadriceps atrophy. Which characteristic of a NMES strengthening program is not accurate?

1. frequency of stimulation: 30 - 75 bursts per second
2. on/off times: 10 - 15 seconds on, 50 - 120 seconds off
3. frequency of sessions: three times per week
4. **number of contractions per session: 20 - 30**

Correct Answer: 4

Explanation: A session consisting of 20-30 contractions using neuromuscular electrical stimulation is excessive. In addition to the session being extremely lengthy due to the necessary on:off time, the patient would experience severe fatigue. (Robinson p. 141)

Clinical Practice: Physical Agents
Content Outline: Intervention

Question Number: 27

A physical therapist makes a conscious effort to demonstrate particular kinds of behavior that are significant and attainable for an eight-year-old patient. This type of behavior therapy is termed:

1. flooding
2. operant conditioning
3. role playing
4. **modeling**

Correct Answer: 4

Explanation: Modeling is a behavior modification technique in which the patient is taught to initiate the desired behavior of another. (Wallace p. 364)

Clinical Practice: Education/Communication
Content Outline: Intervention

Question Number: 28

A physical therapist employed in a rehabilitation hospital reviews the medical record of a 26-year-old patient recently admitted to the facility. The medical record indicates that the patient sustained a spinal cord injury four weeks ago in a diving accident. Which medical diagnosis would result in the patient being most susceptible to autonomic dysreflexia?

1. **T4 paraplegia**
2. T12 paraplegia
3. cauda equina injury
4. posterior cord syndrome

Correct Answer: 1

Explanation: Autonomic dysreflexia is a condition that occurs in patients with spinal cord injuries above the T6 level. The condition is triggered when a noxious stimuli is present followed by an increase in autonomic responses. Symptoms include headache, blotching of the skin, dilation of the pupils, nausea, and a dangerous increase in blood pressure. (O'Sullivan p. 883)

Clinical Practice: Neuromuscular System
Content Outline: Evaluation, Diagnosis, Prognosis, and Outcomes

Question Number: 29
A physical therapist employed in an acute care hospital reviews a patient's medical information prior to initiating an exercise program. Which condition would not be considered a contraindication for exercise?

1. acute systemic illness
2. systolic blood pressure drop of 25 mm Hg
3. **resting systolic blood pressure of 170 mm Hg**
4. active pericarditis

Correct Answer: 3
Explanation: Exercise is not contraindicated for a resting systolic blood pressure until it exceeds 200 mm Hg. (Rothstein p. 677)

Clinical Practice: Cardiopulmonary System
Content Outline: Evaluation, Diagnosis, Prognosis, and Outcomes

Question Number: 30   *Item Includes Graphic*
A patient rehabilitating from knee surgery exhibits significant weakness in the involved extremity. During the most recent therapy session the patient was able to complete an independent straight leg raise as shown. What muscle is emphasized in the exercise?

1. vastus medialis
2. **rectus femoris**
3. vastus lateralis
4. sartorius

Correct Answer: 2
Explanation: Performing a straight leg raise requires dynamic hip flexion and an isometric contraction of the quadriceps. The rectus femoris is the prime mover during the straight leg raise exercise. The muscle is a component of the quadriceps femoris muscle group and is innervated by the femoral nerve. (Kisner p. 550)

Clinical Practice: Musculoskeletal System
Content Outline: Intervention

Question Number: 31
A physical therapist establishes goals for a patient following total hip replacement surgery. Which of the following goals is the most clearly defined?

1. patient will increase lower extremity strength through the use of ankle cuff weights within three weeks
2. patient will understand the importance of surgical precautions at all times
3. patient will perform an independent transfer
4. **patient will demonstrate a three-point gait pattern using axillary crutches within one week**

Correct Answer: 4
Explanation: A properly written goal should include an audience, behavior, condition, and degree. (Quinn p. 104)

Clinical Practice: Administration
Content Outline: Intervention

Question Number: 32
A patient coverage form indicates selective debridement is to be performed on a patient rehabilitating from a lower extremity burn. Based on the coverage form, the most likely intervention would be:

1. whirlpool
2. wet-to-dry dressings
3. **enzymatic debridement**
4. wound irrigation

Correct Answer: 3
Explanation: Selective debridement involves removing devitalized tissues using methods such as sharp, autolytic, and enzymatic debridement. Enzymatic debridement is considered to be selective since the topical preparation of the enzymes used (collagenolytic, proteolytic) will greatly influence the treatment outcome. The remaining options are considered forms of non-selective debridement. (Sussman p. 201)

Clinical Practice: Integumentary System
Content Outline: Intervention

Question Number: 33

A physical therapist treats a patient with chronic back pain using transcutaneous electrical nerve stimulation. When administering sensory level stimulation, which statement most accurately describes the desired amplitude?

1. non-perceptible
2. **perceptible tingling**
3. visible muscle contraction
4. noxious stimuli

Correct Answer: 2

Explanation: Conventional transcutaneous electrical nerve stimulation is characterized by high frequency and low amplitude. The amplitude should be perceptible, however, should not induce muscle contraction. (Nelson p. 308)

Clinical Practice: Physical Agents
Content Outline: Intervention

Question Number: 34

A physical therapist designs an aerobic exercise program for a 54-year-old male rehabilitating from a Colles' fracture. The patient is otherwise healthy and has previously participated in a formal exercise program. Which of the following values would fall within the patient's age-adjusted target heart range?

1. 89 bpm
2. **127 bpm**
3. 166 bpm
4. 187 bpm

Correct Answer: 2

Explanation: The age-adjusted maximal heart rate can be calculated by 220-54=166. The target heart rate range is often expressed as 60%-90% of the age-adjusted maximal heart rate. In this case the range is 99.6 to 149.4 bpm. (Rothstein p. 675)

Clinical Practice: Cardiopulmonary System
Content Outline: Intervention

Question Number: 35

A physical therapist examines the workstation of a patient with a cumulative trauma disorder. When seated at a video display terminal, how far should the screen be positioned from the patient?

1. 6 inches
2. 10 inches
3. **20 inches**
4. 32 inches

Correct Answer: 3

Explanation: The video display terminal should be approximately 20 inches from the patient's head. (Hertfelder p. 138)

Clinical Practice: Education/Communication
Content Outline: Examination

Question Number: 36

A physical therapist entering the hospital physical therapy clinic at 8:00 a.m. finds the waiting room bustling with activity. Which of the following items should be given the highest priority?

1. a patient 15 minutes early for a scheduled appointment
2. a durable medical equipment vendor promoting a new sales line
3. a young man scheduled to job shadow
4. **a patient seated in a chair crying**

Correct Answer: 4

Explanation: The Code of Ethics indicates that therapists must respect the rights and dignity of all individuals. (Code of Ethics)

Clinical Practice: Administration
Content Outline: Intervention

Question Number: 37

A physical therapist is responsible for supervising a physical therapist assistant at an off site location. Which of the following would not necessitate a supervisory visit by the physical therapist?

1. a change in the patient's medical status
2. a modification in the treatment plan of care
3. a request by the physical therapist assistant
4. **an alteration in the patient's level of motivation**

Correct Answer: 4
Explanation: Physical therapist assistants often deal with changes in a patient's level of motivation. If necessary, the physical therapist assistant can modify a specific intervention procedure within the established plan of care based on the observed change. (Guide to Physical Therapist Practice p. 693)

Clinical Practice: Administration
Content Outline: Standards of Care

Question Number: 38
A physical therapist prepares the proximal radioulnar joint for mobilization by placing it in the loose packed position. This position is best described as:

1. 10 degrees flexion, 10 degrees pronation
2. 20 degrees flexion, 45 degrees supination
3. 45 degrees flexion, 20 degrees supination
4. **70 degrees flexion, 35 degrees supination**

Correct Answer: 4
Explanation: The loose packed position of the radioulnar joint is 70 degrees flexion and 35 degrees supination, while the close packed position is 5 degrees supination. (Magee p. 322)

Clinical Practice: Musculoskeletal System
Content Outline: Intervention

Question Number: 39
A physical therapist employed in an outpatient private practice receives a referral for a patient diagnosed with spondylolisthesis. Which of the following scenarios would be most consistent with the medical diagnosis?

1. **a 13-year-old female gymnast with no significant medical history**
2. a 17-year-old female tennis player with a 15 degree lateral curvature of the spine
3. a 28-year-old male machinist with a history of recurrent low back pain
4. a 67-year-old male with a previous diagnosis of ankylosing spondylitis

Correct Answer: 1
Explanation: Spondylolisthesis refers to a condition where one vertebra slips forward on the one below it due to a bilateral fracture of the pars interarticularis. This condition most commonly occurs at L4/L5 or L5/S1. Children ages 10-15 who are involved in activities such as gymnastics, weightlifting, volleyball, and pole vaulting are particularly susceptible to spondylolisthesis. (Starkey p. 359)

Clinical Practice: Musculoskeletal System
Content Outline: Examination

Question Number: 40
A physical therapist completes a ventral glide of the distal tibiofibular articulation. This type of mobilization technique would be most beneficial to improve:

1. ankle plantar flexion
2. **ankle dorsiflexion**
3. subtalar inversion
4. subtalar eversion

Correct Answer: 2
Explanation: Ventral and dorsal glides of the distal tibiofibular articulation increase the mobility of the ankle mortise and therefore are used to improve ankle dorsiflexion. (Kisner p. 250)

Clinical Practice: Musculoskeletal System
Content Outline: Intervention

Question Number: 41
A physician instructs a 26-year-old male to utilize a knee derotation brace for all athletic activities. Which condition would most warrant the use of the derotation brace?

1. medial meniscus repair
2. anterior cruciate ligament reconstruction
3. **anterior cruciate ligament insufficiency**
4. posterior cruciate ligament reconstruction

Correct Answer: 3
Explanation: Derotation braces are most effective in patients with ligamentous instability, usually involving the anterior and posterior cruciate ligaments. The braces have demonstrated little practical application for patients following ligamentous reconstruction. (Anderson p. 54)

Clinical Practice: Musculoskeletal System
Content Outline: Intervention

Question Number: 42

A physical therapist obtains a gross measurement of hamstrings length by passively extending the lower extremity of a patient in short sitting. The most common substitution to exaggerate hamstrings length is:

1. weight shift to the contralateral side
2. anterior rotation of the pelvis
3. **posterior rotation of the pelvis**
4. hiking of the contralateral hip

Correct Answer: 3

Explanation: Posterior rotation of the pelvis or extension of the spine can create the illusion of excessive hamstrings length in short sitting. The tripod sign is the term often associated with this type of substitution. (Magee p. 636)

Clinical Practice: Musculoskeletal System
Content Outline: Examination

Question Number: 43

A physical therapist positions a patient in sidelying in preparation for postural drainage activities. Which lung segment would be indicated based on the patient's position?

1. posterior basal segment of the lower lobes
2. apical segment of the upper lobes
3. **lateral basal segment of the lower lobes**
4. anterior segment of the upper lobes

Correct Answer: 3

Explanation: The lateral basal segment of the lower lobes requires positioning in sidelying with an inclination of 20 inches of the foot of the bed if tolerated. (Frownfelter p. 341)

Clinical Practice: Cardiopulmonary System
Content Outline: Examination

Question Number: 44

A patient with acute back pain is given a transcutaneous electrical nerve stimulation unit to use at home. The physical therapist provides detailed instructions on the care and use of the unit. Which of the following activities is not the responsibility of the patient?

1. modulate current intensity
2. application of new electrodes
3. change battery
4. **alter pulse rate and width**

Correct Answer: 4

Explanation: It is necessary for patients to adjust current intensity, however, they should not be permitted to modify any of the internal parameters that regulate the characteristics and pattern of electrical stimulation. (Robinson p. 60)

Clinical Practice: Physical Agents
Content Outline: Intervention

Question Number: 45

A patient with chronic pulmonary dysfunction is placed on a corticosteroid medication to reduce mucosal edema and inflammation. The most common side effect of corticosteroids is:

1. palpitations
2. arrhythmias
3. **increased blood pressure**
4. tachycardia

Correct Answer: 3

Explanation: Increased blood pressure (hypertension) is a side effect that is associated with heavy or prolonged use of corticosteroids. Other side effects include osteoporosis, muscle atrophy, cataracts, and hyperglycemia. (Ciccone p. 408)

Clinical Practice: Cardiopulmonary System
Content Outline: Evaluation, Diagnosis, Prognosis, and Outcomes

Question Number: 46

A physical therapist inspects a wound that has large quantities of exudate and therefore requires frequent dressing changes. If the therapist applies a dressing that cannot handle the quantity of exudate present, the most likely outcome is:

1. **maceration**
2. granulation
3. epithelialization
4. infection

Correct Answer: 1

Explanation: Maceration refers to a softening of connective tissue fibers due to excessive moisture. The result is a loss of pigmentation and a wound that is highly susceptible to breakdown or enlargement. (Sussman p. 148)

Clinical Practice: Integumentary System
Content Outline: Evaluation, Diagnosis, Prognosis, and Outcomes

Question Number: 47
A patient ambulating in the physical therapy gym suddenly grabs his therapist's arm and indicates that he feels faint. The most appropriate immediate action is:

1. assess the patient's pulse rate
2. ask the patient if he has ever previously fainted
3. loosen tight clothing
4. **assist the patient to a sitting position**

Correct Answer: 4
Explanation: The physical therapist's primary responsibility is to preserve patient safety. By assisting the patient to a chair, the therapist can adequately assess the patient without compromising patient safety. (Code of Ethics)

Clinical Practice: Patient Care Skills
Content Outline: Standards of Care

Question Number: 48
A male physical therapist provides exercise instructions to a female of Portuguese descent. During the treatment session, the patient does not make eye contact with the therapist. The most appropriate action is to:

1. tell the patient to pay attention
2. ask the patient if she would prefer a female therapist
3. **continue with the exercise instructions**
4. discontinue the exercise instructions

Correct Answer: 3
Explanation: It is important for physical therapists to recognize potential cultural differences associated with various patient populations. Therapists should not attempt to impose their cultural views, attitudes, or practices on others. (Nosse p. 94)

Clinical Practice: Education/Communication
Content Outline: Intervention

Question Number: 49
A physical therapist employed in a rehabilitation hospital creates a professional development plan as part of his annual performance appraisal. Which of the following would be the most appropriate plan to facilitate the therapist's development?

1. attend continuing education courses approved by the American Physical Therapy Association
2. attend continuing education courses featuring nationally recognized experts
3. attend a minimum of two continuing education courses annually
4. **attend continuing education courses related to primary patient care responsibilities**

Correct Answer: 4
Explanation: Physical therapists should attend continuing education courses that will directly benefit the patient population they are serving. Although in some cases this is not practical or desirable, it is always an important factor to consider. (Guide for Professional Conduct)

Clinical Practice: Education/Communication
Content Outline: Standards of Care

Question Number: 50
A patient has difficulty accepting the reality of his condition following lower extremity amputation. Which physical therapist action would not be helpful to promote acceptance?

1. refer the patient to a peer support group
2. **avoid treating the patient in a busy area such as the physical therapy gym**
3. allow the patient to observe sports programs for the physically challenged
4. offer the patient the opportunity to express feelings of grief and anxiety

Correct Answer: 2
Explanation: Treating a patient with a lower extremity amputation in the physical therapy gym will assist the patient with the adjustment process and allow for support from staff and other patients that have also had amputations. (Seymour p. 62)

Clinical Practice: Education/Communication
Content Outline: Intervention

Computer-Based Exam One – Section Two

Question Number: 51

A physical therapist reviews the results of an arterial blood gas analysis for a 28-year-old male. Which value would be considered within normal limits for oxygen saturation?

1. 84%
2. 88%
3. 92%
4. **97%**

Correct Answer: 4

Explanation: Oxygen saturation measures the percentage of hemoglobin saturated with oxygen. Normal ranges for oxygen saturation correspond to 95-98%. (Goodman - Differential Diagnosis p. 149)

Clinical Practice: Cardiopulmonary System
Content Outline: Examination

Question Number: 52

A physical therapist conducts an upper quarter screening examination on a patient diagnosed with rotator cuff tendonitis. With the patient in sitting, the most appropriate action to facilitate palpation of the rotator cuff is:

1. passive abduction of the humerus
2. active medial and lateral rotation of the humerus
3. **passive extension of the humerus**
4. active extension and flexion of the elbow

Correct Answer: 3

Explanation: Passive extension of the humerus makes it possible to palpate a portion of the rotator cuff by moving it out from under the acromion process. (Hoppenfeld p. 13)

Clinical Practice: Musculoskeletal System
Content Outline: Examination

Question Number: 53

A patient sustains a burst fracture of a thoracic vertebra secondary to a hyperflexion injury. The physician's note indicates the fracture is stable. Which of the following would not be considered appropriate immediate physical therapy management?

1. bed mobility exercises
2. **active spinal range of motion exercises**
3. postural education
4. instruction in donning and doffing a spinal brace

Correct Answer: 2

Explanation: There is not enough information presented to determine if active spinal range of motion exercises are appropriate for the patient. The remaining options offer valuable treatment alternatives that are considerably less aggressive. (Paz p. 253)

Clinical Practice: Musculoskeletal System
Content Outline: Intervention

Question Number: 54

A physical therapist assesses a patient's heart rate by measuring the time necessary for 30 beats. Assuming the therapist measures this value as 22 seconds, the patient's heart rate should be recorded as:

1. **82 beats per minute**
2. 86 beats per minute
3. 90 beats per minute
4. 95 beats per minute

Correct Answer: 1

Explanation: The easiest method to determine the beats per minute is to establish an equation using the supplied information and solve for beats per minute. The question tells you that 22 seconds = 30 beats, therefore it can be concluded that the number of beats in one second = 1.36 (30/22=1.36). By multiplying 1.36 beats per second by 60 seconds, it becomes possible to obtain a value in beats per minute (1.36*60=81.6). (Pierson p. 53)

Clinical Practice: Cardiopulmonary System
Content Outline: Examination

Question Number: 55

A physical therapist treats a patient following a lower extremity amputation. The patient is currently one week post amputation and has a post-operative rigid dressing. Which of the following is not a benefit of the rigid dressing?

1. limits the development of post-operative edema in the residual limb
2. allows for earlier ambulation with the attachment of a pylon and foot
3. allows for earlier fitting of a definitive prosthesis
4. **allows for daily wound inspection and dressing changes**

Correct Answer: 4
Explanation: A rigid dressing, usually made from plaster of Paris or fiberglass, does not allow for wound inspection or dressing changes. The rigid dressing is applied within a few days after surgery and remains on the residual limb until proper shaping occurs. (Seymour p. 126)

Clinical Practice: Patient Care Skills
Content Outline: Evaluation, Diagnosis, Prognosis, and Outcomes

Question Number: 56
A physical therapist prepares to formally assess the balance of a patient with a neurological disorder. The most appropriate method to assess the vestibular component of balance would be:

1. assess cutaneous sensation
2. **apply a perturbation to alter the body's center of mass**
3. examine proprioception in a weight bearing posture
4. quantify visual acuity and depth perception

Correct Answer: 2
Explanation: The vestibular system reports information to the brain regarding the position and movement of the head with respect to gravity and inertia. The vestibular system maintains clear vision during head motion and generates postural reflexes to assist with balance. General assessment often includes perturbations that require the body to make automatic adjustments that restore normal alignment. (Goodman-Pathology p. 1137)

Clinical Practice: Neuromuscular System
Content Outline: Examination

Question Number: 57
A physical therapist inspects the skin of a child recently admitted to the hospital after sustaining a scald burn from hot water on his torso. The burn is moist and red with several areas of blister formation. The burn covers an area approximately 8 cm^2 and blanches with direct pressure. The most likely burn classification is:

1. superficial
2. **superficial partial-thickness**
3. deep partial-thickness
4. full-thickness

Correct Answer: 2
Explanation: A superficial partial-thickness burn involves the epidermis and the upper portion of the dermis. The involved area may be extremely painful and exhibit blisters. Healing occurs with minimal to no scarring. (Rothstein p. 1115)

Clinical Practice: Integumentary System
Content Outline: Examination

Question Number: 58
A physical therapist prepares to examine a patient's triceps using a reflex hammer. The most appropriate positioning of the patient's arm during the testing procedure is:

1. **shoulder extension and elbow flexion**
2. shoulder flexion and elbow extension
3. shoulder extension and elbow extension
4. shoulder flexion and elbow flexion

Correct Answer: 1
Explanation: To properly assess a deep tendon reflex the therapist must place the tendon to be tested on slight stretch. Shoulder extension and elbow flexion would be the most appropriate position to meet this requirement. The triceps reflex is best elicited with the patient sitting or standing with the arm supported by the physical therapist. The therapist strikes the triceps tendon with a reflex hammer where it crosses the olecranon fossa. (Bickley p. 540)

Clinical Practice: Neuromuscular System
Content Outline: Examination

Question Number: 59
A physical therapist measures the blood pressure of a one-month-old infant. Which of the following measurements would be the most typical based on the infant's chronological age?

1. 55/40 mm Hg
2. 65/45 mm Hg
3. **85/60 mm Hg**
4. 120/80 mm Hg

Correct Answer: 3
Explanation: A newborn's blood pressure typically ranges from 70-90 mm Hg systolic and 45-65 mm Hg diastolic. (Minor p. 42)

Clinical Practice: Cardiopulmonary System
Content Outline: Examination

Question Number: 60

A physical therapist instructs a patient in an upper extremity proprioceptive neuromuscular facilitation pattern by telling the patient to begin by grasping an imaginary sword positioned in a scabbard on their left hip using their right hand. This type of command would be most appropriate to initiate:

1. D1 extension
2. D1 flexion
3. D2 extension
4. **D2 flexion**

Correct Answer: 4

Explanation: The D2 flexion pattern begins with the arm in extension, adduction, and medial rotation. The patient moves the entire arm into flexion, abduction and lateral rotation. The patient may increase the difficulty of this exercise by incorporating resistance to this pattern using tubing, weights, theraband, or manual resistance. (Kisner p. 382)

Clinical Practice: Neuromuscular System
Content Outline: Intervention

Question Number: 61

A patient status post meniscectomy has had difficulty attending physical therapy sessions since being diagnosed with lymphoma. The patient has had an unremarkable recovery, however, has diminished strength and trace edema. After missing an appointment the patient telephoned the physical therapist and explained that he is not able to focus on therapy and needed to cancel two remaining appointments. The most appropriate therapist action is:

1. explain to the patient the consequences of discontinuing physical therapy
2. reduce the frequency of physical therapy visits
3. attempt to convince the patient to continue physical therapy
4. **discharge the patient from physical therapy**

Correct Answer: 4

Explanation: The therapist should accept the patient's decision given the recent diagnosis of lymphoma. The decision is made easier since the patient's recovery from the arthroscopic procedure has been unremarkable. Diminished quadriceps strength and trace edema in the involved knee are not atypical for a patient three weeks status post arthroscopic meniscectomy. As a result, there would be minimal consequences of missing the two remaining physical therapy sessions. (Standards of Practice)

Clinical Practice: Administration
Content Outline: Evaluation, Diagnosis, Prognosis, and Outcomes

Question Number: 62

A physician examines a 36-year-old male with shoulder pain. As part of the examination the physician orders x-rays. Which medical condition could be confirmed using this type of diagnostic imaging?

1. bicipital tendonitis
2. **calcific tendonitis**
3. supraspinatus impingement
4. subacromial bursitis

Correct Answer: 2

Explanation: Calcific tendonitis is often visible on x-ray due to the relative density of calcium. The greater the density of the tissue, the more visible it will appear on x-ray. The supraspinatus and infraspinatus tendons are common sites for calcific tendonitis at the shoulder. (Magee p. 299)

Clinical Practice: Musculoskeletal System
Content Outline: Evaluation, Diagnosis, Prognosis, and Outcomes

Question Number: 63

A physical therapist designs a research study that will examine the effect of high voltage galvanic electrical stimulation on edema following arthroscopic knee surgery. The most appropriate method to collect data is:

1. anthropometric measurements
2. **circumferential measurements**
3. goniometric measurements
4. volumetric measurements

Correct Answer: 2

Explanation: Circumferential measurements using a flexible tape measure allow physical therapists to obtain a gross estimate of edema in the knee. Pre-test and post-test measurements provide information on the effect of the electrical stimulation on the edema. Special tests designed to identify the presence of edema in the knee include the patellar tap test, the indentation test, and the fluctuation test. (Magee p. 726)

Clinical Practice: Musculoskeletal System
Content Outline: Examination

Question Number: 64

A male physical therapist employed in an outpatient orthopedic clinic examines a patient diagnosed with cerebral palsy. The therapist has limited experience with cerebral palsy and is concerned about his ability to provide appropriate treatment. The most appropriate therapist action is:

1. inform the patient of your area of expertise
2. **co-treat the patient with another more experienced therapist**
3. treat the patient
4. refuse to treat the patient

Correct Answer: 2
Explanation: Physical therapists must make decisions that are consistent with their professional training. Since the therapist is concerned about his ability to provide appropriate treatment, he is in need of some form of external assistance. By co-treating the patient, the therapist receives external assistance and at the same time improves his skills with a particular patient population. (Guide for Professional Conduct)

Clinical Practice: Administration
Content Outline: Standards of Care

Question Number: 65

A patient with a 40 degree limitation in right shoulder flexion and a 35 degree limitation in lateral rotation is unable to perform a number of activities of daily living. Which activity would be the most difficult for the patient using the right upper extremity?

1. tucking in shirt
2. **combing hair**
3. eating
4. washing the left shoulder

Correct Answer: 2
Explanation: A patient requires 30-70 degrees of horizontal adduction, 105-120 degrees of abduction, and 90 degrees of lateral rotation to independently comb their hair. (Magee p. 237)

Clinical Practice: Musculoskeletal System
Content Outline: Evaluation, Diagnosis, Prognosis, and Outcomes

Question Number: 66

A patient status post Achilles tendon repair is examined in physical therapy. The physician referral includes a very specific post-operative protocol. If the therapist plans on deviating from the established protocol, the most appropriate action is to:

1. secure the patient's surgical report
2. complete a thorough examination
3. carefully document any modification
4. **contact the referring physician**

Correct Answer: 4
Explanation: In order to deviate from an established protocol it is necessary to receive approval from the referring physician. (Guide for Professional Conduct)

Clinical Practice: Education/Communication
Content Outline: Standards of Care

Question Number: 67

A physical therapist develops a plan of care for a patient status post knee surgery. As part of the plan of care the therapist elects to utilize a continuous passive motion machine. Which treatment objective would not be addressed using this intervention?

1. increase vascular dynamics
2. **prevent muscle atrophy**
3. prevent contractures
4. decrease pain

Correct Answer: 2
Explanation: Muscle atrophy would not be prevented using a continuous passive motion machine since the device incorporates only passive range of motion and does not require any form of muscle contraction. (Kisner p. 54)

Clinical Practice: Physical Agents
Content Outline: Evaluation, Diagnosis, Prognosis, and Outcomes

Question Number: 68

As a component of a cognitive assessment, a physical therapist asks a patient to count from one to twenty-five by increments of three. Which cognitive function does this task most accurately assess?

1. **attention**
2. constructional ability
3. abstract ability
4. judgment

Correct Answer: 1
Explanation: Counting from one to twenty-five by increments of three assesses the patient's ability to concentrate. The task is quite basic and as a result deals more with attention than any higher level cognitive ability. (Bickley p. 556)

Clinical Practice: Neuromuscular System
Content Outline: Examination

Question Number: 69
A physical therapist using ultraviolet light determines a patient's minimal erythemal dose using a four-windowed shield. If measured appropriately, reddening of the skin caused by ultraviolet exposure for the minimal erythemal dose should disappear within:

1. 12 hours
2. 24 hours
3. 48 hours
4. 96 hours

Correct Answer: 2
Explanation: A minimal erythemal dose is the time required for mild reddening of the skin that appears within eight hours of treatment and disappears within 24 hours. (Michlovitz p. 271)

Clinical Practice: Physical Agents
Content Outline: Intervention

Question Number: 70
A physical therapist completes an accessibility analysis at a local business. In order to meet minimum accessibility standards, the bathroom sink should have a knee clearance height of at least:

1. 23 inches
2. 29 inches
3. 35 inches
4. 39 inches

Correct Answer: 2
Explanation: There should be a minimum of 29 inches between floor level and the lowest portion the sink apron. (Minor p. 485)

Clinical Practice: Patient Care Skills
Content Outline: Examination

Question Number: 71
A physical therapy manager randomly selects patient medical records and examines the physical therapy notes. The therapist concludes that several of the notes are incomplete and use unacceptable medical abbreviations. The most appropriate action is to:

1. post a summary of documentation standards in the physical therapy gym
2. continue to randomly monitor physical therapy notes
3. reprimand therapists whose notes were identified as unsatisfactory
4. implement a peer review system

Correct Answer: 4
Explanation: A peer review system can be an extremely effective method to improve the quality of documentation. This type of system offers physical therapists the opportunity to assess selected documentation in relation to established documentation standards. (Scott – Legal Aspects p. 49)

Clinical Practice: Administration
Content Outline: Intervention

Question Number: 72
An 86-year-old female is partial weight bearing on the left lower extremity after a total hip replacement. Her upper extremity strength is 3+/5 and she resides alone. Which assistive device would be the most appropriate for the patient?

1. Lofstrand crutches
2. axillary crutches
3. large base quad cane
4. walker

Correct Answer: 4
Explanation: A walker provides the patient with the necessary stability without relying on significant upper extremity strength. The walker allows for varying degrees of weight bearing on the involved lower extremity. (Minor p. 288)

Clinical Practice: Patient Care Skills
Content Outline: Intervention

Question Number: 73

A patient refuses physical therapy services after being transported to the gym. The physical therapist explains the potential consequences of refusing treatment, however, the patient does not reconsider. The most appropriate initial therapist action is:

1. treat the patient
2. convince the patient to have therapy
3. contact the referring physician
4. **document the incident in the medical record**

Correct Answer: 4

Explanation: It is necessary not only to document that the patient refused physical therapy services, but also to inform the patient of the potential consequences of their action. (Scott - Foundations p. 176)

Clinical Practice: Education/Communication
Content Outline: Standards of Care

Question Number: 74

A patient with a suspected scaphoid fracture is referred to physical therapy. Which clinical sign is most indicative of a scaphoid fracture?

1. localized edema along the dorsum of the hand
2. crepitus with active range of motion
3. **localized bony tenderness in the anatomic snuff box**
4. pain with resisted wrist extension

Correct Answer: 3

Explanation: A scaphoid fracture can occur as a result of a fall on an outstretched hand. Localized tenderness in the anatomic snuff box is the most typical presentation. This injury can be serious due to the potential for avascular necrosis. The fracture is usually treated with prolonged immobilization of the wrist and thumb. (Hertling p. 271)

Clinical Practice: Musculoskeletal System
Content Outline: Evaluation, Diagnosis, Prognosis, and Outcomes

Question Number: 75

A patient in traction for six weeks following a femur fracture is referred to physical therapy. The patient presents with limited range of motion and diminished lower extremity strength. The most appropriate treatment option is:

1. **hot packs and proprioceptive neuromuscular facilitation**
2. cryotherapy and continuous passive motion
3. electrical stimulation and isometric exercises
4. ultrasound and isokinetic exercises

Correct Answer: 1

Explanation: Hot packs and proprioceptive neuromuscular facilitation (PNF) allow the physical therapist to address both the range of motion and strength deficits. The therapist can select from a variety of PNF techniques in order to identify an appropriate treatment option. Treatment will be based on the patient's current stage of healing and the results of the objective examination. (Hall p. 234)

Clinical Practice: Musculoskeletal System
Content Outline: Evaluation, Diagnosis, Prognosis, and Outcomes

Question Number: 76

A patient on prolonged bed rest attempts to get out of bed. Upon attaining a standing position the patient complains of lightheadedness and blurred vision. The most appropriate explanation is:

1. **decrease in blood pressure**
2. decrease in respiratory rate
3. increase in pulse rate
4. adverse reaction to medication

Correct Answer: 1

Explanation: A patient on prolonged bed rest is extremely susceptible to postural hypotension when assuming a standing position. Lightheadedness and blurred vision result from diminished cardiac output due to reduced venous return from the lower extremities. (Pierson p. 336)

Clinical Practice: Patient Care Skills
Content Outline: Intervention

Question Number: 77

A patient's job requires him to move boxes weighing 35 pounds from a transport cart to an elevated conveyor belt. The patient can complete the activity, however, is unable to prevent hyperextension of the spine. The most appropriate physical therapist action is:

1. implement a pelvic stabilization program
2. design an abdominal strengthening program
3. review proper body mechanics
4. **use an elevated platform when placing boxes on the belt**

Correct Answer: 4

Explanation: In order to eliminate hyperextension of the spine it may be necessary to modify the workstation. The most reasonable modification would be to utilize an elevated platform in order to minimize the height of the conveyor belt. (Kisner p. 673)

Clinical Practice: Patient Care Skills
Content Outline: Intervention

Question Number: 78

A physical therapist completes an examination on a 36-year-old female diagnosed with multiple sclerosis. After completing the examination, the therapist should first:

1. develop long-term goals
2. develop short-term goals
3. **develop a problem list**
4. justify the need for physical therapy services

Correct Answer: 3

Explanation: A physical therapist needs to develop a problem list for each patient as part of the initial examination. The justification of services as well as the short and long-term goals will come from this problem list. (Umphred p. 606)

Clinical Practice: Administration
Content Outline: Evaluation, Diagnosis, Prognosis, and Outcomes

Question Number: 79

A 21-year-old male patient informs a physical therapist that additional therapy visits will not be covered by his medical insurance provider. The patient is 12 weeks status post anterior cruciate ligament reconstruction and has had an unremarkable post-operative progression. The most appropriate therapist action is:

1. offer to treat the patient pro bono
2. devise an affordable payment plan
3. request additional visits from the third party payer
4. **discharge the patient with a home exercise program**

Correct Answer: 4

Explanation: A patient 12 weeks status post anterior cruciate ligament reconstruction who has experienced an unremarkable recovery should be able to function independently using a well designed home exercise program. The program should incorporate activities such as jogging, strengthening, and agility drills. (Kisner p. 541)

Clinical Practice: Administration
Content Outline: Evaluation, Diagnosis, Prognosis, and Outcomes

Question Number: 80

A physical therapist prepares to examine a patient status post stroke with left hemisphere involvement. Which patient behavior would not be characteristic of this condition?

1. difficulty sequencing movements
2. difficulty producing language
3. **difficulty with mathematical reasoning and judgment**
4. difficulty processing information in a sequential, linear manner

Correct Answer: 3

Explanation: A patient with left hemisphere involvement and resultant right hemiplegia has difficulty processing information in a linear manner, sequencing movements, and producing language. (O'Sullivan p. 536)

Clinical Practice: Neuromuscular System
Content Outline: Evaluation, Diagnosis, Prognosis, and Outcomes

Question Number: 81

A physical therapist monitors the blood pressure response to exercise of a 52-year-old male on a stationary bicycle. The therapist notes a relatively linear increase in systolic blood pressure with increasing exercise intensity. The change in the patient's systolic blood pressure with exercise is best explained by:

1. increased cardiac output
2. decreased peripheral resistance
3. increased oxygen saturation
4. decreased myocardial oxygen consumption

Correct Answer: 1

Explanation: The linear increase in systolic blood pressure with increasing exercise intensity is due to an increase in cardiac output. Cardiac output refers to the volume of blood pumped into the systemic circulation per minute. (American College of Sports Medicine p. 118)

Clinical Practice: Cardiopulmonary System
Content Outline: Intervention

Question Number: 82

A 64-year-old female patient is admitted to the hospital with a stage III decubitus ulcer over her right ischial tuberosity. The patient's past medical history includes severe chronic obstructive pulmonary disease. The most appropriate position for the patient is:

1. supine with pillows under the knees
2. prone with pillows under the knees
3. left sidelying with pillows between the knees
4. right sidelying with pillows between the knees

Correct Answer: 3

Explanation: Left sidelying is an appropriate position to avoid placing stress on the ulcer over the right ischial tuberosity and does not compromise respiration. Lying in prone can make respiration difficult for a patient with a history of severe chronic obstructive pulmonary disease. Positioning in right sidelying or supine would place too much pressure on the ulcer. (Frownfelter p. 740)

Clinical Practice: Integumentary System
Content Outline: Intervention

Question Number: 83

A physical therapist performs a manual muscle test on a patient's shoulder medial rotators. Which muscle would not be involved in this specific test?

1. pectoralis major
2. teres major
3. latissimus dorsi
4. teres minor

Correct Answer: 4

Explanation: The teres minor acts to laterally rotate, abduct, and extend the shoulder. The muscle is innervated by the axillary nerve. (Magee p. 236)

Clinical Practice: Musculoskeletal System
Content Outline: Examination

Question Number: 84

A patient in an acute care hospital has a catheter inserted into the internal jugular vein. The catheter travels through the superior vena cava and into the right atrium. The device permits removal of blood samples, administration of medication, and monitoring of central venous pressure. The device is best termed:

1. arterial line
2. central venous pressure catheter
3. Hickman catheter
4. Swanz-Ganz catheter

Correct Answer: 3

Explanation: A Hickman catheter (indwelling right atrial catheter) inserts into the right atrium of the heart. The catheter permits removal of blood samples, administration of medication, and monitoring of central venous pressure. Potential complications include sepsis and blood clots. (Pierson p. 284)

Clinical Practice: Cardiopulmonary System
Content Outline: Examination

Question Number: 85
A patient informs her physical therapist that she noticed a small lump on her right breast while dressing. The patient was referred to physical therapy with lateral epicondylitis and has no significant past medical history. The most appropriate therapist action is:

1. inspect the lump
2. **instruct the patient to make an immediate appointment with her physician**
3. inform the patient she may have cancer
4. document the patient's comment in the medical record

Correct Answer: 2
Explanation: 90% of breast cancer is discovered through self-identification. Research has demonstrated that in the United States one in nine women may be affected by breast cancer over the course of their life. As a result, it is imperative that the physical therapist impress upon the patient the importance of consulting with her physician. (Goodman - Differential Diagnosis p. 350)

Clinical Practice: Education/Communication
Content Outline: Intervention

Question Number: 86
A physical therapist attempts to confirm the fit of a wheelchair for a patient recently admitted to a skilled nursing facility. After completing the assessment, the therapist determines the wheelchair has excessive seat width. Which adverse effect results from excessive seat width?

1. difficulty changing position within the wheelchair
2. insufficient trunk support
3. **difficulty propelling the wheelchair**
4. increased pressure to the distal posterior thigh

Correct Answer: 3
Explanation: A patient will have difficulty propelling a wheelchair if the seat width is excessive. The patient will have to stabilize at the shoulders and excessively abduct the upper extremities to reach the wheels. This produces a less functional push. (O'Sullivan p. 1076)

Clinical Practice: Patient Care Skills
Content Outline: Intervention

Question Number: 87
A patient uses a self-administered assessment tool as a method to record daily progress. What type of reliability would be the most essential using this tool?

1. reliability of parallel forms
2. internal consistency
3. **intratester**
4. intertester

Correct Answer: 3
Explanation: Since the self-administered tool is being used to record daily progress, the tool will have to be completed on numerous occasions. As a result it is particularly important for the patient to be reliable with repeated measurements over time. Intratester refers to one tester, while intertester refers to two or more testers. (Payton p. 68)

Clinical Practice: Research
Content Outline: Standards of Care

Question Number: 88
A physical therapist observes a patient status post transfemoral amputation lying in supine with a pillow positioned under the residual limb. This position results in the patient being most susceptible to a:

1. knee flexion contracture
2. knee extension contracture
3. **hip flexion contracture**
4. hip extension contracture

Correct Answer: 3
Explanation: Elevation of a transfemoral residual limb can lead to the development of a hip flexion contracture. Contractures greater than 15 degrees can hinder prosthetic fit and mobility. (Seymour p. 145)

Clinical Practice: Patient Care Skills
Content Outline: Evaluation, Diagnosis, Prognosis, and Outcomes

Question Number: 89
A physical therapist administers the Mini-Mental State Examination to a patient recently admitted to an acute care medical facility. The minimum patient score necessary in order to avoid being classified as possessing a cognitive impairment would be:

1. **24**
2. 28
3. 30
4. 34

Correct Answer: 1

Explanation: The Mini-Mental State Examination can be used to screen for cognitive dysfunction or dementia. The tool examines components of orientation, registration, attention/calculation, recall and language. Possible scores range from 0-30 with 24 being the minimum score necessary in order to avoid being classified as possessing a cognitive impairment. A score less than 20 may be associated with dementia, delirium, schizophrenia, or an affective disorder. (Physical Therapist's Clinical Companion p. 113)

Clinical Practice: Neuromuscular System
Content Outline: Examination

Question Number: 90
A physical therapist identifies excessive lordosis in a patient during a posture screening. Which of the following is most likely associated with this type of finding?

1. **increased anterior pelvic tilt and lengthened hip extensors**
2. decreased anterior pelvic tilt and shortened hip flexors
3. increased posterior pelvic tilt and shortened hip extensors
4. decreased posterior pelvic tilt and lengthened hip flexors

Correct Answer: 1
Explanation: Lordosis refers to an abnormal anterior convexity of the spine. Lordosis most commonly results in shortened hip flexors and lengthened hip extensors. (Kendall p. 80)

Clinical Practice: Musculoskeletal System
Content Outline: Evaluation, Diagnosis, Prognosis, and Outcomes

Question Number: 91
A physical therapist receives a referral to instruct a patient in stair training using axillary crutches. The patient is rehabilitating from a tibial fracture and is currently partial weight bearing on the involved extremity. The most important action prior to initiating the training session is:

1. apply a gait belt
2. maintain proper body mechanics for yourself and the patient
3. assess vital signs
4. **examine the patient's limitations and capabilities**

Correct Answer: 4
Explanation: It is essential to determine the patient's limitations and capabilities prior to initiating an activity such as stair training. Critical areas to assess include uninvolved lower extremity strength, upper extremity strength, and ability to follow instructions. (Pierson p. 234)

Clinical Practice: Patient Care Skills
Content Outline: Intervention

Question Number: 92
A physical therapist orders a wheelchair for a patient with C4 tetraplegia. Which wheelchair would be the most appropriate for the patient?

1. manual wheelchair with friction surface handrims
2. manual wheelchair with handrim projections
3. **power wheelchair with sip-and-puff controls**
4. power wheelchair with joystick controls

Correct Answer: 3
Explanation: A patient with C4 tetraplegia has innervation to the diaphragm and is therefore capable of using a sip-and-puff control for wheelchair locomotion. (O'Sullivan p. 897)

Clinical Practice: Neuromuscular System
Content Outline: Intervention

Question Number: 93
A physical therapist employed in an inpatient rehabilitation center works with a patient rehabilitating from a total knee replacement. Which treatment activity would be the most appropriate to delegate to a physical therapy aide?

1. monitoring vital signs
2. measuring knee range of motion with a goniometer
3. **observing a patient complete a mat exercise program**
4. recording modality parameters in the medical record

Correct Answer: 3
Explanation: A physical therapy aide is a non-licensed worker trained under the direction and supervision of a physical therapist. Aides provide support services that do not require clinical decision making. Aides may function only with continuous on-site supervision by the physical therapist or in some states the physical therapist assistant. (Guide to Physical Therapist Practice p. 42)

Clinical Practice: Administration
Content Outline: Standards of Care

Question Number: 94

A physical therapist develops a plan of care for a patient status post unilateral transtibial amputation. Assuming an uncomplicated recovery, what is the most appropriate number of weeks for prosthetic training?

1. **2 weeks**
2. 4 weeks
3. 6 weeks
4. 8 weeks

Correct Answer: 1

Explanation: A patient that presents with a unilateral transtibial amputation should require approximately two weeks for prosthetic training. This training may include donning and doffing, prosthetic management, transfers, ambulation, and stair training. (Garrison p. 48)

Clinical Practice: Patient Care Skills
Content Outline: Evaluation, Diagnosis, Prognosis, and Outcomes

Question Number: 95

An electrical equipment safety committee develops a policy to limit electrical hazards arising from ground faults. Which action would be the most appropriate to meet the committee's objective?

1. report all equipment defects or failures
2. **manually test each ground fault circuit interrupter on a monthly basis**
3. follow manufacturer recommendations for electrical equipment care and service
4. mandate an introductory inservice on all new electrical equipment

Correct Answer: 2

Explanation: Policies are used to guide or in some instances, standardize certain behaviors within an organization. It is important to recognize that the question asks specifically about a policy related to electrical hazards arising from ground faults. (Scott – Legal Aspects p. 147)

Clinical Practice: Administration
Content Outline: Intervention

Question Number: 96

A 50-year-old male diagnosed with Parkinson's disease is referred to physical therapy. The patient presents with rigidity, postural tremors, and bradykinesia. He is unable to perform basic activities of daily living without assistance from family members. The most appropriate treatment objective is:

1. improve lower extremity strength
2. improve respiratory capacity
3. **improve initiation of movement**
4. improve sensory awareness

Correct Answer: 3

Explanation: A common goal in the treatment of Parkinson's disease is to improve initiation and quality of movement. During the early stages of the disease physical therapy intervention should emphasize movement in order to maximize functional independence. (Umphred p. 675)

Clinical Practice: Neuromuscular System
Content Outline: Evaluation, Diagnosis, Prognosis, and Outcomes

Question Number: 97

A 21-year-old female is examined in physical therapy after sustaining a grade I ankle sprain two days ago in a marching band competition. The patient's description of the mechanism of injury is consistent with inversion and plantar flexion. Which of the following ligaments would most likely be affected?

1. **anterior talofibular ligament**
2. calcaneofibular ligament
3. tibiofibular ligament
4. deltoid ligament

Correct Answer: 1

Explanation: The anterior talofibular ligament is the first ligament of the lateral ankle complex to stretch during plantar flexion and inversion. The calcaneofibular ligament and the posterior talofibular ligament are not typically involved in a grade I sprain. (Magee p. 767)

Clinical Practice: Musculoskeletal System
Content Outline: Examination

Question Number: 98
A physical therapist discusses common cognitive and behavioral changes associated with stroke with family members of a patient with right hemisphere damage and resultant left hemiplegia. Which term does not accurately describe the most typical patient presentation?

1. poor judgment
2. impulsive
3. quick
4. **overly cautious**

Correct Answer: 4
Explanation: Patients with right hemisphere damage often demonstrate impulsivity, quickness, spatial-perceptual deficits, and are unrealistic regarding their impairments. A patient with left hemisphere damage often demonstrates overly cautious behavior and may appear disorganized and anxious. (Umphred p. 755)

Clinical Practice: Neuromuscular System
Content Outline: Evaluation, Diagnosis, Prognosis, and Outcomes

Question Number: 99
A physical therapist gathers a variety of equipment prior to administering a series of sensory tests. Which form of sensation would be examined by utilizing a tuning fork?

1. joint position
2. **vibration**
3. stereognosis
4. barognosis

Correct Answer: 2
Explanation: Vibration sense can be assessed by placing a tuning fork vibrating at 128 Hz over a bony prominence. Failure to identify vibration would be indicative of a positive test. Vibration sense is often the first sensation to be compromised in the presence of a peripheral neuropathy. (Bickley p. 584)

Clinical Practice: Neuromuscular System
Content Outline: Examination

Question Number: 100
A physical therapist discusses the process of learning to drive an adapted van with a patient rehabilitating from a spinal cord injury. What is the highest spinal cord injury level where this activity would be a realistic independent functional outcome?

1. C4
2. **C6**
3. T1
4. T3

Correct Answer: 2
Explanation: A patient with a diagnosis of C6 tetraplegia is the highest level of injury where adaptive driving is a realistic independent functional outcome. The van would need to have numerous adaptations such as modifications to the steering system, driver's compartment, and installation of a wheelchair lift. (Umphred p. 492)

Clinical Practice: Neuromuscular System
Content Outline: Evaluation, Diagnosis, Prognosis, and Outcomes

Computer-Based Exam One – Section Three

Question Number: 101
A physical therapist completing daily documentation at a charting station is asked by a nurse to transfer a patient recently admitted to the intensive care unit. The most appropriate method to confirm the patient's identity prior to completing the transfer is:

1. contact the attending physician
2. check the patient's medical record
3. ask the patient their name
4. **examine the patient's identification bracelet**

Correct Answer: 4
Explanation: An identification bracelet serves as the most appropriate method to confirm a patient's identity. The bracelet is typically applied at the beginning of a hospital stay and is not removed until discharge. (Pierson p. 103)

Clinical Practice: Administration
Content Outline: Intervention

Question Number: 102

A patient classifies the intensity of exercise as a 16 using Borg's (20-point) Rate of Perceived Exertion Scale. This classification best corresponds to:

1. 40 percent of the maximum heart rate range
2. 55 percent of the maximum heart rate range
3. 70 percent of the maximum heart rate range
4. **85 percent of the maximum heart rate range**

Correct Answer: 4

Explanation: Exercise graded as a 16 using Borg's (20-point) Rate of Perceived Exertion Scale is classified as "hard" with regard to exercise intensity. This level corresponds to exercising at a maximum heart rate range of 80% to 89%. (Brannon p. 316)

Clinical Practice: Cardiopulmonary System
Content Outline: Intervention

Question Number: 103

A male patient rehabilitating from a lower extremity injury is referred to physical therapy for gait analysis. The physical therapist begins the session by observing the patient at free speed walking. The normal degree of toe-out at this speed is:

1. 3 degrees
2. **7 degrees**
3. 10 degrees
4. 12 degrees

Correct Answer: 2

Explanation: The degree of toe-out is measured by determining the angle formed by each foot's line of progression and a line intersecting the center of the heel and the second toe. The degree of toe-out decreases as the speed of walking increases. (Levangie p. 446)

Clinical Practice: Musculoskeletal System
Content Outline: Examination

Question Number: 104

A physical therapist completes an upper quarter screening examination on a patient with a suspected cervical spine lesion. Which objective finding is not consistent with C5 involvement?

1. **muscle weakness in the supinator and wrist extensors**
2. diminished sensation in the deltoid area
3. muscle weakness in the deltoid and biceps
4. diminished biceps and brachioradialis reflex

Correct Answer: 1

Explanation: Muscle weakness of the supinator and wrist extensors is associated with C6 involvement. (Magee p. 16)

Clinical Practice: Neuromuscular System
Content Outline: Evaluation, Diagnosis, Prognosis, and Outcomes

Question Number: 105

A physical therapist completes a dorsal glide of the humeroradial articulation with a patient in supine. When performing this mobilization technique, the therapist should stabilize the:

1. distal humerus from the lateral side of the patient's arm
2. **distal humerus from the medial side of the patient's arm**
3. proximal humerus from the lateral side of the patient's arm
4. proximal humerus from the medial side of the patient's arm

Correct Answer: 2

Explanation: The humeroradial articulation is formed by the convex capitulum articulating with the concave radial head. A dorsal glide is used to increase elbow extension. The lateral orientation of the radius would necessitate the therapist stabilizing the patient's distal humerus from the medial side of the patient's arm. (Kisner p. 237)

Clinical Practice: Musculoskeletal System
Content Outline: Intervention

Question Number: 106

A physician provides a group of physical therapists with an overview of diagnostic imaging techniques commonly used in clinical practice. Which imaging technique would not be considered invasive?

1. arthrography
2. myelography
3. discography
4. **computerized tomography**

Correct Answer: 4

Explanation: Computerized tomography is an imaging technique that uses cross-sectional images based on x-ray attenuation. Computer enhancement allows the imaging to have significantly better contrast resolution when compared to conventional x-rays. (Magee p. 54)

Clinical Practice: Musculoskeletal System
Content Outline: Examination

Question Number: 107
A physical therapist uses vibration in conjunction with percussion as part of a postural drainage program. When should vibration occur?

1. **during expiration**
2. during inspiration
3. after a maximal expiration
4. before a maximal inspiration

Correct Answer: 1
Explanation: Vibration is a technique used to aid in the clearance of secretions from the lungs. Vibration is performed during expiration only, whereas percussion is performed during both inspiration and expiration. (Hillegass p. 651)

Clinical Practice: Cardiopulmonary System
Content Outline: Intervention

Question Number: 108
A physical therapist treats a patient diagnosed with adhesive capsulitis with continuous ultrasound and mobilization. The patient has significant range of motion deficits and has been unable to return to work as a general contractor. Which objective finding provides the best support for the current treatment regimen?

1. a decrease in the patient's pain level using a visual analog pain scale
2. improved patient compliance with an established home exercise program
3. **a 10 degree increase in passive glenohumeral abduction range of motion**
4. a subjective report of warmth in the shoulder during and after ultrasound treatment

Correct Answer: 3
Explanation: Continuous ultrasound can be used to increase periarticular extensibility in a patient diagnosed with adhesive capsulitis. A 10 degree increase in passive glenohumeral abduction range of motion following ultrasound application and mobilization demonstrates that the patient is making objective progress. (Cameron p. 196)

Clinical Practice: Administration
Content Outline: Intervention

Question Number: 109
A physical therapist discusses risk factors associated with coronary artery disease with a patient in a cardiac rehabilitation program. Which risk factor would be the most relevant for the patient?

1. age
2. **elevated serum cholesterol**
3. family history
4. gender

Correct Answer: 2
Explanation: The most relevant risk factor for a patient in a cardiac rehabilitation program would be an elevation in serum cholesterol. This is a modifiable risk whereas age, family history, and gender are all non-modifiable risk factors. (Brannon p. 387)

Clinical Practice: Education/Communication
Content Outline: Examination

Question Number: 110
A patient rehabilitating from a spinal cord injury has significant lower extremity spasticity which often results in the patient's feet becoming dislodged from the wheelchair footrests. The most appropriate modification to address this problem is:

1. hydraulic reclining unit
2. elevating footrests
3. **heel loops and/or toe loops**
4. detachable swing-away legrests

Correct Answer: 3
Explanation: A patient with significant lower extremity spasticity would require toe loops if the tone was in an extensor pattern and heel loops if the tone was in a flexor pattern. The loops assist to stabilize the lower extremities on the footplates of the wheelchair. (O'Sullivan p. 907)

Clinical Practice: Neuromuscular System
Content Outline: Intervention

Question Number: 111
A physical therapist utilizes a manual assisted cough technique on a patient with a midthoracic spinal cord injury. When completing this technique with the patient in supine, the most appropriate location for the therapist's hand placement is:

1. diaphragm
2. **epigastric area**
3. xiphoid process
4. umbilicus region

Correct Answer: 2
Explanation: A physical therapist should provide manual contact over the epigastric area and apply pressure inwards and upwards in order to assist the patient to perform a cough. (O'Sullivan p. 894)

Clinical Practice: Cardiopulmonary System
Content Outline: Intervention

Question Number: 112
A patient 72 hours status post stroke is referred to physical therapy. As part of the patient care program, the physical therapist makes positioning recommendations to the nursing staff. How often should turning occur?

1. every 30 minutes
2. **every two hours**
3. every four hours
4. every six hours

Correct Answer: 2
Explanation: During the initial stages of rehabilitation a patient status post stroke should be repositioned in bed on a regular basis. A safe interval to avoid tissue damage would be every two hours. (Pierson p. 84)

Clinical Practice: Patient Care Skills
Content Outline: Intervention

Question Number: 113
A patient is referred to physical therapy after sustaining a lower extremity injury. The physical therapist examines the patient and identifies several postural abnormalities including genu varum. Which of the following motions or postures is not often correlated with genu varum?

1. **lateral patellar subluxation**
2. excessive hip abduction
3. ipsilateral hip lateral rotation
4. medial tibial torsion

Correct Answer: 1
Explanation: Excessive hip abduction, ipsilateral hip lateral rotation, and medial tibial torsion are associated with genu varum. Lateral patellar subluxation, excessive hip adduction, ipsilateral hip medial rotation, and lateral tibial torsion are associated with genu valgum. (Magee p. 667)

Clinical Practice: Musculoskeletal System
Content Outline: Evaluation, Diagnosis, Prognosis, and Outcomes

Question Number: 114
A physical therapist prepares to use soft tissue massage as part of a treatment plan for a patient with an adductor strain. The most appropriate therapist action prior to initiating treatment is:

1. utilize proper draping
2. **explain the treatment procedure and obtain patient consent**
3. ask another therapist to be present during the treatment session
4. describe the benefits of soft tissue massage on muscle strains

Correct Answer: 2
Explanation: Physical therapists should provide patients with a thorough explanation of the purpose and hypothesized benefits of a selected treatment intervention. Failure to obtain informed consent can be considered a form of substandard care. (Scott - Promoting Legal Awareness p. 114)

Clinical Practice: Education/Communication
Content Outline: Standards of Care

Question Number: 115
A physical therapist moves a patient from sidelying to supine after the patient was unable to maintain the manual muscle test position for the hip abductors. Assuming the patient is able to complete full range of motion in the horizontal plane, the most appropriate muscle grade is:

1. fair
2. fair minus
3. **poor**
4. poor minus

Correct Answer: 3
Explanation: A poor grade is characterized by the ability to move through complete range of motion in a gravity eliminated plane. (Kendall p. 189)

Clinical Practice: Musculoskeletal System
Content Outline: Examination

Question Number: 116

A two-year-old child diagnosed with bilateral congenital hip dislocation is referred to physical therapy. The child wears a hip harness designed to stabilize the hip in an attempt to allow the joint capsule to tighten and allow the acetabulum to be properly molded. The most likely position of the hip in the harness is:

1. **hip flexion and abduction**
2. hip flexion and adduction
3. hip extension and abduction
4. hip extension and adduction

Correct Answer: 1
Explanation: Hip flexion and abduction provide the optimal position for tightening of the joint capsule and molding of the acetabulum. The most common type of hip harness for children with congenital hip dysplasia is the Pavlick harness. (Goodman - Pathology p. 846)

Clinical Practice: Patient Care Skills
Content Outline: Intervention

Question Number: 117

A physical therapist completes a lower quarter screening examination on a patient diagnosed with trochanteric bursitis. Assuming a normal end-feel, which of the following classifications would be most consistent with hip extension?

1. soft
2. **firm**
3. hard
4. empty

Correct Answer: 2
Explanation: The end-feel most often associated with hip extension is firm due to tension in the anterior joint capsule and the iliofemoral ligament. (Norkin p. 196)

Clinical Practice: Musculoskeletal System
Content Outline: Examination

Question Number: 118

A physician utilizes diagnostic imaging to show motion in a joint through x-ray. This type of imaging is best termed:

1. computed tomography
2. **fluoroscopy**
3. discography
4. radionuclide scanning

Correct Answer: 2
Explanation: Fluoroscopy refers to examination by means of the fluoroscope. A fluoroscope allows an examiner to observe the actions of joints, organs, or entire systems of the body. The instrument requires a specific body segment to be placed between a fluorescent screen and an x-ray tube. X-rays from the tube pass through the body and project images on the screen. (Magee p. 52)

Clinical Practice: Musculoskeletal System
Content Outline: Examination

Question Number: 119

A physical therapist develops a plan of care for a 21-year-old patient rehabilitating from a traumatic brain injury. The patient's level of cognitive functioning is best described as Rancho Los Amigos level IV. Which treatment approach would be least effective?

1. offer the patient treatment options
2. **focus on teaching new skills associated with activities of daily living**
3. establish a daily treatment routine
4. redirect the patient when distractions occur

Correct Answer: 2
Explanation: A physical therapist would not be able to teach new skills to a patient at "level IV-confused-agitated." This patient is typically unable to cooperate during treatment, demonstrates poor attention, and memory. A patient would benefit from learning new skills at level VII. (Rothstein p. 450)

Clinical Practice: Neuromuscular System
Content Outline: Evaluation, Diagnosis, Prognosis, and Outcomes

Question Number: 120

A physical therapist reviews the medical record of a patient recently admitted to the intensive care unit. A note from the patient's physician indicates an order for arterial blood gas analysis six times daily. Which type of indwelling line would be used to collect the necessary samples?

1. intravenous line
2. **arterial line**
3. central venous line
4. pulmonary artery line

Correct Answer: 2

Explanation: An arterial line consists of a catheter in an artery connected to pressure tubing, a transducer, and a monitor. The device can be used for continuous direct blood pressure readings and for access to the arterial blood supply. The radial and brachial arteries are the most common sites for an arterial line. (Paz p. 787)

Clinical Practice: Patient Care Skills
Content Outline: Intervention

Question Number: 121

A patient with Alzheimer's disease is referred to physical therapy for instruction in an exercise program. The most appropriate initial step is:

1. provide verbal and written instructions
2. frequently repeat multiple step directions
3. **assess the patient's cognitive status**
4. avoid using medical terminology

Correct Answer: 3

Explanation: It is essential for the therapist to determine the patient's cognitive status prior to providing formal exercise instruction. The patient's cognitive status will have a significant impact on a variety of factors including the ability to interpret instructions, the ability to perform exercises correctly, and the ability to recall elements of the exercise program. (Bickley p. 556)

Clinical Practice: Neuromuscular System
Content Outline: Examination

Question Number: 122

A patient positioned in standing with their arm positioned at their side with 90 degrees of elbow flexion completes shoulder medial and lateral rotation exercises using a piece of elastic tubing. Which plane of the body is utilized with this activity?

1. coronal
2. frontal
3. sagittal
4. **transverse**

Correct Answer: 4

Explanation: The transverse plane is horizontal and divides the body into upper and lower portions. Medial and lateral rotation occur in the transverse plane around a vertical axis. (Levangie p. 6)

Clinical Practice: Musculoskeletal System
Content Outline: Intervention

Question Number: 123

A physical therapist uses a self-care assessment to examine change over time in rehabilitation programs. The assessment uses a seven-point scale to examine 18 items. The collected information is based on observations of patient performance. This type of assessment most closely describes:

1. **Functional Independence Measure**
2. Functional Status Index
3. Physical Self-Maintenance Scale
4. Katz Index of Activities of Daily Living

Correct Answer: 1

Explanation: The Functional Independence Measure (FIM) tests a subject in multiple areas to determine the overall degree of disability experienced by an adult rehabilitation patient. The FIM is commonly used to examine changes in disability status that occur over time. (Van Deusen p. 425)

Clinical Practice: Administration
Content Outline: Examination

Question Number: 124

A physical therapist working on a pulmonary rehabilitation unit works with a patient on therapeutic positioning. The patient has experienced a lengthy inpatient hospitalization and was only recently referred to physical therapy. The patient has significant weakness of the diaphragm and is hypertensive. The most appropriate patient position to initiate treatment is:

1. prone
2. supine
3. Trendelenburg
4. **reverse Trendelenburg**

Correct Answer: 4

Explanation: The reverse Trendelenburg position refers to a position in which the patient's head is elevated on an inclined plane in relation to the feet. This position can help to reduce hypertension and facilitate movement of the diaphragm. (Hillegass p. 658)

Clinical Practice: Patient Care Skills
Content Outline: Intervention

Question Number: 125

A physical therapist performs rescue breathing on a patient that collapsed in the physical therapy gym. Which of the following is not accurate when performing rescue breathing on an adult?

1. maintain open airway with head-tilt/chin-lift
2. give one breath every five seconds
3. pinch nose shut
4. **continue for 30 seconds; approximately six breaths**

Correct Answer: 4

Explanation: Rescue breathing is a cardiopulmonary resuscitation technique designed for a patient that exhibits a pulse, but is not breathing. This technique is typically performed on adults for a full cycle of 60 seconds with breaths occurring every five seconds. (American Heart Association p. 75)

Clinical Practice: Cardiopulmonary System
Content Outline: Standards of Care

Question Number: 126

A physical therapist observes a line from an I.V. that is tangled around a patient's bed rail. What type of medical asepsis is indicated prior to coming in contact with the I.V. line?

1. gloves
2. gloves, gown
3. gloves, gown, mask
4. **none**

Correct Answer: 4

Explanation: The physical therapist can reposition the I.V. line through direct hand contact. (Pierson p. 287)

Clinical Practice: Patient Care Skills
Content Outline: Standards of Care

Question Number: 127

A physical therapist treats a 45-year-old female diagnosed with adhesive capsulitis. The therapist administers small amplitude, rhythmic oscillations at the limit of the available range of motion. This description best describes:

1. grade I oscillations
2. grade II oscillations
3. grade III oscillations
4. **grade IV oscillations**

Correct Answer: 4

Explanation: Grade IV oscillations are used primarily as stretching maneuvers. (Kisner p. 224)

Clinical Practice: Musculoskeletal System
Content Outline: Intervention

Question Number: 128

The physical therapy department sponsors a community education program on diabetes mellitus. Which of the following is not characteristic of type I insulin-dependent diabetes?

1. age of onset less than 25 years of age
2. **gradual onset**
3. controlled through insulin and diet
4. islet cell antibodies present at onset

Correct Answer: 2
Explanation: Type I insulin-dependent diabetes usually has an abrupt onset and accounts for 5-10 percent of all cases. This type of diabetes requires insulin injections and is more common in children and young adults. Type II diabetes usually occurs in patients over 40 years of age, has a gradual onset, and can usually be controlled with diet and exercise. (Goodman - Differential Diagnosis p. 307)

Clinical Practice: Education/Communication
Content Outline: Evaluation, Diagnosis, Prognosis, and Outcomes

Question Number: 129
A physical therapist presents an inservice to the rehabilitation staff that compares traditional gait terminology with Rancho Los Amigos terminology. Which pair of descriptive terms describes the same general point in the gait cycle?

1. midstance to heel off and initial swing
2. **heel strike and initial contact**
3. foot flat to midstance and loading response
4. toe off and midswing

Correct Answer: 2
Explanation: Heel strike and initial contact are both terms that describe the moment that the heel contacts the ground and stance phase begins. (Rothstein p. 791)

Clinical Practice: Musculoskeletal System
Content Outline: Examination

Question Number: 130
A physical therapist selects a therapeutic ultrasound generator with a frequency of 3.0 MHz. Which condition would most warrant the use of this frequency?

1. lumbar paravertebral muscle spasm
2. hip contracture
3. quadriceps strain
4. **anterior talofibular ligament sprain**

Correct Answer: 4
Explanation: A higher frequency results in greater attenuation of energy in superficial structures. As a result, an ultrasound generator with a frequency of 3.0 MHz may be more desirable than a generator with a frequency of 1.0 MHz when treating a superficial structure. (Cameron p. 207)

Clinical Practice: Physical Agents
Content Outline: Intervention

Question Number: 131
A physical therapist notices that a patient with a transfemoral amputation consistently takes a longer step with the prosthetic limb. The most likely cause of the deviation is:

1. weak abdominal muscles
2. **hip flexion contracture**
3. weak residual limb
4. fear and insecurity

Correct Answer: 2
Explanation: An uneven step length can be caused by a hip flexion contracture on the prosthetic side. The hip flexion contracture (or insufficient socket flexion) will cause a decrease in hip extension during late stance that will result in a shorter step length on the uninvolved side. (Rothstein p. 838)

Clinical Practice: Patient Care Skills
Content Outline: Evaluation, Diagnosis, Prognosis, and Outcomes

Question Number: 132
After observing a patient during an exercise session, a physical therapist concludes that the patient commonly uses the Valsalva maneuver. Which activity would have the greatest probability of producing the Valsalva maneuver?

1. **lifting a 40 lb. package from the floor to a counter at waist level**
2. walking at 4 mph on a treadmill
3. stationary cycling at 80 revolutions per minute
4. using an upper extremity ergometer at 40 revolutions per minute

Correct Answer: 1
Explanation: The Valsalva maneuver is an attempt to forcibly exhale with the glottis, nose, and mouth closed. This action produces an increase in intrathoracic and intra-abdominal pressures that lead to decreased venous blood flow to the heart. Patients most commonly utilize the Valsalva maneuver during heavy resistance exercise. (Kisner p. 98)

Clinical Practice: Cardiopulmonary System
Content Outline: Intervention

Question Number: 133

A physical therapist completes a chart review prior to examining a patient involved in a serious motor vehicle accident. The chart indicates the patient sustained multiple lower extremity fractures including a femur fracture which was treated with open reduction and internal fixation. The patient is currently taking Demerol. Which side effect is most relevant when taking this medication?

1. peripheral edema
2. dependency
3. tachycardia
4. blood pressure variability

Correct Answer: 2
Explanation: Demerol is a trademark for preparations of meperidine which is a synthetic narcotic analgesic. Inappropriate utilization of opioids, such as Demerol, often results in physical dependence. (Ciccone p. 199)

Clinical Practice: Musculoskeletal System
Content Outline: Examination

Question Number: 134

A physical therapist employed in a rehabilitation hospital utilizes a variety of transfer techniques to move patients of various functional abilities. Which type of transfer would not be classified as dependent?

1. sliding transfer
2. hydraulic lift
3. sliding board transfer
4. two-person lift

Correct Answer: 3
Explanation: A sliding board transfer requires a patient to possess upper extremity strength and sitting balance. The patient is able to perform this transfer with assistance or independently. (Minor p. 248)

Clinical Practice: Patient Care Skills
Content Outline: Intervention

Question Number: 135

A patient four days status post transtibial amputation is transported to physical therapy for a scheduled treatment session. Assuming an uncomplicated recovery, the most appropriate patient transfer to utilize from a wheelchair to a mat table is:

1. two-man lift
2. hydraulic lift
3. standing pivot
4. sliding board

Correct Answer: 3
Explanation: A patient status post transtibial amputation should be able to perform a standing pivot transfer using the uninvolved lower extremity. (Seymour p. 160)

Clinical Practice: Patient Care Skills
Content Outline: Intervention

Question Number: 136

A physical therapist treats a patient rehabilitating from an Achilles tendon repair using cryotherapy. Which cryotherapeutic agent would provide the greatest magnitude of tissue cooling?

1. frozen gel packs
2. ice massage
3. fluori-methane spray
4. cold water bath

Correct Answer: 2
Explanation: Ice massage is a form of cryotherapy most commonly used over small areas such as a muscle belly or tendon. Ice massage is often administered using ice cups. Due to the direct contact of the ice and the target area, five to ten minutes is the typical treatment time. (Cameron p. 150)

Clinical Practice: Physical Agents
Content Outline: Intervention

Question Number: 137

A patient scheduled for posterior cruciate ligament reconstruction in two weeks is examined in physical therapy. The patient has diminished quadriceps strength and walks with a noticeable limp. The involved knee has mild edema and a 15 degree flexion contracture. The most appropriate treatment priority is:

1. improve quadriceps strength
2. improve fluidity of gait
3. reduce edema
4. **improve range of motion**

Correct Answer: 4
Explanation: A physical therapist should work with the patient to restore normal range of motion in the involved knee prior to surgery. By improving range of motion, the patient will likely be able to improve the fluidity of gait and diminish abnormal loading of the patellofemoral joint. (Kisner p. 510)

Clinical Practice: Musculoskeletal System
Content Outline: Evaluation, Diagnosis, Prognosis, and Outcomes

Question Number: 138

A physical therapist positions a patient in supine in preparation for goniometric measurements. When measuring medial rotation of the shoulder, the therapist should position the fulcrum:

1. over the lateral epicondyle of the humerus
2. perpendicular to the floor
3. along the midaxillary line
4. **over the olecranon process**

Correct Answer: 4
Explanation: When measuring medial rotation of the shoulder, the physical therapist should position the proximal arm of the goniometer so that it is parallel or perpendicular to the floor and the distal arm aligned with the ulna, using the olecranon and ulnar styloid as a reference. According to the American Academy of Orthopaedic Surgeons normal shoulder medial rotation is 0-70 degrees. (Norkin p. 84)

Clinical Practice: Musculoskeletal System
Content Outline: Examination

Question Number: 139

A physical therapist examines a patient diagnosed with left-sided heart failure. Which finding is not typically associated with this condition?

1. pulmonary edema
2. persistent cough
3. **dependent edema**
4. muscular weakness

Correct Answer: 3
Explanation: Dependent edema is a characteristic of right-sided heart failure along with liver enlargement, weight gain, and cyanosis. Left-sided heart failure can occur as a result of hypertension, coronary artery disease, infective endocarditis, and various connective tissue disorders. (Rothstein p. 654)

Clinical Practice: Cardiopulmonary System
Content Outline: Evaluation, Diagnosis, Prognosis, and Outcomes

Question Number: 140

A patient with a grade III inversion ankle sprain is examined in physical therapy. The patient sustained the injury approximately 36 hours ago while playing in a basketball game. The most appropriate treatment is:

1. **ice pack and intermittent compression**
2. whirlpool (29 degrees Celsius) and passive exercise
3. ultrasound and electrical stimulation
4. ice massage and mobilization

Correct Answer: 1
Explanation: A grade III inversion ankle sprain involves a severe disruption of the lateral ligaments of the ankle complex. Since the injury occurred only 36 hours ago, the patient is in the acute phase of inflammation and as a result should be treated with rest, ice, compression, and elevation. (Anderson p. 503)

Clinical Practice: Physical Agents
Content Outline: Intervention

Question Number: 141

A physical therapist monitors a patient with a single lead electrocardiogram. After carefully examining the obtained data, the therapist classifies the rhythm as sinus bradycardia. Which description is most indicative of this condition?

1. waveforms are irregular with a fluctuating rate
2. waveforms are irregular with a diminished rate
3. waveforms are normal with a rate greater than 100 beats per minute
4. **waveforms are normal with a rate less than 60 beats per minute**

Correct Answer: 4
Explanation: Sinus bradycardia is a classification of cardiac rhythm where the waveform is normal and the heart rate is between 40 and 59 beats per minute. (Brannon p. 195)

Clinical Practice: Cardiopulmonary System
Content Outline: Examination

Question Number: 142

A physical therapist washes his hands thoroughly after treating a patient with a suspected infection. Which statement regarding hand washing is not accurate?

1. **wash all hand and wrist jewelry**
2. wash your hands, wrists, and two to three inches of your distal forearms
3. wash for at least 30 seconds
4. select warm water to allow soap to lather easily

Correct Answer: 1
Explanation: All hand and wrist jewelry should be removed prior to commencing hand washing. (Pierson p. 29)

Clinical Practice: Patient Care Skills
Content Outline: Standards of Care

Question Number: 143

A physician orders a series of pulmonary function tests for a patient with pectus excavatum. Which test result is not typical for a patient with this condition?

1. forced vital capacity is decreased
2. vital capacity is decreased
3. **forced expiratory volume/forced vital capacity ratio is decreased**
4. total lung capacity is decreased

Correct Answer: 3
Explanation: Pectus excavatum is a congenital malformation of the chest and is characterized by an obvious depression of the sternum. This type of restrictive disorder is characterized by reduced lung volumes secondary to limited lung expansion. (Brannon p. 126)

Clinical Practice: Cardiopulmonary System
Content Outline: Evaluation, Diagnosis, Prognosis, and Outcomes

Question Number: 144

A physical therapist collects data as part of a preseason athletic screening program designed to identify individuals susceptible to heat illness. Which of the following measures would be the most valuable to collect?

1. height
2. weight
3. **percent body fat**
4. vital capacity

Correct Answer: 3
Explanation: Research has demonstrated that overweight individuals may generate up to 18% greater heat production than underweight individuals. (Anderson p. 539)

Clinical Practice: Education
Content Outline: Examination

Question Number: 145

A physical therapist participating in a team conference describes a patient's present cognitive functioning as a level IV, "confused-agitated" according to the Rancho Los Amigos Levels of Cognitive Functioning Scale. Which statement does not accurately describe this level?

1. patient is in a heightened state of awareness
2. verbalizations are often incoherent or inappropriate
3. patient does not discriminate among persons or objects
4. **patient responds to simple commands fairly consistently**

Correct Answer: 4
Explanation: A patient with a head injury classified as level VI, "confused-appropriate" would be able to follow simple directions on a consistent basis. This is not attainable for a patient at level IV, "confused-agitated." (Rothstein p. 450)

Clinical Practice: Neuromuscular System
Content Outline: Evaluation, Diagnosis, Prognosis, and Outcomes

Question Number: 146
A physical therapist employed in an acute care hospital works with a patient on bed mobility activities. The therapist would like to incorporate a strengthening activity for the hip extensors that will improve the patient's ability to independently reposition in bed, however, the patient does not have adequate strength to perform bridging. The most appropriate exercise activity is:

1. anterior pelvic tilts
2. heel slides
3. straight leg raises
4. **isometric gluteal sets**

Correct Answer: 4
Explanation: Bridging occurs when a patient in hooklying lifts their buttocks and low back from a fixed surface. The activity can be used to facilitate pelvic motion and for strengthening of the hip extensors. Isometric gluteal sets are an appropriate precursor to bridging since the activity incorporates the hip extensors. (O'Sullivan p. 416)

Clinical Practice: Patient Care Skills
Content Outline: Intervention

Question Number: 147
A patient on supplemental oxygen participates in a series of active exercises. During the exercise session the patient's oxygen saturation falls to the lower limit of her established acceptable range of 92-95%. When asked by the physical therapist how she is feeling the patient reports that she feels fine. The most appropriate therapist action is:

1. **continue the exercise session**
2. increase the amount of oxygen
3. discontinue the exercise session
4. contact the patient's physician

Correct Answer: 1
Explanation: Supplemental oxygen is most commonly administered by a nasal cannula at flow rates between one and six liters per minute. Since the oxygen saturation rate has not fallen below the patient's established acceptable range and the patient reports feeling fine it is reasonable to continue with the exercise session. (Hillegass p. 601)

Clinical Practice: Cardiopulmonary System
Content Outline: Intervention

Question Number: 148
A physical therapist performs segmental breathing exercises with a patient following atelectasis. Which manual contact would be the most appropriate to emphasize lingula expansion?

1. **place the hands on the left side of the chest below the axilla**
2. place the hands below the clavicle on the anterior chest wall
3. place the hands over the posterior aspect of the lower ribs
4. place the hands on the right side of the chest below the axilla

Correct Answer: 1
Explanation: The goal of segmental breathing is to improve oxygenation to a particular area of the lungs. The position of the lingula corresponds to a position below the axilla on the left side of the body. Breathing should be directed into the hands in an attempt to oxygenate the lingula. (Tan p. 697)

Clinical Practice: Cardiopulmonary System
Content Outline: Intervention

Question Number: 149
A physical therapist performs prosthetic training with a patient status post transfemoral amputation. Which initial instruction would be the most appropriate when ascending the stairs?

1. utilize your arms to propel your legs to the next step simultaneously
2. **place your body weight on the prosthetic side and lead with your uninvolved leg**
3. place your body weight on the uninvolved side and lead with your prosthetic leg
4. avoid using stairs with your prosthesis

Correct Answer: 2
Explanation: A patient with a unilateral transfemoral amputation will ascend stairs leading with the uninvolved lower extremity. This allows for greater stability as the uninvolved lower extremity uses its strength to lift the patient to the next step with the prosthetic side to follow. (Seymour p. 168)

Clinical Practice: Patient Care Skills
Content Outline: Intervention

Question Number: 150
A patient with C5 tetraplegia exercises on a mat table. Suddenly, the patient begins to demonstrate signs and symptoms of autonomic dysreflexia including headache and sweating above the level of the lesion. The most appropriate assessment to validate the presence of autonomic dysreflexia is:

1. pulse rate
2. **blood pressure**
3. respiratory rate
4. oxygen saturation

Correct Answer: 2
Explanation: Blood pressure often rises dramatically with autonomic dysreflexia. This condition should be treated as a medical emergency. (Umphred p. 496)

Clinical Practice: Neuromuscular System
Content Outline: Examination

Computer-Based Exam One – Section Four

Question Number: 151
A patient rehabilitating from a spinal cord injury informs a therapist that he will walk again. Which type of injury would make functional ambulation the most unrealistic?

1. **complete T9 paraplegia**
2. posterior cord syndrome
3. Brown-Sequard's syndrome
4. cauda equina injury

Correct Answer: 1
Explanation: Patients with complete lesions higher than T12 are not able to maintain the high energy cost of functional ambulation. (Umphred p. 521)

Clinical Practice: Neuromuscular System
Content Outline: Evaluation, Diagnosis, Prognosis, and Outcomes

Question Number: 152
As part of a sensory assessment, a physical therapist measures two-point discrimination throughout the upper extremity. Which skin region would you expect to have the smallest measured distance between two perceived points?

1. lateral arm
2. posterior forearm
3. over first dorsal interosseous muscle
4. **distal phalanx of the thumb**

Correct Answer: 4
Explanation: Due to the vast number of sensory receptors present, the fingertips are able to recognize two stimuli at approximately 1-2 millimeters apart. (Bennett p. 141)

Clinical Practice: Neuromuscular System
Content Outline: Examination

Question Number: 153
A physical therapist monitors a 29-year-old male with a C6 spinal cord injury positioned on a tilt table. After elevating the tilt table to 30 degrees, the patient begins to complain of nausea and dizziness. The patient's blood pressure is measured as 70/35 mm Hg. The patient's signs and symptoms are most indicative of:

1. spinal shock
2. postural hypertension
3. autonomic dysreflexia
4. **orthostatic hypotension**

Correct Answer: 4
Explanation: Orthostatic hypotension is a condition that can occur frequently in patients status post spinal cord injury. The patient experiences a loss of sympathetic influence that causes vasoconstriction in combination with diminished muscle pumping. This results in a significant drop in blood pressure due to the vertical position change. (Umphred p. 495)

Clinical Practice: Neuromuscular System
Content Outline: Evaluation, Diagnosis, Prognosis, and Outcomes

Question Number: 154
A physical therapist attempts to examine the relationship between scores on a functional independence measure and another measurement whose validity is known. This type of example best describes:

1. face validity
2. predictive validity
3. **concurrent validity**
4. content validity

Correct Answer: 3
Explanation: Concurrent validity refers to the relationship between test scores and either criterion states or measurements whose validity is known. (Payton p. 73)

Clinical Practice: Research
Content Outline: Standards of Care

Question Number: 155
A physical therapist reporting at a discharge team meeting indicates that a patient rehabilitating from a spinal cord injury should be able to perform household ambulation using knee-ankle-foot orthoses and crutches upon discharge. The patient's quadriceps strength is currently 2+/5. The most likely spinal cord injury level is:

1. L1
2. **L3**
3. L5
4. S1

Correct Answer: 2
Explanation: A patient diagnosed with L3 paraplegia is the highest level of injury that may allow for functional household and community ambulation using knee-ankle-foot orthoses and an assistive device. Complete lesions above the L3 level do not possess quadriceps innervation and the energy cost of ambulation usually makes the task prohibitive. (Umphred p. 523)

Clinical Practice: Neuromuscular System
Content Outline: Evaluation, Diagnosis, Prognosis, and Outcomes

Question Number: 156
A physical therapist reviews physical therapy treatment records as part of a department quality assurance program. Which treatment objective would be the most likely to be reimbursed by a third party payer?

1. promote compliance with exercise activities
2. prevent scar tissue and contractures
3. maintain range of motion
4. **improve cardiovascular endurance**

Correct Answer: 4
Explanation: Physical therapists are often required to demonstrate how physical therapy services improve patient status. Maintenance and prevention, although often necessary components of a treatment program, are less likely to be reimbursed by third party payers. (Anemaet p. 37)

Clinical Practice: Administration
Content Outline: Evaluation, Diagnosis, Prognosis, and Outcomes

Question Number: 157
A patient rehabilitating from a traumatic head injury is lethargic since being placed on Phenobarbital. The primary purpose of the medication is to:

1. decrease agitation
2. **prevent seizures**
3. reduce spasticity
4. limit central nervous system damage

Correct Answer: 2
Explanation: Phenobarbital is classified as a barbituate and is prescribed to prevent adult seizures. The mechanism of action of the drug is unclear and its side effects include sedation, vitamin deficiencies, nystagmus, and ataxia. (Ciccone p. 112)

Clinical Practice: Neuromuscular System
Content Outline: Examination

Question Number: 158
A physical therapist seeks patient consent prior to administering a selected treatment procedure. Which element is most essential when obtaining informed consent?

1. specify treatment parameters
2. **provide the patient with a reasonable opportunity to refuse**
3. offer alternative treatment options
4. justify the need for the selected treatment procedure

Correct Answer: 2
Explanation: Although each of the presented options is appropriate, it is essential to provide all patients with a reasonable opportunity to refuse treatment. Failure to perform this essential element can be considered a form of negligence. (Scott - Promoting Legal Awareness p. 113)

Clinical Practice: Administration
Content Outline: Standards of Care

Question Number: 159
A physical therapist prepares to treat a patient with continuous ultrasound. Which general rule best determines the length of treatment when using ultrasound?

1. 2 minutes for an area that is 2-3 times the size of the transducer face
2. **5 minutes for an area that is 2-3 times the size of the transducer face**
3. 5 minutes is the maximum treatment time regardless of the treatment area
4. 10 minutes is the maximum treatment time regardless of the treatment area

Correct Answer: 2
Explanation: A gross estimate of treatment time can be estimated by allotting 5 minutes of time for each area that is 2-3 times the size of the transducer face. (Michlovitz p. 200)

Clinical Practice: Physical Agents
Content Outline: Intervention

Question Number: 160
A physical therapist attempts to prevent alveolar collapse in a patient following thoracic surgery. Which breathing technique would be the most beneficial to achieve the established goal?

1. diaphragmatic breathing
2. pursed-lip breathing
3. **incentive spirometry**
4. segmental breathing

Correct Answer: 3
Explanation: An incentive spirometer provides visual or in some cases auditory feedback as the patient takes a maximum inspiration. Incentive spirometry increases the amount of air that is inspired and as a result can be used as a treatment to prevent alveolar collapse in a post-operative patient. (Kisner p. 753)

Clinical Practice: Cardiopulmonary System
Content Outline: Intervention

Question Number: 161
A physical therapist instructs a patient in a three-point gait pattern. Which assistive device would be most appropriate when performing the gait pattern?

1. bilateral canes
2. quad cane
3. one axillary crutch
4. **Lofstrand crutches**

Correct Answer: 4
Explanation: A three-point gait pattern requires the use of bilateral ambulation aids or a walker. Since the gait pattern allows for varying degrees of weight bearing through the involved extremity, the use of bilateral canes is not permitted. (Pierson p. 233)

Clinical Practice: Patient Care Skills
Content Outline: Intervention

Question Number: 162
A physical therapist reviews the surface anatomy of the hand in preparation for a patient status post wrist arthrodesis. Which bony structure does not articulate with the lunate?

1. **trapezium**
2. radius
3. capitate
4. scaphoid

Correct Answer: 1
Explanation: The trapezium is located in the distal carpal row on the radial side. This bone articulates with the first metacarpal. (Hoppenfeld p. 66)

Clinical Practice: Musculoskeletal System
Content Outline: Examination

Question Number: 163
A physical therapist conducts a sensory assessment on numerous areas of a patient's face. The cranial nerve most likely assessed using this type of testing procedure is:

1. facial
2. oculomotor
3. **trigeminal**
4. trochlear

Correct Answer: 3
Explanation: The afferent component of the trigeminal nerve (cranial nerve V) can be assessed by examining sensation of the face and jaw. The efferent component is assessed by examining the muscles of mastication. (Magee p. 69)

Clinical Practice: Neuromuscular System
Content Outline: Examination

Question Number: 164
A physical therapist examines a three-year-old child diagnosed with asthma. The child's condition has resulted in limitations of daily activity and occasional bed rest for one or more days. Which type of physical therapy intervention would be the most beneficial?

1. parent education and involvement
2. relaxation training
3. exercise to improve or maintain range of motion
4. instruction in diaphragmatic breathing and effective coughing techniques

Correct Answer: 1
Explanation: Parent education and involvement is required for a child with asthma in order to control the asthma and avoid acute episodes. This can be accomplished by altering the environment, monitoring activities, and assisting the child with making appropriate decisions regarding exercise. (Ratliffe p. 394)

Clinical Practice: Cardiopulmonary System
Content Outline: Evaluation, Diagnosis, Prognosis, and Outcomes

Question Number: 165
A physical therapist treats a patient in a medical intensive care unit. The therapist notices that intravenous solution appears to be infusing into the tissues surrounding the dorsum of the patient's hand. The most appropriate therapist action is:

1. contact nursing
2. reposition the intravenous line
3. remove the intravenous line
4. document the incident in the medical record

Correct Answer: 1
Explanation: An intravenous line that is infusing fluid into tissue has likely become dislodged from a vein. It is necessary to contact nursing in order for the intravenous line to be removed and perhaps reinserted. (Pierson p. 287)

Clinical Practice: Education/Communication
Content Outline: Intervention

Question Number: 166
A physical therapist completes a cognitive function test on a patient status post stroke. As part of the test, the therapist examines the patient's abstract ability. Which of the following tasks would be the most appropriate?

1. repetition of a series of letters
2. reproduce a figure from a picture
3. discuss how two objects are similar
4. verbalize a position statement

Correct Answer: 3
Explanation: Abstract thinking is commonly tested using two specific methods. The first method is by asking the patient to interpret the meaning of a proverb such as "a rolling stone gathers no moss." The other method is by asking the patient to describe how two items such as a cat and a mouse are similar. (Bickley p. 566)

Clinical Practice: Neuromuscular System
Content Outline: Examination

Question Number: 167
A patient fails to attain established physical therapy goals within the number of visits approved by the patient's third party payer. The patient has made progress in therapy, however, has been slowed somewhat by an adverse reaction to medication. The most appropriate physical therapist action is:

1. request additional visits from the referring physician
2. request additional visits from the third party payer
3. inform the patient that physical therapy services may not be fully covered by the third party payer
4. discharge the patient from physical therapy with a home exercise program

Correct Answer: 2
Explanation: A physical therapist should attempt to secure approval for additional physical therapy visits when there is ample evidence that the patient is progressing towards the established goals. (Standards of Practice)

Clinical Practice: Administration
Content Outline: Intervention

Question Number: 168
A physical therapist documents in the medical record that a patient has moved from Stage 5 to Stage 6 of Brunnstrom's Stages of Recovery. This type of transition is characterized by:

1. absence of associated reactions
2. **disappearance of spasticity**
3. voluntary movement begins outside of synergy patterns
4. normal motor function

Correct Answer: 2
Explanation: Stage 6 is characterized by the disappearance of spasticity and the ability to complete individual joint movements. In stage 5, spasticity is still present although it continues to decrease. Normal motor function would not be present until stage 7. (Brunnstrom p. 47)

Clinical Practice: Neuromuscular System
Content Outline: Evaluation, Diagnosis, Prognosis, and Outcomes

Question Number: 169
A physical therapist attempts to auscultate over the aortic valve on a patient status post myocardial infarction. The most appropriate area to auscultate is:

1. **second right intercostal space at the right sternal border**
2. second left intercostal space at the left sternal border
3. fourth left intercostal space along the lower left sternal border
4. fifth left intercostal space at the midclavicular line

Correct Answer: 1
Explanation: The aortic valve is a semilunar valve that separates the left ventricle and the aorta. The valve opens at the end of diastole, causing the second heart sound. (Rothstein p. 621)

Clinical Practice: Cardiopulmonary System
Content Outline: Examination

Question Number: 170
A physical therapist preparing a hot pack notices the water in the hot pack unit is cloudy. The most probable explanation is:

1. power failure
2. **seepage from a hot pack**
3. ineffective heating element
4. thermostat set too low

Correct Answer: 2
Explanation: Hot packs usually consist of a canvas case filled with hydrophilic silicate. A disruption in the case may cause small quantities of the silicate to be released into the water. (Cameron p. 168)

Clinical Practice: Physical Agents
Content Outline: Intervention

Question Number: 171
A physical therapist designs a home exercise program for a patient rehabilitating from a lower extremity injury. Which step would be the most appropriate to maximize patient compliance?

1. limit the exercise program to 10 minutes
2. select a maximum of five different exercises
3. **select exercises consistent with the patient's rehabilitation goals**
4. avoid physically demanding exercises

Correct Answer: 3
Explanation: Many factors can influence patient compliance with a home exercise program, however, regardless of the construction of the program it is essential that the program is designed to be consistent with the patient's rehabilitation goals. (Kisner p. 20)

Clinical Practice: Education/Communication
Content Outline: Evaluation, Diagnosis, Prognosis, and Outcomes

Question Number: 172
A physical therapist performs gait training activities with an eight-year-old child who utilizes a reciprocating gait orthosis. Which medical diagnosis is most often associated with the use of this type of orthotic device?

1. cerebral palsy
2. Down syndrome
3. Legg-Calve-Perthes disease
4. **spina bifida**

Correct Answer: 4

Explanation: A reciprocating gait orthosis is a type of hip-knee-ankle-foot orthosis that incorporates a cable connecting the two hip joint mechanisms. The orthosis is most commonly utilized with children diagnosed with spina bifida. (Tecklin p. 194)

Clinical Practice: Patient Care Skills
Content Outline: Intervention

Question Number: 173

A physical therapist instructs a patient rehabilitating from thoracic surgery to produce an effective cough. Which patient position would be the most appropriate to initiate treatment?

1. standing
2. **sitting**
3. sidelying
4. hooklying

Correct Answer: 2

Explanation: Coughing is an effective method to assist with airway clearance following thoracic surgery. A sitting position is typically the easiest position to produce a cough. (Kisner p. 758)

Clinical Practice: Cardiopulmonary System
Content Outline: Intervention

Question Number: 174

A 65-year-old female falls while attempting to shovel snow in her driveway and sustains a nondisplaced humerus fracture. The patient has no significant past medical history and has lived alone since the death of her spouse approximately six years ago. The most appropriate setting for physical therapy is:

1. inpatient rehabilitation hospital
2. skilled nursing facility
3. **outpatient orthopedic practice**
4. home health services

Correct Answer: 3

Explanation: An otherwise healthy patient that was living independently prior to sustaining the injury is a good candidate for outpatient physical therapy services. Although the patient's spouse is not living, she may be able to rely on friends or community transport to drive her to scheduled therapy sessions. (Nosse p. 24)

Clinical Practice: Administration
Content Outline: Evaluation, Diagnosis, Prognosis, and Outcomes

Question Number: 175

A patient with a transtibial amputation ambulates in the physical therapy gym. The patient exhibits an extended knee throughout early stance phase on the prosthetic side. The most appropriate solution to resolve the patient's difficulty is:

1. inset the foot
2. soften the heel wedge
3. move the foot anteriorly
4. **dorsiflex the foot**

Correct Answer: 4

Explanation: The prosthesis should be set with slight ankle dorsiflexion which will allow for subsequent knee flexion during the initial stance phase. A prosthesis with the foot in excessive plantar flexion tends to promote full knee extension during the initial stance phase. (Rothstein p. 831)

Clinical Practice: Patient Care Skills
Content Outline: Intervention

Question Number: 176

A physical therapist examines a patient with right hemiplegia. As part of the examination the therapist positions the patient in supine. The most appropriate therapist action to facilitate spontaneous right hip abduction is to:

1. apply manual resistance to the right hip adductors
2. apply manual resistance to the left hip adductors
3. apply manual resistance to the right hip abductors
4. **apply manual resistance to the left hip abductors**

Correct Answer: 4

Explanation: Raimiste's phenomenon is an associated reaction that is considered a form of overflow or irradiation. Manual resistance applied by the therapist to the left hip abductors would therefore produce a similar response on the affected limb (right hip abduction). (O'Sullivan p. 532)

Clinical Practice: Neuromuscular System
Content Outline: Intervention

Question Number: 177
A physical therapist provides pre-operative instructions for a patient scheduled for hip replacement surgery. As part of the session, the therapist discusses the importance of preventing deep venous thrombosis following surgery. Which finding is the best indicator that the patient is at minimal risk of acquiring a deep venous thrombosis?

1. ability to perform ankle pumps and muscle setting exercises
2. **ability to ambulate on a frequent schedule**
3. ability to achieve full hip range of motion within the allowable limits
4. ability to utilize pneumatic compression devices and elastic stockings

Correct Answer: 2
Explanation: All of the presented options can be helpful to diminish the risk of acquiring a deep venous thrombosis, however, ambulating on a frequent schedule is an activity that requires a significant increase in lower extremity circulation and is an indication that the patient is returning to a more active state. (Kisner p. 717)

Clinical Practice: Cardiopulmonary System
Content Outline: Intervention

Question Number: 178
A physical therapist applies silver sulfadiazine to a wound after hydrotherapy treatment. What type of aseptic equipment is necessary when applying the topical agent?

1. gloves
2. **sterile gloves**
3. gloves, gown
4. sterile gloves, gown

Correct Answer: 2
Explanation: Silver sulfadiazine is an antimicrobial drug used for the prevention and treatment of wound sepsis. Since the topical agent is applied directly to the wound, it is necessary to use sterile gloves. (Ciccone p. 564)

Clinical Practice: Integumentary System
Content Outline: Intervention

Question Number: 179
A patient diagnosed with Cushing's syndrome is referred to physical therapy. Which of the following signs and symptoms is not consistent with this syndrome?

1. distension of the abdomen
2. swelling in the facial area
3. **adrenal hypoplasia**
4. cardiac hypertrophy

Correct Answer: 3
Explanation: Cushing's syndrome is produced by an excess of free circulating cortisol from the adrenal cortex. Other signs and symptoms of Cushing's syndrome include amenorrhea, high blood pressure, osteoporosis, and susceptibility to bruising. (Goodman - Differential Diagnosis p. 294)

Clinical Practice: Neuromuscular System
Content Outline: Evaluation, Diagnosis, Prognosis, and Outcomes

Question Number: 180
A physical therapist performs an initial examination on an 84-year-old female in the physical therapy gym. The patient answers the therapist's questions in a very soft voice and appears to be intimidated by the bustling environment. The most appropriate therapist action is:

1. ask the patient if she understands why she was referred to physical therapy
2. tell the patient to relax and speak louder
3. **complete the examination in a private treatment room**
4. ask the patient about her rehabilitation goals

Correct Answer: 3
Explanation: A physical therapist should make every attempt to ensure that a patient is comfortable with the surroundings. A private treatment room offers a secure, quiet location that can be much less intimidating than a physical therapy gym. (Purtilo p. 289)

Clinical Practice: Education/Communication
Content Outline: Standards of Care

Question Number: 181

A group of physical therapists designs a research study which examines the reliability of the Functional Independence Measure (FIM). To measure reliability the therapists utilize a test-retest design. What is the most significant source of error with this type of research design?

1. change in subject behavior as a result of being measured
2. tendency to rate too strictly or leniently
3. change in test forms due to sampling of items
4. **change in subject situation over time**

Correct Answer: 4

Explanation: Reliability in this particular example refers to the degree of consistency of the Functional Independence Measure to produce similar scores on repeated testing occasions. Since a test-retest design incorporates an interval of time between each of the testing sessions, it is possible for items such as a change in patient status to significantly alter the results. (Domholdt p. 232)

Clinical Practice: Research
Content Outline: Standards of Care

Question Number: 182

A patient status post knee surgery receives instructions on the use of a continuous passive motion machine. Which of the following would be the most essential to ensure patient safety?

1. instructions on progression of range of motion
2. utilization of proximal and distal stabilization straps
3. recommendations for cryotherapy following treatment sessions
4. **orientation to remote on/off switch**

Correct Answer: 4

Explanation: A continuous passive motion machine is a piece of equipment that moves a desired joint through a selected range of motion in a constant pattern. The machine is commonly used to avoid the negative effects of immobilization. Orientation to the on/off switch is essential to maintain patient safety. (Kisner p. 54)

Clinical Practice: Physical Agents
Content Outline: Intervention

Question Number: 183

A physical therapist instructs a patient rehabilitating from a rotator cuff repair in a home exercise program. The patient is a 27-year-old male who is illiterate. The most appropriate action to promote compliance with the exercise program is:

1. ask the patient to memorize the exercises
2. use short sentences consisting of simple words
3. **draw pictures to describe the exercises**
4. do not utilize a home exercise program

Correct Answer: 3

Explanation: A physical therapist must adapt his/her educational media to best meet the needs of each individual. Drawing pictures is an appropriate modification that should allow the patient to refer to the handout at home. (Kisner p. 22)

Clinical Practice: Education/Communication
Content Outline: Intervention

Question Number: 184

A physical therapist treats a patient status post femur fracture with external fixation. While monitoring the patient during an exercise session, the therapist observes clear drainage from a distal pin site. The most appropriate therapist action is:

1. discontinue the exercise session and contact the referring physician
2. use a gauze pad to absorb the drainage and notify nursing
3. **use a gauze pad to absorb the drainage and continue with the exercise session**
4. document the finding and discontinue the exercise session

Correct Answer: 3

Explanation: External fixation devices provide stabilization to fracture sites through the use of pins that are inserted into bone fragments. Clear drainage from a pin site is not uncommon and should not be viewed as a sign of infection or any other serious medical complication. (Pierson p. 292)

Clinical Practice: Integumentary System
Content Outline: Intervention

Question Number: 185

A patient attempts to complete a transfer from a wheelchair to a mat table. The most appropriate method to protect the patient while completing the transfer is:

1. have the patient use non-skid socks
2. **utilize proper guarding technique**
3. insist the patient use a gait belt
4. instruct the patient how to fall

Correct Answer: 2
Explanation: It is essential for physical therapists to utilize proper guarding techniques for both dependent and independent transfers. (Pierson p. 129)

Clinical Practice: Patient Care Skills
Content Outline: Intervention

Question Number: 186

A physical therapist completes a gait assessment on a patient diagnosed with knee pain of unknown etiology. The therapist identifies excessive foot pronation during midstance through toe off. The most likely cause of the deviation is:

1. pes cavus
2. uncompensated lateral rotation of the tibia
3. **compensated forefoot varus deformity**
4. dorsiflexor weakness

Correct Answer: 3
Explanation: Other possible causes of excessive foot pronation from midstance through toe off include compensated rearfoot varus deformity, uncompensated forefoot valgus deformity, pes planus, and decreased ankle dorsiflexion. (Magee p. 869)

Clinical Practice: Musculoskeletal System
Content Outline: Evaluation, Diagnosis, Prognosis, and Outcomes

Question Number: 187

A physical therapist reviews the medical record of a patient with a suspected head injury. During testing using the Glasgow Coma Scale, the patient exhibited spontaneous eye opening, was able to follow selected motor commands, and was considered to be "oriented" based on verbal responses. The most likely score assigned to the patient would be:

1. 6
2. 12
3. **15**
4. 18

Correct Answer: 3
Explanation: The Glasgow Coma Scale is scored on a 3-15 ordinal scale. The test examines the primary areas: eye opening, best motor response, and best verbal response. A higher score represents a greater level of consciousness. (Magee p. 93)

Clinical Practice: Neuromuscular System
Content Outline: Examination

Question Number: 188

A physical therapist uses a subjective pain scale to assess pain intensity in a patient with multiple sclerosis. The pain scale consists of a 10 cm line with each end anchored by one extreme of perceived pain intensity. The patient is asked to mark on the line the point that best describes their present pain level. This type of scale is best termed:

1. descriptor differential scale
2. verbal rating scale
3. **visual analog scale**
4. numerical rating scale

Correct Answer: 3
Explanation: A visual analog scale is a form of a subjective pain scale that is commonly used in physical therapy. The scale provides physical therapists with the opportunity to compare changes in pain intensity over time. (Van Deusen p. 127)

Clinical Practice: Neuromuscular System
Content Outline: Examination

Question Number: 189

A physical therapist assesses end-feel while completing passive plantar flexion range of motion. The therapist classifies the end-feel as firm. Which of the following structures would not contribute to the firm end-feel?

1. tension in the anterior joint capsule
2. tension in the tibialis anterior
3. tension in the anterior talofibular ligament
4. **tension in the calcaneofibular ligament**

Correct Answer: 4

Explanation: Tension in the calcaneofibular ligament is often associated with the normal end-feel of dorsiflexion. (Norkin p. 261)

Clinical Practice: Musculoskeletal System
Content Outline: Examination

Question Number: 190

A physical therapist would like to use phonophoresis as a component of a patient's plan of care, but is concerned about the potential of the ultrasound to exacerbate the patient's current inflammation. The most effective method to address the therapist's concern is:

1. utilize ultrasound with a frequency of 1 MHz
2. limit treatment time to five minutes
3. **incorporate a pulsed 20% duty cycle**
4. select an ultrasound intensity less than 1.5 W/cm^2

Correct Answer: 3

Explanation: Duty cycle refers to the portion of the total treatment time that ultrasound is being generated. A 20% duty cycle would be used for nonthermal effects and would therefore not significantly increase tissue temperature. (Cameron p. 208)

Clinical Practice: Physical Agents
Content Outline: Intervention

Question Number: 191

A physical therapist attempts to assess the integrity of the first cranial nerve. Which test would provide the therapist with the desired information?

1. the patient protrudes the tongue while an examiner checks lateral deviation
2. the patient completes a vision examination
3. the patient performs a shoulder shrug against resistance
4. **the patient is asked to identify familiar odors with the eyes closed**

Correct Answer: 4

Explanation: Cranial nerve I refers to the olfactory nerve which is a sensory nerve concerned with sense of smell. To test the integrity of the nerve, a physical therapist typically assesses a patient's ability to identify familiar odors by sense of smell. (Bickley p. 567)

Clinical Practice: Neuromuscular System
Content Outline: Examination

Question Number: 192

A patient eight days status post anterior cruciate ligament reconstruction using a patellar tendon autograft is examined in physical therapy. Which of the following exercises would be the most appropriate based on the patient's post-operative status?

1. limited range isokinetics at 30 degrees per second
2. unilateral leg press
3. **mini-squats in standing**
4. active knee extension in short sitting

Correct Answer: 3

Explanation: A mini-squat is a closed chain exercise typically performed in standing that enables the patient to vary the force through the involved extremity by simply shifting their weight. This exercise significantly limits the amount of knee flexion and as a result does not place a great deal of stress through the reconstructed knee. (Kisner p. 554)

Clinical Practice: Musculoskeletal System
Content Outline: Intervention

Question Number: 193

A physical therapy department in an acute care hospital utilizes physical therapy aides to perform a variety of patient care services. What health care professional is directly responsible for the actions of the physical therapy aide?

1. **the physical therapist of record**
2. the physical therapist assistant of record
3. the director of physical therapy
4. the director of rehabilitation

Correct Answer: 1

Explanation: Physical therapy aides work under the direction and supervision of a physical therapist. As a result, the physical therapist of record is the responsible health care professional. (Guide to Physical Therapist Practice p. 42)

Clinical Practice: Administration
Content Outline: Standards of Care

Question Number: 194
A physical therapist prepares to administer iontophoresis over the anterior surface of a patient's knee. The therapist would like to keep the current density low in order to avoid skin irritation. Which of the listed parameters would best accomplish the therapist's objective?

1. **current amplitude of 4 mA; electrode with an area of 12 cm^2**
2. current amplitude of 4 mA; electrode with an area of 4 cm^2
3. current amplitude of 3 mA; electrode with an area of 6 cm^2
4. current amplitude of 3 mA; electrode with an area of 4 cm^2

Correct Answer: 1
Explanation: Current density with iontophoresis equals current amplitude (mA) divided by electrode size (cm^2). Option 1 has the lowest current density (4 mA / 12 cm^2 = .33 mA/cm^2). (Cameron p. 235)

Clinical Practice: Physical Agents
Content Outline: Intervention

Question Number: 195
A 67-year-old male with longstanding cardiac pathology is referred to physical therapy. The medical record indicates the patient is taking Nitrostat. The primary indication for this medication is:

1. to strengthen the heart's pumping force
2. **to produce a general vasodilation of vascular structures**
3. to increase excretion of sodium and water
4. to decrease electrical conduction

Correct Answer: 2
Explanation: Nitrates are administered to produce a general vasodilation throughout the body. Nitrates decrease the amount of blood returning to the heart as well as the amount of work the heart must perform. Through this process there is a decrease in the myocardial oxygen demand. (Ciccone p. 328)

Clinical Practice: Cardiopulmonary System
Content Outline: Examination

Question Number: 196
A physical therapist administers conventional transcutaneous electrical nerve stimulation (TENS) to treat a patient with acute low back pain. Which of the following parameters would best achieve this goal?

1. phase duration of 200 microseconds with a frequency of 4 pulses per second
2. phase duration of 500 microseconds with a frequency of 100 pulses per second
3. **phase duration of 40 microseconds with a frequency of 100 pulses per second**
4. phase duration of 40 microseconds with a frequency of 5 pulses per second

Correct Answer: 3
Explanation: Conventional TENS is characterized by short phase duration, high frequency, and relatively low current amplitude. The primary effects of conventional TENS last only while the stimulus is being applied. (Belanger p. 30)

Clinical Practice: Physical Agents
Content Outline: Intervention

Question Number: 197
A physical therapist provides pre-operative instructions to a patient scheduled for lower extremity amputation. Which of the following is the most common cause of lower extremity amputation?

1. tumor
2. trauma
3. **peripheral vascular disease**
4. cardiac disease

Correct Answer: 3
Explanation: Peripheral vascular disease is the most prevalent cause of lower extremity amputations. This disease has a strong association with smoking and/or diabetes. (Palmer p. 41)

Clinical Practice: Cardiopulmonary
Content Outline: Examination

Question Number: 198

A physical therapist completes documentation after administering an ultrasound treatment. Which treatment parameter would be the least important to document?

1. **patient position**
2. treatment time
3. intensity
4. duty cycle

Correct Answer: 1

Explanation: Although each option includes information that may at times be necessary to document, patient position is perhaps the least important. The other listed options provide essential information that define the specific parameters of the ultrasound treatment. (Michlovitz p. 207)

Clinical Practice: Education/Communication
Content Outline: Intervention

Question Number: 199

A physical therapist completes a coordination assessment on a 67-year-old patient with central nervous system involvement. After reviewing the results of the assessment, the therapist concludes the clinical findings are indicative of cerebellar dysfunction. Which finding is not associated with cerebellar dysfunction?

1. dysmetria
2. **hypertonia**
3. ataxia
4. nystagmus

Correct Answer: 2

Explanation: Hypotonicity, not hypertonicity, is a common finding in patients with cerebellar involvement. It can occur unilaterally or bilaterally and will most significantly affect muscles that surround proximal joints. (Goodman - Pathology p. 984)

Clinical Practice: Neuromuscular System
Content Outline: Evaluation, Diagnosis, Prognosis, and Outcomes

Question Number: 200

A patient status post open knee meniscectomy is referred to physical therapy for neuromuscular electrical stimulation. The most beneficial frequency of treatment to promote strengthening is:

1. one time per week
2. two times per week
3. **three times per week**
4. once every two weeks

Correct Answer: 3

Explanation: Research indicates that three sessions per week of neuromuscular electrical stimulation produces the most desirable clinical outcome. (Robinson p. 141)

Clinical Practice: Physical Agents
Content Outline: Evaluation, Diagnosis, Prognosis, and Outcomes

EXAM TWO: COMPUTER-BASED
Answer Key

Computer-Based Exam Two – Section One

Question Number: 1
A physical therapist compiles a table which identifies joint position at the hip, knee, ankle, and metatarsophalangeal joints for each subunit of the stance phase of gait. Which of the following is not accurate in describing normal joint position at the end of terminal stance?

1. 15 degrees of hip hyperextension
2. 0 degrees of knee extension
3. 0 degrees of ankle dorsiflexion
4. **10 degrees of metatarsophalangeal hyperextension**

Correct Answer: 4
Explanation: Normal position of the lower extremity at the end of terminal stance is as follows: hip 10-20 degrees of hyperextension; knee 0 degrees; ankle 0 degrees of dorsiflexion; metatarsophalangeal 30 degrees of hyperextension. (Levangie p. 448)

Clinical Practice: Musculoskeletal System
Content Outline: Examination

Question Number: 2
A physical therapist instructs a patient diagnosed with C6 tetraplegia in functional activities. Which of the following activities would be least appropriate?

1. independent raises for skin protection
2. manual wheelchair propulsion
3. assisted to independent transfers with a sliding board
4. **independent self-range of motion of the lower extremities**

Correct Answer: 4
Explanation: A patient with C7 tetraplegia is the highest spinal injury level that will consistently attain independence with self-range of motion of the lower extremities. (Umphred p. 493)

Clinical Practice: Neuromuscular System
Content Outline: Evaluation, Diagnosis, Prognosis, and Outcomes

Question Number: 3
A physical therapist participates in a research study to determine the effect of noise level on the ability to perform a physical skill. In the study, noise is the:

1. **independent variable**
2. dependent variable
3. criterion variable
4. extraneous variable

Correct Answer: 1
Explanation: The independent variable, often termed the experimental variable, is manipulated by the researcher to determine the effect on the dependent variable. (Payton p. 11)

Clinical Practice: Research
Content Outline: Standards of Care

Question Number: 4
A physical therapist uses paraffin as a means of superficial heat for a patient with a hand injury. When using the dip and wrap method, the most appropriate number of times to dip the hand would be:

1. 1-3
2. 2-4
3. 4-6
4. **6-10**

Correct Answer: 4
Explanation: A patient is usually required to immerse the hand in paraffin 6-10 times in order to form a solid wax glove around the fingers, wrist, and hand. (Michlovitz p. 120)

Clinical Practice: Physical Agents
Content Outline: Intervention

Question Number: 5

A physical therapist interviews a patient recently involved in a motor vehicle accident. The patient sustained multiple lower extremity injuries as a result of the accident and appears to be very depressed. In an attempt to encourage active dialogue the therapist asks open-ended questions. Which of the following would not be considered an open-ended question?

1. How does your knee feel today?
2. What are your goals for physical therapy?
3. **Do you have trouble sleeping at night?**
4. Tell me about your present condition?

Correct Answer: 3
Explanation: Open-ended questions allow patients to answer with a myriad of responses, while closed-ended questions can often be answered with a yes or no response. (Goodman - Differential Diagnosis p. 38)

Clinical Practice: Education/Communication
Content Outline: Intervention

Question Number: 6

A group of physical therapists employed in an acute care hospital is responsible for developing departmental guidelines for electrical equipment care and safety. What is the minimum required testing interval for electrical equipment?

1. 3 months
2. 6 months
3. 9 months
4. **12 months**

Correct Answer: 4
Explanation: Electrical equipment should be inspected according to the specified intervals outlined by the manufacturer. Although often these intervals may be more frequent than every 12 months, it is unacceptable for any electrical equipment to be uninspected for more than a 12 month period. (Nelson p. 48)

Clinical Practice: Administration
Content Outline: Intervention

Question Number: 7   *Item Includes Graphic*

A physical therapist positions a patient as shown in order to assess their claim of complete paresis of the right lower extremity. The therapist then instructs the patient to perform a rapid straight leg raise with their left lower extremity. Which finding would best dispute the patient's claim?

1. The patient is unable to lift their left heel from the therapist's hand.
2. The patient experiences radiating pain into the right lower extremity.
3. **The patient exerts a downward force into the therapist's hand with their right heel.**
4. The patient experiences radiating pain into their left lower extremity.

Correct Answer: 3
Explanation: A rapid straight leg raise with the left lower extremity will typically result in the patient pushing their right heel down into the therapist's hand. The described testing procedure is consistent with Hoover's test which is often employed as a gross test for malingering. (DeMyer p. 695)

Clinical Practice: Neuromuscular System
Content Outline: Examination

Question Number: 8

A patient rehabilitating from a lower extremity injury has been non-weight bearing for three weeks. A recent physician entry in the medical record indicates the patient is cleared for weight bearing up to 25 pounds. The most appropriate device to use when instructing the patient on her new weight bearing status is:

1. an inclinometer
2. **a scale**
3. an anthropometer
4. a tape measure

Correct Answer: 2
Explanation: A standard bathroom scale can effectively be used to educate patients on weight bearing status. (Minor p. 289)

Clinical Practice: Education/Communication
Content Outline: Intervention

Question Number: 9
A patient is referred to physical therapy for instruction in an exercise program. Which of the following conditions is not an absolute contraindication to exercise training?

1. acute myocarditis
2. acute infection
3. **hypertrophic cardiomyopathy**
4. deep venous thrombosis

Correct Answer: 3
Explanation: Hypertrophic cardiomyopathy is considered a relative contraindication to exercise testing, while the remaining options are absolute contraindications. (American College of Sports Medicine p. 50)

Clinical Practice: Cardiopulmonary System
Content Outline: Intervention

Question Number: 10
A physical therapist observes a patient complete hip abduction and adduction exercises in standing. Which axis of movement is utilized with these partcular motions?

1. coronal
2. vertical
3. **anterior-posterior**
4. longitudinal

Correct Answer: 3
Explanation: Abduction and adduction typically occur in a frontal plane around an anterior-posterior axis. (Levangie p. 5)

Clinical Practice: Musculoskeletal System
Content Outline: Intervention

Question Number: 11
A physical therapist treats a 56-year-old male status post transfemoral amputation with a hip flexion contracture. As part of the treatment regimen the therapist performs passive stretching exercises to the involved hip. The most appropriate form of passive stretching is:

1. **moderate tension over a prolonged period of time**
2. moderate tension over a brief period of time
3. maximal tension over a prolonged period of time
4. maximal tension over a brief period of time

Correct Answer: 1
Explanation: Moderate tension over a prolonged period of time would be the most appropriate form of stretching for the hip flexors. In addition, this type of stretch will be better tolerated by the patient. (Kisner p. 184)

Clinical Practice: Musculoskeletal System
Content Outline: Intervention

Question Number: 12
A patient is treated using pulsed wave ultrasound at 1.2 W/cm^2 for seven minutes. The specific parameters of the pulsed wave are 2 msec on time and 8 msec off time for one pulse period. The duty cycle should be recorded as:

1. 10 %
2. **20 %**
3. 25 %
4. 50 %

Correct Answer: 2
Explanation: Duty cycle is defined as the ratio of the on time to the total time. Duty cycle = 2 msec / (2 msec + 8 msec) = .20(100) = 20%. (Nelson p. 28)

Clinical Practice: Physical Agents
Content Outline: Intervention

Question Number: 13
A physical therapist instructs a patient with a unilateral amputation to ascend and descend stairs. Which amputation level would you expect to have the most difficulty performing the described task?

1. transmetatarsal
2. transtibial
3. **transfemoral**
4. Symes

Correct Answer: 3
Explanation: A patient with a transfemoral amputation would have the greatest difficulty in ascending and descending stairs. Due to the higher lever of the amputation and subsequent shorter lever arm the patient requires greater energy expenditure, balance, and coordination when using a prosthesis. (O'Sullivan p. 669)

Clinical Practice: Patient Care Skills
Content Outline: Evaluation, Diagnosis, Prognosis, and Outcomes

Question Number: 14
A physical therapist examines the output from a single lead electrocardiogram of a patient with first degree atrioventricular heart block. The defining characteristic of this condition is:

1. heightened T wave
2. **prolonged PR interval**
3. bizarre QRS complex
4. shortened ST segment

Correct Answer: 2
Explanation: Atrioventricular blocks are caused by an abnormal delay or failure of conduction through the AV node or the atrioventricular bundle. Appearance of all waves on the electrocardiogram will be normal, however, the PR interval will be prolonged. (Brannon p. 212)

Clinical Practice: Cardiopulmonary System
Content Outline: Examination

Question Number: 15
A physical therapist obtains a complete medical history prior to administering cryotherapy. Which condition would not be considered a contraindication to cryotherapy?

1. Raynaud's phenomenon
2. cryoglobinemia
3. **cancer**
4. cold urticaria

Correct Answer: 3
Explanation: Cryotherapy is not contraindicated for patient's with cancer, however, secondary impairments such as diminished sensation may make cryotherapy an unacceptable treatment option in certain situations. (Michlovitz p. 101)

Clinical Practice: Physical Agents
Content Outline: Intervention

Question Number: 16
A patient rehabilitating from a trimalleolar fracture is cleared for 20 pounds of weight bearing. During a scheduled therapy session, the patient admits he has not used crutches during the past week. The most appropriate physical therapist action is:

1. instruct the patient to ask the physician to modify his weight bearing status
2. **inform the patient of the potential consequence of placing too much weight on the involved leg**
3. contact the patient's insurance provider
4. discharge the patient from physical therapy due to noncompliance

Correct Answer: 2
Explanation: The most important factor is to promote patient compliance in order to avoid the complications associated with premature weight bearing on a fracture. (Pierson p. 189)

Clinical Practice: Education/Communication
Content Outline: Intervention

Question Number: 17
A 26-year-old male rehabilitating from a fractured tibia sustained in a skiing accident is referred to physical therapy for instruction and fitting of an assistive device. The most appropriate number of patient visits to accomplish the stated objective is:

1. **1**
2. 3
3. 5
4. 7

Correct Answer: 1
Explanation: A 26-year-old with a lower extremity injury without other complicating factors should have little difficulty utilizing an assistive device following a single training session. (Pierson p. 188)

Clinical Practice: Patient Care Skills
Content Outline: Evaluation, Diagnosis, Prognosis, and Outcomes

Question Number: 18

A child with a unilateral hip disarticulation works on advanced gait training activities. Which of the following activities would be the most difficult for the patient?

1. rising from a wheelchair
2. ascending stairs with a handrail
3. descending stairs with a handrail
4. **ascending a curb**

Correct Answer: 4

Explanation: A child with a hip disarticulation would have the greatest difficulty with ascending a curb during prosthetic training since there are no external supports (rails) to assist with the activity. (O'Sullivan p. 669)

Clinical Practice: Patient Care Skills
Content Outline: Intervention

Question Number: 19

A patient with a C6 spinal cord injury is examined in physical therapy. Which objective finding would be the strongest indication the spinal cord injury is not complete?

1. intact sensation on the lateral portion of the shoulder
2. absent triceps reflex
3. **diminished sensation over the hypothenar eminence**
4. weakness of the biceps muscle

Correct Answer: 3

Explanation: The dermatome that corresponds to the hypothenar eminence is at the C8 level. As a result, the finding of diminished sensation (not absent) at a level below C6 may indicate the injury is incomplete. (Goodman - Pathology p. 779)

Clinical Practice: Neuromuscular System
Content Outline: Evaluation, Diagnosis, Prognosis, and Outcomes

Question Number: 20

A physical therapist monitors a patient's vital signs while completing 20 minutes of jogging at 5 mph on a treadmill. As the session approaches its conclusion the therapist incorporates a cool down period. The anticipated blood pressure response during the post-exercise period is:

1. a progressive increase in systolic blood pressure
2. **a progressive decrease in systolic blood pressure**
3. a progressive increase in diastolic blood pressure
4. a progressive decrease in diastolic blood pressure

Correct Answer: 2

Explanation: Systolic blood pressure tends to increase with increasing exercise intensity and progressively decrease during the cool down and post-exercise period. (American College of Sports Medicine p. 118)

Clinical Practice: Cardiopulmonary System
Content Outline: Intervention

Question Number: 21

A patient diagnosed with ankylosing spondylitis exhibits a forward stooped posture. As part of the patient's care plan the physical therapist selects a number of active exercises that promote improved posture. Which proprioceptive neuromuscular facilitation pattern would be the most appropriate to achieve the therapist's objective?

1. D1 extension
2. D1 flexion
3. D2 extension
4. **D2 flexion**

Correct Answer: 4

Explanation: A D2 flexion pattern incorporates flexion, abduction, and lateral rotation of the shoulder and therefore promotes upright posture. The verbal command to complete this pattern would be open your hand and pull up and away from your body. (Sullivan p. 300)

Clinical Practice: Neuromuscular System
Content Outline: Intervention

Question Number: 22
A patient rehabilitating from a CVA exhibits a flexor synergy pattern in the upper extremity. The strongest component of the pattern is:

1. shoulder lateral rotation
2. forearm supination
3. **elbow flexion**
4. scapular elevation

Correct Answer: 3
Explanation: Elbow flexion is usually the first and the strongest component of the flexor synergy. (Brunnstrom p. 10)

Clinical Practice: Neuromuscular System
Content Outline: Evaluation, Diagnosis, Prognosis, and Outcomes

Question Number: 23
A manager develops a policy on physical therapy utilization of continuing education resources. Which of the following would be the most appropriate action to enhance the quality of patient care?

1. offer continuing education resources to senior therapists in relation to their years of experience
2. divide the continuing education resources evenly among therapy staff
3. establish a committee to review requests for continuing education resources
4. **prioritize requests for continuing education resources based on established patient care standards**

Correct Answer: 4
Explanation: Continuing education resources should be allocated in a manner that will provide the greatest tangible benefit for the current patient population. (Walter p. 128)

Clinical Practice: Administration
Content Outline: Standards of Care

Question Number: 24
A physical therapist familiarizes himself with potential sources of negligence in physical therapy. Which activity is most frequently cited as the basis for a malpractice claim?

1. sexual misconduct
2. failure to follow physician's orders
3. **failure to monitor the condition of the patient**
4. improper utilization of universal precautions

Correct Answer: 3
Explanation: Negligence results when a therapist provides care that falls below a standard established by law. Failure to monitor the condition of a patient is often the basis for health care malpractice claims. (Scott - Promoting Legal Awareness p. 32)

Clinical Practice: Administration
Content Outline: Standards of Care

Question Number: 25
A physical therapist examines the gait of a patient with a transtibial amputation. The patient exhibits delayed and limited knee flexion after heel strike on the prosthetic side. The most likely cause of the deviation is:

1. foot positioned in plantar flexion
2. **heel wedge is too soft**
3. socket positioned posteriorly
4. socket is too large

Correct Answer: 2
Explanation: If the heel wedge of a prosthesis is too soft it will not allow the prosthesis to advance as needed over the foot in order to create a flexion moment at the knee. (Rothstein p. 831)

Clinical Practice: Patient Care Skills
Content Outline: Evaluation, Diagnosis, Prognosis, and Outcomes

Question Number: 26
A physical therapist examines a patient status post CVA. The patient has severe difficulty in verbal expression and mild difficulty in understanding complex syntax. This type of communication disorder is best termed:

1. **Broca's aphasia**
2. conduction aphasia
3. global aphasia
4. Wernicke's aphasia

Correct Answer: 1
Explanation: Broca's aphasia usually occurs from a lesion to the left inferior frontal lobe. A patient with Broca's aphasia can understand what is said to them, however, recovery of verbal output is slow and fragmented. (Rothstein p. 441)

Clinical Practice: Neuromuscular System
Content Outline: Evaluation, Diagnosis, Prognosis, and Outcomes

Question Number: 27
A physical therapist completing a balance assessment positions a patient in standing prior to administering the Romberg test. When administering the Romberg test it would be most important for the therapist to determine:

1. the width of the base of support necessary in order to maintain standing
2. the amount of time the patient is able to maintain the test position
3. **the amount of sway present during the testing period**
4. the complexity of tasks the patient is able to perform with eyes open and eyes closed

Correct Answer: 3
Explanation: The Romberg test can be used to examine the influence of proprioceptive, visual, and vestibular input on balance. The test is administered with the patient in standing with the feet together and arms crossed over the chest. Initially the test should be performed with the patient's eyes open and then closed, if applicable. The therapist should attempt to subjectively quantify the amount of postural sway present during four trials lasting approximately one minute each. (Montgomery p. 191)

Clinical Practice: Neuromuscular System
Content Outline: Examination

Question Number: 28
A physical therapist reviews the medical record of a patient diagnosed with peripheral vascular disease prior to initiating treatment. Which objective finding would most severely limit the patient's ability to participate in an ambulation exercise program?

1. **signs of resting claudication**
2. decreased peripheral pulses
3. cool skin
4. blood pressure of 165/90 mm Hg

Correct Answer: 1
Explanation: Peripheral vascular disease refers to a condition involving the arterial, venous, or lymphatic systems that results in compromised circulation to the extremities. Resting claudication is typically considered a contraindication to active exercise in patients with peripheral vascular disease. (Kisner p. 715)

Clinical Practice: Cardiopulmonary System
Content Outline: Evaluation, Diagnosis, Prognosis, and Outcomes

Question Number: 29
A patient with limited elbow and forearm range of motion is referred to physical therapy. When mobilizing the humeroradial articulation, the treatment plane is considered to be:

1. in the concave radial head, parallel to the long axis of the radius
2. **in the concave radial head, perpendicular to the long axis of the radius**
3. in the convex radial head, parallel to the long axis of the radius
4. in the convex radial head, perpendicular to the long axis of the radius

Correct Answer: 2
Explanation: The humeroradial joint consists of the convex capitulum articulating with the concave radial head. The resting position of the joint is full extension and supination. (Kisner p. 236)

Clinical Practice: Musculoskeletal System
Content Outline: Intervention

Question Number: 30
A physical therapist treats a patient diagnosed with spinal stenosis. As part of the treatment program the patient lies prone on a treatment plinth with a hot pack draped over the low back. The most effective method to monitor the patient while using the hot pack is:

1. check on the patient at least every ten minutes
2. **supply the patient with a bell to ring if the hot pack becomes too hot**
3. instruct the patient to remove the hot pack if it becomes too hot
4. select an alternate superficial heating modality

Correct Answer: 2
Explanation: A bell supplies the patient with a method to communicate with the therapist in a safe and efficient manner without alarming other patients. (Michlovitz p. 116)

Clinical Practice: Physical Agents
Content Outline: Intervention

Question Number: 31

A physical therapist asks a patient to complete a pain questionnaire. The questionnaire utilizes an ascending numeric scale ranging from "0" equaling no pain to "10" equaling excruciating pain. This type of measurement scale is best described as:

1. nominal
2. **ordinal**
3. interval
4. ratio

Correct Answer: 2
Explanation: An ordinal measurement scale uses independent categories that have a qualitative relationship regarding the order of ranking. (Payton p. 59)

Clinical Practice: Research
Content Outline: Standards of Care

Question Number: 32

A patient with T10 paraplegia is discharged from a rehabilitation hospital following 12 weeks of intense rehabilitation. Which of the following pieces of equipment would be the most essential to assist the patient with functional mobility?

1. ambulation with Lofstrand crutches
2. ambulation with Lofstrand crutches and ankle-foot orthoses
3. ambulation with Lofstrand crutches and knee-ankle-foot orthoses
4. **wheelchair**

Correct Answer: 4
Explanation: Patients with a lesion above T12 are not functional ambulators due to the extreme energy demands and therefore utilize a wheelchair as their primary mode of mobility. (Umphred p. 521)

Clinical Practice: Patient Care Skills
Content Outline: Intervention

Question Number: 33

A physical therapist conducts an inservice on exercise guidelines for a group of senior citizens. As part of the inservice the therapist discusses the benefits of improving cardiovascular status through a low intensity activity such as a walking program. What frequency of exercise would be the most desirable to achieve the stated objective?

1. twice per day
2. one time per week
3. three times per week
4. **five times per week**

Correct Answer: 4
Explanation: According to the American College of Sports Medicine, exercise performed at a moderate intensity should be performed most days of the week. If exercise is at a vigorous level, it should be performed at least three times per week. Since the cited exercise is low intensity, five times per week is the most appropriate option. (American College of Sports Medicine p. 226)

Clinical Practice: Cardiopulmonary System
Content Outline: Intervention

Question Number: 34

A physical therapist identifies the pisiform after palpating along the proximal row of carpals. Which carpal bone articulates with the pisiform?

1. trapezium
2. trapezoid
3. lunate
4. **triquetrum**

Correct Answer: 4
Explanation: The pisiform is located within the flexor carpi ulnaris tendon and lies immediately superior to the triquetrum. (Hoppenfeld p. 71)

Clinical Practice: Musculoskeletal System
Content Outline: Examination

Question Number: 35

A physical therapist employed in an acute care hospital reviews the medical record of a patient diagnosed with congestive heart failure. The therapist would like to implement a formal exercise program, but is concerned about the patient's exercise tolerance. Which condition is most responsible for the patient's limited exercise tolerance?

1. diminished lung volumes
2. arterial oxygen desaturation
3. **insufficient stroke volume during ventricular systole**
4. excessive rise in blood pressure

Correct Answer: 3

Explanation: Congestive heart failure is characterized by an inability of the heart to adequately deliver oxygenated blood to tissue. Specifically, the heart cannot eject a sufficient stroke volume during ventricular systole. Stroke volume is the difference between end diastolic volume and end systolic volume. (American College of Sports Medicine p. 186)

Clinical Practice: Cardiopulmonary System
Content Outline: Intervention

Question Number: 36

A physical therapist measures a patient for a wheelchair. When measuring back height, which method is most accurate?

1. measure from the seat of the chair to the base of the axilla and subtract two inches
2. **measure from the seat of the chair to the base of the axilla and subtract four inches**
3. measure from the seat of the chair to the acromion process and subtract two inches
4. measure from the seat of the chair to the acromion process and subtract four inches

Correct Answer: 2

Explanation: A physical therapist should measure from the seat of the chair to the patient's axilla and subtract four inches. This procedure will allow the back height to fall below the inferior angle of the scapula. Average back height in an adult size wheelchair is 16 to 16.5 inches. (Pierson p. 149)

Clinical Practice: Patient Care Skills
Content Outline: Intervention

Question Number: 37

A patient diagnosed with infrapatellar tendonitis completes a series of functional activities. After completing the activities the physical therapist instructs the patient to use ice massage over the anterior surface of the knee. The most appropriate treatment time is:

1. 3 - 5 minutes
2. **5 - 10 minutes**
3. 10 - 15 minutes
4. 15 - 20 minutes

Correct Answer: 2

Explanation: Ice massage serves as an effective method of cryotherapy over local areas such as tendons, bursae or muscle bellies. Due to the limited size of the treatment area, 5-10 minutes of ice massage is usually adequate. (Michlovitz p. 99)

Clinical Practice: Physical Agents
Content Outline: Intervention

Question Number: 38

A patient sustains a deep partial-thickness burn to the anterior surface of the right upper extremity and a superficial partial-thickness burn to the anterior surface of the trunk. According to the rule of nines, the patient has burns over:

1. 18.5 percent of the body
2. **22.5 percent of the body**
3. 27 percent of the body
4. 36 percent of the body

Correct Answer: 2

Explanation: The "rule of nines" is commonly utilized to assess the percentage of the body surface affected by a burn. Anterior surface of the right upper extremity = 4.5%, anterior surface of the trunk = 18%. (Rothstein p. 1119)

Clinical Practice: Integumentary System
Content Outline: Examination

Question Number: 39
A physical therapist reviews the medical record of a patient scheduled for debridement. The record indicates that the patient sustained a chemical burn eight days ago in an industrial accident. The burn area was measured as 13 cm by 33 cm. This measurement most closely corresponds to:

1. 2 inches by 7 inches
2. 3 inches by 11 inches
3. **5 inches by 13 inches**
4. 6 inches by 21 inches

Correct Answer: 3
Explanation: 1 inch is equivalent to 2.54 centimeters, therefore 13 cm = 5.12 inches and 33 cm = 12.99 inches. (Bickley p. 62)

Clinical Practice: Integumentary System
Content Outline: Examination

Question Number: 40
A physical therapist examines a patient's scapulohumeral rhythm as the arm is actively abducted to 30 degrees. Which description best summarizes the action of the scapula and clavicle during this movement?

1. scapula 20 degrees rotation, clavicle 25-35 degrees elevation
2. scapula 10 degrees rotation, clavicle 15-25 degrees elevation
3. **scapula minimal movement, clavicle 0-5 degrees elevation**
4. scapula 30 degrees rotation, clavicle 5 degrees elevation

Correct Answer: 3
Explanation: The 2:1 ratio of humerus to scapula movement does not pertain to the initial phase of movement. (Magee p. 225)

Clinical Practice: Musculoskeletal System
Content Outline: Examination

Question Number: 41
A physical therapist uses functional electrical stimulation as part of a treatment regimen designed to improve quadriceps strength. Which on:off time ratio would result in the most rapid onset of muscle fatigue?

1. 3:1
2. 1:4
3. **5:1**
4. 1:6

Correct Answer: 3
Explanation: Fatigue will vary directly with the ratio of on:off time. A ratio of 5:1 will therefore promote the greatest amount of muscle fatigue. (Robinson p. 42)

Clinical Practice: Physical Agents
Content Outline: Intervention

Question Number: 42
A national health care corporation agrees to provide physical therapy services for a group of 25,000 autoworkers. The corporation is prepaid for services on a per member per month basis. This arrangement is best described as:

1. credentialing
2. fee for service
3. accrual
4. **capitation**

Correct Answer: 4
Explanation: Capitation refers to a method of payment for services on a per member, per month basis. In this type of system the provider receives payment whether or not services are utilized. (Sultz p. 256)

Clinical Practice: Administration
Content Outline: Standards of Care

Question Number: 43
A physical therapist employed in an outpatient clinic observes a patient complete a series of exercises. During the treatment session the patient mentions to the therapist that he is experiencing angina. After resting for 20 minutes the patient's condition is unchanged, however, he insists it is something that he can work through. The most appropriate therapist action is:

1. allow the patient to resume exercise and continue to monitor the patient's condition
2. reduce the intensity of the exercise and continue to monitor the patient's condition
3. discontinue the treatment session and encourage the patient to make an appointment with his physician
4. **discontinue the treatment session and call an ambulance**

Correct Answer: 4
Explanation: Angina that does not dissipate after the termination of exercise should be considered a medical emergency. As a result, the most appropriate therapist action is to discontinue the treatment session and call an ambulance. (American College of Sports Medicine p. 186)

Clinical Practice: Patient Care Skills
Content Outline: Intervention

Question Number: 44
A 55-year-old male status post myocardial infarction is referred to physical therapy. The patient has a history of cardiac disease and is moderately obese. The patient's age-predicted maximal heart rate should be recorded as:

1. 190
2. 185
3. **165**
4. 155

Correct Answer: 3
Explanation: Age-predicted maximal heart rate is determined by the formula 220 - patient's age (55) = 165. (Brannon p. 254)

Clinical Practice: Cardiopulmonary System
Content Outline: Intervention

Question Number: 45
A physical therapist transports a patient in a wheelchair to the parallel bars in preparation for ambulation activities. The patient is status post abdominal surgery and has not ambulated in over two weeks. The most appropriate action to facilitate ambulation is:

1. assist the patient to standing
2. monitor the patient's vital signs
3. **demonstrate ambulation in the parallel bars**
4. secure an additional staff member to offer assistance

Correct Answer: 3
Explanation: Demonstration is an essential component of any educational session particularly when initially instructing a patient. The parallel bars offer a secure and stable base for the patient to attempt ambulation. (Minor p. 289)

Clinical Practice: Education/Communication
Content Outline: Intervention

Question Number: 46
A physical therapist prepares to transfer a patient from a wheelchair to a treatment table. The patient cannot stand independently, but is able to bear some weight through the lower extremities. The most appropriate transfer technique is:

1. sliding board transfer
2. hydraulic lift
3. **dependent standing pivot**
4. two-person lift

Correct Answer: 3
Explanation: A dependent standing pivot transfer is used when a patient can bear some weight through the lower extremities, however, cannot transfer independently. (Minor p. 246)

Clinical Practice: Patient Care Skills
Content Outline: Intervention

Question Number: 47

A risk management committee composed of various members of the rehabilitation team is charged with identifying methods to prevent employee exposure to blood and body fluids. The most appropriate initial action is:

1. provide follow-up to staff if exposed to blood and body fluids
2. provide free hepatitis B immunizations to staff
3. **develop an infection control policy that conforms to O.S.H.A. guidelines**
4. educate staff about the policies

Correct Answer: 3
Explanation: All health care facilities must have a formal infection control policy that is consistent with O.S.H.A. requirements. (Pierson p. 314)

Clinical Practice: Administration
Content Outline: Intervention

Question Number: 48

A physical therapist attempts to classify the amount of assistance a patient requires to complete a sit to stand transfer. After completing the transfer, the therapist estimates that he was required to exert approximately 20% of the physical work in order to ensure the transfer was completed safely. The most appropriate classification of the level of assistance would be:

1. independent
2. standby assistance
3. **minimal assistance**
4. moderate assistance

Correct Answer: 3
Explanation: A transfer classified as minimal assistance usually requires up to 25% of the physical work to be performed by the physical therapist. (Montgomery p. 190)

Clinical Practice: Patient Care Skills
Content Outline: Intervention

Question Number: 49

A physical therapist examines a patient with a suspected injury to the thoracodorsal nerve. Which objective finding would be consistent with this injury?

1. shoulder medial rotation weakness
2. **shoulder extension weakness**
3. paralysis of the rhomboids
4. forward displacement of the lateral end of the clavicle

Correct Answer: 2
Explanation: The latissimus dorsi is innervated by the thoracodorsal nerve. Weakness in this muscle would produce impaired strength during shoulder extension. (Kendall p. 279)

Clinical Practice: Neuromuscular System
Content Outline: Evaluation, Diagnosis, Prognosis, and Outcomes

Question Number: 50

A patient explains to her therapist that she was instructed to bear up to five pounds of weight on her involved extremity. The patient's weight bearing status would be best described as:

1. non-weight bearing
2. toe touch weight bearing
3. **partial weight bearing**
4. weight bearing as tolerated

Correct Answer: 3
Explanation: Toe touch weight bearing permits the toes of the involved extremity to touch the ground for balance, but not for weight bearing. Partial weight bearing permits the transfer of a small amount of weight through the involved extremity. (Pierson p. 298)

Clinical Practice: Patient Care Skills
Content Outline: Intervention

Computer-Based Exam Two – Section Two

Question Number: 51
A physical therapist completing a lower quarter screening examination attempts to palpate the tendon of the anterior tibialis. The most appropriate therapist action to facilitate palpation is:

1. ask the patient to actively move the foot into dorsiflexion and eversion
2. **ask the patient to actively move the foot into dorsiflexion and inversion**
3. passively move the patient's foot into dorsiflexion and eversion
4. passively move the patient's foot into dorsiflexion and inversion

Correct Answer: 2
Explanation: The anterior tibialis acts to dorsiflex the ankle joint and assist in inversion of the foot. The muscle is innervated by the deep peroneal nerve. (Kendall p. 201)

Clinical Practice: Musculoskeletal System
Content Outline: Examination

Question Number: 52
A physical therapist uses a transcutaneous electrical nerve stimulation unit to generate sensory-level stimulation. Which stimulation characteristic is not accurate when describing this technique?

1. duration of treatment: 20-30 minutes
2. amplitude: perceptible tingling
3. **phase duration: 150-200 microseconds**
4. frequency: 50-150 Hz

Correct Answer: 3
Explanation: Sensory-level stimulation is characterized by a relatively short phase duration of 20-100 microseconds. (Robinson p. 285)

Clinical Practice: Physical Agents
Content Outline: Intervention

Question Number: 53
A 67-year-old female status post total knee arthroplasty due to severe degenerative joint disease is referred to physical therapy. During the examination the patient reports to the therapist that she has significant difficulty negotiating stairs. How much knee range of motion would be required to perform this activity?

1. approximately 0-60 degrees of knee flexion
2. **approximately 0-90 degrees of knee flexion**
3. approximately 0-110 degrees of knee flexion
4. approximately 0-125 degrees of knee flexion

Correct Answer: 2
Explanation: Knee flexion of approximately 90 degrees is required for stair climbing. (Levangie p. 469)

Clinical Practice: Patient Care Skills
Content Outline: Intervention

Question Number: 54
A physical therapist completes a balance assessment on a patient recently admitted to a skilled nursing facility. The therapist concludes that the patient is able to maintain their balance without support in standing, however, cannot maintain balance during weight shifting or with any form of external perturbation. The most appropriate balance grade would be:

1. normal
2. good
3. **fair**
4. poor

Correct Answer: 3
Explanation: The patient's ability to maintain balance in standing and inability to maintain balance with weight shifting or outside challenges is typical of a patient with fair balance. A poor grade would indicate that the patient requires some form of assistance to maintain balance. (Montgomery p. 190)

Clinical Practice: Neuromuscular System
Content Outline: Examination

Question Number: 55

A patient rehabilitating from a CVA requires an orthosis due to occasional dragging of the toe during swing phase. The patient presents with weakness of the dorsiflexors and has good medial/lateral stability at the ankle. The most appropriate option for the patient is:

1. solid ankle-foot orthosis
2. tone reducing foot orthosis
3. **posterior leaf spring orthosis**
4. custom articulating ankle-foot orthosis with anterior trim lines

Correct Answer: 3

Explanation: A posterior leaf spring orthosis is a type of ankle-foot orthosis that provides a dorsiflexion assist during swing phase. The trim line is posterior to the malleoli and does not provide any medial or lateral ankle support. (O'Sullivan p. 1031)

Clinical Practice: Neuromuscular System
Content Outline: Intervention

Question Number: 56

A physical therapist completes a standing flexion test to identify possible innominate distortion in a patient referred to physical therapy with chronic back pain. The most appropriate structure to palpate while completing the test is:

1. spinous process of L5
2. anterior superior iliac spines
3. **posterior superior iliac spines**
4. pubic tubercles

Correct Answer: 3

Explanation: The standing flexion test is designed to identify innominate distortion. The physical therapist should palpate the inferior portion of the posterior superior iliac spines as the patient actively flexes the spine. (Hertling p. 711)

Clinical Practice: Musculoskeletal System
Content Outline: Examination

Question Number: 57

A physical therapist completes a respiratory assessment on a patient with T2 paraplegia. As a component of the assessment, the therapist measures the amount of chest excursion during inspiration. The most appropriate patient position to conduct the measurement is:

1. sitting
2. **supine**
3. prone
4. sidelying

Correct Answer: 2

Explanation: The supine position creates support and resistance to the diaphragm. There is a direct correlation between the amount of chest expansion and intercostal strength. (Umphred p. 499)

Clinical Practice: Cardiopulmonary System
Content Outline: Examination

Question Number: 58

A physical therapist prescribes a wheelchair for a patient with bilateral lower extremity amputations. The most important feature of a wheelchair designed for the patient should be:

1. friction surface handrims
2. **the drive wheels are set behind the vertical back supports**
3. reclining back with elevating legrests
4. removable armrests

Correct Answer: 2

Explanation: A patient with bilateral lower extremity amputations requires offset rear wheels to accommodate for the change in the center of gravity. An anti-tipping device is another method which will prevent the wheelchair and patient from falling backwards. (O'Sullivan p. 637)

Clinical Practice: Patient Care Skills
Content Outline: Intervention

Question Number: 59
A physical therapist examines a 26-year-old female whose subjective complaints include morning stiffness of her hands and visible swelling. The patient indicates that the stiffness seems to diminish with activity. This description best describes:

1. carpal tunnel syndrome
2. osteoporosis
3. **rheumatoid arthritis**
4. osteoarthritis

Correct Answer: 3
Explanation: Rheumatoid arthritis is a chronic systemic disease characterized by inflammatory changes in joints and related structures. Symptoms of rheumatoid arthritis include morning stiffness, limited range of motion, and pain with movement. The disease is 2-3 times more common in women than men. (Pauls p. 90)

Clinical Practice: Musculoskeletal System
Content Outline: Evaluation, Diagnosis, Prognosis, and Outcomes

Question Number: 60   *Item Includes Graphic*
A physical therapist working in an outpatient physical therapy clinic guards a patient descending a curb with axillary crutches. Based on the photograph, the most likely patient scenario is:

1. **partial weight bearing secondary to a left lateral ankle sprain**
2. partial weight bearing secondary to a right lateral ankle sprain
3. toe touch weight bearing secondary to a left lateral ankle sprain
4. toe touch weight bearing secondary to a right lateral ankle sprain

Correct Answer: 1
Explanation: When descending a curb with axillary crutches the involved lower extremity and crutches are moved from the curb to the ground, while the upper extremities and the uninvolved lower extremity are used to slowly lower the body. As a result, the patient's involved ankle must be on the left. The amount of weight being transmitted through the foot using this specific technique is most consistent with a partial weight bearing gait. (Pierson p. 233)

Clinical Practice: Patient Care Skills
Content Outline: Intervention

Question Number: 61
A physical therapist reviews a patient's medical history before initiating soft tissue massage. Which condition would not be considered a contraindication for this intervention?

1. osteomyelitis
2. **tendonitis**
3. septic arthritis
4. psoriasis

Correct Answer: 2
Explanation: A variety of massage techniques are appropriate to incorporate into a treatment program for a patient with tendonitis. (De Domenico p. 68)

Clinical Practice: Physical Agents
Content Outline: Intervention

Question Number: 62
A physical therapist prepares a patient recovering from a total hip replacement for discharge from the hospital. The patient is 65-years-old and resides alone. Assuming an uncomplicated recovery, which of the following pieces of adaptive equipment would not be necessary for home use?

1. long handled shoehorn
2. raised toilet seat
3. **sliding board**
4. tub bench

Correct Answer: 3
Explanation: A patient scheduled for discharge home following total hip replacement surgery should be able to perform transfers independently without using a sliding board. (Minor p. 248)

Clinical Practice: Patient Care Skills
Content Outline: Intervention

Question Number: 63
A patient with increased sympathetic output is examined in physical therapy. Which treatment technique would not be beneficial in decreasing the level of sympathetic activity?

1. connective tissue massage
2. rotating the lower trunk in hooklying
3. **slow reversal hold of the quadriceps and hamstrings**
4. gentle manual pressure to the abdomen

Correct Answer: 3
Explanation: Slow reversal hold is a technique that is utilized to improve stability around a joint and control a particular movement. Techniques that are used in order to decrease sympathetic activity include massage, rocking, slow rolling, maintained pressure, and slow breathing. (Sullivan p. 60)

Clinical Practice: Neuromuscular System
Content Outline: Intervention

Question Number: 64
A physical therapist records the end-feel associated with forearm supination as firm in the medical record. Which of the following is not consistent with an end-feel categorized as firm?

1. muscular stretch
2. capsular stretch
3. **soft tissue approximation**
4. ligamentous stretch

Correct Answer: 3
Explanation: Soft tissue approximation is associated with a soft end-feel. An example of a soft end-feel is created by contact between the soft tissue of the posterior leg and the posterior thigh during knee flexion. (Norkin p. 8)

Clinical Practice: Musculoskeletal System
Content Outline: Examination

Question Number: 65
A physical therapist examines several superficial reflexes on a patient diagnosed with an upper motor neuron lesion. When assessing the cremasteric reflex the most appropriate stimulus is:

1. stroke the skin of the lower abdominal quadrant
2. **stroke the skin of the upper and inner thigh**
3. prick the skin of the perianal region
4. prick the skin of the glans penis

Correct Answer: 2
Explanation: The therapist should stroke the skin in the area of the upper and inner thigh in order to elicit the superficial cremasteric reflex. The anticipated response is elevation of the testicle on the same side as the stimulus. (DeMyer p. 333)

Clinical Practice: Neuromuscular System
Content Outline: Examination

Question Number: 66
A 35-year-old male diagnosed with ankylosing spondylitis is referred to physical therapy for instruction in a home exercise program. Which general treatment objective would be the most beneficial for the patient?

1. strengthening of the rectus abdominus
2. strengthening of the internal and external obliques
3. strengthening of the quadratus lumborum
4. **strengthening of the back extensors**

Correct Answer: 4
Explanation: Ankylosing spondylitis is a form of systemic rheumatic arthritis that results in inflammation of the axial skeleton with subsequent back pain. The condition often is associated with an increase in thoracic kyphosis and loss of the lumbar curve. As a result, extension exercises are often an important component of a comprehensive treatment plan. (Pauls p. 74)

Clinical Practice: Musculoskeletal System
Content Outline: Intervention

Question Number: 67
A 73-year-old male patient receiving outpatient physical therapy begins to experience acute angina. The patient indicates he uses nitroglycerin to alleviate the angina. The most appropriate mode of administration is:

1. oral
2. buccal
3. **sublingual**
4. topical

Correct Answer: 3
Explanation: Sublingual administration of nitroglycerin is most appropriate with an acute angina attack due to the rapid absorption into the systemic circulation. (Ciccone p. 329)

Clinical Practice: Cardiopulmonary System
Content Outline: Examination

Question Number: 68
A physical therapist attempts to assess the motor component of the axillary nerve by conducting a resistive test. Which muscle would be the most appropriate to utilize?

1. **teres minor**
2. teres major
3. subscapularis
4. supraspinatus

Correct Answer: 1
Explanation: The teres minor and deltoid muscles are innervated by the axillary nerve. (Kendall p. 403)

Clinical Practice: Musculoskeletal System
Content Outline: Examination

Question Number: 69
A physical therapist performs a dorsal glide to the distal radioulnar joint on a patient 12 weeks status post fracture. This technique is best used to increase:

1. wrist flexion
2. wrist extension
3. **forearm supination**
4. forearm pronation

Correct Answer: 3
Explanation: The concave ulnar notch of the radius articulates with the convex head of the ulna to form the distal radioulnar joint. A dorsal glide of the distal radius is used to increase supination. (Edmond p. 66)

Clinical Practice: Musculoskeletal System
Content Outline: Intervention

Question Number: 70
A physical therapist prepares to conduct a manual muscle test of the hip flexors. Assuming a grade of poor, the most appropriate testing position is:

1. prone
2. **sidelying**
3. supine
4. standing

Correct Answer: 2
Explanation: A grade of poor indicates that the hip flexors can produce movement with gravity-eliminated, but cannot function against gravity. As a result the recommended testing position is in sidelying. (Kendall p. 214)

Clinical Practice: Musculoskeletal System
Content Outline: Examination

Question Number: 71
A physical therapist administers the Functional Reach Test to a patient rehabilitating from a neurological disorder. Which bony landmark would be the most appropriate to utilize when formally measuring the distance the patient reached during each trial?

1. distal tip of the third digit
2. **third metacarpal**
3 radial styloid process
4. ulnar styloid process

Correct Answer: 2
Explanation: Measurements should be taken from the head of the third metacarpal before and after the patient reaches as far forward as possible without taking a step. The Functional Reach Test has been found to exhibit intrarater reliability of r =.98 and interrater reliability of r =.92. (Montgomery p. 190)

Clinical Practice: Neuromuscular System
Content Outline: Examination

Question Number: 72
A physical therapist applies a bandage to secure a dressing on the forearm. Which of the following would indicate that the bandage was applied too loosely?

1. the distal segment appears to be pale
2. edema develops in the distal segment
3. **the bandage changes position with active movement**
4. the patient complains of pain in the segment distal to the bandage

Correct Answer: 3
Explanation: A bandage can be used for a variety of reasons including securing a dressing, maintaining a barrier between the dressing and the environment, or providing pressure to control swelling. (Pierson p. 307)

Clinical Practice: Integumentary System
Content Outline: Intervention

Question Number: 73

A physical therapist measures elbow flexion while a patient grasps the handgrip of a walker in standing. The therapist records elbow flexion as 35 degrees. Which statement best describes the height of the walker?

1. the walker height is too low for the patient
2. **the walker height is too high for the patient**
3. the walker height is appropriate for the patient
4. not enough information is given to assess walker height

Correct Answer: 2
Explanation: The walker should be positioned at a height that allows for 20-30 degrees of elbow flexion when the handgrip is grasped. (Minor p. 313)

Clinical Practice: Patient Care Skills
Content Outline: Intervention

Question Number: 74

A patient with bilateral transtibial amputations works on ambulation activities prior to being discharged from a rehabilitation hospital. Which type of assistive device would be the most appropriate to utilize during the training session?

1. cane
2. two canes
3. **two forearm crutches**
4. walker

Correct Answer: 3
Explanation: Bilateral forearm crutches allow the patient to take adequate step length and exhibit a normal gait pattern without unnecessarily jeopardizing patient safety. (O'Sullivan p. 668)

Clinical Practice: Patient Care Skills
Content Outline: Intervention

Question Number: 75

A physical therapist continually makes errors when completing daily documentation. Which of the following statements would be the most appropriate advice to the therapist when an error occurs?

1. use correction fluid as needed on your documentation
2. **place a single line through the error, write "error", date and initial it**
3. use pencil when completing your documentation
4. use erasable ink when completing your documentation

Correct Answer: 2
Explanation: The accepted method for correcting a mistake is to place a single line through the error, write "error", date, and initial it. Other forms of correcting mistakes may be construed as negligence. (Shamus – Effective Documentation p. 10)

Clinical Practice: Education/Communication
Content Outline: Intervention

Question Number: 76

A 22-year-old male rehabilitating from a motor vehicle accident is referred to physical therapy for gait training. The patient sustained multiple injuries including a fractured tibia and a traction injury to the brachial plexus. The patient is partial weight bearing and has good upper extremity strength. The most appropriate assistive device is:

1. axillary crutches
2. **Lofstrand crutches**
3. walker with platform attachment
4. cane

Correct Answer: 2
Explanation: Lofstrand crutches avoid transmitting pressure to the brachial plexus area and accommodate for the weight bearing status of the involved lower extremity. The patient's age and upper extremity strength make Lofstrand crutches the most appropriate device. (Pierson p. 194)

Clinical Practice: Patient Care Skills
Content Outline: Intervention

Question Number: 77
A physical therapist asks a patient to complete a visual analog scale designed to assess pain intensity. The scale consists of a 10 cm line with descriptive labels at each end. Which terminology would be the most appropriate for the first label?

1. **no pain**
2. mild pain
3. weak pain
4. faint pain

Correct Answer: 1
Explanation: The first label on a visual analog scale should always refer to "no pain" or the "absence of pain." The second label is most often termed "most severe pain." (Magee p. 7)

Clinical Practice: Education/Communication
Content Outline: Examination

Question Number: 78
A physical therapist working on a medical-surgical rotation attends an inservice on HIV transmission. Which general precaution would be the most effective to prevent the transmission of HIV?

1. use protective barriers when performing invasive procedures
2. **consider all clients as potentially infected**
3. wear gloves when touching blood or body fluids
4. frequently wash hands and skin surfaces

Correct Answer: 2
Explanation: By considering all patients as potentially infected, therapists greatly reduce the transmission risk of HIV. (Pierson p. 275)

Clinical Practice: Patient Care Skills
Content Outline: Standards of Care

Question Number: 79
A physical therapist treats an infant diagnosed with torticollis with marked lateral flexion of the neck to the right. As part of the infant's plan of care the therapist performs passive stretching activities to improve the patient's range of motion. The most appropriate stretch for the patient is:

1. lateral flexion to the right and rotation to the right
2. lateral flexion to the left and rotation to the left
3. lateral flexion to the right and rotation to the left
4. **lateral flexion to the left and rotation to the right**

Correct Answer: 4
Explanation: Torticollis is a condition caused by a contracture of the sternocleidomastoid muscle. This condition is characterized by lateral flexion of the head toward the affected side and rotation toward the unaffected side. Stretching activities should be performed in the opposite direction. (Long p. 190)

Clinical Practice: Musculoskeletal System
Content Outline: Intervention

Question Number: 80
A physical therapist instructs a patient to close her eyes and hold out her hand. The therapist places a series of different weights in the patient's hand one at a time. The patient is then asked to identify the comparative weight of the objects. This method of sensory testing is used to examine:

1. **barognosis**
2. graphesthesia
3. recognition of texture
4. stereognosis

Correct Answer: 1
Explanation: Barognosis is a cortical sensation that is responsible for recognition of the weight of an object. It is responsible for the ability to differentiate weight between two or more objects. (O'Sullivan p. 147)

Clinical Practice: Neuromuscular System
Content Outline: Examination

Question Number: 81
A physical therapist assesses the pulse rate of a patient exercising on a treadmill. The therapist notes that the rhythm of the pulse is often irregular. The most appropriate action to ensure an accurate measurement of pulse rate is:

1. select a different pulse site
2. **measure the pulse rate for 60 seconds**
3. use a different stethoscope
4. document the irregular pulse rate in the patient's medical record

Correct Answer: 2
Explanation: An irregular rhythm often requires a physical therapist to assess the pulse for 60 seconds. (Pierson p. 52)

Clinical Practice: Cardiopulmonary System
Content Outline: Examination

Question Number: 82
A physical therapist prepares to treat a patient with paraplegia on a floor mat. The patient has fair upper extremity strength and trunk control. The most appropriate method to transfer the patient from a wheelchair to the floor is:

1. dependent standing pivot
2. sliding board transfer
3. **two-person lift**
4. hydraulic lift

Correct Answer: 3
Explanation: A two-person lift is often used to transfer a patient with some trunk control between a wheelchair and the floor. One therapist controls the trunk and head, while the other manages the patient's legs. The therapist controlling the trunk and the head verbalizes the commands and the patient is moved as a unit. (Minor p. 242)

Clinical Practice: Patient Care Skills
Content Outline: Intervention

Question Number: 83
A physical therapist participates in a community fitness program by conducting anthropometric measurements designed to determine percent body fat. Which site is not typically utilized when measuring skinfolds?

1. iliac crest
2. subscapular
3. triceps
4. **lateral calf**

Correct Answer: 4
Explanation: The triceps and the subscapular skinfolds are the two most common sites utilized when measuring body composition using a skinfold caliper. Other possible sites include the iliac crest, anterior chest, just below and lateral to the umbilicus, and the anterior thigh. (Arnerican College of Sports Medicine p. 107)

Clinical Practice: Musculoskeletal System
Content Outline: Examination

Question Number: 84
A physical therapist prepares to administer ultrasound to a patient with lateral epicondylitis. When applying ultrasound the amount of heat absorbed is least dependent upon:

1. the intensity
2. the duration of exposure
3. **the choice of coupling agent**
4. the size of the area sonated

Correct Answer: 3
Explanation: A number of factors play a significant role in determining the amount of heat absorbed using ultrasound, however, the choice of coupling agent has a relatively small impact when compared to the other presented options. (Michlovitz p. 198)

Clinical Practice: Physical Agents
Content Outline: Intervention

Question Number: 85
A physical therapist employed in a rehabilitation hospital utilizes the services of a physical therapy aide. Which variable best determines the extent to which physical therapy aides are involved in patient care activities?

1. the number of years of experience
2. the scope of formal training
3. **the discretion of the physical therapist**
4. the quantity of continuing education courses

Correct Answer: 3
Explanation: Physical therapy aides are non-licensed health care workers who are trained under the direction of a physical therapist. The physical therapist of record is directly responsible for the actions of the physical therapy aide. (Guide to Physical Therapist Practice p. 42)

Clinical Practice: Administration
Content Outline: Standards of Care

Question Number: 86
The treatment plan for a patient with hemiplegia is based on the theory of reinforcing normal movement through key points of control and avoiding all reflex movement patterns and associated reactions. This approach most closely resembles:

1. **Bobath**
2. Kabat
3. Trendelenburg
4. Brunnstrom

Correct Answer: 1
Explanation: The Bobath concept for neurological rehabilitation is often termed neurodevelopmental treatment (NDT). This theory of rehabilitation emphasizes influencing normal movement through handling of the patient and does not utilize abnormal movement patterns or reflexes. (Scott - Foundations p. 156)

Clinical Practice: Neuromuscular System
Content Outline: Intervention

Question Number: 87
A physical therapist prepares to treat a patient with cystic fibrosis using postural drainage. The most appropriate patient position when treating the superior segments of the lower lobes is:

1. sitting, leaning over a folded pillow at a 30 degree angle
2. head down on left side, 1/4 turn backward
3. supine with two pillows under the knees
4. **prone with two pillows under the hips**

Correct Answer: 4
Explanation: To perform postural drainage to the superior segments of the lower lobes a physical therapist should clap over the middle of the back at the tip of the scapula on either side of the spine with the patient in prone and two pillows positioned under the hips. (Rothstein p. 535)

Clinical Practice: Cardiopulmonary System
Content Outline: Intervention

Question Number: 88
A patient rehabilitating from a knee injury completes an isokinetic examination. The patient produces 88 ft/lbs. of torque with the hamstrings at 120 degrees per second. Assuming normal quadriceps/hamstrings ratio, which of the following most accurately reflects the predicted quadriceps value?

1. 67 ft/lbs.
2. 109 ft/lbs.
3. **136 ft/lbs.**
4. 183 ft/lbs.

Correct Answer: 3
Explanation: The most commonly accepted ratio of quadriceps to hamstrings strength is 3:2. As the speed of movement increases above 200 degrees per second the ratio approaches 1:1. (Hamill p. 236)

Clinical Practice: Musculoskeletal System
Content Outline: Intervention

Question Number: 89
A physical therapist elects to treat a patient with a second degree ankle sprain using a contrast bath. Which temperatures would be the most appropriate when preparing the cool and warm water?

1. 9 degrees Celsius and 34 degrees Celsius
2. **14 degrees Celsius and 38 degrees Celsius**
3. 19 degrees Celsius and 45 degrees Celsius
4. 23 degrees Celsius and 48 degrees Celsius

Correct Answer: 2
Explanation: The cooler water temperature should range from 12-20 degrees Celsius, while the warmer water temperature should range from 27-40 degrees Celsius. (Michlovitz p. 161)

Clinical Practice: Physical Agents
Content Outline: Intervention

Question Number: 90
A physical therapist uses a 3.0 MHz ultrasound beam at 1.5 W/cm^2 to treat a patient diagnosed with carpal tunnel syndrome. The majority of ultrasound energy will be absorbed within a depth of:

1. **1 - 2 cm**
2. 2 - 3 cm
3. 3 - 4 cm
4. 4 - 5 cm

Correct Answer: 1
Explanation: 3.0 MHz frequency is used to treat tissues up to 1-2 cm from the skin surface, while 1.0 MHz frequency is more appropriate for deeper structures. (Michlovitz p. 177)

Clinical Practice: Physical Agents
Content Outline: Intervention

Question Number: 91
A physical therapist serves as an accessibility consultant for a local retail store. What is the minimum width required for a patient using a wheelchair to safely traverse through a doorway?

1. 28 inches
2. 30 inches
3. **32 inches**
4. 34 inches

Correct Answer: 3
Explanation: According to the Americans with Disabilities Act the minimum doorway width is 32 inches. (Minor p. 472)

Clinical Practice: Education/Communication
Content Outline: Examination

Question Number: 92
A physical therapist reviews the medical record of a 52-year-old male status post myocardial infarction. The patient is currently in the coronary care unit and is scheduled to begin cardiac rehabilitation tomorrow. Which potential complication of a myocardial infarction is the patient most susceptible to?

1. heart failure
2. **arrhythmias**
3. thrombus formation
4. heart structural damage

Correct Answer: 2
Explanation: Arrhythmias occur in approximately 90% of individuals following myocardial infarction. Each of the listed options are possible complications following myocardial infarction, however, they are not as prevalent as arrhythmias. (Brannon p. 102)

Clinical Practice: Cardiopulmonary System
Content Outline: Evaluation, Diagnosis, Prognosis, and Outcomes

Question Number: 93
A physical therapist discusses numerous aspects of a bladder management program with a patient diagnosed with a spinal cord injury. Which value is most reflective of the patient's recommended daily fluid intake?

1. 1000 mL
2. **2000 mL**
3. 4000 mL
4. 8000 mL

Correct Answer: 2
Explanation: A patient that has sustained a spinal cord injury must intake approximately 2000 mL of fluid daily. This amount is required to avoid dehydration and prevent overdistention of the bladder. Scheduled catheterizations along with monitoring of fluid intake are required for a successful bladder program. (O'Sullivan p. 880)

Clinical Practice: Neuromuscular System
Content Outline: Examination

Question Number: 94
A physical therapist positions a patient in prone on a treatment plinth in preparation for a hot pack. When preparing the hot pack for the low back, the therapist should utilize:

1. 2 - 4 towel layers
2. 4 - 6 towel layers
3. **6 - 8 towel layers**
4. 8 - 10 towel layers

Correct Answer: 3
Explanation: Six to eight towel layers placed between a hot pack and the treatment surface is generally adequate to allow transmission of heat without jeopardizing patient safety. (Michlovitz p. 116)

Clinical Practice: Physical Agents
Content Outline: Intervention

Question Number: 95
A physical therapist attempts to determine if a wheelchair is the appropriate size for a patient recently admitted to a rehabilitation program. As part of the assessment, the therapist examines the distance from the front edge of the seat to the posterior aspect of the lower leg. If the seat depth is appropriate, how much space should exist between these two landmarks?

1. 2 inches
2. 4 inches
3. 6 inches
4. 8 inches

Correct Answer: 1
Explanation: Two inches between the front edge of the seat and the posterior aspect of the lower leg demonstrates appropriate seat depth. Normal seat depth in an adult size wheelchair is 16 inches. (Pierson p. 95)

Clinical Practice: Patient Care Skills
Content Outline: Examination

Question Number: 96
A patient confined to a wheelchair arranges for a local contractor to build a ramp that will allow entry into the patient's house. What is the maximum recommended grade for the ramp?

1. 6.2 %
2. 8.3 %
3. 9.5 %
4. 10.4 %

Correct Answer: 2
Explanation: According to the Americans with Disabilities Act the grade of a ramp should be no greater than 8.3%. The information can also be expressed as for every inch of rise, there should be a minimum of 12 inches of run. (Minor p. 471)

Clinical Practice: Education/Communication
Content Outline: Examination

Question Number: 97
A physical therapist examines a 23-year-old male diagnosed with a lower brachial plexus injury sustained four weeks ago. Which of the following mechanisms of injury is the most probable based on the patient's diagnosis?

1. high velocity motorcycle accident
2. excessive hyperabduction of the arm caused during a free fall
3. a direct forceful blow to the anterior shoulder complex
4. excessive traction and lateral flexion of the head and neck during the birthing process

Correct Answer: 2
Explanation: Lower brachial plexus injuries can occur during the birthing process, however, due to the patient's age and acuity of the injury, the most likely mechanism of injury is through excessive hyperabduction of the upper extremity. Upper brachial plexus injuries can occur through high velocity accidents where there is excessive separation of the neck and shoulder. (Saidoff p. 236)

Clinical Practice: Neuromuscular System
Content Outline: Examination

Question Number: 98
A 16-year-old female accompanied by her mother receives exercise instructions. During the treatment session the mother makes several comments to her daughter that appear to be extremely upsetting and result in the daughter losing concentration. The most appropriate physical therapist action is:

1. document the mother's comments in the medical record
2. ask the patient if her mother is verbally abusive
3. ask the mother to return to the waiting area
4. discontinue the treatment session

Correct Answer: 3
Explanation: The physical therapist's primary concern should be to establish an environment that is conducive to instructing the patient in an exercise program. Failure to address the negative interaction between the mother and daughter may limit the effectiveness of the session. (Purtilo p. 263)

Clinical Practice: Education/Communication
Content Outline: Intervention

Question Number: 99
A physical therapist working on a medical/surgical rotation returns from a morning inservice and finds a number of items that require her attention. Which of the following items should be given the highest priority?

1. **a patient requiring pre-operative instruction**
2. an incomplete exercise flow sheet
3. an unfinished wheelchair order form
4. a written note from a staff dietician

Correct Answer: 1
Explanation: The most important priority is to provide pre-operative patient instruction. The other stated activities are important, however, can be deferred without immediate consequence. (Code of Ethics)

Clinical Practice: Administration
Content Outline: Intervention

Question Number: 100
A physical therapist employed in a busy outpatient orthopedic clinic attempts to determine a schedule for calibration and maintenance of an ultrasound unit. The most important factor for the therapist to consider when determining an appropriate schedule is:

1. beam nonuniformity ratio
2. **frequency of use**
3. cost associated with calibration and maintenance
4. availability of qualified personnel to inspect the unit

Correct answer: 2
Explanation: The frequency of use of an ultrasound device is extremely important when determining a schedule for calibration and maintenance. Ultrasound units used frequently may be calibrated many times within a year, while a unit used sparingly would likely warrant a longer interval. (Belanger p. 237)

Clinical Practice: Physical Agents
Content Outline: Intervention

Computer-Based Exam Two – Section Three

Question Number: 101
A case manager discusses placement options for a 78-year-old female rehabilitating from a total hip replacement. The patient has moderate dementia, however, was living independently prior to surgery. The patient's spouse is deceased and she denies having any family or friends in the area. The most appropriate location for continued therapy services is:

1. **skilled nursing facility**
2. outpatient private practice
3. home physical therapy services
4. outpatient rehabilitation facility

Correct Answer: 1
Explanation: The patient's cognitive status combined with her post-operative condition make it unrealistic for the patient to return to her home. A skilled nursing facility would enable the patient to receive continued therapy services and at the same time provide a safe living environment. (Curtis p. 95)

Clinical Practice: Administration
Content Outline: Evaluation, Diagnosis, Prognosis, and Outcomes

Question Number: 102
A male patient referred to physical therapy with low back pain attempts to complete an abdominal strengthening exercise. The patient is unable to complete a curl-up with his arms across his chest. The most appropriate modification is:

1. place the hands behind the head
2. arch the back to lock the spine
3. anteriorly rotate the pelvis
4. **place the arms at the side**

Correct Answer: 4
Explanation: Placing the arms at the side of the body makes the exercise easier to perform and as a result is an acceptable modification. (Kisner p. 663)

Clinical Practice: Musculoskeletal System
Content Outline: Intervention

Question Number: 103
A physical therapist examines a patient rehabilitating from a middle cerebral artery stroke. Which condition is not typically associated with this type of stroke?

1. **urinary incontinence**
2. contralateral hemiplegia
3. aphasia
4. homonymous hemianopsia

Correct Answer: 1
Explanation: Urinary incontinence is a clinical symptom often associated with a vascular infarct to the anterior cerebral artery. (Umphred p. 745)

Clinical Practice: Neuromuscular System
Content Outline: Evaluation, Diagnosis, Prognosis, and Outcomes

Question Number: 104
A patient sustains a deep laceration on the anterior surface of the forearm. The physical therapist attempts to stop the bleeding by direct pressure over the wound, but is unsuccessful. The most appropriate action is to:

1. **apply pressure to the brachial artery pressure point**
2. apply pressure to the femoral artery pressure point
3. apply pressure to the radial artery pressure point
4. apply pressure to the ulnar artery pressure point

Correct Answer: 1
Explanation: The brachial artery can be compressed against the medial aspect of the humerus in an attempt to control the bleeding. (Anaemet p. 569)

Clinical Practice: Integumentary System
Content Outline: Standards of Care

Question Number: 105
A physical therapist discusses the importance of a well balanced diet with a patient diagnosed with type II diabetes. The most appropriate action to emphasize the importance of diet is:

1. provide a handout from the American Diabetes Association which outlines an appropriate diet
2. ask other patients that have made dietary changes to speak to the patient
3. **arrange for a consultation with a dietician**
4. provide copies of recent research articles which cite the benefit of a well balanced diet

Correct Answer: 3
Explanation: Although many therapists possess a basic background in nutrition, a patient with type II (non-insulin dependent) diabetes is an ideal candidate to refer to a dietician. (Tierney p. 1005)

Clinical Practice: Education/Communication
Content Outline: Intervention

Question Number: 106
A patient of Iranian descent wearing a traditional turban is examined in physical therapy after sustaining a whiplash type injury in a motor vehicle accident. The physical therapist would like the patient to remove the turban, however, is concerned that the patient may become insulted. The most appropriate action is to:

1. modify the examination in order to avoid removing the turban
2. explain to the patient the difficulty of conducting the examination with the turban on
3. **ask the patient if he would feel comfortable removing the turban during the examination**
4. instruct the patient to remove the turban

Correct Answer: 3
Explanation: In order to conduct an appropriate examination of the cervical spine, a physical therapist should attempt to expose the entire cervical region. Asking the patient permission to remove the turban provides the patient with an opportunity to refuse the request. (Haggard p. 39)

Clinical Practice: Education/Communication
Content Outline: Standards of Care

Question Number: 107
A physical therapist suspects a female patient recently referred to physical therapy may be a victim of domestic abuse. The most appropriate initial action is:

1. provide the patient with a phone number to a domestic abuse center
2. report your suspicions to the local authorities
3. **ask the patient if she has experienced any form of domestic abuse**
4. document the domestic abuse in the medical record

Correct Answer: 3
Explanation: Physical therapists have a duty to identify and report suspected patient abuse to local authorities, however, it is often advisable to seek confirming information prior to initiating formal action. (Scott - Professional Ethics p. 162)

Clinical Practice: Education/Communication
Content Outline: Standards of Care

Question Number: 108
A physical therapist administers a contrast bath to a patient rehabilitating from a lateral ankle sprain. The therapist begins the first cycle by immersing the involved ankle in warm water for three minutes and then promptly moves the ankle into cold water. How long should the therapist leave the ankle in the cold water?

1. 30 seconds
2. **1 minute**
3. 3 minutes
4. 5 minutes

Correct Answer: 2
Explanation: The ratio of heat to cold when using a contrast bath is most commonly expressed as 3:1 or 4:1. (Cameron p. 203)

Clinical Practice: Physical Agents
Content Outline: Intervention

Question Number: 109
A patient rehabilitating from a fractured acetabulum is referred to physical therapy for ambulation activities. The patient has been on bed rest for three weeks and appears to be somewhat apprehensive about weight bearing. The most appropriate device to use when initiating ambulation activities is:

1. **parallel bars**
2. walker
3. axillary crutches
4. straight cane

Correct Answer: 1
Explanation: The parallel bars provide the patient with the most stable environment to begin ambulation activities. (Pierson p. 193)

Clinical Practice: Patient Care Skills
Content Outline: Intervention

Question Number: 110
A 12-year-old boy sitting in the physical therapy waiting area suddenly grasps his throat and appears to be in distress. The boy slowly stands, but is obviously unable to breathe. The physical therapist recognizing the signs of an airway obstruction should administer:

1. **abdominal thrusts**
2. chest thrusts
3. back blows
4. back blows in combination with abdominal thrusts

Correct Answer: 1
Explanation: An airway obstruction in a child or an adult is best treated by using subdiaphragmatic abdominal thrusts. (American Heart Association p. 162)

Clinical Practice: Cardiopulmonary System
Content Outline: Standards of Care

Question Number: 111
A physical therapist assesses a patient's upper extremity deep tendon reflexes as part of a screening examination. The most appropriate location to elicit the brachioradialis reflex is the:

1. radial tuberosity
2. antecubital fossa
3. biceps tendon
4. **styloid process of the radius**

Correct Answer: 4
Explanation: The brachioradialis reflex is best elicited by using the flat end of the reflex hammer over the distal end of the radius. This reflex can be used to examine the integrity of the C6 nerve root. (Gross p. 221)

Clinical Practice: Neuromuscular System
Content Outline: Examination

Question Number: 112
A physical therapist working on an acute care floor in a hospital reviews the medical record of a patient with suspected renal involvement. Which laboratory test would be the most useful to assess the patient's present renal function?

1. platelet count
2. hemoglobin
3. **blood urea nitrogen**
4. hematocrit

Correct Answer: 3
Explanation: Blood urea nitrogen is a common measure used to examine renal function. A rise in blood urea nitrogen levels can be indicative of an impairment in renal tubule excretion. (Goodman - Differential Diagnosis p. 252)

Clinical Practice: Cardiopulmonary System
Content Outline: Examination

Question Number: 113
A physical therapist attends an inservice on incomplete spinal cord injuries. As part of the inservice the speaker describes several frequently observed syndromes of neurological involvement. Which syndrome does not include an alteration in motor function?

1. central cord syndrome
2. anterior cord syndrome
3. Brown-Sequard's syndrome
4. **posterior cord syndrome**

Correct Answer: 4
Explanation: Posterior cord syndrome results from an injury to the posterior column of the spinal cord. This injury is rare and does not affect motor function, light touch, and pain. (Goodman - Pathology p. 779)

Clinical Practice: Neuromuscular System
Content Outline: Evaluation, Diagnosis, Prognosis, and Outcomes

Question Number: 114
A physical therapist prepares to assist a patient with a sliding board transfer from a wheelchair to a mat table. Which of the following would be the most appropriate initial instruction to the patient?

1. place the sliding board under your buttocks
2. move your buttocks toward the mat table
3. complete a series of push-ups
4. **secure the wheelchair brakes**

Correct Answer: 4
Explanation: Securing the wheelchair brakes is always the most appropriate action when initiating a transfer from a wheelchair. (Minor p. 248)

Clinical Practice: Patient Care Skills
Content Outline: Intervention

Question Number: 115
A physical therapist completes a respiratory assessment on a patient in an acute care hospital. The examination reveals decreased breath sounds and decreased fremitus. This finding is most indicative of:

1. **pleural effusion**
2. pulmonary edema
3. consolidation
4. atelectasis

Correct Answer: 1
Explanation: Decreased breath sounds and decreased fremitus are most likely caused by pleural effusion or pneumothorax. Pulmonary edema, consolidation, and atelectasis are often associated with decreased breath sounds and increased fremitus. (Irwin p. 172)

Clinical Practice: Cardiopulmonary System
Content Outline: Evaluation, Diagnosis, Prognosis, and Outcomes

Question Number: 116
A patient with several motor and sensory abnormalities exhibits signs of autonomic nervous system dysfunction. Which of the following is not an indicator of increased sympathetic involvement?

1. anxiety, distractibility
2. mottled, cold, shiny skin
3. **constriction of the pupils**
4. rapid, shallow breathing

Correct Answer: 3
Explanation: Increased sympathetic involvement would tend to produce dilation of the pupils and not constriction. (Sullivan p. 60)

Clinical Practice: Neuromuscular System
Content Outline: Evaluation, Diagnosis, Prognosis, and Outcomes

Question Number: 117
A patient diagnosed with Guillain-Barre syndrome works on weight shifting activities while standing in the parallel bars. The primary objective of this activity is to improve:

1. mobility
2. stability
3. **controlled mobility**
4. skill

Correct Answer: 3
Explanation: Controlled mobility is the third stage of motor control where proximal segments move over a distal weight bearing part. Control should be attained first in a small range and gradually expanded as warranted based on the patient response. (Sullivan p. 77)

Clinical Practice: Neuromuscular System
Content Outline: Evaluation, Diagnosis, Prognosis, and Outcomes

Question Number: 118
A physical therapist records the parameters of an electrical stimulation treatment in a patient's medical record. The standard unit of measure when recording AC frequency is:

1. volt
2. **hertz**
3. coulomb
4. pulses per second

Correct Answer: 2
Explanation: Acceptable terminology for the frequency of alternating current is cycles per second or hertz. Pulses per second is utilized to describe the frequency of pulsed current. (Robinson p. 14)

Clinical Practice: Physical Agents
Content Outline: Intervention

Question Number: 119
A physical therapist working in cardiac rehabilitation progresses a patient involved in a phase II program through an established exercise protocol. The patient weighs 70 kg and has progressed without difficulty through the rehabilitation program. The protocol indicates the patient should be performing activities requiring 3 - 4 METs. An example of an appropriate activity would be:

1. level walking at 1.5 mph
2. jogging at 5 mph
3. cycling at 10 mph
4. **walking on a treadmill at 3 mph**

Correct Answer: 4
Explanation: One metabolic equivalent is the amount of oxygen consumed at rest and is equal to approximately 3.5 milliliters of oxygen per kilogram of body weight per minute. Other recreational activities requiring 3-4 METs include cycling at 6 mph and golfing while pulling a bag cart. (Brannon p. 3)

Clinical Practice: Cardiopulmonary System
Content Outline: Intervention

Question Number: 120
A physical therapist instructs a patient with a lower motor neuron disorder to perform a swing-to gait pattern. The most appropriate initial step when instructing the patient is:

1. secure another staff member to assist with guarding
2. **demonstrate a swing-to gait pattern**
3. describe the various stages of weight bearing
4. provide a written handout describing the gait pattern

Correct Answer: 2
Explanation: Demonstration provides the opportunity for the patient to observe a specific action being performed correctly and as a result often enhances learning and decreases anxiety. (Minor p. 289)

Clinical Practice: Education/Communication
Content Outline: Intervention

Question Number: 121
A recent entry in the medical record indicates a patient exhibits dysdiadochokinesia. Based on the patient's documented deficit, which activity would be the most difficult for the patient?

1. **alternate supination and pronation of the forearm**
2. perform a standing squat
3. march in place
4. walk along a straight line

Correct Answer: 1
Explanation: Dysdiadochokinesia is defined as the inability to perform rapidly alternating movements. (Umphred p. 724)

Clinical Practice: Neuromuscular System
Content Outline: Intervention

Question Number: 122

A physical therapist utilizes continuous ultrasound to supply thermal effects to a patient rehabilitating from a lower extremity injury. During the treatment session, the patient suddenly becomes startled and reports feeling an electrical shock from the ultrasound machine. The most appropriate therapist action is to:

1. decrease the intensity of the ultrasound
2. modify the duty cycle
3. discontinue ultrasound treatment
4. **unplug the machine and label - defective, do not use**

Correct Answer: 4

Explanation: Any equipment that is potentially defective should be formally inspected prior to being used to treat patients. (Nelson p. 48)

Clinical Practice: Physical Agents
Content Outline: Intervention

Question Number: 123

A patient in a rehabilitation hospital begins to verbalize about the uselessness of life and the possibility of committing suicide. The most appropriate physical therapist action is:

1. suggest the patient be placed on a locked unit
2. ask nursing to check on the patient every 15 minutes
3. **discuss the situation with the patient's case manager**
4. review the patient's past medical history for signs and symptoms of mental illness

Correct Answer: 3

Explanation: Any formal or informal indication that a patient may be suicidal should be taken seriously. The case manager communicates with all of the members of the rehabilitation team and is therefore the most appropriate of the presented options. (Bailey p. 317)

Clinical Practice: Education/Communication
Content Outline: Intervention

Question Number: 124

A physical therapy department embarks on a quality assurance program. Results from a random sample of patient charts reveal that 40% of the charts do not include a discharge summary. A logical next step to the quality assurance program would be:

1. dismiss the findings because discharge summaries are not directly related to the quality of patient care
2. discipline the staff members who did not complete the discharge summaries and continue to monitor the situation
3. dismiss the findings because a random sample does not provide accurate information
4. **notify the staff that discharge summaries are to be completed on all patients and continue to monitor the situation**

Correct Answer: 4

Explanation: Quality assurance refers to activities or programs designed to achieve a desired degree or grade of care. Findings from quality assurance initiatives should be communicated directly to staff in a manner that is constructive, instead of punitive. (Walter p. 242)

Clinical Practice: Administration
Content Outline: Intervention

Question Number: 125 *Item Includes Graphic*

A physical therapist positions a patient as shown prior to testing for clonus. The most appropriate action to complete the test is:

1. **provide a quick stretch to the plantar flexors**
2. provide a quick stretch to the dorsiflexors
3. provide a quick stretch to the plantar flexors while extending the knee
4. provide a quick stretch to the dorsiflexors while extending the knee

Correct Answer: 1

Explanation: Clonus refers to rhythmic oscillation of a body part resulting from a quick stretch. The test is ideally performed by producing the stretch to the plantar flexors with the gastrocnemius in a relaxed position. (DeMyer p. 311)

Clinical Practice: Neuromuscular System
Content Outline: Examination

Question Number: 126
A physical therapist employed in a rehabilitation hospital examines a patient that exhibits several signs and symptoms of anemia. Which question would be the most useful to gather additional information related to anemia?

1. Does it hurt to take a deep breath?
2. **Do you experience heart palpitations or shortness of breath at rest or with mild exertion?**
3. Do you frequently experience dizziness, headaches or blurred vision?
4. Are you susceptible to bruising?

Correct Answer: 2
Explanation: Anemia refers to a condition in which there is reduced delivery of oxygen to the tissues due to a reduction in the number of circulating red blood cells. Heart palpitations along with dyspnea are often associated with this condition. (Goodman - Differential Diagnosis p. 182)

Clinical Practice: Education/Communication
Content Outline: Examination

Question Number: 127
A physical therapist performs bronchial drainage to the anterior basal segments of the lower lobes. During the treatment session the patient suddenly complains of dizziness and mild dyspnea. The most appropriate therapist action is:

1. reassure the patient that the response is normal
2. assess the patient's vital signs
3. **elevate the patient's head**
4. call for assistance

Correct Answer: 3
Explanation: Bronchial drainage of the anterior basal segments of the lower lobes requires the patient to be positioned in supine with the bottom of the bed elevated 18-20 inches. Since this position results in the head being significantly below the feet, the patient would be susceptible to dizziness and dyspnea. (Hillegass p. 650)

Clinical Practice: Patient Care Skills
Content Outline: Intervention

Question Number: 128
A terminally ill patient completes a formal document that names his daughter as the individual to make health care decisions in the event that he is unable. This type of advanced directive is termed:

1. living will
2. directives to physicians
3. **durable power of attorney**
4. euthanasia

Correct Answer: 3
Explanation: Durable power of attorney for health care decisions is a legal document that delegates decision making to a specified individual in the event another individual is found to be incompetent to make a decision. (Scott - Professional Ethics p. 150)

Clinical Practice: Administration
Content Outline: Standards of Care

Question Number: 129
A physical therapist recognizes that a child has great difficulty flexing the neck while in a supine position. Failure to integrate which reflex could explain the child's difficulty?

1. **symmetrical tonic labyrinthine**
2. Moro
3. asymmetrical tonic neck
4. symmetrical tonic neck

Correct Answer: 1
Explanation: The symmetrical tonic labyrinthine reflex creates full extension of the body and extremities when positioned in supine. Extension serves to limit the child's ability to flex the neck. (Ratliffe p. 26)

Clinical Practice: Neuromuscular System
Content Outline: Intervention

Question Number: 130
The medical record indicates a patient has been diagnosed with chronic respiratory alkalosis. The most consistent laboratory finding with this condition is:

1. **elevated arterial blood pH, low $PaCO_2$**
2. low arterial blood pH, elevated $PaCO_2$
3. elevated arterial blood pH, elevated $PaCO_2$
4. low arterial blood pH, low $PaCO_2$

Correct Answer: 1
Explanation: Respiratory alkalosis is caused by alveolar hyperventilation. Signs and symptoms include dizziness, syncope, tingling, and numbness. (Rothstein p. 529)

Clinical Practice: Cardiopulmonary System
Content Outline: Examination

Question Number: 131
A physical therapist completes an examination on a self-referred patient. The patient complains of general fatigue, shortness of breath, and occasional dizziness. Results of a physical examination reveal localized lower extremity weakness and diminished balance. The most appropriate action is to:

1. implement a low-level exercise program
2. identify appropriate strengthening exercises
3. establish short and long-term goals
4. **refer the patient to a physician**

Correct Answer: 4
Explanation: A self-referred patient that presents with multi-system involvement should be examined by a physician prior to engaging in a formal physical therapy program. (Guide for Professional Conduct)

Clinical Practice: Administration
Content Outline: Evaluation, Diagnosis, Prognosis, and Outcomes

Question Number: 132
A patient recently diagnosed with a deep venous thrombophlebitis is placed on Heparin. The primary side effect associated with Heparin is:

1. hypotension
2. depression
3. **excessive anticoagulation**
4. thrombocytopenia

Correct Answer: 3
Explanation: Heparin, the primary drug used to treat deep venous thrombophlebitis, is administered parenterally. The most common side effect of the drug is increased bleeding. (Ciccone p. 377)

Clinical Practice: Cardiopulmonary System
Content Outline: Examination

Question Number: 133
A 29-year-old male diagnosed with ankylosing spondylitis reports progressive stiffening of the spine and associated pain for more than five years. The patient's most typical standing posture demonstrates:

1. posterior thoracic rib hump
2. **flattened lumbar curve, exaggerated thoracic curve**
3. excessive lumbar curve, flattened thoracic curve
4. lateral curvature of the spine with fixed rotation of the vertebrae

Correct Answer: 2
Explanation: Ankylosing spondylitis is a form of systemic rheumatic arthritis that is associated with an increase in thoracic kyphosis and loss of the lumbar curve. Ankylosing spondylitis occurs three times more often in males than females with a typical age of onset of 20-40 years. (Pauls p. 74)

Clinical Practice: Musculoskeletal System
Content Outline: Intervention

Question Number: 134
A physical therapist examines the residual limb of a patient following ambulation activities with a patellar tendon bearing prosthesis. The therapist identifies excessive redness over the patella. The most likely cause is:

1. **settling due to limb shrinkage**
2. socket not properly aligned
3. excessive withdrawal in sitting
4. excessive number of residual limb socks

Correct Answer: 1
Explanation: A patient would likely have reddening over the patella if the residual limb has shrunk and/or if there is inadequate ply of socks used. In both cases, the residual limb would sit lower in the prosthesis and the patella would hit the patellar tendon bearing surface. (O'Sullivan p. 635)

Clinical Practice: Patient Care Skills
Content Outline: Evaluation, Diagnosis, Prognosis, and Outcomes

Question Number: 135

A 55-year-old patient, six months status post CVA with right hemiparesis, attends physical therapy on an outpatient basis. As the patient lies supine on the mat, the physical therapist applies resistance to right elbow flexion. The therapist notes mass flexion of the right lower extremity as the resistance is applied. The therapist should document this as:

1. Raimiste's phenomenon
2. Souque's phenomenon
3. coordination synkinesis
4. **homolateral synkinesis**

Correct Answer: 4

Explanation: Homolateral synkinesis is an associated reaction that can occur after neurological damage. Resistance to flexion of the affected upper extremity will cause flexion in the lower extremity. (O'Sullivan p. 532)

Clinical Practice: Neuromuscular System
Content Outline: Intervention

Question Number: 136

A physical therapist attempts to determine if a patient is a candidate for aquatic therapy. Which condition would not be considered a contraindication to aquatic therapy?

1. infectious disease
2. urinary tract infection
3. fever
4. **Raynaud's disease**

Correct Answer: 4

Explanation: Raynaud's disease is a peripheral vascular disorder characterized by abnormal vasoconstriction of the extremities upon exposure to cold or emotional distress. Although Raynaud's disease can be considered a contraindication for selected forms of cryotherapy, it is not contraindicated for aquatic therapy. (Michlovitz p. 102)

Clinical Practice: Physical Agents
Content Outline: Intervention

Question Number: 137

A physical therapist examines a patient diagnosed with adhesive capsulitis. The examination reveals the patient has significant capsular tightness in the anterior-inferior aspect. The most likely range of motion limitation is:

1. adduction and medial rotation
2. **abduction and lateral rotation**
3. flexion and medial rotation
4. extension and lateral rotation

Correct Answer: 2

Explanation: Anterior capsular tightness at the glenohumeral joint may result in limited lateral rotation and extension, while inferior capsular tightness is associated with limited abduction. (Edmond p. 25)

Clinical Practice: Musculoskeletal System
Content Outline: Evaluation, Diagnosis, Prognosis, and Outcomes

Question Number: 138

A patient is asked to complete a pain questionnaire. The patient selects words such as cramping, dull, and aching to describe the pain. What related structure is most consistent with the pain description?

1. nerve root
2. **muscle**
3. fracture
4. sympathetic nerve

Correct Answer: 2

Explanation: Muscle pain is often characterized as cramping, dull, and aching, while nerve root pain is more often termed sharp or shooting. Subjective pain descriptors can provide valuable information related to a patient's condition. (Magee p. 8)

Clinical Practice: Musculoskeletal System
Content Outline: Evaluation, Diagnosis, Prognosis, and Outcomes

Question Number: 139

A physical therapist examines a patient with suspected vascular compression in the shoulder region. Which special test would be least beneficial to confirm the therapist's suspicions?

1. Adson maneuver
2. Halstead maneuver
3. **Froment's sign**
4. Wright Test

Correct Answer: 3
Explanation: Froment's sign is a special test where a patient attempts to grasp a piece of paper between the thumb and index finger. A positive test is indicated by flexion of the terminal phalanx of the thumb caused by paralysis of the adductor pollicis longus. The test is used to assess the integrity of the ulnar nerve. (Magee p. 398)

Clinical Practice: Musculoskeletal System
Content Outline: Examination

Question Number: 140
A 29-year-old female status post Colles' fracture is referred to physical therapy. The patient has moderate edema in her fingers and the dorsum of her hand and complains of pain during active range of motion. The most appropriate method to quantify the patient's edema is:

1. **volumetric measurements**
2. circumferential measurements
3. girth measurements
4. anthropometric measurements

Correct Answer: 1
Explanation: Volumetric measurements are often used to quantify the presence of edema in the wrist and hand. Comparison with the uninvolved extremity provides a baseline measure, however, it is important to note there may be a small difference between the dominant and non-dominant hand. (Magee p. 402)

Clinical Practice: Musculoskeletal System
Content Outline: Examination

Question Number: 141
A physical therapist is scheduled to treat a patient requiring droplet precautions. What type of protective equipment would be necessary prior to entering the patient's room?

1. gloves
2. **mask**
3. gloves and mask
4. gloves, gown, and mask

Correct Answer: 2
Explanation: Droplet precautions require individuals coming within three feet of the patient to wear a mask, but does not require the use of a gown or gloves. Droplet precautions are designed to prevent transmission of infectious agents that are transmitted primarily through coughing, sneezing, or talking. (Center for Disease Control)

Clinical Practice: Patient Care Skills
Content Outline: Standards of Care

Question Number: 142
A physical therapist administers tapotement as part of a treatment plan for a patient diagnosed with bronchiectasis. Which of the following massage strokes is not an example of tapotement?

1. **kneading**
2. clapping
3. hacking
4. beating

Correct Answer: 1
Explanation: Kneading is a form of petrissage that utilizes intermittent rolling and pressing of muscles to increase circulation and reduce edema. (Tan p. 52)

Clinical Practice: Physical Agents
Content Outline: Intervention

Question Number: 143
A physical therapist collects data as part of a research project that requires direct observation of children performing selected gross motor activities. The therapist is concerned about the influence of an observer on the children's performance. The most effective strategy to control for this source of error is to:

1. provide initial and refresher observer training
2. increase observer awareness of the influence of their background
3. **have an observer spend time with the children before direct observation**
4. ask the children to ignore the presence of the observer

Correct Answer: 3
Explanation: Spending time with the children prior to direct observation will allow them to feel more at ease and as a result their performance may be more reflective of their current abilities. (Payton p. 104)

Clinical Practice: Research
Content Outline: Intervention

Question Number: 144
A patient reports to a physical therapist that she completely tore one of the ligaments in her ankle. If the patient's comment is accurate, the injury to the ligament is most likely classified as a:

1. grade I sprain
2. **grade III sprain**
3. grade I strain
4. grade III strain

Correct Answer: 2
Explanation: A third degree sprain involves a complete rupture or break in the continuity of a ligament. The injury usually results in significant joint play hypermobility. (Hertling p. 349)

Clinical Practice: Musculoskeletal System
Content Outline: Evaluation, Diagnosis, Prognosis, and Outcomes

Question Number: 145
A physical therapist preparing to administer phonophoresis on a patient diagnosed with impingement syndrome palpates the insertion of the supraspinatus. What bony landmark best corresponds to this site?

1. lesser tubercle of the humerus
2. **greater tubercle of the humerus**
3. supraspinatus fossa of the scapula
4. deltoid tuberosity of the humerus

Correct Answer: 2
Explanation: The supraspinatus originates on the supraspinatus fossa of the scapula and inserts on the greater tubercle of the humerus. The muscle is innervated by the suprascapular nerve. (Reese p. 57)

Clinical Practice: Physical Agents
Content Outline: Intervention

Question Number: 146
A patient status post motor vehicle accident is referred to physical therapy. The patient has multiple injury sites including the hand, wrist, elbow, and knee. As part of the patient care plan, the physical therapist attempts to increase tissue temperature at each of the involved sites. The most appropriate thermal agent is:

1. diathermy
2. ultrasound
3. **hydrotherapy**
4. hot packs

Correct Answer: 3
Explanation: Hydrotherapy is the most appropriate thermal agent due to the varied location and size of the treatment area. (Cameron p. 174)

Clinical Practice: Physical Agents
Content Outline: Intervention

Question Number: 147
A physical therapist presents an inservice on graded oscillation techniques. Which grades of oscillation are the most appropriate for stretching maneuvers?

1. I, II
2. I, III
3. II, III
4. **III, IV**

Correct Answer: 4
Explanation: Grades I and II oscillations are used primarily to treat joints limited by pain, while grades III and IV oscillations are used as stretching maneuvers. (Kisner p. 224)

Clinical Practice: Musculoskeletal System
Content Outline: Intervention

Question Number: 148
A physical therapist examines the breath sounds of a 55-year-old male diagnosed with pulmonary disease. The therapist identifies rales during both inspiration and expiration. This finding is most representative of:

1. pleural effusion
2. pulmonary fibrosis
3. **impaired secretion clearance**
4. localized stenosis

Correct Answer: 3
Explanation: Low-pitched, non-rhythmical sounds occurring throughout the ventilatory cycle often are indicative of fluid in the large airways due to impaired secretion clearance. (Irwin p. 292)

Clinical Practice: Cardiopulmonary System
Content Outline: Evaluation, Diagnosis, Prognosis, and Outcomes

Question Number: 149
A rehabilitation manager conducts an inservice on Medicare rules and regulations. Which of the following practice settings would not receive primary reimbursement through Medicare Part A?

1. hospital
2. home health care
3. **outpatient**
4. skilled nursing

Correct Answer: 3
Explanation: Outpatient physical therapy services are primarily reimbursed though Medicare Part B. Medicare Part A provides benefits for hospitals, outpatient diagnostic services, extended care facilities, and short-term care at home required by an illness for which the patient was hospitalized. (Sultz p. 220)

Clinical Practice: Administration
Content Outline: Standards of Care

Question Number: 150
A physical therapist reviews the medical record of a patient recently referred to physical therapy. The record indicates the patient has polycythemia. Which of the following laboratory results would be expected based on the patient's condition?

1. **increased hematocrit and hemoglobin levels**
2. decreased hematocrit and hemoglobin levels
3. increased hematocrit and decreased hemoglobin levels
4. decreased hematocrit and increased hemoglobin levels

Correct Answer: 1
Explanation: Polycythemia is a condition characterized by an excessive number of erythrocytes and an increased concentration of hemoglobin. (Goodman - Differential Diagnosis p. 184)

Clinical Practice: Cardiopulmonary System
Content Outline: Evaluation, Diagnosis, Prognosis, and Outcomes

---

Computer-Based Exam Two – Section Four

Question Number: 151
A physical therapist instructs a patient's spouse to remove and reapply a bandage. Which of the following instructional methods would be the most appropriate to ensure the task is performed appropriately?

1. have the patient instruct the spouse how to remove and reapply the bandage
2. provide written instructions on how to remove and reapply the bandage
3. **instruct the spouse to remove and reapply the bandage and observe her performance**
4. instruct the spouse to contact the physical therapy department if she has specific questions on how to remove or reapply the bandage

Correct Answer: 3
Explanation: The physical therapist should observe the removal and reapplication of the bandage in order to determine if the spouse is capable of performing the task. Although this will not ensure the task is done appropriately in the future, it will identify if the spouse needs remedial assistance. (Hall p. 37)

Clinical Practice: Education/Communication
Content Outline: Intervention

Question Number: 152
A physical therapist completes a study which examines the effect of goniometer size on the reliability of passive shoulder joint measurements. The therapist concludes that goniometric measurements of passive shoulder range of motion can be highly reliable when taken by a single therapist, regardless of the size of the goniometer. This study demonstrates the use of:

1. interrater reliability
2. **intrarater reliability**
3. internal validity
4. external validity

Correct Answer: 2
Explanation: Intrarater reliability refers to the amount of agreement between repeated measurements of the same joint position by the same therapist. (Norkin p. 41)

Clinical Practice: Research
Content Outline: Examination

Question Number: 153

A physical therapist employed in an acute care hospital examines a patient rehabilitating from surgery. The patient has diabetes, however, has no other significant past medical history. Which of the following situations would most warrant immediate medical attention?

1. **signs of confusion and lethargy**
2. systolic blood pressure increase of 20 mm Hg during exercise
3. lack of significant clinical findings following the examination
4. discovery of significant past medical history unknown to the physician

Correct Answer: 1
Explanation: Signs of confusion and lethargy in a patient with diabetes can be indicative of a significant alteration in a patient's glycemic state. The condition, if untreated, can rapidly progress towards a life threatening situation. (Goodman - Differential Diagnosis p. 356)

Clinical Practice: Patient Care Skills
Content Outline: Evaluation, Diagnosis, Prognosis, and Outcomes

Question Number: 154

A patient with a peripheral nerve injury is examined in physical therapy. The patient's primary symptoms result from an injury to the superficial peroneal nerve. The most likely area of sensory alteration is:

1. sole of the foot
2. plantar surface of the toes
3. **lateral aspect of the leg and dorsum of the foot**
4. triangular area between the first and second toes

Correct Answer: 3
Explanation: The superficial peroneal nerve innervates the peroneus longus and brevis. A peripheral nerve injury affecting the superficial peroneal nerve often results in sensory alterations along the lateral aspect of the leg and dorsum of the foot. (Magee p. 811)

Clinical Practice: Neuromuscular System
Content Outline: Evaluation, Diagnosis, Prognosis, and Outcomes

Question Number: 155

A physical therapist reviews a physician examination which indicates diminished sensation in the L3 dermatome. The most appropriate location to confirm the physician's findings is:

1. dorsum of foot
2. **anterior thigh**
3. lateral thigh
4. lateral calf

Correct Answer: 2
Explanation: The L3 dermatome corresponds to portions of the back, upper buttock, anterior thigh and knee, and the medial lower leg. (Magee p. 16)

Clinical Practice: Neuromuscular System
Content Outline: Evaluation, Diagnosis, Prognosis, and Outcomes

Question Number: 156

A 32-year-old female complains of pain in her left wrist and forearm. The patient reports an insidious onset of pain two weeks ago. Physical examination reveals weakness and point tenderness along the distal radius and pain with resisted thumb extension and abduction. The most appropriate special test to gain additional insight into the patient's condition is:

1. Froment's sign
2. Phalen's test
3. **Finkelstein test**
4. Bunnel-Littler test

Correct Answer: 3
Explanation: The Finkelstein test is designed to identify the presence of de Quervain's tenosynovitis in the thumb. A positive test is indicated by pain over the abductor pollicis longus and the extensor pollicis brevis tendons at the wrist. (Magee p. 396)

Clinical Practice: Musculoskeletal System
Content Outline: Examination

Question Number: 157

A physical therapist and a physical therapist assistant work as a team in an orthopedic private practice. Which activity would be inappropriate for the physical therapist assistant?

1. application of a superficial modality
2. **completing a discharge summary**
3. leading a group exercise program
4. performing an isokinetic test

Correct Answer: 2

Explanation: Physical therapist assistants often complete documentation in the medical record, however, the physical therapist is responsible for establishing a discharge plan and documenting the discharge summary. (Guide to Physical Therapist Practice p. 42)

Clinical Practice: Administration
Content Outline: Standards of Care

Question Number: 158

A physical therapist conducts an examination on a patient diagnosed with Parkinson's disease. Which of the following clinical findings would you expect the therapist to identify?

1. aphasia
2. ballistic movements
3. severe muscle atrophy
4. **cogwheel rigidity**

Correct Answer: 4

Explanation: Signs and symptoms of Parkinson's disease include cogwheel rigidity, resting tremor, poor initiation of movement, shuffling gait, and flat affect. (Paz p. 321)

Clinical Practice: Neuromuscular System
Content Outline: Evaluation, Diagnosis, Prognosis, and Outcomes

Question Number: 159

A physical therapist prepares a patient with burns over 65 percent of the body for hydrotherapy. Due to the extent of the patient's burns, the therapist plans to use full-body immersion. The most appropriate piece of equipment to satisfy the therapist's objective is:

1. fluidotherapy
2. highboy tank
3. lowboy tank
4. **Hubbard tank**

Correct Answer: 4

Explanation: An average size Hubbard tank is eight feet long, six feet wide, and four feet deep. The tanks often hold over 400 gallons of water and are designed for full-body immersion. (Cameron p. 201)

Clinical Practice: Physical Agents
Content Outline: Intervention

Question Number: 160

A patient elevated on a tilt table to 60 degrees suddenly begins to demonstrate signs and symptoms of orthostatic hypotension. The most appropriate physical therapist action is to:

1. lower the tilt table 10 degrees and monitor the patient's vital signs
2. lower the tilt table 20 degrees and monitor the patient's vital signs
3. lower the tilt table 40 degrees and monitor the patient's vital signs
4. **lower the tilt table completely and monitor the patient's vital signs**

Correct Answer: 4

Explanation: The tilt table should be lowered to a horizontal position when a patient begins to demonstrate signs and symptoms of orthostatic hypotension. Signs and symptoms of this condition include a 20 mm Hg or greater decrease in systolic blood pressure, dizziness, and nausea. (Pierson p. 328)

Clinical Practice: Patient Care Skills
Content Outline: Standards of Care

Question Number: 161

A physical therapist examines a patient with a limited straight leg raise of 40 degrees due to inadequate hamstrings length. Which proprioceptive neuromuscular facilitation technique would be most appropriate to increase the patient's hamstrings length?

1. **contract-relax**
2. rhythmic initiation
3. rhythmic stabilization
4. rhythmic rotation

Correct Answer: 1

Explanation: Contract-relax is a proprioceptive neuromuscular facilitation technique utilized to increase range of motion on one side of a joint. This technique utilizes isometric as well as isotonic contractions. (Sullivan p. 66)

Clinical Practice: Neuromuscular System
Content Outline: Intervention

Question Number: 162
A physical therapist administers effleurage to the posterior neck and shoulder region of a patient with myofascial pain. Which therapeutic effect is most likely to occur when using effleurage?

1. stimulation of muscle activity and deep circulation
2. mobilization and removal of lung secretions
3. mobilization of muscle tissue
4. **stimulation of superficial blood and lymph flow**

Correct Answer: 4
Explanation: Effleurage is defined as a slow, stroking movement performed with increasing pressure in the direction of flow within the veins and lymph vessels. (De Domenico p. 35)

Clinical Practice: Physical Agents
Content Outline: Intervention

Question Number: 163
A physical therapist attempts to obtain a history from a patient that has recently immigrated to the United States. The patient does not speak English and seems to be intimidated by the hospital environment. The most appropriate action is to:

1. ask the patient to communicate in writing
2. ask another physical therapist to complete the examination
3. move the patient to a private treatment room
4. **request an interpreter**

Correct Answer: 4
Explanation: In order to effectively communicate with a patient that does not speak English it is often essential to utilize an interpreter. (Haggard p. 39)

Clinical Practice: Education/Communication
Content Outline: Intervention

Question Number: 164
A physical therapist prepares to perform volumetric measurements as a means of quantifying edema. Which patient would appear to be the most appropriate candidate for this type of objective measure?

1. **a 38-year-old female with a Colles' fracture**
2. a 27-year-old male with bicipital tendonitis
3. a 48-year-old male with a rotator cuff tear
4. a 57-year-old male with pulmonary edema

Correct Answer: 1
Explanation: Volumetric measurements are commonly used to measure edema in the distal extremities. The measurement is typically performed by examining the amount of water displaced from a cylinder following immersion of an affected body part. (Magee p. 311)

Clinical Practice: Musculoskeletal System
Content Outline: Examination

Question Number: 165
A physical therapist educates a patient status post transfemoral amputation on the importance of frequent skin checks. The most appropriate resource for the patient to utilize when inspecting the posterior aspect of the residual limb is:

1. **hand mirror**
2. video camera
3. nurse
4. prosthetist

Correct Answer: 1
Explanation: The use of a mirror during skin inspection of the residual limb will ensure that the patient can independently see all areas that are not easily visible. (O'Sullivan p. 630)

Clinical Practice: Integumentary System
Content Outline: Intervention

Question Number: 166
A patient status post stroke ambulates with a large base quad cane. The patient presents with left neglect and diminished proprioception. The most appropriate method to ensure patient safety is:

1. provide continuous verbal cues
2. utilize visual cues and demonstration
3. **offer manual assistance on the left side**
4. offer manual assistance on the right side

Correct Answer: 3

Explanation: The physical therapist can offer manual contact and assistance with lower extremity placement while standing on the patient's affected side. This will also help to alert the patient as to the environment on the left. (O'Sullivan p. 552)

Clinical Practice: Neuromuscular System
Content Outline: Intervention

Question Number: 167
A physical therapist completes a work site analysis for a patient with T3 paraplegia. The patient is employed in the marketing department of an advertising agency and relies on a wheelchair for daily locomotion. Which of the following is likely to be the most significant architectural barrier for the patient?

1. hardwood floors
2. **an entrance ramp (six inches of ramp length for every one-inch of step height)**
3. one quarter-inch thresholds at each door
4. pedestal type sinks

Correct Answer: 2

Explanation: An entrance ramp that has six inches of ramp length for each inch of vertical rise exceeds the 12:1 inch minimum ratio identified in the Americans with Disabilities Act. (Minor p. 471)

Clinical Practice: Education/Communication
Content Outline: Intervention

Question Number: 168
A three-year-old child throws frequent temper tantrums, usually contrived to gain attention. The physical therapist, recognizing the child's objective, refuses to acknowledge the action. This type of behavior therapy is best termed:

1. aversive conditioning
2. **extinction**
3. operant conditioning
4. emotive imagery

Correct Answer: 2

Explanation: By refusing to acknowledge the child's tantrums the physical therapist avoids reinforcing the behavior. As a result, the tantrums may decrease in frequency and eventually disappear. (Wortman p. 136)

Clinical Practice: Education/Communication
Content Outline: Evaluation, Diagnosis, Prognosis, and Outcomes

Question Number: 169
A physical therapist consults with a psychiatrist after examining a patient with a lengthy history of mental health issues. The psychiatrist describes the patient's current difficulty as short-lived, recurrent, unpredictable episodes of intense anxiety. This description best describes:

1. psychosomatic disorder
2. dissociative disorder
3. **panic disorder**
4. obsessive-compulsive disorder

Correct Answer: 3

Explanation: Panic disorders may affect up to 3-5% of the population with a 2:1 prevalence in females. This disorder may be associated with signs and symptoms such as dyspnea, tachycardia, dizziness, nausea, and feelings of impending doom. (Tierney p. 906)

Clinical Practice: Education
Content Outline: Evaluation, Diagnosis, Prognosis, and Outcomes

Question Number: 170
A physical therapist selects an assistive device for a patient rehabilitating from a recent illness. Which assistive device provides the least stability?

1. **Lofstrand crutches**
2. walker
3. parallel bars
4. axillary crutches

Correct Answer: 1

Explanation: Lofstrand crutches are wooden or metal crutches with a full or half-cuff that fits over a patient's forearms. Patients grasp the crutches using a handgrip that extends from the vertical axis of the crutch. Lofstrand crutches allow for greater ease of movement than axillary crutches, but provide less stability. (Minor p. 296)

Clinical Practice: Patient Care Skills
Content Outline: Intervention

Question Number: 171
A 61-year-old male referred to physical therapy complains of an excessive cough, sputum production, and shortness of breath. The patient indicates that he has been bothered by some combination of these symptoms for over 10 years. The patient's present condition is most indicative of:

1. idiopathic hypoventilation
2. chronic hypoxemia
3. Parkinson's disease
4. **chronic bronchitis**

Correct Answer: 4
Explanation: Chronic bronchitis is identified by the presence of a cough and pulmonary secretion expectoration for at least three months, two years in a row. This disease is often associated with cigarette smoking. (Paz p. 131)

Clinical Practice: Cardiopulmonary System
Content Outline: Evaluation, Diagnosis, Prognosis, and Outcomes

Question Number: 172
A physical therapist reviews a physician's note on an 18-year-old male diagnosed with impingement syndrome. The note indicates standard radiographs were utilized as part of the examination. Which finding would not be identifiable using a standard radiograph?

1. chronic calcific tendonitis
2. acromioclavicular arthritis
3. **partial-thickness tear of the rotator cuff**
4. unfused acromial apophysis

Correct Answer: 3
Explanation: Soft tissue structures such as muscles and tendons do not possess the density necessary to be seen on x-ray. (Magee p. 52)

Clinical Practice: Musculoskeletal System
Content Outline: Examination

Question Number: 173
A physical therapist obtains a history of a self-referred patient to physical therapy. During the history the therapist identifies several subjective reports that suggest the possibility of cancer. Which finding is not typically associated with cancer?

1. difficulty swallowing
2. change in bowel or bladder habits
3. persistent cough
4. **change in vision**

Correct Answer: 4
Explanation: Seven early danger signs of cancer include change in bowel or bladder habits, a sore that does not heal, unusual bleeding or discharge, thickening or lump in breast or elsewhere, indigestion or difficulty swallowing, obvious change in a wart or mole, and a nagging cough or hoarseness. (Goodman - Differential Diagnosis p. 402)

Clinical Practice: Neuromuscular System
Content Outline: Evaluation, Diagnosis, Prognosis, and Outcomes

Question Number: 174
A patient appears to be somewhat anxious after learning her treatment will include soft tissue massage. The most appropriate massage stroke to begin treatment is:

1. **effleurage**
2. kneading
3. petrissage
4. tapotement

Correct Answer: 1
Explanation: Effleurage is a massage stroke that is often utilized as a transitional stroke or as a means of introducing massage. (De Domenico p. 35)

Clinical Practice: Physical Agents
Content Outline: Intervention

Question Number: 175
Physical therapists and physical therapist assistants work together in a variety of health care settings. Which statement regarding the physical therapist assistant is not accurate?

1. Physical therapist assistants can make entries in the patient medical record.
2. **Physical therapist assistants are licensed in all 50 states.**
3. Physical therapist assistants are affiliate members of the American Physical Therapy Association.
4. Physical therapist assistants must work under direction and supervision of a physical therapist.

Correct Answer: 2
Explanation: There are several states that do not license physical therapist assistants. (Pagliarulo p. 59)

Clinical Practice: Administration
Content Outline: Intervention

Question Number: 176
A patient two days status post arthrotomy of the knee completes a quadriceps setting exercise while lying supine on a mat table. During the exercise the patient begins to experience severe pain. The most appropriate physical therapist action is:

1. have the patient perform the exercise in sidelying
2. have the patient flex the knee prior to initiating the exercise
3. place a pillow under the ankle
4. **discontinue the exercise**

Correct Answer: 4
Explanation: Severe pain in a patient rehabilitating from a surgical procedure is an acceptable reason to immediately discontinue an exercise. (Kisner p. 83)

Clinical Practice: Musculoskeletal System
Content Outline: Evaluation, Diagnosis, Prognosis, and Outcomes

Question Number: 177
A patient diagnosed with a cervical strain is examined in physical therapy. As part of the examination, the physical therapist attempts to palpate the transverse process of C1. Which instructions describe the most appropriate method to palpate C1?

1. place your fingers on the inion and move laterally and inferiorly
2. place your fingers immediately inferior to the patient's earlobes until you identify a bony prominence
3. **place your fingers in the space between the mastoid process and the angle of the mandible and move medially**
4. place your fingers on the superior nuchal line and move laterally and inferiorly

Correct Answer: 3
Explanation: C1, commonly termed the atlas, has the broadest transverse process in the cervical spine and is therefore easily identifiable. (Hoppenfeld p. 107)

Clinical Practice: Musculoskeletal System
Content Outline: Examination

Question Number: 178
A physical therapist enters a private treatment area and observes a patient collapsed on the floor. The patient appears to be moving slightly, however, seems to be in need of medical assistance. The most immediate therapist action is:

1. **check for unresponsiveness**
2. monitor airway, breathing, and circulation
3. position the patient
4. phone emergency medical services

Correct Answer: 1
Explanation: The first step in performing a primary survey is to determine responsiveness. (American Heart Association p. 5)

Clinical Practice: Patient Care Skills
Content Outline: Standards of Care

Question Number: 179

A physical therapist presents an inservice on ergonomics for administrative personnel. As part of the presentation the therapist discusses positioning when seated at a computer terminal. Which of the following recommendations would be most helpful?

1. position your thighs parallel with the floor
2. position your knees one-inch above your hips
3. position your knees two-inches above your hips
4. position your knees one-inch below your hips

Correct Answer: 1
Explanation: Other recommendations when seated at a computer terminal include: top of screen at eye level, minimum viewing distance of 12 inches, height of work surface at 23-28 inches, and width of work surface at 30 inches. (Hertfelder p. 138)

Clinical Practice: Education/Communication
Content Outline: Examination

Question Number: 180

A patient four weeks status post anterior dislocation of the glenohumeral joint is treated in physical therapy. The patient's arm was immobilized for three weeks following the injury. Currently the patient has limited active range of motion in flexion, abduction, and lateral rotation. Which of the following treatment options would be least appropriate for the patient?

1. D2 flexion proprioceptive neuromuscular facilitation muscle strengthening
2. strengthening of the scapular stabilizers
3. posterior glenohumeral joint mobilization
4. use of single-channel electromyographic biofeedback

Correct Answer: 1
Explanation: D2 flexion proprioceptive neuromuscular facilitation muscle strengthening should be avoided due to its emphasis on a pattern of shoulder flexion, abduction, and lateral rotation. This type of resistive exercise would likely place too much pressure on a shoulder that is only four weeks status post anterior dislocation. (Kisner p. 353)

Clinical Practice: Neuromuscular System
Content Outline: Intervention

Question Number: 181

A physical therapist examines the posture of a 16-year-old distance runner. The therapist identifies excessive genu valgum. Which of the following would be the most probable associated finding?

1. decreased Q angle
2. excessive subtalar pronation
3. posterior pelvic tilt
4. ipsilateral pelvic rotation

Correct Answer: 2
Explanation: Excessive subtalar pronation is a common finding in patients with genu valgum. This type of alignment results in patients bearing excessive weight on the inner side of the foot. (Magee p. 901)

Clinical Practice: Musculoskeletal System
Content Outline: Examination

Question Number: 182

A physical therapist completes a functional leg length assessment as part of a lower quarter screening examination. The therapist determines the right lower extremity is shorter than the left lower extremity. Which of the following would be most indicative of functional shortening?

1. lateral rotation of the right hip
2. supination of the right foot
3. posterior rotation of the right innominate
4. extension of the right knee

Correct Answer: 3
Explanation: Functional shortening refers to a shortening that is not a result of a structural change, but rather is associated with a compensation for a positional change. Posterior rotation of the right innominate on the sacrum results in functional shortening of the right lower extremity. (Magee p. 591)

Clinical Practice: Musculoskeletal System
Content Outline: Examination

Question Number: 183
A physical therapist attends an inservice entitled "Principles of Exercise for the Obstetric Patient." During the session, the speaker identifies several conditions that are considered to result in high risk pregnancies. Which of the following conditions would not be considered high risk?

1. **diastasis recti**
2. incompetent cervix
3. pre-eclampsia
4. multiple gestation

Correct Answer: 1
Explanation: Diastasis recti refers to a separation of the two halves of the rectus abdominus muscle in the midline at the linea alba. This condition is often associated with pregnancy during the second and third trimesters, however, is not considered to place a pregnancy at high risk. (Kisner p. 685)

Clinical Practice: Musculoskeletal System
Content Outline: Evaluation, Diagnosis, Prognosis, and Outcomes

Question Number: 184
A 48-year-old female rehabilitating from a fractured femur asks questions about her expected functional level following rehabilitation. Assuming an uncomplicated recovery, the most accurate prediction of functional level would be based on the patient's:

1. frequency of physical therapy visits
2. previous medical history
3. **previous functional level**
4. compliance with a home exercise program

Correct Answer: 3
Explanation: A relatively young patient rehabilitating from a fractured femur should have a near complete recovery. As a result, the patient's previous functional level should serve as the best predictor of her future functional level. (Hertling p. 104)

Clinical Practice: Education/Communication
Content Outline: Evaluation, Diagnosis, Prognosis, and Outcomes

Question Number: 185
A physical therapist utilizes neuromuscular electrical stimulation by attaching an electrode over the motor point of the peroneus longus. The most appropriate location to attach the electrode is:

1. along the lateral border of the popliteal fossa
2. **on the anterolateral surface of the lower leg**
3. proximal to the first metatarsophalangeal joint
4. immediately inferior to the lateral malleolus

Correct Answer: 2
Explanation: The peroneus longus originates on the head and upper two-thirds of the lateral surface of the fibula and inserts on the base of the first metatarsal and the lateral aspect of the medial cuneiform. The muscle acts to evert the foot at the subtalar joint and assists in plantar flexion at the ankle. (Robinson p. 161)

Clinical Practice: Physical Agents
Content Outline: Intervention

Question Number: 186
A physical therapist attempts to assess the dynamic balance of an elderly patient. Which screening tool would be most helpful to test balance and gait?

1. Functional Independence Measure
2. **Tinetti Performance Oriented Mobility Assessmennt**
3. Rankin Scale
4. Barthel Index

Correct Answer: 2
Explanation: The Tinetti Performance Oriented Mobility Assessmennt measures balance and gait using a 2-3 point ordinal scale. The test takes 5-15 minutes to administer with a total possible score of 28. Patients scoring less than 19 are considered to be at high risk for falling. (Physical Therapists Clinical Companion p. 123)

Clinical Practice: Neuromuscular System
Content Outline: Evaluation, Diagnosis, Prognosis, and Outcomes

Question Number: 187

A physical therapist instructs a patient how to fall safely to the floor when using axillary crutches. Which of the following should be the first to occur in the case of a forward fall?

1. reach towards the floor
2. turn your face towards one side
3. **release the crutches**
4. flex the trunk and head

Correct Answer: 3

Explanation: A patient should release the crutches in an attempt to utilize the upper extremities to break the forward fall. (Pierson p. 249)

Clinical Practice: Patient Care Skills
Content Outline: Intervention

Question Number: 188

A physical therapist attempts to strengthen the lumbricales on a patient with a low metatarsal arch. Which exercise would be the most appropriate?

1. resisted extension of the metatarsophalangeal joint
2. **resisted flexion of the metatarsophalangeal joint**
3. resisted abduction of the metatarsophalangeal joint
4. resisted adduction of the metatarsophalangeal joint

Correct Answer: 2

Explanation: The lumbricales act to flex the metatarsophalangeal joints and assist in extending the interphalangeal joints of the second through fifth digits. The lumbricales are innervated by the tibial nerve. (Kendall p. 196)

Clinical Practice: Musculoskeletal System
Content Outline: Intervention

Question Number: 189

A 46-year-old male rehabilitating from a radial head fracture misses his third consecutive physical therapy treatment session. The therapist called the patient after the second missed appointment, but did not receive a return phone call. The most appropriate physical therapist action is:

1. contact the patient's insurance provider
2. design a home exercise program for the patient
3. schedule the patient with another physical therapist
4. **discharge the patient from physical therapy**

Correct Answer: 4

Explanation: A patient consistently missing scheduled appointments should be discharged from physical therapy unless there are extraordinary circumstances. (Shamus – Effective Documentation p. 219)

Clinical Practice: Administration
Content Outline: Intervention

Question Number: 190

A physical therapist treats a patient with a decubitus ulcer using whirlpool. After treating the wound for 10 treatment sessions the wound still shows little evidence of granulation. The most appropriate action is:

1. begin aggressive debridement
2. recommend a wound culture
3. apply aseptic ointment to the wound
4. **discontinue whirlpool treatments**

Correct Answer: 4

Explanation: The physical therapist has an obligation to discontinue an ineffective intervention. In addition, the question does not provide enough evidence to justify any of the remaining options. (Sussman p. 199)

Clinical Practice: Integumentary System
Content Outline: Evaluation, Diagnosis, Prognosis, and Outcomes

Question Number: 191

A physical therapist completes a review of a patient's medical record prior to beginning a physical examination. The record indicates the patient was recently placed on an antidepressant medication. The most common side effect associated with antidepressants is:

1. **sedation**
2. dysarthria
3. seizures
4. blood pressure variability

Correct Answer: 1

Explanation: Antidepressant medications can produce a broad range of side effects including sedation. Tricyclics are an example of a category of antidepressant medication that commonly results in sedation. (Ciccone p. 91)

Clinical Practice: Neuromuscular System
Content Outline: Examination

Question Number: 192
A physical therapist instructs a patient rehabilitating from a low back injury in a series of five pelvic stabilization exercises. The patient indicates he understands the exercises, however, frequently becomes confused and is unable to perform them correctly. The most appropriate therapist action is:

1. repeat the exercise instructions
2. **reduce the number of exercises in the series**
3. select a different treatment option
4. conclude the patient is not a candidate for physical therapy

Correct Answer: 2
Explanation: A physical therapist should attempt to simplify the exercise session in order to reduce the patient's confusion. The most appropriate method to simplify the program is to reduce the number of exercises. (Haggard p. 107)

Clinical Practice: Education/Communication
Content Outline: Intervention

Question Number: 193
A physical therapist employed in a rehabilitation hospital prepares to perform a stand pivot transfer with a 42-year-old male rehabilitating from a motor vehicle accident. Prior to initiating the transfer, the therapist notices that the patient is wearing only a pair of hospital issued non-skid socks on his feet. The most appropriate therapist action is to:

1. ask another therapist for assistance and complete a dependent transfer
2. have the patient complete a sliding board transfer
3. perform the stand pivot transfer without socks
4. **perform the stand pivot transfer with the patient wearing the hospital-issued socks**

Correct Answer: 4
Explanation: Therapists should not permit patients to perform transfer activities with standard socks, however, since the hospital-issued socks are "non-skid" this becomes an acceptable option. (Pierson p. 190)

Clinical Practice: Patient Care Skills
Content Outline: Intervention

Question Number: 194
A physical therapist designs an exercise program consisting of closed-chain activities for a patient rehabilitating from a medial meniscus repair. An appropriate closed-chain exercise to include in the rehabilitation program is:

1. submaximal velocity spectrum isokinetic exercise
2. **bilateral mini-squats in standing**
3. short-arc terminal knee extension
4. prone leg curls with a two pound cuff weight

Correct Answer: 2
Explanation: Closed-chain activities require the distal segment to be in contact with the ground or some other surface. (Kisner p. 554)

Clinical Practice: Musculoskeletal System
Content Outline: Intervention

Question Number: 195
A patient with a T3 spinal cord injury exercising on a treatment table in supine begins to exhibit signs and symptoms of autonomic dysreflexia including a dramatic increase in blood pressure. The most immediate action to address the patient's blood pressure response is to:

1. elevate the patient's legs
2. call for assistance
3. **sit the patient upright**
4. check urinary drainage system

Correct Answer: 3
Explanation: Moving the patient from supine to a sitting position will serve to reduce the patient's blood pressure. Checking the patient's urinary drainage system could be useful to reduce the patient's blood pressure, but only if it served as the noxious stimulus triggering the sympathetic response. (Pierson p. 335)

Clinical Practice: Neuromuscular System
Content Outline: Standards of Care

Question Number: 196
A physical therapist observes a change in the muscle tone of an infant's extremities as a result of head rotation. Which developmental reflex would facilitate this type of response?

1. **asymmetrical tonic neck reflex**
2. symmetrical tonic neck reflex
3. symmetrical tonic labyrinthine reflex
4. crossed extension reflex

Correct Answer: 1

Explanation: The asymmetrical tonic neck reflex normally occurs in infants from birth to 6 months of age when the head is rotated to one side. This reflex causes extension of the extremities toward the side of rotation. (Ratliffe p. 26)

Clinical Practice: Neuromuscular System
Content Outline: Intervention

Question Number: 197
A physical therapist palpates medially along the spine of the scapula. Which spinous process is at the same level as the vertebral end of the spine?

1. T2
2. T3
3. T4
4. T5

Correct Answer: 2

Explanation: In the resting position the scapula covers ribs two through seven, while the spine of the scapula is opposite the spinous process of T3. (Hoppenfeld p. 11)

Clinical Practice: Musculoskeletal System
Content Outline: Examination

Question Number: 198
A physical therapist instructs a patient in an exercise designed to increase pelvic floor awareness and strength. The exercise requires the patient to tighten the pelvic floor as if attempting to stop the flow of urine. The patient is instructed to hold the isometric contraction for 5 seconds and complete 10 repetitions. The most appropriate initial position for the exercise is:

1. supine
2. sitting
3. tall kneeling
4. standing

Correct Answer: 1

Explanation: Kegel exercises are often utilized as part of a treatment program for incontinence. Supine and sidelying are the easiest positions to begin the training session. (Kisner p. 697)

Clinical Practice: Musculoskeletal System
Content Outline: Intervention

Question Number: 199
An attorney contacts you by phone and requests specific information on a patient he claims to represent. Questions asked include the extent of the patient's disability and his willingness to return to work. The most appropriate response is:

1. answer the questions asked by the attorney
2. request the attorney provide a completed release of patient medical information form
3. tell the attorney not to bother you at work
4. send the attorney a copy of the patient's medical records

Correct Answer: 2

Explanation: The attorney would not be entitled to the patient's medical information without a completed release of patient medical information form. (Scott - Professional Ethics p. 86)

Clinical Practice: Administration
Content Outline: Standards of Care

Question Number: 200
A patient four weeks status post anterior cruciate ligament reconstruction questions a physical therapist as to why he is still partial weight bearing. An acceptable rationale is:

1. the patient does not have full active knee extension
2. the patient has good quadriceps strength
3. the patient has fair hamstrings strength
4. the patient has diminished superficial cutaneous sensation

Correct Answer: 1

Explanation: A patient status post anterior cruciate ligament reconstruction surgery may continue to use an assistive device for weight bearing if they do not possess full active knee extension. Ambulation on a flexed knee can result in excessive irritation of the patellofemoral joint. (Kisner p. 537)

Clinical Practice: Musculoskeletal System
Content Outline: Intervention

APPENDIX

Sample Examination Scoring Summary

	Available Questions	Correct Questions	% Correct
Paper and Pencil Sample Examination One	200	134	67%
Paper and Pencil Sample Examination Two	200	142	71%
Computer-Based Testing Sample Examination One	200		
Computer-Based Testing Sample Examination Two	200		

*The Content Outline Examination was designed to provide candidates with a better appreciation of the breadth and depth of the current Physical Therapist Examination. Due to the unique composition of the examination (20 questions in each content outline category) the examination was not included in the Sample Examination Scoring Summary.

Resource List

American Physical Therapy Association
1111 North Fairfax Street
Alexandria, Virginia 22314
Phone: (800) 999-2782
Web site: www.apta.org

Federation of State Boards of Physical Therapy
509 Wythe Street
Alexandria, Virginia 22314
Phone: (703) 299-3100
Web site: www.fsbpt.org

Scorebuilders
P.O. Box 7242
Scarborough, Maine 04070-7242
Toll Free: (866) PTEXAMS
Phone: (207) 885-0304
Web site: www.scorebuilders.com
Fax: (207) 883-8377

Physical Therapy State Licensing Agencies

Alabama

Alabama Board of Physical Therapy
100 N. Union Street
Suite 627
Montgomery, AL 36130-5040

(334) 242-4064
www.pt.state.al.us

Arizona

Arizona State Board of Physical Therapy
1400 West Washington
Suite 230
Phoenix, AZ 85007

(602) 542-3095
www.ptboard.state.az.us

California

Physical Therapy Board of California
1418 Howe Avenue
Suite 16
Sacramento, CA 95825

(916) 561-8200
www.ptb.ca.gov

Connecticut

Connecticut Dept of Public Health
410 Capitol Avenue
P.O.Box 340308
Hartford, CT 06134-0308

(860) 509-7562
www.dph.state.ct.us

Alaska

State PT & OT Board Div of Occup Licensing
333 Willoughby Avenue, 9th Floor
P.O. Box 110806
Juneau, AK 99811

(907) 465-2580
www.dced.state.ak.us/occ/pphy.htm

Arkansas

Arkansas State Board of Physical Therapy
9 Shackleford Plaza
Suite 3
Little Rock, AR 72211

(501) 228-7100
www.arptb.org

Colorado

Colorado Division of Registrations
1560 Broadway
Suite 1340
Denver, CO 80202

(303) 894-2440
www.dora.state.co.us

Delaware

Division of Professional Regulation
861 Silver Lake Blvd.
Suite 203 Cannon Building
Dover, DE 19904-2467

(302) 744-4506
www.state.de.us/research/profreg/physical.htm

District of Columbia

District of Columbia Board of Physical Therapy
Dept of Health
825 N. Capital Street, NE
Room 2224
Washington, DC 20002

(478) 207-1686

Georgia

Georgia Board of Physical Therapy
237 Coliseum Drive
Macon, GA 31217

(478) 207-1686
www.sos.state.ga.us/plb/pt/

Idaho

Idaho State Board of Medicine
1755 Westgate Drive
Suite 140
Boise, ID 83704

(208) 327-7000
www.bom.state.id.us

Indiana

Indiana Physical Therapy Committee
402 W. Washington Street
Room W041
Indianapolis, IN 46204

(317) 234-2051
www.in.gov/hpb/boards/ptc/

Florida

Florida Dept of Health
Board of Physical Therapy Practice
4052 Bald Cypress Way
Bin #C05
Tallahassee, FL 32399-3255

(850) 245-4373
www.doh.state.fl.us/mqa/physical/pt_home.html

Hawaii

Hawaii Dept of Commerce & Consumer Affairs
P.O. Box 3469
Honolulu, HI 96801

(808) 586-2694
www.state.hi.us/dcca/pvl/

Illinois

Illinois Dept of Professional Regulation
320 West Washington
3rd Floor
Springfield, IL 62786

(217) 782-8556
www.dpr.state.il.us

Iowa

Iowa Board of Physical Therapy Examiners
Iowa Dept of Public Health
321 East 12th Street, 5th Floor
Des Moines, IA 50319-0075

(515) 281-4413
www.idph.state.ia.us/licensure/

Kansas

Kansas State Board of Healing Arts
PT Examining Committee
235 S. Topeka Blvd
Topeka, KS 66603

(785) 296-7413
www.ink.org/public/boha

Louisiana

Louisiana State Board of PT Examiners
104 Fairland Drive
Lafayette, LA 70507-3834

(337) 262-1043
www.laptboard.org

Maryland

Maryland Board of PT Examiners
4201 Patterson Avenue #223
Baltimore, MD 21215-2299

(410) 764-4752
www.dhmh.state.md.us/bphte

Michigan

Physical Therapy State Boards
P.O. Box 30670
Lansing, MI 48909

(517) 335-0918
www.michigan.gov/bhser

Mississippi

Mississippi State Board of Physical Therapy
570 East Woodrow Wilson Blvd.
Room 162
Jackson, MS 39216

(601) 576-7260

Kentucky

Kentucky State Board of PT
9110 Leesgate Road, #6
Louisville, KY 40222-5159

(502) 327-8497
www.pt.ky.gov

Maine

Maine Board of Examiners in PT
35 State House Station
Augusta, ME 04330

(207) 624-8600
www.state.me.us/pfr/led/ledhome2.htm

Massachusetts

Massachusetts Board of Allied Health
Division of Registration
239 Causeway Street, Suite 500
Boston, MA 02114

(617) 727-3071
www.state.ma.us/reg/boards/ah

Minnesota

Minnesota Board of Physical Therapy
2829 University Avenue, SE, #315
Minneapolis, MN 55414-3222

(612) 627-5406
www.physicaltherapy.state.mn.us

Missouri

Advisory Comm for Prof PTs & PTAs
P.O. Box 4
3605 Missouri Boulevard
Jefferson City, MO 65102

(573) 751-0098
www.ded.state.mo.us/regulatorylicensing/

Montana

Montana Board of Physical Therapy Examiners
301 South Park, 4th Floor
P.O. Box 200513
Helena, MT 59620-0513

(406) 841-2395
www.discoveringmontana.com/dli/ptp

Nevada

Nevada Board of Physical Therapy Examiners
810 South Durango Drive, Suite 109
Las Vegas, NV 89145

(702) 876-5535
www.ptboard.nv.gov

New Jersey

New Jersey State Board of Physical Therapy
P.O. Box 45014
Newark, NJ 07101

(973) 504-6455
www.state.nj.us/lps/ca/home.htm

New York

New YorkState Board for PT
89 Washington Avenue
Education Bldg, East Mezzanine
Albany, NY 12234

(518) 474-3817
www.op.nysed.gov/pt.htm

Nebraska

Nebraska Board of Physical Therapy
301 Centennial Mall
P.O. Box 94986
Lincoln, NE 68509

(402) 471-2299
www.hhs.state.ne.us/crl/rcs/pt/pt.htm

New Hampshire

PT Governing Boad of New Hampshire
Office of Allied Health Prof
2 Industrial Park Drive
Concord, NH 03301

(603) 271-8389

New Mexico

New Mexico Physical Therapy Board
2055 S. Pacheco
Suite 400
Santa Fe, NM 87505

(505) 476-7085
www.rld.state.nm.us/rid/b&c/ptb/index.htm

North Carolina

North Carolina Board of Physical Therapy
18 W. Colony Place #140
Durham, NC 27705

(919) 490-6393
www.ncptboard.org

North Dakota

North Dakota State Examination Committee
106 Eastern Avenue
Grafton, ND 58237

(701) 352-0125
www.governor.state.nd.us/boards/

Oklahoma

Board of Medical Licensing
PT Advisory Committee
5104 North Francis, Suite C
Oklahoma City, OK 73118

(405) 848-6841
www.okmedicalboard.org

Pennsylvania

Pennsylvania State Board of PT
P.O. Box 2649
Harrisburg, PA 17105

(717) 783-7134
www.dos.state.pa.us/bpoa/cwp/

Rhode Island

Rhode Island Physical Therapy Board
Department of Health
3 Capitol Hill, Room 104
Providence, RI 02908-5097

(401) 222-1272
www.health.state.ri.us

South Dakota

South Dakota Board of Medical Examiners
1323 S. Minnesota Avenue
Sioux Falls, SD 57105

(605) 334-8343
www.state.sd.us/doh/medical/pt.htm

Ohio

Ohio State Board of Physical Therapy
77 S. High Street
16th Floor
Columbus, OH 43215-6108

(614) 466-3774
www.otptat.ohio.gov/

Oregon

Oregon Physical Therapy Licensing Board
800 NE Oregon Street
Suite 407
Portland, OR 97232

(503) 731-4047
www.ptboard.state.or.us

Puerto Rico

Office of Regulation and Certification
Call Box 10200
Santurce, PR 00908

(787) 725-8161 x209

South Carolina

South Carolina Board of PT Examiners
110 Centerview Drive
P.O. Box 11329
Columbia, SC 29211

(803) 896-4655
www.llr.state.sc.us

Tennessee

Division of Health Related Boards
Bd of Occupational & Physical Therapy
426 5th Ave North, 1st Floor
Nashville, TN 37247

(615) 532-5136
www.state.tn.us/health

Texas

Texas Board of PT Examiners
333 Guadalupe, Suite 2-510
Austin, TX 78701

(512) 305-6900
www.ecptote.state.tx.us

Vermont

Physical Therapy Advisors
Office of Professional Regulations
26 Terrace Street, Drawer 09
Montpelier, VT 05609-1106

(802) 828-2191
www.vtprofessionals.org

Virginia

Board of Physical Therapy
Dept of Health Professions, 5th Floor
6603 West Broad Street
Richmond, VA 23230

(804) 662-9924
www.dhp.state.va.us

West Virginia

West Virginia Board of Physical Therapy
153 W. Main Street
Suite 103
Clarksburg, WV 26301

(304) 627-2251
www.wvbopt.com

Wyoming

Wyoming Board of Physical Therapy
2020 Carey Avenue
Suite 201
Cheyenne, WY 82002

(307) 777-3507
www.soswy.state.wy.us/director/

Utah

Division of Professional Licensing
P.O. Box 146741
Salt Lake City, UT 84114

(801) 530-6621
www.dopl.utah.gov/licensing/

Virgin Islands

Virgin Islands Board of PT Examiners
48 Sugar Estate
St. Thomas, VI 00802

(340) 774-0117

Washington

Washington Board of Physical Therapy
1112 SE Quince Street
P.O. Box 47868
Olympia, WA 98504-7868

(360) 236-4700
www.doh.wa.gov

Wisconsin

Wisconsin Dept of Regulation & Licensing
1400 E. Washington Avenue
Room 178
P.O. Box 8935
Madison, WI 53708-8935

(608) 266-2112

Prometric Testing Centers

Alabama
Birmingham
Decatur
Dothan
Mobile
Montgomery

Alaska
Anchorage

Arizona
Goodyear (2)
Phoenix (2)
Tucson

Arkansas
Arkadelphia
Fort Smith
Little Rock

California
Alameda
Anaheim (2)
Atascadero
Camarillo
Culver City (3)
Diamond Bar
Gardena
Glendale (2)
Irvine
Rancho Cucamonga
Redlands
Sacramento (2)
San Diego (3)

Colorado
Colorado Springs
Greenwood Village (2)
Longmont

Connecticut
Glastonbury (2)
Hamden

District of Columbia
Washington, D.C. (2)

Delaware
Wilmington

Florida
Coral Springs (2)
Fort Myers
Gainesville
Jacksonville
Maitland
Miami (2)
Orlando (2)
Sarasota (2)
Tallahassee
Tampa (2)

Georgia
Atlanta (5)
Augusta
Macon
Marietta (2)
Savannah
Valdosta

Guam
Hagatna (2)

Hawaii
Honolulu

Idaho
Garden City

Illinois
Carbondale
Chicago (5)
Homewood
Lombard
Northbrook
Peoria

Springfield
Sycamore

Indiana
Evansville
Fort Wayne
Indianapolis (2)
Lafayette
Mishawaka
Terre Haute

Iowa
Ames
Bettendorf
Urbandale

Kansas
Topeka
Wichita

Kentucky
Lexington
Louisville

Louisiana
Baton Rouge
Bossier City
New Orleans (2)

Maine
Orono
South Portland

Maryland
Baltimore
Bethesda
Columbia
Lanham
Pikesville
Salisbury
Towson

Massachusetts
Boston (4)
Burlington (2)
East Longmeadow
Worcester (2)

Michigan
Ann Arbor (2)
Grand Rapids
Lansing
Livonia
Portage
Sault Ste Marie
Troy

Minnesota
Duluth
Edina (2)
Rochester
Woodbury

Mississippi
Jackson
Tupelo

Missouri
Ballwin
Hazelwood
Jefferson City
Lees Summit
Springfield
St. Joseph

Montana
Billings
Helena

Nebraska
Columbus
Lincoln
Omaha

Nevada
Las Vegas
Reno

New Hampshire
Portsmouth

New Jersey
Clark (2)
Deptford
Edison
Fairlawn (2)
Hamilton Township
Toms River

New Mexico
Albuquerque

New York
Albany
Brooklyn Heights (2)
Buffalo
Garden City
Ithaca
Lynbrook
Melville (2)
New York City (10)
Queens
Rochester
Staten Island
Vestal
Wappingers Falls
White Plains

North Carolina
Asheville
Charlotte (2)
Greensboro
Greenville
Raleigh (2)
Wilmington

North Dakota
Bismarck
Fargo

Ohio
Cincinnati (2)
Columbus (2)
Dayton

Maumee
Mentor
Niles
Stow
Strongsville

Oklahoma
Oklahoma City
Tulsa

Oregon
Eugene
Milwaukee
Portland

Pennsylvania
Allentown
Clark Summit
Erie
Harrisburg
Lancaster
Montgomeryville (2)
Philadelphia (2)
Pittsburgh
York

Puerto Rico
Guaynabo (2)

Rhode Island
Warwick

South Carolina
Charleston
Columbia
Greenville

South Dakota
Sioux Falls

Tennessee
Chattanooga
Clarksville
Franklin
Knoxville

Madison
Memphis

Texas
Abilene
Amarillo
Austin (2)
Beaumont
Corpus Christi
Dallas (4)
El Paso
Fort Worth
Houston (5)
Lubbock
McAllen
Midland
San Antonio (2)
Tyler
Waco

Utah
Ogden
Orem
Salt Lake City

Vermont
Williston

Virginia
Fairfax (2)
Glen Allen (2)
Lynchburg
Newport News (2)
Roanoke

Virgin Islands
St. Croix

Washington
Seattle (3)
Spokane

West Virginia
Morgantown
S. Charleston

Wisconsin
Madison
Milwaukee (2)

Wyoming
Casper

Bibliography

American Cancer Society, www.cancer.org., 2004

American College of Obstetricians and Gynecologists: Exercise during Pregnancy and the Postpartum Period (Technical Bulletin No 189), copyright ACOG, 1994

American College of Sports Medicine: ACSM's Guidelines for Exercise Testing and Prescription, Sixth Edition, Lippincott Williams & Wilkins, 2000

American Heart Association: BLS for Healthcare Providers, American Heart Association, 2001

American Red Cross: CPR/AED for the Professional Rescuer, American Red Cross, 2002

Anemaet W, Moffa-Trotter M: Home Rehabilitation: Guide to Clinical Practice, Mosby, 2000

Anderson MK, Hall SJ, Martin M: Fundamentals of Sports Injury Management, Second Edition, Lippincott Williams & Wilkins, 2000

Arends R: Learning to Teach, Second Edition, McGraw-Hill Inc., 1991

Bahr R, Maehlum S: Clinical Guide to Sports Injuries, Human Kinetics, 2004

Bailey D, Robinson D: Therapeutic Approaches in Mental Health/Psychiatric Nursing, FA Davis Company, 1997

Behrens BJ, Michlovitz S: Physical Agents: Theory and Practice for the Physical Therapist Assistant, FA Davis Company, 1996

Belanger A: Evidence-Based Guide to Therapeutic Physical Agents, Lippincott Williams & Wilkins, 2003

Bennett S, Karnes J: Neurological Disabilities: Assessment and Treatment, Lippincott-Raven Publishers, 1998

Bergen A, Presperin J, Tallman T: Positioning for Function: Wheelchairs and Other Assistive Technologies, Valhalla Rehabilitation Publications, 1990

Bickley L, Szilagyi P: Bates' Guide to Physical Examination and History Taking, Eighth Edition, Lippincott Williams & Wilkins, 2003

Bly L: Motor Skill Acquisition in the First Year, Therapy Skill Builders, 1994

Bobath B: Adult Hemiplegia: Evaluation and Treatment, Heinemann Medical Books Limited, 1978

Boissonnault W: Examination in Physical Therapy Practice: Screening for Medical Disease, WB Saunders Company, 1995

Brannon F, Foley M, Starr J, Saul L: Cardiopulmonary Rehabilitation: Basic Theory and Application, FA Davis Company, 1998

Brotzman SB, Wilk KE: Clinical Orthopedic Rehabilitation, Mosby, 2003

Brunnstrom S: Movement Therapy in Hemiplegia, Harper and Row Publishers Inc., 1970

Cameron M: <u>Physical Agents in Rehabilitation: From Research to Practice</u>, WB Saunders Company, 2003

Campbell M: <u>Rehabilitation for Traumatic Brain Injury: Physical Therapy Practice in Context</u>,
   Churchill Livingstone, 2000

Campbell S: <u>Decision Making in Pediatric Neurologic Physical Therapy</u>, Churchill Livingstone, 1999

Campbell S: <u>Physical Therapy for Children</u>, Second Edition, WB Saunders Company, 2000

Carr J, Shepard R: <u>Neurological Rehabilitation: Optimizing Motor Performance</u>, Butterworth-Heinemann,
   1998

Carr J, Shepard R: <u>Stroke Rehabilitation: Guidelines for Exercise and Training to Optimize Motor Skill</u>,
   Elsevier Science Limited, 2003

Centers for Disease Control and Prevention: <u>Guidelines for Isolation Precautions in Hospitals</u>, Atlanta, GA
   <u>www.cdc.gov</u>, 2004

Ciccone C: <u>Pharmacology in Rehabilitation</u>, Third Edition, FA Davis Company, 2002

Clark C, Bonfiglio M: <u>Orthopaedics: Essentials of Diagnosis and Treatment</u>, Churchill Livingstone, 1994

Clarkson HM: <u>Musculoskeletal Assessment</u>, Second Edition, Lippincott Williams & Wilkins, 2000

<u>Code of Ethics</u>, American Physical Therapy Association, 2004

Curtis K: <u>The Physical Therapist's Guide to Health Care</u>, Slack Inc., 1999

Davis C: <u>Patient Practitioner Interaction</u>, Third Edition, Slack Inc., 1998

De Domenico G, Wood E: <u>Beard's Massage</u>, WB Saunders Company, 1997

DeMyer W: <u>Technique of the Neurologic Examination</u>, McGraw-Hill Companies, 2004

Denegar C: <u>Therapeutic Modalities for Athletic Injuries</u>, Human Kinetics, 2000

DePoy E, Gitlin L: <u>Introduction to Research: Multiple Strategies for Health and Human Services</u>, Mosby-
   Year Book, Inc., 1994

DeTurk W, Cahalin L: <u>Cardiovascular and Pulmonary Physical Therapy: An Evidence-Based Approach</u>,
   McGraw-Hill Companies, 2004

Domholdt E: <u>Physical Therapy Research Principles and Application</u>, Second Edition, WB Saunders
   Company, 2000

Donatelli R, Wooden M: <u>Orthopedic Physical Therapy</u>, Third Edition, Churchill Livingstone, 2001

Drench M, Noonan A, Sharby N, Ventura S: <u>Psychosocial Aspects of Healthcare</u>, Prentice Hall, 2002

Dutton M: <u>Orthopaedic Examination, Evaluation, and Intervention</u>, McGraw-Hill Inc., 2004

Edelman C, Mandle C: <u>Health Promotion: Throughout the Lifespan</u>, Mosby, 2002

Falkenstein N, Weiss-Lessard S: <u>Hand Rehabilitation: A Quick Reference Guide and Review</u>, Mosby,
   1999

Falvo DR: <u>Effective Patient Education</u>, Third Edition, Jones and Bartlett Publishers, 2004

Frownfelter D, Dean E: <u>Principles and Practice of Cardiopulmonary Physical Therapy</u>, Third Edition, Mosby-Year Book, Inc., 1996

Garrison S: <u>Physical Medicine and Rehabilitation Basics</u>, J.B. Lippincott Company, 1995

Giles S: <u>PTEXAM: The Complete Study Guide</u>, Scorebuilders, 2005

Goodman C, Boissonnault W, Fuller K: <u>Pathology: Implications for the Physical Therapist</u>, Second Edition, WB Saunders Company, 2003

Goodman C, Snyder T: <u>Differential Diagnosis in Physical Therapy</u>, Third Edition, WB Saunders Company, 2000

Greathouse JS: <u>Radiographic Positioning & Procedures</u>, Delmar Publishers, 1998

Gross J, Fetto J, Rosen E: <u>Musculoskeletal Examination</u>, Second Edition, Blackwell Science, Inc., 2002

<u>Guide for Conduct of the Physical Therapist Assistant</u>, American Physical Therapy Association, 2004

<u>Guide for Professional Conduct</u>, American Physical Therapy Association, 2004

<u>Guide to Physical Therapist Practice</u>, Second Edition, American Physical Therapy Association, 2004

Haggard A: <u>Handbook of Patient Education</u>, Aspen Publishers, 1989

Hall C, Brody L: <u>Therapeutic Exercise: Moving Toward Function</u>, Lippincott Williams & Wilkins, 1999

Hamill J, Knutzen K: <u>Biomechanical Basis of Human Movement</u>, Lippincott Williams & Wilkins, 1995

Hertfelder S, Gwin C: <u>Work in Progress: Occupational Therapy in Work Programs</u>, American Occupational Therapy Association, 1989

Hertling D, Kessler R: <u>Management of Common Musculoskeletal Disorders</u>, Third Edition, Lippincott Williams & Wilkins, 1996

Hillegass E, Sadowsky H: <u>Cardiopulmonary Physical Therapy</u>, Second Edition, WB Saunders Company, 2001

Hislop HJ, Montgomery J: <u>Daniels and Worthingham's Muscle Testing: Techniques of Manual Examination</u>, 7th Ed, WB Saunders Company, 2002

Hodgkin JE, Celli B, Connors G: <u>Pulmonary Rehabilitation: Guidelines to Success</u>, Third Edition, Lippincott Williams & Wilkins, 2000

Hoppenfeld S: <u>Physical Examination of the Spine and Extremities</u>, Appleton-Century-Crofts, 1982

Houglum P: <u>Therapeutic Exercise for Athletic Injuries</u>, Human Kinetics, 2001

Ignatavicius D, Workman L: <u>Medical Surgical Nursing: A Nursing Process Approach, Volume I</u>, Second Edition, WB Saunders Company, 1995

Irwin S, Tecklin J: <u>Cardiopulmonary Physical Therapy: A Guide to Practice</u>, Fourth Edition, Mosby, 2004

Jacobs M, Austin N: <u>Splinting The Hand and the Upper Extremity: Principles and Process</u>, Lippincott Williams & Wilkins, 2003

Kahn J: <u>Principles and Practice of Electrotherapy</u>, Churchill Livingstone, 2000

Kendall F, McCreary E, Provance P: <u>Muscle Testing and Function</u>, Williams & Wilkins, 1993

Kisner C, Colby L: <u>Therapeutic Exercise Foundations and Techniques</u>, Fourth Edition, FA Davis Company, 2002

Kitchen S: <u>Electrotherapy: Evidence-Based Practice</u>, Churchill Livingstone, 2002

Kloth LC, McCulloch JM: <u>Wound Healing: Alternatives in Management</u>, Third Edition, FA Davis Company, 2002

Knight W: <u>Managed Care: What it is and How it Works</u>, Aspen Publishers, 1998

Konin J, Wiksten D, Isear J, Brader H: <u>Special Tests for Orthopedic Examination</u>, Second Edition, Slack Inc., 2002

Kornblau B, Starling S: <u>Ethics in Rehabilitation: A Clinical Perspective</u>, Slack Inc., 2000

Langford RW, Thompson JD: <u>Mosby's Handbook of Diseases</u>, Second Edition, Mosby, 2000

Levangie P, Norkin C: <u>Joint Structure and Function: A Comprehensive Analysis</u>, Third Edition, FA Davis Company, 2001

Lewis B: <u>Geriatric Physical Therapy: A Clinical Approach</u>, Appleton & Lange, 1994

Lippert LS: <u>Clinical Kinesiology for Physical Therapist Assistants</u>, FA Davis Company, 2000

Long T, Toscano K: <u>Handbook of Pediatric Physical Therapy</u>, Second Edition, Lippincott Williams & Wilkins, 2002

Lundy-Ekman L: <u>Neuroscience Fundamentals for Rehabilitation</u>, WB Saunders Company, 2002

Magee D: <u>Orthopedic Physical Assessment</u>, Fourth Edition, WB Saunders Company, 2002

Malone T, McPoil T, Nitz A: <u>Orthopedic and Sports Physical Therapy</u>, Third Edition, Mosby-Year Book, Inc., 1997

Meyers B: <u>Wound Management: Principles and Practice</u>, Prentice Hall, 2002

Michlovitz S: <u>Thermal Agents in Rehabilitation</u>, Third Edition, FA Davis Company, 1996

Miller-Keane: <u>Encyclopedia and Dictionary of Medicine, Nursing, and Allied Health</u>, WB Saunders, 1997

Minor M, Minor S: <u>Patient Care Skills</u>, Fourth Edition, Appleton & Lange, 1999

Montgomery P, Connolly B: <u>Clinical Applications for Motor Control</u>, Slack Inc., 2003

<u>National Physical Therapy Examinations Candidate Handbook</u>, Federation of State Boards of Physical Therapy, 2004

Neistadt M, Crepeau E: <u>Occupational Therapy</u>, Ninth Edition, Lippincott, 1998

Nelson R, Hayes K, Currier D: <u>Clinical Electrotherapy</u>, Third Edition, Appleton & Lange, 1999

Neumann DA: <u>Kinesiology of the Musculoskeletal System</u>, Mosby, 2002

Norkin C, White D: <u>Measurement of Joint Motion: A Guide to Goniometry</u>, Third Edition, FA Davis Company, 2003

Nosse L, Friberg D: <u>Managerial and Supervisory Principles for Physical Therapists</u>, Second Edition, Lippincott Williams & Wilkins, 2005

<u>Nurse's 3-Minute Clinical Reference</u>, Lippincott Williams & Wilkins, 2003

O'Sullivan S, Schmitz T: <u>Physical Rehabilitation: Assessment and Treatment</u>, Fourth Edition, FA Davis Company, 2001

Ozer M, Payton O, Nelson C: <u>Treatment Planning for Rehabilitation: A Patient Centered Approach</u>, McGraw-Hill Inc., 2000

Pagliarulo M: <u>Introduction to Physical Therapy</u>, Second Edition, Mosby, 2001

Pauls J, Reed K: <u>Quick Reference to Physical Therapy</u>, Aspen Publishers, 1996

Payton O: <u>Research: The Validation of Clinical Practice</u>, Third Edition, FA Davis Company, 1994

Paz J, Panik M: <u>Acute Care Handbook for Physical Therapists</u>, Second Edition, Butterworth-Heinemann, 2002

<u>Physical Therapist's Clinical Companion</u>, Springhouse Corporation, 2000

Pierson F: <u>Principles and Techniques of Patient Care</u>, Third Edition, WB Saunders Company, 2002

Placzek J, Boyce D: <u>Orthopaedic Physical Therapy Secrets</u>, Hanley and Belfus, Inc., 2001

Portney L, Watkins M: <u>Foundations of Clinical Research: Applications to Practice</u>, Prentice Hall, 2000

Prentice W: <u>Therapeutic Modalities for Physical Therapists</u>, Second Edition, McGraw-Hill Inc., 2002

Prentice W, Voight M: <u>Techniques in Musculoskeletal Rehabilitation</u>, McGraw-Hill Inc., 2001

Purtilo R, Haddad A: <u>Health Professional and Patient Interaction</u>, Sixth Edition, WB Saunders Company, 2002

Quinn L, Gordon J: <u>Functional Outcomes: Documentation for Rehabilitation</u>, Elsevier Science, 2003

Rancho Los Amigos National Rehabilitation Center: <u>Normal and Pathological Gait Syllabus</u>, Downey California

Ratliffe K: <u>Clinical Pediatric Physical Therapy: A Guide for the Physical Therapy Team</u>, Mosby, 1998

Reese N, Bandy WD: <u>Joint Range of Motion and Muscle Length Testing</u>, WB Saunders Company, 2002

Reider B: <u>The Orthopaedic Physical Examination</u>, WB Saunders Company, 1999

Richard R, Staley M: <u>Burn Care and Rehabilitation: Principles and Practice</u>, FA Davis Company, 1994

Robinson A, Snyder-Mackler L: Clinical Electrophysiology, Williams & Wilkins, 1995

Rothstein J, Roy S, Wolf S: The Rehabilitation Specialist's Handbook, FA Davis Company, 1998

Sackett DL, Straus SE, Richardson WS, Rosenberg W, Haynes RB: Evidence-Based Medicine: How to Practice and Teach EBM, Churchill Livingstone, 2000

Sahrman S: Diagnosis and Treatment of Movement Impairment Syndromes, Mosby, 2002

Saidoff DC, McDonough AL: Critical Pathways in Therapeutic Intervention: Extremities and Spine, Mosby, 2002

Salter R: Textbook of Disorders and Injuries of the Musculoskeletal System, Third Edition, Williams & Wilkins, 1999

Sandstrom RW, Lohman H, Bramble JD: Health Services: Policy and Systems for Therapists, Prentice Hall, 2003

Saunders H: Evaluation, Treatment, and Prevention of Musculoskeletal Disorders, The Saunders Group, 1993

Scott R: Foundations of Physical Therapy: A 21st Century-Focused View of the Profession, McGraw-Hill Inc., 2002

Scott R: Health Care Malpractice: A Primer of Legal Issues for Professionals, Second Edition, McGraw-Hill Inc., 1999

Scott R: Legal Aspects of Documenting Patient Care, Second Edition, Aspen Publishers, 2000

Scott R: Professional Ethics: A Guide for Rehabilitation Professionals, Mosby, 1998

Scott R: Promoting Legal Awareness in Physical and Occupational Therapy, Mosby, 1997

Seymour R: Prosthetics and Orthotics: Lower Limb and Spinal, Lippincott Williams & Wilkins, 2002

Shamus E, Shamus J: Sports Injury: Prevention & Rehabilitation, McGraw-Hill Inc., 2001

Shamus E, Stern D: Effective Documentation for the Physical Therapy Professional, McGraw-Hill Inc., 2004

Shepard K, Jensen G: Handbook of Teaching for Physical Therapists, Butterworth- Heinemann, 1997

Shumway-Cook A, Woollacott M: Motor Control: Theory and Practical Applications, Second Edition, Lippincott Williams & Wilkins, 2001

Sine R, Liss S: Basic Rehabilitation Techniques: A Self Instructional Guide, Fourth Edition, Aspen Publishers, 2000

Standards of Ethical Conduct for the Physical Therapist Assistant, American Physical Therapy Association, 2004

Standards of Practice for Physical Therapy, American Physical Therapy Association, 2004

Starkey C, Ryan J: Evaluation of Orthopedic and Athletic Injuries, FA Davis Company, 2002

Stephenson R, O'Connor L: <u>Obstetric and Gynecologic Care in Physical Therapy</u>, Second Edition, Slack Incorporated, 2000

Stokes M: <u>Neurological Physiotherapy</u>, Mosby International Limited, 1998

Sullivan P, Markos P: <u>Clinical Decision Making in Therapeutic Exercise</u>, Appleton & Lange, 1995

Sultz H: <u>Health Care USA: Understanding Its Organization and Delivery</u>, Second Edition, Aspen Publishers, 1999

Sussman C, Bates-Jensen B: <u>Wound Care: A Collaborative Practice Manual for Physical Therapists and Nurses</u>, Second Edition, Aspen Publishers, 2001

Tan JC: <u>Practical Manual of Physical Medicine and Rehabilitation</u>, Mosby, 1998

Tecklin J: <u>Pediatric Physical Therapy</u>, Third Edition, Lippincott Williams & Wilkins, 1999

Tierney L: <u>Current Medical Diagnosis and Treatment</u>, 34th Edition, Appleton & Lange, 1995

Triola M: <u>Elementary Statistics</u>, 9th Edition, Pearson Addison Wesley Publishing Company Inc., 2003

Trofino R: <u>Nursing Care of the Burn Injured Patient</u>, FA Davis Company, 1991

Umphred D: <u>Neurological Rehabilitation</u>, Fourth Edition, Mosby, 2001

Van Deusen J: <u>Assessment in Occupational and Physical Therapy</u>, WB Saunders Company, 1997

Walter J: <u>Physical Therapy Management</u>, Mosby, 1993

Watchie J: <u>Cardiopulmonary Physical Therapy: A Clinical Manual</u>, WB Saunders Company, 1995

Waxman S, deGroot J: <u>Correlative Neuroanatomy</u>, Appleton & Lange, 1995

* Things to check

- Norm blood values Pg. 145
  (make cue-card)

- dermatomes/myatomes

- ABG's values (acidosis/alkalosis)
  metabolic vs respir.

- Exercise tests (submax, max, etc)

- lung volumes (terms: tidal volume, vessl cap, etc)

- Brachial plexus

- Types of cord injuries (Post., ant, central, etc)

- Ranchos levels

- ECG readings (QRS, ST, etc.)

Greg

524-1394

Notes